HEALTH ASSESSMENT

TENTH EDITION

Janet R. Weber, RN, EdD

Professor Emeritus
Department of Nursing
Southeast Missouri State University
Cape Girardeau, Missouri

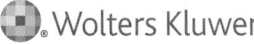 Wolters Kluwer

Philadelphia • Baltimore • New York • London
Buenos Aires • Hong Kong • Sydney • Tokyo

Vice President, Nursing Segment: Julie K. Stegman
Director, Nursing Education and Nursing Practice Content: Jamie Blum
Senior Acquisitions Editor: Jonathan Joyce
Senior Development Editor: Meredith L. Brittain
Marketing Manager: Greta H. Swanson
Editorial Assistant: Molly Kennedy
Senior Production Project Manager: Sadie Buckallew
Manager, Graphic Arts and Design: Steve Druding
Art Director: Jennifer Clements
Manufacturing Coordinator: Margie Orzech
Prepress Vendor: S4Carlisle Publishing Services

10th edition

Copyright © 2022 Wolters Kluwer.

9 8 7 6 5 4 3 2 1

Printed in Singapore

Library of Congress Cataloging-in-Publication Data

ISBN-13: 978-1-975161-24-8

ISBN-10: 1-975161-24-6

Cataloging-in-Publication data available on request from the Publisher.

To my loving husband, Bill,
for encouragement, patience, and confidence

To my precious sons and grandson:
Joe, *for encouraging me to always try a little harder*
Wes, *for making me laugh and realize what is most important in life*
Eli, *for reminding me to play, giggle, and have fun*

To my Mom,
for showing me how to be still and grow old wisely

To my friend Jane Kelley,
for your knowledge and enduring research for the book

To all my students,
who taught me how to write to help them learn

To all practicing nurses,
whom I admire as they inspire me to continue to write

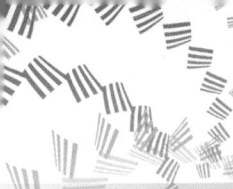

CONTRIBUTOR

Jane H. Kelley, RN, PhD
Retired Professor
School of Nursing
Indiana Wesleyan University
Louisville, Kentucky

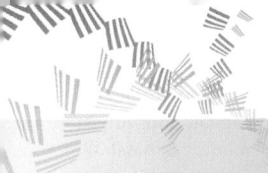

PREFACE

Purpose

The tenth edition of the *Nurses' Handbook of Health Assessment* provides both students and practicing nurses an easy-to-use guide with up-to-date references to assist with interviewing clients and performing a physical assessment. This guide provides the nurse tools to assess clients, various questions to elicit information in the client interview, and instructions on how to correctly perform a physical examination. Normal versus abnormal findings are provided, with precise descriptions to assist the nurse with accurate documentation.

This handbook may be used as a standalone textbook or as a convenient shortened guide to accompany *Health Assessment in Nursing*, Seventh Edition, which contains more in-depth, comprehensive assessment rationales and concepts. The handbook's small size and spiral binding facilitate its use at the client's bedside or in a learning laboratory as a step-by-step guide while performing the examination.

Because this handbook can also be used as a freestanding text, in this edition more in-depth content, abnormal findings, and illustrative photos have been added. This includes additional content on safety, assessment tests, clinical tips for examination procedures, and more photos of abnormal pathologic findings.

Key Features

The key features of this handbook include **full-color anatomy and physiology** images, illustrations of **normal and abnormal** physiologic findings, **risk factors**, the **three-column format** of assessment procedures, and the **spiral binding** that allows the handbook to stay open on any flat surface. This edition includes **additional new photos of abnormal findings and additional assessment tests.**

Along with a chapter on older adults, the more common **geriatric variations** that occur with advancing age are summarized at the end of each body system assessment chapter, identified by 🄑. **Pediatric variations** are also presented at the end of each body system assessment chapter and are identified by 🄟. In addition, **cultural variations** appear at the end of each chapter and are identified by 🄒.

Organization

This tenth edition of *Nurses' Handbook of Health Assessment* is organized similar to the seventh edition of the Weber and Kelley *Health Assessment in Nursing* textbook.

Unit 1 (Nursing Data Collection, Documentation, and Analysis; Chapters 1 through 3) focuses on nursing data collection, analysis, and making accurate clinical judgments. Chapter 1 explains the purpose of obtaining a nursing health history and describes basic guidelines and frameworks for interviewing a client. Chapter 2 describes the basic skills and techniques needed for performing the physical assessment. Chapter 3 describes the validation, analysis, documentation, and verbal communication of data collected and clinical judgments made.

Unit 2 (Integrative Holistic Nursing Assessment; Chapters 4 through 9) covers assessment of the client's developmental level, mental status, risk for substance abuse, general overall health status, vital signs, pain level, potential for being a victim of violence, and nutritional status. This unit precedes the nursing assessment of physical systems located in Unit 3 because these integrative assessments may affect physical assessment findings, and vice versa.

Unit 3 (Nursing Assessment of Physical Systems; Chapters 10 through 23) encompasses assessment of all the physical body systems. Each chapter consists of the following:
- Overview of relevant anatomy and physiology
- Illustrations of relevant anatomic or physiologic processes
- Focus questions to collect subjective data specific to the body system being assessed
- Risk factors related to chapter content
- Equipment needed for the examination
- Preparation of the client for each physical assessment
- Physical assessment procedure (three-column format: procedure, normal findings, and abnormal findings)
- Pediatric variations
- Geriatric variations
- Cultural variations
- Teaching tips for select client concerns

Unit 4 (Nursing Assessment of Special Groups; Chapters 24 through 26) focuses on nursing assessment of childbearing women, newborns and infants, and older adults.

The appendices at the end of the handbook contain useful tools to complete a holistic assessment. The first two appendices are an interview guide based on functional health patterns followed by a physical assessment guide to pull it all together. These are followed by an example of how to document the entire adult assessment. Other reference tools needed for health assessment that are found in the appendices include: assessment of family functional health patterns, developmental information collaborative problem list, and a convenient Spanish translation guide to conduct an interview and explain the physical assessment.

Student Resources Available on thePoint®

- Assessment Tool: Nursing Health History Guide
- Assessment Tool: Physical Assessment Guide
- Concepts in Action Animations
- Watch and Learn Video Clips
- Heart and Breath Sounds

Instructor Resources Available on thePoint®

- Image Bank

Janet R. Weber, RN, EdD

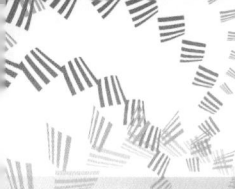

CONTENTS

Nursing Data Collection, Documentation, and Analysis

1 OBTAINING A NURSING HEALTH HISTORY: GUIDELINES AND FRAMEWORKS

A nursing health assessment can be defined as the systematic collection of subjective data stated by the client and objective data observed by the nurse used to make nursing judgments (client concerns, collaborative problems, and referrals).

This chapter focuses on the subjective collection of data, which are sensations or symptoms (e.g., pain, hunger), feelings (e.g., happiness, sadness), perceptions, desires, preferences, beliefs, ideas, values, and personal information that can be elicited and verified only by the client. To elicit accurate subjective data, effective interview skills are needed by the nurse.

Guidelines for obtaining the client nursing health history are discussed in addition to the phases of the client interview and communication techniques. Both a generic and functional health pattern framework that may be used by the nurse to interview the client are presented.

Guidelines for Obtaining a Nursing Health History

A nursing health history usually precedes the physical assessment and guides the nurse as to which body systems must be assessed. It also assists the nurse in establishing a nurse–client relationship and allows client participation in identifying problems and goals. Standard 1 in the *Nursing: Scope and Standards of Practice* (American Nurses Association [ANA], 2015) states, "The registered nurse collects pertinent data and information relative to the health care consumer's health or the situation" (p. 53). These guidelines are essential for the nurse to follow when collecting client data and making professional judgments. Standard 2 states, "The registered nurse analyzes assessment data to determine actual or potential diagnoses, problems and issues."

PHASES OF THE NURSING INTERVIEW

Professional interpersonal and interviewing skills are necessary to obtain a valid nursing health history. The nursing interview is a communication process that focuses on the client's developmental, psychological, physiological, sociocultural, and spiritual responses that can be treated with nursing and collaborative interventions. The nursing interview has three basic phases: introductory phase, working phase, and summary and closure phase.

Introductory Phase

Introduce yourself and describe your role (e.g., RN, student). Address the client by surname. Next, explain the purpose of the interview to the client (i.e., to collect data, to understand the client's needs, and to plan nursing care). Discuss the types of questions that will be asked, reason for taking notes, electronic documentation, and assure client that confidential information will remain confidential using Health Insurance Portability and Accountability Act (HIPAA) guidelines enacted by the U.S. Department of Health and Human Services (www.hhs.gov) to ensure confidentiality of client information. Ensure client comfort and privacy, and conduct the interview at eye level to show respect. This promotes trust to help the client feel comfortable with disclosing personal information. Convey a sense of priority and interest in the client.

Working Phase

Facilitate the client's comments about major biographic data, reason for seeking health care, history of present health concern, past health history, family history, review of body systems for current health problems, lifestyle and health practices, developmental level, and functional health pattern responses. Use critical thinking skills to listen for and observe cues and to interpret and validate the information received from the client. Collaborate with the client to identify client concerns and goals. The approach used for facilitation may be either free flowing or more structured with specific questions, depending on available time and type of data needed.

Summary and Closure Phase

Summarize the information obtained during the working phase and validate the problems and goals with the client. You may begin to discuss possible plans to resolve the problems (client concerns and collaborative problems). Allow the client time to express feelings, concerns, and questions.

SPECIFIC COMMUNICATION TECHNIQUES

Specific communication techniques are used to facilitate the interview. The following sections include specific guidelines for phrasing questions and statements to promote an effective and productive interview.

Types of Questions to Use

- Use open-ended questions to elicit the client's feelings and perceptions. These questions begin with "What," "How," or "Which" and require more than a one-word response.
- Use closed-ended questions to obtain facts and zero in on specific information. The client can respond with one or two words. These questions begin with "Is," "Are," "Will," "When," or "Did" and help avoid rambling by the client.
- Use a laundry list (scrambled words) approach to obtain specific answers. For example, "Is the pain severe, dull, sharp, mild, cutting, or piercing?" "Does the pain occur once every year, day, month, or hour?" This reduces the likelihood of the client perceiving and providing an expected answer.

• Explore all data that deviate from normal with the following questions: "What alleviates or aggravates the problem?" "How long has it occurred?" "How severe is it?" "Does it radiate?"

"When does it occur?" "Is its onset gradual or sudden?" The mnemonic COLDSPA may be used to further explore the client's symptoms (see Box 1-1).

BOX 1-1 SAMPLE APPLICATION OF COLDSPA: EXPLORING THE SYMPTOMS OF BACK PAIN

Mnemonic	General Question	Adapted Question
Character	Describe the sign or symptom (feeling, appearance, sound, smell, or taste if applicable).	"What does the pain feel like?"
Onset	When did it begin?	"When did this pain start?"
Location	Where is it? Does it radiate? Does it occur anywhere else?	"Where does it hurt the most? Does it radiate or go to any other part of your body?"
Duration	How long does it last? Does it recur?	"How long does the pain last? Does it come and go or is it constant?"
Severity	How bad is it? How much does it bother you?	"How intense is the pain? Rate it on a scale of 1 to 10."
Pattern	What makes it better or worse?	"What makes your back pain worse or better? Are there any treatments you've tried that relieve the pain?"
Associated factors/ how it affects the client	What other symptoms occur with it? How does it affect you?	"What do you think caused it to start? Do you have any other problems that seem related to your back pain? How does this pain affect your life and daily activities?"

Types of Statements to Use

- Rephrase or repeat your perception of the client's response to reflect or clarify the information shared. For example, "You feel you have a serious illness?"
- Encourage verbalization of client by saying "Um hum," "Yes," or "I agree," or nodding.
- Describe what you observe in the client. For example, "It seems you have difficulty on the right side."

Additional Helpful Hints

- Accept the client; display a nonjudgmental attitude.
- Use silence to help the client and yourself reflect and reorganize thoughts.
- Provide the client with information during the interview as questions and concerns arise.
- Note that not all clients can read. Basic care terms can be communicated best by using pictures.

Communication Styles to Avoid

- Excessive or insufficient eye contact (varies with cultures).
- Doing other things while taking the history and being mentally distant or physically far away from the client (>60.9–91.4 cm [2–3 ft]).
- Biased or leading questions—for example, "You don't feel bad, do you?"
- Relying on memory to recall all the information or recording all the details.
- Rushing the client.
- Reading questions from the history form, distracting attention from the client.

  Specific Age Variations

When interviewing the pediatric client from birth to early adolescence (through age 14 years), validate information from the history for reliability with the responsible significant others (e.g., parent, grandparent). Use the following guidelines when interviewing the pediatric client:

- Use language that is familiar for the appropriate age.
- Involve the parent and/or significant other when interviewing the child to achieve accurate information.
- Allow the child to sit with parent, or in parent's lap, if desired.

When interviewing the older adult client, remember that age affects and often slows all body systems within a person to varying degrees.

Use the following guidelines when interviewing the older adult client:

- Use a gentle, genuine approach.
- Use simple, straightforward questions in lay terms. Let the client set the pace of the conversation. Be patient and listen well. Allow ample time.
- Introduce yourself, but remember that an older client may forget your name—you may have to write it for the client later in the interview.
- Use direct eye contact and sit at client's eye level. Establish and maintain privacy (especially important).
- Assess hearing acuity; with loss, speak slowly, face the client, and speak on the side on which hearing is more adequate. Speak louder only if you confirm the client has a hearing deficit. Turn off any background noises.
- Wear a nametag and provide written notes for the client to refer to in the future.

Emotional Variations

Not all clients are calm and friendly. It is important to assess the client's mood in order to adapt your approach to promote an effective interaction with the client.

- *Angry client:* Approach in a calm, reassuring, in-control manner. Allow ventilation of client's feelings. Avoid arguing and provide personal space.
- *Anxious client:* Approach with simple, organized information. Explain your role and purpose.
- *Manipulative client:* Provide structure and set limits.
- *Depressed client:* Express interest and understanding in a neutral manner.
- *Sensitive issues* (e.g., sexuality, dying, spirituality): Be aware of your own thoughts and feelings. These factors may affect the client's health and need to be discussed with someone. Such personal, sensitive topics may be referred when you do not feel comfortable discussing these topics.

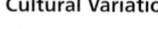 ### Cultural Variations

Cultural variations in communication and self-disclosure styles may seriously affect the information obtained. Be aware of possible variations in the communication styles of yourself and client. If misunderstanding or difficulty in communicating is evident, seek help from a "culture broker" who is skilled at cross-cultural communication. See Box 1-2 for observations and questions to ask clients from another culture.

BOX 1-2 EXAMPLE OF OBSERVATIONS AND QUESTIONS TO ASK A CLIENT FROM ANOTHER CULTURE

1. What is your full name?
2. What is your legal name?
3. By what name do you wish to be called?
4. What is your primary language?
5. Do you speak a specific dialect?
6. What other languages do you speak?
7. Do you find it difficult to share your thoughts, feelings, and ideas with family? Friends? Health care providers?
8. Do you mind being touched by friends? Strangers? Health care workers?
9. How do you wish to be greeted? Handshake? Nod of the head, etc.?
10. Are you usually on time for appointments?
11. Are you usually on time for social engagements?
12. Observe the client's speech pattern. Is the speech pattern low or high context? Remember, clients from highly contexted cultures place greater value on silence.
13. Observe the client when physical contact is made. Do they withdraw from the touch or become tense?
14. How close does the client stand when talking with family members? With health care providers?
15. Does the client maintain eye contact when talking with the nurse/physician, etc.?

Frequently noted cultural variations include the following:

- Reluctance to reveal personal information to strangers for various culturally-based reasons.
- Variation in willingness to express emotional distress or pain openly.
- Variation in ability to receive information and/or listen.
- Variation in meaning conveyed by use of language (e.g., by nonnative speakers, by use of slang).
- Variation in use and meaning of nonverbal communication: eye contact, stance, gestures, demeanor (e.g., eye contact may be perceived as rude, aggressive, or immodest by some cultures, but lack of eye contact may be perceived as evasive, insecure, or inattentive by other cultures; slightly bowed stance may indicate respect in some groups; size of personal space affects one's comfortable interpersonal distance; touch may be perceived as comforting or threatening).

- Variation in disease/illness perception: culture-specific syndromes or disorders are accepted by some groups (e.g., *susto* in Latin America). *Susto* (fright, emotional shock, soul loss) is perceived to have either a physical or a supernatural cause resulting in loss of appetite, weight, strength, and motivation to carry out even simple tasks (from culture-bound syndrome; Nogueira et al., 2015).
- Variation in past, present, or future time orientation (e.g., the dominant U.S. culture is future oriented; other cultures vary).
- Variation in family decision-making process: person other than the client or the client's parent may be the major decision maker regarding appointments, treatments, or follow-up care for client.

Assessing Non–English-Speaking Clients

- Use a bilingual interpreter familiar with the client's culture and with health care, when possible (e.g., a nurse culture broker).
- Consider the relationship of the interpreter to the client. If the interpreter is a child or is of the opposite sex, different age, or different social status, interpretation may be impaired.

Frameworks for Collecting Client Data

NURSING MODEL VERSUS MEDICAL MODEL FOR DATA COLLECTION

Although all health care professionals perform assessments to make professional judgments related to clients, the purpose of a nursing health history and physical examination differs greatly from that of a medical or other type of health care assessment (e.g., dietary assessment or examination for physical therapy). A nursing framework helps to organize information and promotes the collection of holistic data and to identify client concerns, collaborative problems, and/or referrals. Two frameworks will be introduced in this handbook: a "Generic" and a "Functional Health Pattern" framework.

GENERIC NURSING FRAMEWORK

The Generic Nursing Framework provides a foundation for identifying client concerns and provides a focus for the physical examination. Taking a health history should begin with an explanation to the client of why the information is being requested, for example, "so that I will be able to plan individualized nursing care with you." This generic format has eight sections. See Box 1-3 for a description of each section.

BOX 1-3 GENERIC NURSING HISTORY FORMAT SUMMARY

Biographic Data
Name
Address
Phone
Gender
Provider of history (client or other)
Birth date
Place of birth
Race or ethnic background
Primary and secondary languages (spoken and read)
Marital status
Religious or spiritual practices
Educational level
Occupation
Significant others or support persons (availability)

Reasons for Seeking Health Care
Reason for seeking health care (major health problem or concern)
Feelings about seeking health care (fears and past experiences)

History of Present Health Concern Using COLDSPA
Character (How does it feel, look, smell, sound, etc.?)
Onset (When did it begin; is it better, worse, or the same since it began?)

Location (Where is it? Does it radiate?)
Duration (How long does it last? Does it recur?)
Severity (How bad is it on a scale of 1 [barely noticeable] to 10 [worst pain ever experienced]?)
Pattern (What makes it better? What makes it worse?)
Associated factors (What other symptoms do you have with it? Will you be able to continue doing your work or other activities [leisure or exercise]?)

Past Health History
Problems at birth
Childhood illnesses
Immunizations to date
Adult illnesses (physical, emotional, and mental)
Surgeries
Accidents
Prolonged pain or pain patterns
Allergies
Physical, emotional, social, or spiritual weaknesses
Physical, emotional, social, or spiritual strengths

Family Health History
Age of parents (Living? Deceased date?)

(Continued on following page)

BOX 1-3 GENERIC NURSING HISTORY FORMAT SUMMARY (*continued*)

Parents' illnesses and longevity
Grandparents' illnesses and longevity
Ages and longevity
Children's ages and illnesses or handicaps and longevity

Review of Systems for Current Health Problems
Skin, hair, and nails: Color, temperature, condition, rashes, lesions, excessive sweating, hair loss, dandruff
Head and neck: Headache, stiffness, difficulty swallowing, enlarged lymph nodes, sore throat
Ears: Pain, ringing, buzzing, drainage, difficulty hearing, exposure to loud noises, dizziness, drainage
Eyes: Pain, infections, impaired vision, redness, tearing, halos, blurring, black spots, flashes, double vision
Mouth, throat, nose, and sinuses: Mouth pain, sore throat, lesions, hoarseness, nasal obstruction, sneezing, coughing, snoring, nosebleeds
Thorax and lungs: Pain, difficulty breathing, shortness of breath with activities, orthopnea, cough, sputum, hemoptysis, respiratory infections
Breasts and regional lymphatics: Pain, lumps, discharge from nipples, dimpling or changes in breast size, swollen and tender lymph nodes in axilla

Heart and neck vessels: Chest pain or pressure, palpitations, edema, last blood pressure, last electrocardiogram (ECG)
Peripheral vascular: Leg or feet pain, swelling of feet or legs, sores on feet or legs, color of feet and legs
Abdomen: Pain, indigestion, difficulty swallowing, nausea and vomiting, gas, jaundice, hernias
Male genitalia: Painful urination, frequency or difficulty starting or maintaining urinary system, blood in urine, sexual problems, penile lesions, penile pain, scrotal swelling, difficulty with erection or ejaculation, exposure to sexually transmitted infections (STIs)
Female genitalia: Pelvic pain, voiding pain, sexual pain, voiding problems (dribbling, incontinence), age of menarche or menopause (date of last menstrual period), pregnancies and types of problems, abortions, STIs, hormone replacement therapy (HRT), birth control methods
Anus, rectum, and prostate: Pain with defecation, hemorrhoids, bowel habits, constipation, diarrhea, blood in stool
Musculoskeletal: Painful, swollen, red, stiff joints; strength of extremities; ability to care for self, ability to work
Neurologic: Mood, behavior, depression, anger, headaches, concussions, loss of strength or sensation, coordination, difficulty with speech, memory problems, strange thoughts or actions, difficulty reading or learning

Lifestyle and Health Practices
Description of a typical day (AM to PM)
Nutrition and weight management
24-hour dietary intake (foods and fluids)
Who purchases and prepares meals
Activities on a typical day
Exercise habits and patterns
Sleep and rest habits and patterns
Use of medications and other substances (caffeine, nicotine, alcohol, and recreational drugs)
Self-concept
Self-care responsibilities

Social activities for fun and relaxation
Social activities contributing to society
Relationships with family, significant others, and pets
Values, religious affiliation, and spirituality
Past, current, and future plans for education
Type of work, level of job satisfaction, and work stressors
Finances
Stressors in life, coping strategies used
Residency, type of environment, neighborhood, and environmental risks
Developmental Level (See Chapter 4)

GORDON'S FUNCTIONAL HEALTH PATTERN ASSESSMENT MODEL

Marjory Gordon's Functional Health Pattern Assessment Framework (2020) is particularly useful in collecting health data to identify client concerns. Gordon has defined 11 functional health patterns that provide for a holistic client database. A pattern is a sequence of related behaviors that assists the nurse in collecting and categorizing data. These 11 functional health patterns can be used for nursing assessment in any practice areas for clients of all ages and in the assessment of families and communities. For the purpose of this handbook, assessment is focused on the individual. However, guideline questions for families organized according to functional health patterns are included in Appendix 1. Box 1-4 presents a brief overview of the subjective and objective assessment focus data needed for each functional health pattern (Gordon, 2014).

BOX 1-4   SUBJECTIVE AND OBJECTIVE ASSESSMENT FOCUS FOR FUNCTIONAL HEALTH PATTERNS

1. Health Perception–Health Management Pattern
   Subjective data: Perception of health status and health practices used by client to maintain health
   Objective data: Appearance, grooming, posture, expression, vital signs, height, weight
2. Nutritional–Metabolic Pattern
   Subjective data: Dietary habits, including food and fluid intake
   Objective data: General physical survey, including examination of skin, mouth, abdomen, and cranial nerves (CN) V, IX, X, and XII
3. Elimination Pattern
   Subjective data: Regularity and control of bowel and bladder habits
   Objective data: Skin examination, rectal examination
4. Activity–Exercise Pattern
   Subjective data: Activities of daily living that require energy expenditure
   Objective data: Examination of musculoskeletal system, including gait, posture, range of motion (ROM) of joints, muscle tone, and strength; cardiovascular examination; peripheral vascular examination; thoracic examination

5. Sexuality–Reproduction Pattern
   Subjective data: Sexual identity, activities, and relationships; expression of sexuality and level of satisfaction with sexual patterns; reproduction patterns
   Objective data: Genitalia examination, breast examination
6. Sleep–Rest Pattern
   Subjective data: Perception of effectiveness of sleep and rest habits
   Objective data: Appearance and attention span
7. Cognitive–Perceptual Pattern
   For the purposes of this handbook, the cognitive pattern has been divided into two parts: (1) the sensory–perceptual pattern, to include the senses of hearing, vision, smell, taste, and touch; and (2) the cognitive pattern, to include knowledge, thought, perception, and language.

   a. Sensory–Perceptual Pattern
      Subjective data: Perception of ability to hear, see, smell, taste, and feel (including light touch, pain, and vibratory sensation)
      Objective data: Visual and hearing examinations, pain perception, CN examination; testing for taste, smell, and touch

b. Cognitive Pattern
Subjective data: Perception of messages, decision-making, thought processes
Objective data: Mental status examination
8. Role–Relationship Pattern
Subjective data: Perception of and level of satisfaction with family, work, and social roles
Objective data: Communication with significant others, visits from significant others and family, family genogram
9. Self-Perception–Self-Concept Pattern
Subjective data: Perception of self-worth, personal identity, feelings

Objective data: Body posture, movement, eye contact, voice and speech pattern, emotions, moods, and thought content
10. Coping–Stress Tolerance Pattern
Subjective data: Perception of stressful life events and ability to cope
Objective data: Behavior, thought processes
11. Value–Belief Pattern
Subjective data: Perception of what is good, correct, proper, and meaningful; philosophical beliefs; values and beliefs that guide choices
Objective data: Presence of religious articles, religious actions and routines, and visits from clergy

Functional Health Pattern Framework

Using a functional health pattern framework assists the nurse with collecting data necessary to identify and validate client concerns. This approach eliminates repetition of medical data already obtained by physicians and other members of the health care team.

The components of a nursing health assessment incorporating a functional health pattern approach (Gordon, 2014) are listed below. Prior to data collection for each functional health pattern, it is important to obtain a client profile and developmental history.
- Client Profile
- Developmental History

- Health Perception–Health Management Pattern
- Nutritional–Metabolic Pattern
- Elimination Pattern
- Activity–Exercise Pattern
- Sexuality–Reproduction Pattern
- Sleep–Rest Pattern
- Sensory–Perceptual Pattern
- Cognitive Pattern
- Role–Relationship Pattern
- Self-Perception–Self-Concept Pattern
- Coping–Stress Tolerance Pattern
- Value–Belief Pattern

References

American Nurses Association. (2015). *Nursing: Scope and standards of practice* (3rd ed.). Author.

Current Nursing. (2020). Functional health patterns. Available at https://www.currentnursing.com/theory/functional_health_patterns.html

Gordon, M. (2014). *Manual of nursing diagnosis* (13th ed.). Jones & Bartlett.

Nogueira, B., Mari, J., & Razzouk, D. (2015). Culture bound syndromes in Spanish speaking Latin America: The case of *nervios, susto,* and *ataque de nervios. Archives of Clinical Psychiatry, 42*(6), 171–178. https://doi.org/10.1590/0101-60830000000070

2 PERFORMING THE PHYSICAL ASSESSMENT: SKILLS AND TECHNIQUES

Physical Assessment Skills

Objective data are data that are directly observed by the nurse, measurements reported by other health care professionals, or observations noted by the family or significant others about the client. See Table 2-1 for a comparison of subjective data (discussed in Chapter 1) and objective data (discussed in this chapter).

The nurse obtains objective data by performing a physical assessment using four basic techniques: *inspection, palpation, percussion,* and *auscultation.* The definition and proper technique for each of these are described in the next section. Always use Standard Precautions as recommended by the Hospital Infection Control Practices Advisory Committee (HICPAC) and the Centers for Disease Control and Prevention (CDC).

TABLE 2-1 Comparing Subjective and Objective Data

	Subjective	Objective
Description	Data elicited and verified by the client	Data directly or indirectly observed through measurement
Sources	Client	Observations and physical assessment findings of the nurse or other health care professionals
	Family and significant others	
	Client record	Documentation of assessments made in client record
	Other health care professionals	Observations made by the client's family or significant others
Methods used to obtain data	Client interview	Observation and physical examination
Skills needed to obtain data	Interview and therapeutic communication skills	Inspection
	Caring ability and empathy	Palpation
		Percussion
	Listening skills	Auscultation
Examples	"I have a headache"	Respirations 16 per minute
	"It frightens me"	Blood pressure 180/100, apical pulse 80 and irregular
	"I am not hungry"	X-ray film reveals fractured pelvis

INSPECTION

Definition

Inspection is using the senses of vision, smell, and hearing to observe the condition of various body parts, including any deviations from normal.

Technique

- Expose body parts being observed while keeping the rest of the client properly draped.
- *Always* look before touching.

- Use good lighting. Tangential sunlight is best. Be alert for the effect of bluish red-tinted or fluorescent lighting that interferes with observing bruises, cyanosis, and erythema.
- Provide a warm room for examination of the client. (An environment that is too cold or hot may alter skin color and appearance.)
- Observe for color, size, location, texture, symmetry, odors, and sounds.

PALPATION

Definition

Palpation is touching and feeling body parts with your hands to determine the following characteristics:
- Texture (roughness/smoothness)
- Temperature (warm/hot/cold)
- Moisture (dry/wet/moist)
- Motion (stillness/vibration)
- Consistency of structures (solid/fluid filled)

Technique

- Keep your fingernails short.
- Use the most sensitive part of the hand to detect various sensations. See Table 2-2.

TABLE 2-2 **Sensitivity of Parts of the Hand**

Hand Part Used	Type of Sensation Felt
Fingertips	Fine discriminations, pulsations
Palmar/ulnar surface	Vibratory sensations (e.g., thrills, fremitus)
Dorsal surface (back of hand)	Temperature

- Perform light palpation before deep palpation.
- Palpate tender areas last.
- Use four different types of palpation, depending on the purpose of the examination. The purpose and technique for each are described in Table 2-3.

PERCUSSION

Definition

Percussion is tapping a portion of the body to elicit evidence of tenderness or sounds that vary with the density of underlying structures. The reliability of this technique is often questioned because of variations in the specificity and sensitivity of percussion.

TABLE 2-3   **Types of Palpation**

Type	Purpose	Technique
Light palpation	To determine surface variations such as pulses, tenderness, surface skin texture, temperature, and moisture	Place your dominant hand lightly on the surface of the structure. There should be very little or no depression (<1 cm). Feel the surface structure using a circular motion.
Moderate palpation	To feel for easily palpable body organs and masses	Depress the skin surface 1–2 cm (0.5–0.75 in.) with your dominant hand, using a circular motion. Note size, consistency, and mobility of structures.

Deep palpation

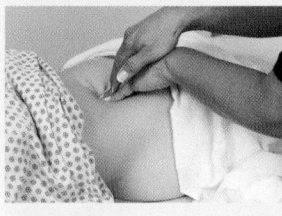

To feel very deep organs or structures that are covered by thick muscle

Place your dominant hand on the skin surface and your nondominant hand on top of your dominant hand to apply pressure. This should result in a surface depression between 2.5 and 5 cm (1 and 2 in.).

Bimanual palpation (use with caution as it may provoke internal injury)

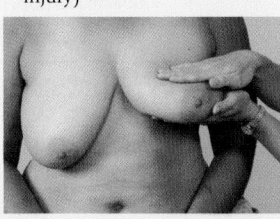

To palpate breasts and deep abdominal organs

Use two hands, placing one on each side of the body part (e.g., uterus, breasts, and spleen) being palpated. Use one hand to apply pressure and the other hand to feel the structure. Note the size, shape, consistency, and mobility of the structures you palpate.

Technique

Use three types of percussion depending on the purpose of the examination. The three types of percussion are explained in Table 2-4. Percussion notes elicited through indirect percussion vary with the density of the underlying structures. Five percussion notes are described in Table 2-5.

TABLE 2-4 **Types of Percussion**

Type	Purpose	Technique
Direct percussion Direct percussion of sinuses	To elicit tenderness or pain	Directly tap a body part with one or two fingertips such as over the sinuses.

Blunt percussion (most commonly used method of percussion)	To detect tenderness over organs (e.g., kidneys)	Place one hand flat on the body surface and use the fist of the other hand to strike the back of the hand flat on the body surface.

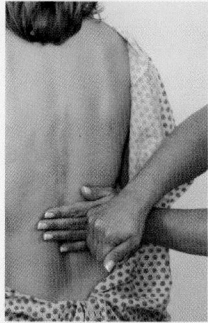

Blunt percussion of the kidneys

(*Continued on following page*)

TABLE 2-4 **Types of Percussion** (*continued*)

Type	Purpose	Technique
Indirect percussion (least used method of percussion because of its low reliability) 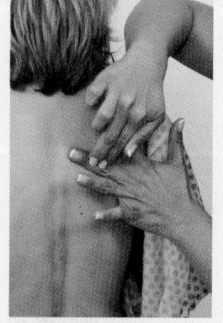 Indirect or mediate percussion of lungs	To elicit one of the following sounds over the chest or abdomen: tympany, resonance, hyper-resonance, dullness, and flatness. As density increases, the sound of the tone becomes quieter. Solid tissue produces a soft tone, fluid produces a louder tone, and air produces an even louder tone (see Table 2-5).	Press middle finger of nondominant hand firmly on body part. Keep other fingers off body part to avoid dampening of the sound elicited. Strike the finger on the body part with the middle finger (with short fingernail) with two quick taps of the dominant hand. Flex dominant wrist (not forearm) quickly. Listen to sound. (Use quick wrist movement, not forearm.)

TABLE 2-5   Sounds (Tones) Elicited by Percussion

Sound	Intensity	Pitch	Length	Quality	Example of Origin
Resonance (heard over part air and part solid)	Loud	Low	Long	Hollow	Normal lung
Hyperresonance (heard mostly over air)	Very loud	Low	Long	Booming	Lung with emphysema
Tympany (heard over air)	Loud	High	Moderate	Drum like	Puffed-out cheek, gastric bubble
Dullness (heard over more solid tissue)	Medium	Medium	Moderate	Thud like	Diaphragm, pleural effusion, liver
Flatness (heard over very dense tissue)	Soft	High	Short	Flat	Muscle, bone, sternum, thigh

AUSCULTATION

Definition

Auscultation is listening for various breath, heart, vasculature, and bowel sounds using a stethoscope.

Technique

Use a good stethoscope that has the following:

- Snug-fitting earplugs
- Tubing not longer than 38.1 cm (15 in.) and internal diameter not greater than 2.5 cm (1 in.)
- Diaphragm and bell.

The diaphragm and bell are used differently to detect various sounds, as shown in Table 2-6.

Basic Guidelines for Physical Assessment

Obtain a nursing history and survey the client's general physical status for an overall impression before performing the physical assessment. This is done to determine which specific body systems should be examined (e.g., if the client complains of chest pain, the nurse should perform a thoracic and cardiac physical examination). A complete examination of all body systems may be done only on admission to the hospital or health care facility;

TABLE 2-6 **Uses for Diaphragm and Bell of Stethoscope**

		Purpose	Technique
	Diaphragm	To detect high-pitched sounds (e.g., breath sounds, normal heart sounds, bowel sounds)	Press firmly on body part
	Bell	To detect low-pitched sounds (e.g., abnormal extra heart sounds, heart murmurs, carotid bruits)	Press lightly over body part

otherwise, the physical assessment may only include one or a few body systems.

Guidelines for performing a physical assessment include the following:

- Wash hands before beginning the examination, after completing the physical examination, or after removing gloves.
- Wear gloves if you will have direct contact with blood or other body fluids, if you have an open wound, when collecting body fluids (e.g., blood, sputum, wound drainage, urine, or stools) for a specimen, when handling contaminated surfaces (e.g., linen, tongue blades, vaginal speculum), and when

performing an examination of the mouth, an open wound, genitalia, vagina, or rectum.

- Maintain privacy and proper draping; make sure the examination area has adequate lighting and a comfortable temperature (provide blanket if necessary).
- Explain the procedure and purpose of each part of the examination to the client.
- Follow a planned examination order for each body system, using the four techniques described earlier. Specific history questions related to each body part being examined may be integrated with the physical examination (e.g., when

examining vision, ask the date of the client's last eye examination, if they have a history of blurring or double vision).

- First inspect, palpate, percuss, and then auscultate, except in the abdominal examination. To avoid alterations in bowel sounds: First auscultate and then percuss the abdomen, before palpating the abdomen.
- Use each technique to compare symmetrical sides of the body and organs.
- Assess both structure *and* function of each body part and organ (e.g., the appearance and condition of the ear, as well as its hearing function).
- When you identify an abnormality, assess for further data on the extent of the abnormality and the client's responses to the abnormality. Is there radiation of pain to other areas? Is there an effect on eating? Bowels? Activities of daily living? (e.g., with left upper quadrant abdominal pain: Is there radiation of the pain?).
- Integrate client education with the physical assessment (e.g., breast self-examination, testicular self-examination, foot care for the client with diabetes).
- Allow time for client questions.

Variations in Physical Assessment of the Pediatric Client

Note: The physical assessment sequence is dependent on the development level of the client. (For a detailed discussion, see Appendix 5, *Developmental Information—Age 1 Month to 18 Years.)*

- Establishing rapport with the child and caregiver is the most essential step in obtaining meaningful physical assessment data.
- Allowing time for interaction with the child before beginning the examination helps to reduce fears.
- Allowing the child to use play medical instruments and/or allowing the child to touch and see instruments used, such as the stethoscope, otoscope, and ophthalmoscope, may reduce anxiety and fear, making use of instruments more accepting by the child.
- In certain age groups, portions of the assessment will require physical restraint of the pediatric client with the help of another adult.

- Intermingling distraction and play throughout the examination assists in maintaining rapport with the pediatric client.
- Involving assistance from the child's parent or guardian may facilitate a more meaningful examination of the younger child.
- Based on the child's responses, prepare to alter the order of the assessment and your approach to the child.
- For infants and small children, the examiner should use a pediatric stethoscope to auscultate the heart and the lungs. If a pediatric stethoscope is not available, use the bell of the adult scope.
- Protest or an uncooperative attitude toward the examiner is a normal finding in children from birth to early adolescence, throughout parts or even all of the assessment process. Appendix 5 describes normal behavior at various developmental levels for the pediatric client.
- If another member of the health care team is needed to help restrain the child, allow the parent to comfort the child *after* the procedure.

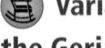 Variations in Physical Assessment of the Geriatric Client

Note: Normal variations related to aging may be observed in all parts of the physical examination.

- To avoid fatiguing the older client, allow rest periods between parts of the physical assessment. Provide a room with a comfortable temperature setting and no drafts, close to the restroom.
- Allow sufficient time for the client to respond to directions and to change positions. Use silence to provide more time for the client to process thoughts and respond.
- If possible, assess geriatric clients in a setting where they have an opportunity to perform normal activities of daily living to determine their optimum potential.
- Conduct the examination in an area with ample space to accommodate wheelchairs and other supportive devices.

3 · VALIDATING, ANALYZING, DOCUMENTING, AND COMMUNICATING DATA

Although validation, documentation, and communication of data often occur concurrently with collection of subjective and objective assessment data, looking at each step separately can help emphasize each step's importance in nursing assessment.

Validating Data

Validation of data is the process of confirming or verifying that the subjective and objective data you have collected are reliable and accurate. The steps of validation include deciding whether the data require validation, determining ways to validate the data, and identifying areas for which data are missing. Failure to validate data may result in premature closure of the assessment or collection of inaccurate data. Errors during assessment cause clinical judgments to be made on unreliable data, which results in diagnostic errors when analyzing data to determine the client's concerns, risks for concerns, collaborative problems, and/or referrals.

Not every piece of data you collect must be verified. Conditions that require data to be rechecked and validated include:

- Discrepancies between the subjective and objective data. For example, a male client tells you that he is very happy despite learning that he has terminal cancer.
- Discrepancies between what the client says at one time versus another time.
- Cues that are highly abnormal and/or inconsistent with other cues. For example, a client has a temperature of 104°F, but is comfortable, and skin is warm to touch and not flushed.

There are several ways to validate data:

- Recheck your own data through a repeat assessment, such as taking the client's temperature again with a different thermometer.
- Clarify data with the client by asking additional questions. Example: A client is holding their abdomen; the nurse may assume they are having abdominal pain, when actually the client is feeling nauseated.
- Verify the data with another health care professional. Example: Ask a more experienced nurse to listen to the abnormal heart sounds you think you have just heard.
- Compare your objective findings with your subjective findings to uncover discrepancies. Example: A client states "I never get any time in the sun," yet has dark, wrinkled, suntanned skin. Validate the client's perception of never getting any time in the sun by asking exactly how much time is spent working, sitting, or doing other activities outdoors. Also, ask what the client wears when engaging in outdoor activities.

Once you have collected the necessary database, identify areas for which more data are needed. For example, if an adult client weighs only 98 lb, you would explore further to see if the client recently lost weight or if this has been the usual weight for an extended time. If a client tells you that they live alone, you may need to identify the existence of a support system, their degree of social involvement with others, and their ability to function independently.

Analyzing Data to Make Informed Clinical Judgments

Steps for making a clinical judgment are outlined in Table 3-1. Data analysis, which is the second step of the nursing process, can be challenging because the nurse is required to use diagnostic reasoning skills to interpret cues accurately to make an informed clinical judgment. This requires critical thinking skills. Because of the complex nature of nursing as both a science and an art, the nurse must think critically—in a rational, self-directed, intelligent, and purposeful manner.

TABLE 3-1 **Steps to Make a Clinical Judgment from Assessment Data**

Step	Description
1	**Identify** abnormal cues and supportive cues (client strengths).
2	**Cluster** cues.
3	**Draw** inferences to propose or hypothesize clinical judgments (opportunity to improve health, risk for and actual client concerns/problems, collaborative problems, and/or referral to primary care provider).
4	**Identify** possible client concerns.
5	**Validate** the client concern with the client, family, significant others, and/or health team members.
6	**Document** clinical judgments.

Subjective and objective data collected are used to identify and cluster client strengths and abnormal cues to assist the nurse in identifying client concerns and/or collaborative problems. A client concern may fall into one of three categories: actual, risk, or opportunity to improve health. An **"actual"** client concern indicates that the client is currently experiencing the issue (e.g., poor skin integrity: reddened area on right buttocks). A **"risk"** for client concern indicates that the client does not currently have the problem but is vulnerable to developing it. An **"opportunity for health promotion"** means that the client is ready or motivated to learn about or take action to improve their health (see Table 3-2).

EXAMPLES OF CLIENT CONCERNS

The most useful format for an **actual client concern** is:
- Client Concern + associated with + underlying cause + as seen in
- *Example:* Fatigue associated with increased job demands and stress as seen in client's statements of feeling exhausted all of the time and lack of energy to perform usual work and home responsibilities (e.g., cooking, cleaning)

The most useful format for a **risk for client concern** is:
- Risk for + client concern + associated with + underlying cause
- *Example:* Risk for infection associated with the presence of dirty knife wound, leukopenia, and lack of client wound care knowledge

The most useful format for an **opportunity to improve health** is:
- Opportunity to improve + client concern + associated with + statement of desire to improve etiology

TABLE 3-2   **Comparison of Opportunity to Improve Health, Risk for Client Concerns, and Actual Client Concerns**

	Opportunity to Improve Health	**Risk for Client Concern**	**Actual Client Concern**
Client status	Client describes motivation and desire to increase well-being and enhance personal health status	Increased susceptibility to a health concern	Actual health problems exist
Format for stating	Opportunity to improve …	"Risk for …"	Health concern and "associated with" clause
Examples	Opportunity to improve communication	Risk for poor body image	Poor body image associated with non-healing facial wounds
	Opportunity to improve self-management of health	Risk for impaired bonding between child and caregiver	Abrupt family role changes associated with hospitalization of client
	Opportunity to improve quality of diversional activities	Risk for poor skin integrity	Poor skin integrity associated with immobility

- *Example:* Opportunity to improve sleep pattern associated with request to improve sleep by learning ways to stay asleep throughout night

COLLABORATIVE PROBLEMS

Collaborative problems are equivalent in importance to client concerns but represent the interdependent or collaborative role of nursing, whereas client concerns represent the independent role of the nurse. Collaborative problems are defined as "certain physiologic complications that nurses monitor to detect their onset or changes in status; nurses manage collaborative problems using physician-prescribed and nursing-prescribed interventions to minimize the complications of events" (Carpenito-Moyet, 2017, p. 21). The definitive treatment for a client concern is developed by the nurse; the definitive treatment for a collaborative problem is developed by both the nurse and the physician. Not all physiologic complications are collaborative problems. If the nurse can prevent the complication or provide the primary treatment, then the problem may very well be a client concern. For example, nurses can prevent and treat pressure injury. Therefore, "risk for poor skin integrity" is the client concern.

Table 3-2 compares the three types of client concerns: (1) opportunities to improve health, (2) risks for client concern, and (3) actual client concerns. The nurse can use this model to decide whether the identified problem can be treated independently as a client concern or whether the nurse will monitor and use both medical and nursing interventions to treat or prevent the problem. Table 3-3 compares and differentiates client concerns and collaborative problems.

If collaborative and nursing interventions are not enough to resolve the problem, the problem requires medical diagnoses and intervention to resolve, so the nurse should refer these situations to the client's primary care provider. Table 3-4 gives examples of client concerns, collaborative problems, and medical diagnoses.

TABLE 3-3 **Comparison of Client Concerns and Collaborative Problems**

Identifying Criteria of a Client Concern	Identifying Criteria of a Collaborative Problem
1. The client problem is physiologic, psychosocial, or spiritual.	1. The client problem is a physiologic complication.
2. The nurse monitors and treats.	2. The nurse monitors for signs and symptoms of the complication and notifies the physician if a change occurs. (In some cases, the nurse may initiate interventions.)
3. The nurse independently orders and implements the primary nursing interventions.	3. The physician orders the primary treatment, and the nurse collaborates to implement additional treatments that are licensed to be implemented and monitors for responses to and effectiveness of treatments.

(*Continued on following page*)

TABLE 3-3 **Comparison of Client Concerns and Collaborative Problems** (*continued*)

Format and Follow-Up for Client Concern	Format and Follow-Up for Collaborative Problems
1. **Client concern** + associated with + cause 2. Write specific client goals. 3. Write specific nursing orders (interventions) including assessments, teaching, counseling, referrals, and direct client care.	1. Use "Risk for complication: _____." 2. Write nursing goals. 3. Write which parameters the nurse must monitor, including how often. Indicate when the physician should be notified. Identify the nursing interventions to prevent the complication and those to be initiated if a change occurs.

TABLE 3-4 **Examples of Client Concerns, Collaborative Problems, and Medical Diagnoses**

Client Concerns	Collaborative Problems	Medical Diagnoses
Unhealthy oral mucous membranes associated with difficulty with hygiene secondary to fixation devices and memory loss	Risk for complication: Aspiration	Fractured jaw
Poor skin integrity associated with poor leg circulation	Risk for complication: Hyperglycemia	Diabetes mellitus
Ineffective airway clearance related to the presence of excessive mucus production	Risk for complication: Hypoglycemia	Pneumonia
	Risk for complication: Hypoxemia	

Documenting Data

Documentation of assessment data is crucial as evidenced by state nurse practice acts, accreditation and/or reimbursement agencies (e.g., The Joint Commission on Accreditation of Healthcare Organizations [TJC], Medicare, Medicaid), professional organizations (local, state, and national), and institutional agencies (acute, transitional, long term, and home care). The primary reason for documentation of assessment data is to promote effective communication among multidisciplinary health team members. The use of electronic health records (EHRs) has improved diagnostic and clinical outcomes, reduced errors, and improved client safety (Health IT, 2019).

GUIDELINES FOR DOCUMENTING DATA

Use these guidelines to document your findings:

- *Make notes* as you perform the assessments and document as concisely as possible. *Avoid documenting with general nondescriptive or nonmeasurable terms* such as normal, abnormal, good, fair, satisfactory, or poor. *Instead, use specific descriptive and measurable terms* (e.g., 3 in. in diameter, red excoriated edges, with purulent yellow drainage) about what you inspected, palpated, percussed, and auscultated. See Table 3-5 for examples of vague versus clear, concise documentation.

- *Keep confidential all documented information in the client record.* Most agencies require nurses to complete Health Insurance Portability and Accountability Act (HIPAA, 1996) training. This training is intended to ensure that use, disclosure of, and requests for protected information are controlled and that the protected information is used only for intended purposes and that use is kept to a minimum. Clients must also be educated on their rights in relation to HIPAA.

- *Document legibly or print clearly in permanent ink.* Errors in documentation are usually corrected by drawing one line through the entry, writing "error," and initialing the entry. Never obliterate the error with white paint or tape, an eraser, or a marking pen. Keep in mind that the health record is a legal document.

- *Use correct grammar and spelling.* **Use only abbreviations that are acceptable and approved by the institution.** Avoid slang, jargon, or labels unless they are direct quotes.

- *Avoid wordiness that creates redundancy.* For example, do not record: "Auscultated gurgly bowel sounds in right upper, right lower, left upper, and left lower abdominal quadrants. Heard

TABLE 3-5 **Examples of Vague Versus Clear and Concise Documentation of Data**

Vague Documentation	Clear and Concise Documentation
Source and reliability of information: Client	Client awake, alert, and oriented to person, place, time, and events. Initiates and maintains conversation. Asks and answers questions that are appropriate.
Memory intact	Recent and remote memory intact
Vital signs good	Temperature 98.6°F, pulse 66 regular, respirations 18, blood pressure 160/88
Skin color normal	Skin pink with consistent pigmentation
Appetite good	Reports no change in appetite (list 24-hour diet recall on a typical day)
Swelling of ankles	Pitting edema 3+ of both ankles that lasts 10 seconds
Hears poorly	"My wife says I always turn the radio and TV up too loud so I guess I am hard of hearing."
Heart rate regular	Heart regular rate and rhythm: S1 and S2 present; S1 loudest at the apex, S2 loudest at base; no S3, S4, murmur, rub, or gallop
Chest sounds clear	Anterior, posterior, and bilateral chest sounds clear to auscultation
Normal bowel sounds	5–20 bowel sounds per minute, active bowel sounds in all four quadrants
Voids a lot	Polyuria, urine output = 3,000 mL/day

36 gurgles per minute." Instead record: "Bowel sounds present in all quadrants at 36 per minute."

- *Use phrases instead of sentences to record data.* For example, avoid recording: "The client's lung sounds were clear both in the right and left lungs." Instead record: "Bilateral lung sounds clear."

- *Record data findings, not how they were obtained.* For example, do not record: "Client was interviewed for past history of high blood pressure, and blood pressure was taken." Instead record: "Client has 3-year history of hypertension treated with medication. BP sitting right arm 140/86, left arm 136/86."

- *Write entries objectively without making premature judgments or diagnoses.* Use quotation marks to identify clearly the client's responses. For example, record: "Client crying in room, refuses to talk, husband has gone home" instead of "Client depressed due to fear of breast biopsy report and not getting along well with husband." Avoid making inferences and diagnostic statements until you have collected and validated all data with client and family.

- *Record the client's understanding and perception of problems.* For example, record: "Client expresses concern regarding being discharged soon after gallbladder surgery because of inability to rest at home with six children."

- *Avoid recording the word "normal" for normal findings.* For example, do not record: "Liver palpation normal." Instead record: "Liver span 10 cm in right MCL and 4 cm in MSL. No tenderness on palpation." Also avoid using the terms *good, fair, poor, sometimes, occasional, frequently, recently,* or *some.* Instead use specific quantitative or qualitative descriptive terms.

- *Record complete information and details for all client symptoms or experiences.* For example, do not record: "Client has pain in lower back." Instead record: "Client reports aching-burning pain in lower back for 2 weeks. Pain worsens after standing for several hours. Rest and ibuprofen used to take edge off pain. No radiation of pain. Rates pain as 7 on scale of 1 to 10."

- *Include additional assessment content when applicable.* For example, include information about the caregiver or last physician contact.

- *Support objective data with specific observations obtained during the physical examination.* For example, when describing the emotional status of the client as depressed, follow it with a description of the ways depression is demonstrated, such as "dressed in dirty clothing, avoids eye contact, unkempt appearance, and slumped shoulders."

VERBAL COMMUNICATION OF DATA USING SBAR

Nurses are often in situations in which they are required to verbally share their subjective and objective assessment findings. The SBAR (Situation, Background, Assessment, and Recommendation) model of communication is one consistent way to communicate assessment data. SBAR, described in Box 3-1, has been found to improve quality and client safety outcomes when used by health team members to communicate or hand off client information (Beckett & Kipnis, 2009). In order to prevent data communication errors, it is important to:

- use a standardized method of data communication such as SBAR (see Box 3-1).
- communicate face to face with good eye contact.
- allow time for the receiver to ask questions.

BOX 3-1 SBAR (SITUATION, BACKGROUND, ASSESSMENT, AND RECOMMENDATION)

Situation: State concisely why you need to communicate the client data that you have assessed (e.g., Mary Lorno, age 18, is experiencing a sudden onset of periumbilical pain).

Background: Describe the events that led to the current situation (e.g., client first noticed periumbilical pain at 10:30 AM. She denies any precipitating factors).

Assessment: State the subjective and objective data you have collected (e.g., *Subjective:* Client rated pain as 7 to 8 on a scale of 0 to 10 at onset and now rates the pain as 3 to 4 on a scale of 0 to 10. She denies nausea, vomiting, and diarrhea. She voices anorexia. Eating and drinking exacerbate the pain, and lying in a knee-chest position diminishes pain. Describes the pain as "stabbing." *Objective:* Client is awake, alert, and oriented. She makes and maintains conversation. Does not appear to be in acute distress. T—98.7, P—72, R—16, BP—112/64. Color pink. Skin warm and dry. Mucous membranes moist. Abdomen flat without visible pulsations. Bowel sounds present and hypoactive. Abdomen tympanic upon percussion. Abdomen is soft. Light palpation reveals minimal tenderness in right lower quadrant [RLQ]. Deep palpation reveals minimal tenderness in RLQ. Rovsing sign is negative. Obturator sign is negative. No rebound tenderness noted.).

Recommendation: Suggest what you believe needs to be done for the client based on your assessment findings. (Example: Suggest that the primary care provider come to further assess the client and intervene).

- provide documentation of the data you are sharing.
- validate what the receiver has heard by questioning or asking them to summarize your report.
- when reporting over a telephone ask the receiver to read back what they heard you report and document the phone call with time, receiver, sender, and information shared.

References

Beckett, C., & Kipnis, G. (2009). Collaborative communication: Integrating SBAR to improve quality/patient safety outcomes. *Journal of Healthcare Quality, 31*(5), 19–28. https://doi.org/10.1111/j.1945-1474.2009.00043.x

Carpenito-Moyet, L. J. (2017). *Nursing diagnosis: Applications to clinical practice* (15th ed.). Lippincott Williams & Wilkins.

Health IT. (2019). *Improved diagnostics and patient outcomes.* https://www.healthit.gov/topic/health-it-and-health-information-exchange-basics/improved-diagnostics-patient-outcomes

U.S. Department of Health and Human Services. (1996). *Health Insurance Portability and Accountability Act of 1996.* https://aspe.hhs.gov/report/health-insurance-portability-and-accountability-act-1996

4

ASSESSING PSYCHOSOCIAL, COGNITIVE, AND MORAL DEVELOPMENT

Growth and Development Overview

The developmental theories presented in this chapter focus on the psychosocial, cognitive, and moral *growth* (addition of new skills) and *development* (improvement of existing skills) of an individual throughout the life span. Psychosocial growth and development is explained using the works of Erikson. Cognitive development is explained using Piaget theory, and moral development is described using Kohlberg theory.

ERIKSON THEORY OF PSYCHOSOCIAL DEVELOPMENT

Erikson (1963) developed the psychosocial theory, which is defined as the intrapersonal and interpersonal responses of a person to external events (Schuster & Ashburn, 1992). Erikson concluded that societal, cultural, and historic factors as well as biophysical processes and cognitive function influence personality development (Erikson, 1968). He declared that the *ego* not only mediates between the *id's* abrupt impulses and the *superego's* moral demands but also can positively affect a person's development as more skills and experience are gained. Erikson believed that personality development continues to evolve throughout the life span. He identified eight stages of the life span through which a person may sequentially develop (see Table 4-1). Each stage (or achievement level) proposed has a central developmental task called a *crisis*. Crises are dilemmas composed of opposing viewpoints (e.g., *basic trust vs. basic mistrust*). If a person resolves the challenge in favor of the more positive of the two viewpoints (e.g., emphasis on *basic trust*), then that person achieves resolution of the developmental task. The person must negotiate a healthy balance between the two concepts in order to move to the next stage and eventually become a well-adjusted adult in

society. For example, a person needs some *basic mistrust* in some situations (e.g., stay a safe distance from blazing flames, cautiously approach an unfamiliar animal). Positive resolution for a crisis in one stage is necessary for positive resolution in the next stage. Erikson proposed that strengths emerge with the positive resolution of each *crisis*. If a task is only partially resolved, then a person experiences difficulty in subsequent developmental tasks. These issues must be remediated to realize one's psychosocial potential. Erikson did not use chronologic boundaries but assigned developmental levels throughout the life span, which each person develops at their own rate based on potential and experiences (see Table 4-1).

PIAGET THEORY OF COGNITIVE DEVELOPMENT

Dr. Piaget (1970) explained the growth and development of intellectual structures. He focused on *how* a person learns and recognized that interrelationships of physical maturity, social interaction, environmental stimulation, and experiences were necessary for cognitive development. To explain his theory, he applied the concepts of *schema* (plural: *schemata*), *assimilation*, *accommodation*, and *equilibration* (equilibrium). A *schema* is a unit of thought that may consist of a thought, emotional memory,

TABLE 4-1 **Erik Erikson's Stages of Psychosocial Development**

Developmental Level	Central Task	Focal Relationships/Issues	Negative Resolution	Positive Resolution (Basic Virtues)
Infant	Basic trust vs. basic mistrust	Mother, primary caregivers, feeding, *"feeling and being comforted,"* sleeping, teething, *"taking in,"* trusting self, others, and environment	Suspicious, fearful	Drive and hope
Toddler	Autonomy vs. shame and doubt	Parents, primary caregivers, toilet training, bodily functions, experimenting with *"holding on and letting go,"* having control without loss of self-esteem	Doubts abilities, feels ashamed for not trying	Self-confidence and willpower
Preschooler	Initiative vs. guilt	Family, play, exploring and discovering, learning how much assertiveness influences others and the environment, developing a sense of moral responsibility	May fear disapproval of own powers	Direction and purpose
School-ager	Industry vs. inferiority	School, teachers, friends, experiencing physical independence from parents, neighborhood, wishing to accomplish, learning to create and produce, accepting when to cease a project, learning to complete a project, learning to co-operate, developing an attitude toward work	May feel sense of failure	Method and competence

(*Continued on following page*)

TABLE 4-1　Erik Erikson's Stages of Psychosocial Development (*continued*)

Developmental Level	Central Task	Focal Relationships/Issues	Negative Resolution	Positive Resolution (Basic Virtues)
Adolescent	Identity vs. role confusion	Peers and groups, experiencing emotional independence from parents, seeking to be the same as others yet unique, planning to actualize abilities and goals, fusing several identities into one	Confused, nonfocused	Devotion and fidelity
Young adult	Intimacy vs. isolation	Friends, lovers, spouses, community, work connections (networking), committing to work relationships, committing to social relationships, committing to intimate relationships	Loneliness, poor relationships	Affiliation and love
Middle-aged adult	Generativity vs. stagnation	Younger generation—often children (whether one's own or those of others), family, community, mentoring others, helping to care for others, discovering new abilities/talents, continuing to create, *"giving back"*	Shallow involvement with the world in general, selfish, little psychosocial growth	Production and care
Older adult	Ego integrity vs. despair[a]	All mankind, reviewing one's life, acceptance of self-uniqueness, acceptance of worth of others, acceptance of death as an entity	Regretful, discontented, pessimistic	Renunciation and wisdom

[a]Based on his experiences/research and as he continued to live longer, Erikson contemplated extending this phase of generativity and suggested that a ninth stage might be added to his theory. He posited that those who positively resolved generativity could move to a higher level that addressed a *premonition of immortality* (i.e., a new sense of self that transcends universe and time).

Information from Erikson, E. H. (1963). *Childhood and society* (2nd ed.). W. W. Norton & Company, Inc.; Erikson, E. H. (1968). *Identity: Youth and crisis.* W. W. Norton & Company, Inc.; Erikson, E. H., Erikson, J. M., & Kivnick, H. Q. (1986). *Vital involvement in old age.* W. W. Norton & Company, Inc.; Erikson, E. H. (Ed.). (1991). *Erikson's stages of personality development. Childhood and society.* W. W. Norton & Company, Inc.; Schuster, C. S., & Ashburn, S. S. (1992). *The process of human development: A holistic life-span approach* (3rd ed.). J. B. Lippincott Company.

movement of a part of the body, or a sensory experience (such as making use of sight, hearing, taste, smell, or touch). *Schemata* can be categorized using either *assimilation* or *accommodation*. *Assimilation* is an adaptive process whereby a stimulus or information is incorporated into an already existing *schema*. Another way of saying this is the person changes reality into what they already know. For example, a toddler, who knows their pet cat to be a "Kitty," sees a dog for the first time and thinks the new animal is called "Kitty." *Accommodation* is the creation of a new *schema* or the modification of an old one to differentiate more accurately a stimulus or a behavior from an existing *schema*. One changes the self to fit reality. The same toddler may meet other cats and modify "Kitty" to "cat" and eventually, with experience and guidance, meet more dogs and create the idea of "dog." *Equilibration* is the balance between assimilation and *accommodation*. When disequilibrium occurs, it provides motivation for the individual to *assimilate* or *accommodate* further. A person who only assimilated stimuli would not be able to detect differences in things; a person who only accommodated stimuli would not be able to detect similarities. Piaget emphasized that *schemata, assimilation, accommodation,* and *equilibration* are all essential for cognitive growth and development. Piaget (1970) postulated that a person may progress through four major stages of intellectual development beginning at birth. Ages are not attached to these stages since each person progresses at their own rate. At each new stage, previous stages of thinking are incorporated and integrated. If a person attained formal operational thinking (see Table 4-2), they declare that qualitative changes in thinking cease and quantitative changes in the content and function of thinking may continue.

KOHLBERG THEORY OF MORAL DEVELOPMENT

Lawrence Kohlberg, a psychologist, developed a theory of moral development. He proposed that morality is a dynamic process that extends over one's lifetime, involving the affective and cognitive domains in determining what is "right" and "wrong." Dr. Kohlberg examined the *reasoning* a person uses to make a decision, as opposed to the *action* that results after that decision is made. Moral development is influenced by cognitive structures, but not in the same way as cognitive development. Kohlberg viewed *justice* (or fairness) as the goal of moral judgment.

TABLE 4-2   **Jean Piaget's Stages of Cognitive Development**

Stage	Approximate Age	Significant Characteristics
Sensorimotor	0–2 years	Thoughts are demonstrated by physical manipulation of objects/stimuli
Substage 1: Making use of ready-made reflexes (pure *assimilation*)	0–1 month	Pure reflex adaptation (e.g., if lips are touched, baby sucks; if object placed in palm, baby grasps)
Substage 2: Primary circular reactions (*assimilation, accommodation,* and *equilibrium* are now used as individual grows and develops)	1–4 months	Actions centered on infant's body and endlessly repeated reflex activities become modified and coordinated with each other with experience. Infant repeats behaviors for sensual pleasure (e.g., kicks repetitively, plays with own hands and fingers, sucking for a long time). Early coordination of selected reflexes (e.g., sucking and swallowing) and schema (e.g., hearing and looking at same object)
Substage 3: Secondary circular reactions	4–8 months	Center of interest is not on own body's action but the environmental consequences of those actions. Behavior becomes *intentional*. Baby repeats behaviors that produce *novel* (e.g., pleasing, interesting) effects on environment (e.g., crying to get caregivers' attention). Increased voluntary coordination of motor skills enabling exploration (e.g., mouthing objects by combining grasping and sucking). Appears to have *cognitive object constancy*—an awareness that an object or person is the same regardless of the angle from which viewed (e.g., baby will anticipate eating when they see bottle of formula even if it is upside down and across the room)

Substage 4: Coordination of secondary circular reactions in new situations	8–12 months	Infant consciously uses an action that is a means to an end and solves simple problems (e.g., will reach for a toy and then will use that toy to retrieve another toy originally out of reach). *Object permanence* appears at approximately 8 months. This is the awareness that an object continues to exist even though one is not in direct contact with that object (e.g., when infant sees someone hide a favorite toy under a blanket, they will attempt to retrieve it from under the blanket). Imitate simple behaviors of others
Substage 5: Tertiary circular reactions	12–18 months	Child now "experiments" (much trial and error) in order to discover new properties of objects and events. Varies approaches to an old situation or applies old approaches to a new problem. Must physically solve a problem to understand cause–effect relationship. Imitates simple novel behaviors
Substage 6: Invention of new means through mental combinations	18–24 months	Invention of new means can occur without actual physical experimentation. Occasional new means through physical experimentation—still much trial and error problem solving. Child begins to *mentally represent* object/events before physically acting (e.g., can solve "detour" problems to go one small distance to another). Engages in early symbolic play. Both immediate and deferred imitation of actions and words noted

(*Continued on following page*)

TABLE 4-2   **Jean Piaget's Stages of Cognitive Development** (*continued*)

Stage	Approximate Age	Significant Characteristics

Preoperational
• Divided into two substages:
 	
• Preconceptual (2–4 years) and intuitive (4–7 years)
• During the preconceptual substage, the child inconsistently assigns any word to several similar stimuli (e.g., child calls all four-legged mammals by their pet cat's name)
	2–7 years	Increasing ability to make a mental representation for something not immediately present using language as a major tool. Eventually, the child is able to give their reasons for beliefs and rationales for action; however, they remain biased and immature. Magical thought (wishing something will make it so) predominates
		• The following characteristics (although they go through modification as the child develops from 2 to 7 years of age) serve as some obstacles to "adult logic":
		  • *Fundamental egocentrism*—never thinks that anything is other than the way they perceive it (e.g., "If I'm going to bed now, every child is going to bed now")
		  • *Centration*—tends to focus on one aspect of an object or experience (e.g., when asked to compare two rows of like objects with one row containing six pennies and the other, a longer row containing three pennies would answer that the longer row is "more")
		  • *Limited transformation*—is not able to comprehend the steps of how an object is changed from one state to another (e.g., could not explain the sequence of events that occurs when an ice cube melts and turns into a puddle of water)

- During the intuitive stage, the child begins to realize the ability of a word to truly represent a specific object, event, or action

- *Action rather than abstraction*—perceives an event as if actually participating in the event again (e.g., when asked about riding in a toy car, may imitate turning the steering wheel when they think about it)
- *Irreversibility*—unable to follow a line of reasoning back to its beginning (e.g., if child is taken on a walk, especially one with a turn, they are unable to retrace their steps and return to the original point)
- *Transductive reasoning*—thinks specific to specific; if two things are alike in one aspect, the child thinks they are alike in all aspects (e.g., child thinks beetle seen on a picnic in the park is the same beetle seen in their backyard)
- *Animism*—believes that inert objects are alive with feelings and can think and function with intent (e.g., child thinks that if vacuum cleaner "eats" the dirt, then it can "eat" them)

| Concrete operational | 7–11 years | Begins to think and reason logically about objects in the environment. Can mentally perform actions that previously had to be carried out in actuality. Reasoning is limited to concrete objects and events ("what is"), but not yet abstract objects and events ("what might be"). *Inductive* reasoning (specific to general) has begun. Can consider viewpoints of others. Understands and uses time on a clock. Understands days of week, months of year. Best understands years within life experience. Can decenter, understands transformations. Can reverse thoughts |

(*Continued on following page*)

TABLE 4-2   **Jean Piaget's Stages of Cognitive Development** (*continued*)

Stage	Approximate Age	Significant Characteristics
		Progressively able to *conserve* (understand that properties of substances will remain the same despite changes made in shape or physical arrangement) numbers, mass, weight, and volume in that order. Begins to understand relationship between distance and speed. Learns to add, subtract, multiply, and divide. Can organize, then classify objects. Progressively capable of money management
Formal operational	11–15+ years	Develops ability to problem-solve about both the real and the possible. Can logically and flexibly think about the past, present, and future. Possesses ability to think about symbols that represent other symbols (e.g., $x = 1$, $y = 2$). Can think abstractly when presented with information in verbal (as opposed to written) form
		Able to envision and systematically test many possible combinations in reaching a conclusion. Able to generate multiple potential solutions while considering the possible positive/negative effects of each solution. Can perform *deductive* reasoning (general to specific). Can hypothesize ("If … then" thinking)
		Can think about thinking (metacognition)

Information from Piaget, J. (1952). *The origins of intelligence in children* (M. Cook, Trans.). International Universities Press; Piaget, J. (1969). *The language and thought of the child* (M. Gabain, Trans.). Meridian Books; Piaget, J., & Inhelder, B. (1969). *The psychology of the child* (H. Weaver, Trans.). Basic Books, Inc.; Piaget, J. (1981). *The psychology of intelligence* (M. Piercy & D. E. Berlyne, Trans.). Littlefield & Adams; Piaget, J. (1982). *Play, dreams and imitation in children* (C. Gattengo & F. M. Hodgson, Trans.). Norton; and Schuster, C. S., & Ashburn, S. S. (1992). *The process of human development: A holistic life-span approach* (3rd ed.). J. B. Lippincott Company.

Kohlberg (Colby et al., 1983) proposed three levels of moral development that encompass six stages (see Table 4-3). He believed that few people progress past the second level. Asserting that moral development extends beyond adolescence, he saw moral decisions and reasoning becoming increasingly differentiated, integrated, and universalized (i.e., independent of culture)

TABLE 4-3 **Lawrence Kohlberg's Stages of Moral Development**

Level	Stage	Average Age	Characteristic Moral Reasoning That May Influence Behavior
Preconventional (premoral)	1. Orientation to punishment and obedience	Preschool through early school age	Finding it difficult to consider two points of view in a moral dilemma, individual ignores, or is unaware of meaning, value, or intentions of others and instead focuses on fear of authority. Will avoid punishment by obeying what told to do by caregiver/supervisor. The physical consequences of individual actions determine "right" or "wrong." Punishment means action was "wrong."
	2. Orientation to instrumental relativism (individual purpose)	Late preschool through late school age	Slowly becoming aware that people can have different perspectives in a moral dilemma. Individual views "right" action as what satisfies personal needs and believes others act out of self-interest. No true feelings of loyalty, justice, or gratitude. Individual conforms to rules out of self-interest or in relation to what others can do in return. Desires reward for "right" action.

(*Continued on following page*)

TABLE 4-3 Lawrence Kohlberg's Stages of Moral Development (*continued*)

Level	Stage	Average Age	Characteristic Moral Reasoning That May Influence Behavior
Conventional (maintain external expectations of others)	3. Orientation to interpersonal concordance (unity and mutuality)	School age through adulthood	Attempting to adhere to perceived norms; desires to maintain approval and affection of friends, relatives, and significant others. Wants to avoid disapproval and be considered a "good person" who is trustworthy, loyal, respectful, and helpful. Capable of viewing a two-person relationship as an impartial observer (beginning to judge the intentions of others—may or may not be correct in doing so)
	4. Orientation to maintenance of social order ("law and order")	Adolescence through adulthood	Attempting to make decisions and behave by strictly conforming to fixed rules and the written law—whether these be of a certain group, family, community, or the nation. "Right" consists of "doing one's duty."
Postconventional (maintain internal principles of self—Piaget's concept of formal operations must be employed at this level)	5. Orientation to social contract legalism	Middlescence through older adulthood (only 10%–20% of the dominant American *culture* attains this stage)	Regarding rules and laws as changeable with due process. "Right" is respecting individual rights while emphasizing the needs of the majority. Outside of legal realm, will honor an obligation to another individual or group, even if the action is not necessarily viewed as the correct thing to do by friends, relatives, or numerous others

| 6. Orientation to universal ethical principle[a] | Middlescence through older adulthood (few people either attain or maintain this stage) | Making decisions and behaving based on internalized rules, on conscience instead of social law and on self-chosen ethical principles that are consistent, comprehensive, and universal. Believes in absolute justice, human equality, reciprocity, and respect for the dignity of every individual person. Willing to act alone and be punished (or actually die) for belief. Such behavior may be seen in times of crisis |

[a]Shortly before his death, Kohlberg added a seventh stage of moral reasoning titled *Orientation to Self-Transcendence and Faith*. Kohlberg proposed that this stage moved beyond the concept of justice; the goal was to achieve a sense of unity with the cosmos, nature, or God. The person attaining this stage views everyone and everything as being connected; thus, any action of a person affects everyone and everything with any consequences of that person's action ultimately returning to him. According to Garsee and Schuster (1992), the person in stage 6 may be willing to *die* for their principles, whereas the person in stage 7 is willing to live for their beliefs.

Information from Colby, A., Kohlberg, L., Gibbs, J., Lieberman, M., Fischer, K., & Saltzstein, H. D. (1983). A longitudinal study of moral judgment. *Monographs of the Society for Research in Child Development, 48*(1–2), 1–124. https://doi.org/10.2307/1165935; Garsee, J. W., & Schuster, C. S. (1992). Moral development. In C. S. Schuster & S. S. Ashburn (Eds.), *The process of human development: A holistic life-span approach.* J.B. Lippincott Company; Kohlberg, L. (1984). *Essays on moral development* (Vol. 2). Harper & Row; Kohlberg, L. (1981). *The philosophy of moral development.* Harper & Row; Kohlberg, L., & Ryncarz, R. (1990). Beyond justice reasoning: Moral development and consideration of a seventh stage. In C. Alexander & E. Langer (Eds.), *Higher stages of human development* (pp. 191–207). Oxford University Press; Levine, C., Kohlberg, L., & Hewer, A. (1985). The current formulation of Kohlberg's theory and a response to critics. *Human Development, 28*(2), 94–100; and Schuster, C. S., & Ashburn, S. S. (1992). *The process of human development: A holistic life-span approach* (3rd ed.). J.B. Lippincott Company.

at each successive stage. A person must enter their moral stage hierarchy in an ordered and irreversible sequence with no relationship to biologic age. He concluded that a person may never attain a higher stage of moral development and thus not ascend this proposed hierarchy of stages. He believed part of this was determined by how much a person is challenged with decisions of a higher order. Kohlberg did not theorize that infants and young toddlers were capable of moral reasoning. He viewed them as being naïve and egocentric.

Nursing Assessment

COLLECTING SUBJECTIVE DATA

Ask the client about the following: age, birthplace, number of years in current country, residence, cultural group, primary language, highest level of education, employment history, means of making a living or maintaining everyday needs (food, shelter, etc.) if retired or unemployed, current health concerns or changes, body weight, major stressors, coping patterns, support systems, difficulty making decisions, current life changes, description of self, strengths, weaknesses, best way to learn, history of psychiatric or psychological problems, treatment and outcome, use of medications (prescribed or over the counter [OTC]), counseling, weight changes, eating patterns, elimination patterns, exercise patterns, sleep patterns, chronic illnesses, treatment and outcome, perception of whom one calls "family," recall of growing up as a child, siblings and relationships, significant genetic predisposition, characteristic trait, or disorder that you believe you have inherited, and lifestyle and health practices.

OBJECTIVE ASSESSMENT OF DEVELOPMENTAL LEVEL: PSYCHOSOCIAL STATUS

The following assessment table offers guidance for the objective assessment of the client's psychosocial, cognitive, and moral development.

ASSESSMENT PROCEDURE	NORMAL FINDINGS	ABNORMAL FINDINGS
Determine the client's psychosocial level by asking the following suggested questions. Does the young adult • still live with parent(s) at home? • accept roles and responsibilities at place of residence? • have experience of growing up in a single-parent home? • have unresolved issues with parent(s)? • have a satisfying sexual relationship with a significant other? • have gainful employment?	Many young adults today still live with parent(s) to continue higher education, become established in a career, or decrease financial hardship (Barroso et al., 2019). Others return home to recover from divorce, obtain support with their children, or regain financial stability. It is important that the young adult assume different roles than those performed during the earlier years of development. Generation Y (born between 1982 and 2001) is much more accepting of same-gender relationships. In the 21st century, a healthy sexual relationship includes practicing "safe sex." The young adult is more likely to possess a sense of positive self-preservation if they can meet some financial expenses. Today, healthy young adults experience mild anxiety while attempting to balance employment, education, and relationships.	If a young adult demonstrates extreme dependence on a parent (e.g., assumes no responsibility for household which they share), they may end up making poor relationship choices, experience gender role confusion and more than mild anxiety, and suffer from low self-esteem. Defense mechanisms including projection (attributing one's unacceptable feelings, thoughts, impulses, or wishes to another person). If the young adult does not possess a sense of healthy sexuality, social and emotional isolation may occur. This person has difficulty establishing healthy relationships with others. The young adult concerned about finances without a career may experience depression, anxiety, poor eating habits, insomnia, or vivid dreams.

(Continued on following page)

ASSESSMENT PROCEDURE	NORMAL FINDINGS	ABNORMAL FINDINGS
Does the middle-aged adult • demonstrate nervous mannerisms? • frequently derive pleasure from selected activities? • cope effectively with stress? • have a satisfying sexual relationship? • believe physical changes of aging have affected any relationships? Does the older adult • engage in sexual activity? • positively cope with loss? • believe any changes in cognition have occurred? • believe any significant changes have occurred in interests/relationships?	Copes with stress in a socially acceptable manner. All people experience stress throughout the life cycle. Mild anxiety (remaining attentive and alert to relevant stimuli) is normal throughout adulthood, providing motivation. Adaptive defense (coping) mechanisms may be used. Positive coping makes use of previously successful actions to decrease stress. Healthy middle-aged adults may vent frustration to significant others and effectively communicate in relationships, seeking assistance as needed. Meets socially accepted norms and maintains a balance of responsibilities and leisure activities. Many older adults are capable of enjoying sexual intimacy. Many older adults make effective use of communication and companionship to have a healthy sense of sexuality (Fig. 4-1). It is not uncommon to occasionally forget (e.g., to lose keys, misplace a pen or glasses, or not recall a person's name). The older adult makes effective use of previous experiences, self, and others to grieve loss. Experiencing more than one loss does not make a subsequent loss less painful.	Each person experiences midlife crisis differently. Those who effectively prioritize issues as they arise create an adaptive midlife transition. Common stressors for middle age include assisting adolescents to be more independent, caring for aging parents, grieving the loss of parents/grandparents, and maintaining career/social status. The unhealthy older adult may avoid relationships and society. Chronic depression is not normal in older adulthood. Current research on effects of stress and symptoms of dementia has not supported this belief. Memory loss is the first symptom of dementia. Other symptoms include difficulty remembering recent events, finding the right words, using good judgment, and maintaining personal hygiene.

ASSESSMENT PROCEDURE	NORMAL FINDINGS	ABNORMAL FINDINGS
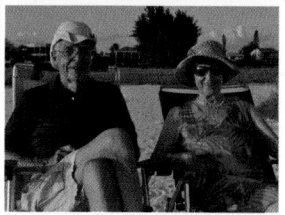 **FIGURE 4-1** Stereotypical images of the older adult as narrow minded, forgetful, sexless, and dependent are untrue for most of the older adult population. This older couple exhibits the vitality, joy, and spontaneity of a young couple. Determine the client's psychosocial developmental level by answering the following questions:		

(Continued on following page)

ASSESSMENT PROCEDURE	NORMAL FINDINGS	ABNORMAL FINDINGS

Does the young adult
- accept self—physically, cognitively, and emotionally?
- have independence from the parental home?
- express love responsibly, emotionally, and sexually?
- have close or intimate relationships with a partner?
- have a social group of friends?
- have a physiology of living and life?
- have a profession or a life's work that provides a means of contribution?
- solve problems of life that accompany independence from the parental home?

Intimacy

The young adult should have achieved self-efficacy during adolescence and is now ready to open up and become intimate with others (Fig. 4-2). Although this stage focuses on the desire for a special and permanent love relationship, it also includes the ability to have close, caring relationships with friends of both genders and a variety of ages. Spiritual love also develops during this stage. Having established an identity apart from the childhood family, the young adult is now able to form adult friendships with their parents and siblings. However, the young adult will always be a son or daughter.

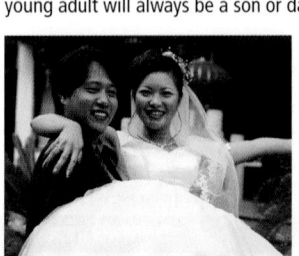

FIGURE 4-2 This young couple has reached Erikson's stage of intimacy. They have developed a loving relationship apart from their original families and fused their identity with one another.

Isolation

If the young adult cannot express emotion and trust enough to open up to others, social and emotional isolation may occur. Loneliness may cause the young adult to turn to addictive behaviors such as alcoholism, drug abuse, or sexual promiscuity. Some people try to cope with this developmental stage by becoming very spiritual or social, playing an acceptable role, but never fully sharing who they are or becoming emotionally involved with others. When adults successfully navigate this stage, they have stable and satisfying relationships with important others.

ASSESSMENT PROCEDURE	NORMAL FINDINGS	ABNORMAL FINDINGS
Does the middle-aged adult • have healthful life patterns? • derive satisfaction from contributing to growth and development of others? • have an abiding intimacy and long-term relationship with a partner? • maintain a stable home? • find pleasure in an established work or profession? • take pride in self and family accomplishments and contributions? • contribute to the community to support its growth and development?	**Generativity** During this stage, the middle-aged adult is able to share self with others and establish nurturing relationships. The adult will be able to extend self and possessions to others. Although traditionalists tend to think of generativity in terms of raising one's children and guiding their lives, generativity can be realized in several ways even without having children. Generativity implies mentoring and giving to future generations (Fig. 4-3). This can be accomplished by producing ideas, products, inventions, paintings, writings, books, films, or any other creative endeavors that are then given to the world for the unrestricted use of its people. Generativity also includes teaching others, children or adults; mentoring young workers; or providing experience and wisdom to assist a new business to survive and grow. Successful movement through this stage results in a fuller and more satisfying life and prepares the mature adult for the next stage.	**Stagnation** Without this important step, the gift is not given and the stage does not come to successful completion. Stagnation occurs when the middle-aged person has not accomplished one or more of the previous developmental tasks and is unable to give to future generations. Severe losses may result in withdrawal and stagnation. Then a person may have total dependency on work, a favorite child, or even a pet and be incapable of giving to others. Goals (e.g., projects, schooling) may never be finished because the person cannot let go. Without a creative outlet, a paralyzing stagnation sets in.

(Continued on following page)

ASSESSMENT PROCEDURE	NORMAL FINDINGS	ABNORMAL FINDINGS

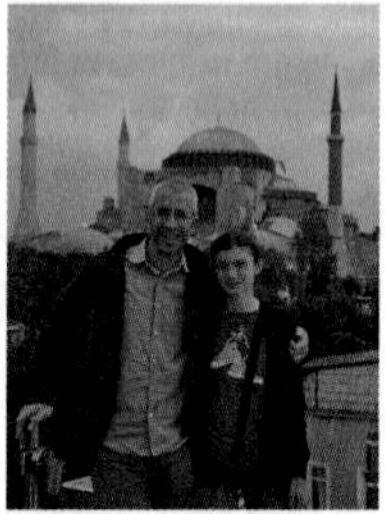

FIGURE 4-3 This father, in his early middle adult years, enjoys traveling with his teenage daughter and sharing with her his knowledge of history and culture.

Does the older adult
- adjust to the changing physical self?
- recognize changes present as a result of aging in relationships and activities?

Integrity

According to Erikson (1950), a person in this stage looks back and either finds that life was good or despairs because goals were not accomplished. This stage can extend over a long time and include excursions into previous stages to complete unfinished business. Successful movement through this stage does not mean that one day a person wakes up and says, "My life has been good"; rather, it encompasses a series of reminiscences in which the person may be able to see past events in a new and more positive light.

Despair

If the older person cannot feel grateful for their life, cannot accept those less desirable aspects as merely part of living, or cannot integrate all of the experiences of life, then the person will spend their last days in bitterness and regret and will ultimately die in despair.

ASSESSMENT PROCEDURE	**NORMAL FINDINGS**	**ABNORMAL FINDINGS**
• maintain relationships with children, grandchildren, and other relatives? • continue interests outside self and home? • complete transition from retirement at work to satisfying alternative activities? • establish relationships with others who are their own age? • adjust to deaths of relatives, spouse, and friends?	This can be a very rich and rewarding time in a person's life, especially if there are others with whom to share memories and who can assist with reframing life experiences (Fig. 4-4). For some people, resolution and acceptance do not come until the final weeks of life, but this still allows for a peaceful death.	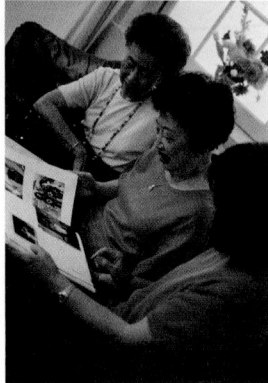 **FIGURE 4-4** Older adulthood can be a rich and rewarding time to review life events.

(*Continued on following page*)

ASSESSMENT PROCEDURE	NORMAL FINDINGS	ABNORMAL FINDINGS
• maintain a maximum level of physical functioning through diet, exercise, and personal care? • find meaning in past life and face inevitable mortality of self and significant others? • integrate philosophical or religious values into self-understanding to promote comfort? • review accomplishments and recognize meaningful contributions they have made to community and relatives?		
Determine the client's cognitive level by asking the following questions. Does the young adult • assume responsibility for independent decision making?	The young adult who has attained formal operational thought continues to use sensorimotor thought and learning. Being alert to both internal and external stimuli assists information processing. Cognitive regression occurs in all individuals throughout the life cycle under conditions of stress. However, it should be regained in a timely manner. Formal operations incorporate deductive reasoning. The young	The young adult who has not attained formal operations will operate at the stage at which cognitive arrest occurred. This person will have difficulty with abstract thinking when information is presented in written form.

ASSESSMENT PROCEDURE	NORMAL FINDINGS	ABNORMAL FINDINGS
• realistically self-evaluate strengths and weaknesses? • identify and explore multiple options and potential outcomes? • seek assistance as necessary? • place decision in long-range context? • make realistic plans for the future? • seek career mentors?	adult can evaluate the validity of reasoning. This person who performs self-evaluation must be able to make objective judgment. All people learn at their own pace and in their own style. The young adult is interested in learning that which is considered relevant and worthy of use. These people are capable of making realistic plans for the future.	This young adult will find it difficult to understand and process the information in some high-school and definitely college-level textbooks.
Does the middle-aged adult • differentiate discrepancies among goals, wishes, and realities? • identify factors that give life meaning and continuity? • effectively share knowledge and experience with others?	The middle-aged adult using formal operational thought is capable of readjusting/modifying goals as necessary. Improving active and developing latent interests and talents increases creativity. The healthy middle-aged person provides mentorship to others due to increased problem-solving abilities and experiences (Fig. 4-5). Seeking new information maintains currency and promotes continued self-development and responsibility. This is especially true regarding rapid progress in technology and emphasis on computerization. The older members of generation X (born between 1965 and 1981) wish to learn to advance	The middle-aged adult who has not attained/maintained formal operational thought experiences difficulty in remaining current at work and meeting expectations in all aspects of life in general. This person has not made adequate realistic plans for the future.

(Continued on following page)

ASSESSMENT PROCEDURE	NORMAL FINDINGS	ABNORMAL FINDINGS
• separate emotional (affective) issues from the cognitive domain for decision making? • seek new ways to improve/add to knowledge? • adapt quickly to change and new knowledge?	in their careers and other responsibilities. The "baby boomers" (born between 1946 and 1964) learn to adapt to fast change. Many of these adults have been called the sandwich generation (Schuster & Ashburn, 1992, p. 786; Parker & Patten, 2013) because they try to meet the needs of their teenagers/adult children (who have often returned to live at home and bring grandchildren) as well as caring for aging parents/grandparents. They are attempting to guide young people who are seeking independence while managing the older persons who are experiencing loss of independence.	The middle-aged client who has not attained formal operational thought may be able to teach other "hands-on" skills that do not require in-depth explanation and rationale.

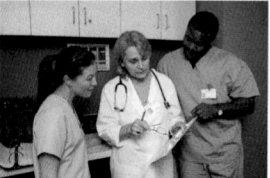

FIGURE 4-5 The middle-aged adult is able to mentor young adults in the workplace because they have increased problem-solving abilities and life experience.

ASSESSMENT PROCEDURE	NORMAL FINDINGS	ABNORMAL FINDINGS
Does the older adult • maintain maximal independence with activities of daily living? • problem-solve ways to find satisfaction with life? • determine realistic plans for future, including own mortality?	The older adult who uses formal operational thinking shares expertise with others, remembering events from earlier years. They teach others about the history and continuities of life. Many older adults prefer gradual transitions rather than abrupt changes. One who has seen much change can demonstrate flexibility and is able to make realistic decisions regarding activities, self-care, living arrangements, transportation, medical regimen, and finances. "Traditionalists" (born before 1946) value achievement and are often fiscally conservative due to experiences with rationing during wars and the great depression. Capable of gradually transferring social/civic responsibilities to others. Solidifies the concepts of life and death. Piaget believed new learning can continue to occur.	The older adult who does not possess formal operational thinking eventually profits from assistance from others, especially in obtaining activities of daily living, correctly taking medication, and maintaining the highest level of wellness.
Determine the client's moral level by asking the following suggested questions. Does the young adult • state priorities to be considered when making a moral decision? • perceive being approved by family?	According to Kohlberg theory, which was based on male behavior, the young adult who has at least reached Piaget's stage of concrete operations may have attained the conventional level of moral reasoning. As the young adult attempts to take on new roles (adult student, exclusive sexual relationship, vocation, marriage, parent), attempts are made to maintain expectations and rules of the family, group, partnership, or society. This young adult obeys the law because doing so signifies respect for authority. Guilt can be a motivator to do the	The young adult who continues to make decisions and behave for sole satisfaction has not attained the conventional level. Continued behavior that negatively affects the comfort zone of others or infringes on the rights of others is not normal (Fig. 4-6). Those persons

(Continued on following page)

ASSESSMENT PROCEDURE	NORMAL FINDINGS	ABNORMAL FINDINGS
• perceive being approved by peers? • perceive being approved by supervisor/teachers/authority figures? • perceive being approved by significant other? • consider self to be a "good person"? Why or why not? • have the ability to judge the intentions of others?	"right" thing. Decisions and behaviors are based on concerns about gaining approval from others. Some young adults who are capable of Piaget's formal operations will vacillate between the conventional and postconventional levels. For example, a young adult may intentionally break the law and join a protest group to stop medical research and experimentation on animals, believing that the principle of being humane to animals justifies the revolt. That same person may, however, exhibit more conventional reasoning when making decisions about "doing one's duty" at work, fulfilling the role of accountable student, and responsibly parenting a child.	experiencing extreme stress overload may demonstrate moral regression. 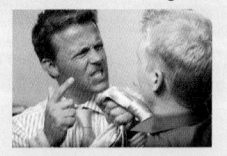 **FIGURE 4-6** The young adult who continually exhibits behavior that negatively affects the comfort zone of others or infringes on the rights of others is not normal.
Does the middle-aged adult • state priorities to be considered when making a moral decision? • focus more on law and order or individual rights when making a decision? • express willingness to stop unhealthy behavior and change lifestyle patterns to foster a higher level of wellness?	Kohlberg found that although many adults are capable of Piaget's stage of formal operations, few demonstrated the postconventional level of behavior and, if healthy, were more than likely at the conventional level. Kohlberg believed that if a person was capable of formal operations and experienced additional positive personal moral choices, then that person could reach a higher level of moral development. Many older middle-aged adults questioned authority and challenged the status quo during their young adult years. There are many healthy middle-aged people who feel that they have learned from mistakes made earlier during young adulthood.	The person who has consistently used maladaptive coping will not reach the postconventional level. Such a person could regress as far as the premoral (or even amoral) level. This person fears authority and hopes to "not get caught."

ASSESSMENT PROCEDURE	NORMAL FINDINGS	ABNORMAL FINDINGS
Does the older adult • state priorities to be considered when making a moral decision? • view rules and laws as changeable using legal means? • make decisions consistently on internalized rules and in terms of conscience? • believe in equality for every person?	Kohlberg believed very few people attain and maintain the highest stage of the postconventional level. During the fifth stage, the person believes in respect for individuals while still emphasizing that the needs of the majority are more important. During the sixth stage, the person believes in absolute justice for every individual and is willing to make a decision or perform an action risking external punishment. It may be that the older adult perceives more authority, time, and courage to "speak one's mind." Today's senior citizens may have developed belief patterns during a time very different from the 21st century. A few older adults, as they ponder their mortality, may enter Kohlberg's seventh stage. Such a person would analyze the "whole picture" and conclude that all organisms are interconnected.	The person who has consistently used maladaptive coping will not reach the postconventional level. Such a person could regress as far as the premoral (or even amoral) level. This person fears authority and hopes to "not get caught." It is difficult to assess anyone as normal or abnormal unless that person is harming self or others. Kohlberg hypothesized that older adults who were still at the preconventional level obey rules to avoid the disapproval of others. Kohlberg believed that older adults at the conventional level adhere to society's rules and laws because they believe this is what others expect of them.

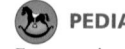 **PEDIATRIC VARIATIONS**

For a review of the stages associated with each developmental theory, see Tables 4-1 to 4-3.

Psychosocial Development (Erikson)

- Trust versus mistrust (birth to 1 year): Ask the parents or caregiver the following questions: How do you usually respond to your infant when they cry? Who usually cares for your infant when you are not around? Does your infant have a special blanket or toy that they often seek out for comfort or sleeping time?
- Autonomy versus shame and doubt (1–3 years): Ask the parents or caregiver the following questions: Does your toddler try to do things for themselves (e.g., feed, dress)? Does your toddler have temper tantrums? How are they handled? Does your toddler frequently use the word "no"? At what age was your toddler completely toilet trained? Does your toddler actively explore the environment?
- Initiative versus guilt (3–6 years): Ask the parents or caregiver the following questions: Does your preschooler have an active imagination? Does your preschooler imitate adult activities? Does your preschooler engage in fantasy play? Does your preschooler frequently ask questions? Does your preschooler enjoy new activities?
- Industry versus inferiority (7–11 years): Ask the parents or caregiver the following questions: What are your school-age child's interests/hobbies? Does your school-age child interact well with teachers, peers? Does your school-age child enjoy accomplishments? Does your school-age child shame self for failures? What is your school-age child's favorite activity?
- Identity versus role diffusion (11–18 years): Ask the parents or caregiver the following questions: Does your adolescent have a peer group? Does your adolescent have a best friend? Does your adolescent exhibit rebellious behavior at home? How does your adolescent see self as fitting in with peers? What does your adolescent want to do with their life?

Cognitive and Language Development (Piaget)

- Sensorimotor stage (birth to 18 months): Ask the parents or caregiver the following questions: Does your child have different types of crying? Explain. Does your infant coo, babble, make consonant sounds, combine syllables such as *mama* or *dada*? What does your infant do when you say "no-no"? What words does your infant use?

- Sensorimotor phase (12–24 months): Ask the parents or caregiver the following questions: Can your toddler name some body parts? Can your toddler state first and last name? Does your toddler imitate adults? Does your toddler put two words together to form a sentence (e.g., "me go")?
- Preoperational thought (2–7 years): Ask the parents or caregiver the following questions: Does your preschooler tell fantasy stories or have an imaginary friend? Does your preschooler have an invisible friend? Can your preschooler make simple classifications (e.g., dogs, cats)? Is your preschooler "chatty"? Does your preschooler frequently ask "why"? Can your preschooler name at least four colors?
- Concrete operations (7–11 years): Ask the parents or caregiver the following questions: Can your school-age child see another's point of view? Does your child collect things (e.g., baseball cards, dolls)? Does your child try to solve problems? How well does your child do in school? How well does your child read?
- Formal operations (11–15 years): Ask the parents or caregiver the following questions: Do you consider your adolescent to be a problem solver? How well does your adolescent do in school? Also ask the adolescent and compare the responses.

Moral Development (Kohlberg)

- Infants: Although Kohlberg theory of moral development begins with toddlerhood, infants cannot be overlooked. Child moral development begins with the value and belief system of the parents and the infant's own development of trust.
- First substage of the preconventional stage (1–2 years): What forms of discipline do you use with your child? How do you praise your child?
- Preconventional stage of moral development (3–10 years): What forms of discipline do you use with your child when they do something not acceptable? How do you reward your child? How do they respond to discipline and rewards?
- Conventional level of the role conformity stage (10–13 years): How does your child try to please others? Who do they try to please the most?
- Postconventional stage of morality (>13 years): Ask the parents or caregiver the following questions: Does your child understand the difference between right and wrong? Do you discuss family values with your child? Do you have family rules? How are they implemented? How are disciplinary measures handled? Has your child ever had problems with lying, cheating, or stealing? Has your child ever required disciplinary action at school? Has your child ever violated the law?

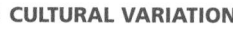 **GERIATRIC VARIATIONS**

Psychosocial Development (Erikson)

Ego integrity versus despair: Does the older adult accept self as unique, accept others, and accept death as an entity?

Cognitive Development (Piaget)

Does the older adult maintain maximal independence with activities of daily living? Problem-solve ways to find satisfaction with life? Determine realistic plans for future, including own mortality?

Moral Development (Kohlberg)

Does the older adult state priorities to be considered when making a moral decision? View rules and laws as changeable using legal means? Make decisions consistently on internalized rules and in terms of conscience? Believe in equality for every individual?

CULTURAL VARIATIONS

It is important to recognize and respect cultural variation. Ask the client: With what cultural group(s) do you most identify? What is your primary language? When do you speak it? Are you fluent in other languages? Language is initially promulgated via culture.

Erikson (1950) acknowledged differences of behavior caused by cultural conditions. Piaget (1981) postulated that cultural factors contribute significantly to differences in cognitive development. Kohlberg (Kohlberg & Gilligan, 1971) noted that cultures teach different beliefs, but that the stage sequence is universal and not affected by cultural difference.

POSSIBLE COLLABORATIVE PROBLEMS—RISK OF

- Anxiety
- Depression
- Suicide
- Neurosis
- Psychosis

Teaching Tips for Selected Client Concerns

Client Concern: Opportunity to improve parenting skills associated with acceptance and excitement of giving birth to first child

Teach new parents ways (bonding, interacting, playing, reading) to promote healthy physical, psychosocial, and cognitive development. Explain the variation in developmental milestones with individual children to alleviate anxiety.

Client Concern: *Caregiver stress associated with caring full time for dependent older parent*

Teach available resources to assist with the financial, physical, and psychosocial care of the older parent. Discuss the importance of engaging in healthy activities of daily living to stay healthy to meet one's own developmental goals.

 Client Concern: *Poor social interactions related to loss of driver's license, and poor vision and hearing*

Assist and teach client ways to access community resources (e.g., Meals on Wheels, senior centers, transportation for the disabled, local church organizations). Refer to organizations (e.g., American Foundation for the Blind, Hearing Loss Association of America) to acquire assistance with obtaining tools (e.g., magnifying glasses, large-print reading materials and checks, hearing devices) to enhance activities of daily living.

 Client Concern: *Poor family coping skills associated with family crisis with attempting to adapt to child's delayed development*

Discuss social development of the child. Assess the parents' knowledge and understanding of the developmental milestones for the child and educate them regarding normal parameters for the developmental stage of their child and the tasks that need to be achieved for the child to move to the next level. Infant's "stranger anxiety" is normal. Teach parents ways to assist infant to warm up to strangers. Encourage verbalization, reassurance, and cuddling. Help parent assess child's readiness to begin school and to discuss any school problems with child. Teach parents the importance of spending quality time with child and ways to promote effective communication with child. Encourage parents to identify parenting strategies that will enhance parenting skills and communication between themselves and the child. Identify strengths, weaknesses, and new coping skills that will improve communication and family dynamics between parents and child throughout the developmental changes of the life span.

References

Barroso, A., Parker, K., & Fry, R. (2019). *Majority of Americans say parents are doing too much for their young adult children.* Pew Research Center: Social & Demographic Trends. https://www.pewsocialtrends.org/2019/10/23/majority-of-americans-say-parents-are-doing-too-much-for-their-young-adult-children/

Colby, A., Kohlberg, L., Gibbs, J., Lieberman, M., Fischer, K., & Saltzstein, H. D. (1983). A longitudinal study of moral judgment. *Monographs of the Society for Research in Child Development, 48*(1–2), 1–124. https://doi.org/10.2307/1165935

Erikson, E. H. (1950). *Childhood and society.* W. W. Norton & Company, Inc.

Erikson, E. H. (1963). *Childhood and society* (2nd ed.). W. W. Norton & Company, Inc.

Erikson, E. H. (1968). *Identity: Youth and crisis.* W. W. Norton & Company, Inc.

Kohlberg, L., & Gilligan, C. (1971). *The adolescent as a philosopher: The discovery of the self in a postconventional world.* Daedalus.

Parker, K., & Patten, E. (2013). *The sandwich generation.* Pew Research Center: Social & Demographic Trends. https://www.pewsocialtrends.org/2013/01/30/the-sandwich-generation/

Piaget, J. (1970). Piaget's theory. In P. H. Mussen (Ed.), *Carmichael's manual of child psychology* (3rd ed.). Wiley.

Piaget, J. (1981). *The psychology of intelligence* (M. Piercy & D. E. Berlyne, Trans.). Littlefield & Adams.

Schuster, C. S., & Ashburn, S. S. (1992). *The process of human development: A holistic life-span approach* (3rd ed.). J. B. Lippincott Company.

Conceptual Foundations

Mental status refers to a client's level of cognitive and emotional functioning. The ability to think clearly and respond appropriately to daily stressors of life is necessary to function effectively in the activities of daily living. One cannot be totally healthy without "mental health." Mental health is an essential part of one's total health and is more than just the absence of mental disabilities or disorders. It is reflected in one's appearance, behavior, speech, thought patterns, and decision making and in one's ability to function in an effective manner in relationships in a variety of settings (home, work, social, recreational). The structure and function of the neurologic system can affect a client's mental and psychosocial status. Cerebral abnormalities may disturb the client's intellectual ability, communication ability, or emotional behaviors. Refer to Chapter 21, Assessing Neurologic System, for a review of the structure and function of the cerebral cortex. Several factors may influence the client's mental health or put them at risk for impaired mental health. These include economic and social factors, unhealthy lifestyle choices, exposure to violence, personality factors, spiritual factors, cultural factors, and/or changes or impairments in the structure and function of the neurologic system.

Nursing Assessment

COLLECTING SUBJECTIVE DATA

Past mental health diagnoses? Counseling services? Head injury, meningitis, encephalitis, stroke? Headaches? Served active duty in armed forces? Difficulty breathing, dizziness, nausea and vomiting, heart palpitations? Eating and bowel habits, family history of mental health disease, Alzheimer disease? Coping patterns? Pattern activities of daily living (energy level, sleep patterns, eating habits)? Use of over-the-counter and prescribed drugs?

Use of alcohol? Use the SBIRT (Screening, Brief Intervention, and Referral to Treatment) (Substance Abuse and Mental Health Services Administration–Health Resources and Services Administration, 2011) tool to identify, reduce, and prevent problematic use, abuse, and dependence on alcohol and illicit drugs. This is the most current recommended tool to use when substance abuse is suspected. The tool is designed for use by physicians, other health workers, and mental health professionals, and it can be used with clients 12 years of age and older. An app describing use of this tool can be found online (search on the key term "SBIRT app").

Use the CAGE or CAGE-AID Assessment Questionnaire (Brown & Rounds, 1995; Ewing, 1984) to detect alcohol and drug dependence in primary care populations. The AUDIT (the Alcohol Use Disorders Identification Test) Questionnaire (Box 5-1) may also be used to assess alcohol-related disorders by asking the client questions and then calculating a score. These questionnaires are available at https://www.drugabuse.gov/nidamed-medical-health-professionals/tool-resources-your-practice/screening-assessment-drug-testing-resources/chart-evidence-based-screening-tools-adults (National Institute on Drug Abuse [NIDA], 2018).

BOX 5-1 THE ALCOHOL USE DISORDERS IDENTIFICATION TEST (AUDIT): INTERVIEW VERSION

Instructions: Read questions as written. Record answers carefully. Begin the AUDIT by saying "Now I am going to ask you some questions about your use of alcoholic beverages during this past year." Explain what is meant by "alcoholic beverages" by using local examples of beer, wine, vodka, etc. Code answers in terms of "standard drinks." Place the correct answer number in the box at the right.

Questions

1. How often do you have a drink containing alcohol? ☐

   (0)   Never
   (1)   1 monthly or less
   (2)   2 to 4 times a month
   (3)   2 to 3 times a week
   (4)   4 or more times a week

If the score for Question 1 is 0, skip to Question 9.

2. How many drinks containing alcohol do you have on a typical day when you are drinking? ☐

   (0)   1 or 2
   (1)   3 or 4
   (2)   5 or 6
   (3)   7, 8, or 9
   (4)   10 or more

3. How often do you have six or more drinks on one occasion? ☐

   (0)   Never
   (1)   Less than monthly
   (2)   Monthly
   (3)   Weekly
   (4)   Daily or almost daily

Skip to Questions 9 and 10 if total score for Questions 2 and 3 is 0.

4. How often during the last year have you found that you were not able to stop drinking once you had started? ☐

   (0)   Never
   (1)   Less than monthly
   (2)   Monthly
   (3)   Weekly
   (4)   Daily or almost daily

(Continued on following page)

BOX 5-1 THE ALCOHOL USE DISORDERS IDENTIFICATION TEST (AUDIT): INTERVIEW VERSION (*continued*)

5. How often during the last year have you failed to do what was normally expected from you because of drinking? □
   - (0) Never
   - (1) Less than monthly
   - (2) Monthly
   - (3) Weekly
   - (4) Daily or almost daily

6. How often during the last year have you needed a first drink in the morning to get yourself going after a heavy drinking session the night before? □
   - (0) Never
   - (1) Less than monthly
   - (2) Monthly
   - (3) Weekly
   - (4) Daily or almost daily

7. How often during the last year have you had a feeling of guilt or remorse after drinking? □
   - (0) Never
   - (1) Less than monthly
   - (2) Monthly
   - (3) Weekly
   - (4) Daily or almost daily

8. How often during the last year have you been unable to remember what happened the night before because you had been drinking? □
   - (0) Never
   - (1) Less than monthly
   - (2) Monthly
   - (3) Weekly
   - (4) Daily or almost daily

9. Have you or someone else been injured as a result of your drinking? □
   - (0) No
   - (2) Yes, but not in the last year
   - (4) Yes, during the last year

10. Has a relative or friend or a doctor or another health worker been concerned about your drinking or suggested you cut down? □
    - (0) No
    - (2) Yes, but not in the last year
    - (4) Yes, during the last year

    Total Score: □

Scoring: The AUDIT is easy to score. Each of the questions has a set of responses to choose from, and each response has a score ranging from 0 to 4. The interviewer enters the score (the number within parentheses) corresponding to the patient's response into the box beside each question. All the response scores should then be added and recorded in the box labeled "Total."

Total scores of 8 or more are recommended as indicators of hazardous and harmful alcohol use, as well as possible alcohol dependence. (A cutoff score of 10 will provide greater specificity but at the expense of sensitivity.) Because the effects of alcohol vary with average body weight and differences in metabolism, establishing the cutoff point for all women and men older than 65 years one point lower at a score of 7 will increase sensitivity for these population groups.

Selection of the cutoff point should be influenced by national and cultural standards and by clinician judgment, which also determine recommended maximum consumption allowances. Technically speaking, higher scores simply indicate greater likelihood of hazardous and harmful drinking. However, such scores may also reflect greater severity of alcohol problems and dependence, as well as a greater need for more intensive treatment.

More detailed interpretation of a patient's total score may be obtained by determining on which questions points were scored. In general, a score of 1 or more on Question 2 or Question 3 indicates consumption at a hazardous level. Points scored above 0 on Questions 4 to 6 (especially weekly or daily symptoms) imply the presence or incipience of alcohol dependence.

Points scored on Questions 7 to 10 indicate that alcohol-related harm is already being experienced. The total score, consumption level, signs of dependence, and present harm all should play a role in determining how to manage a patient. The final two questions should also be reviewed to determine whether patients give evidence of a past problem (i.e., "yes, but not in the past year"). Even in the absence of current hazardous drinking, positive responses on these items should be used to discuss the need for vigilance by the patient.

Reproduced with permission from Babor, T. F., Higgins-Biddle, J. C., Saunders, J. B., & Monteiro, M. G. (2019). *AUDIT: The Alcohol Use Disorders Identification Test: Guidelines for use in primary health care* (2nd ed.). World Health Organization. https://www.who.int/publications-detail/audit-the-alcohol-use-disorders-identification-test-guidelines-for-use-in-primary-health-care

If alcohol withdrawal is suspected, use Box 5-2, Clinical Institute Withdrawal Assessment Scale.

Use of recreational drugs such as marijuana, tranquilizers, barbiturates, or cocaine? Relationship patterns with others?

Marital status? Educational level? Socioeconomic level? Exposure to environmental toxins? Cultural practices? Religious practices? Support systems? Feelings about the future?

BOX 5-2 CLINICAL INSTITUTE WITHDRAWAL ASSESSMENT SCALE

The Clinical Institute Withdrawal Assessment for Alcohol, commonly abbreviated as CIWA or CIWA-Ar (revised version), is a 10-item scale used in the assessment and management of alcohol withdrawal. Each item on the scale is scored independently, and the summation of the scores correlates with the severity of alcohol withdrawal. The scores are designed to prompt specific management decisions such as the administration of benzodiazepines. The 10 items evaluated on the scale are common symptoms and signs of alcohol withdrawal and are as follows:

Symptoms and Assessment	Scores
Nausea and vomiting. Ask "Do you feel sick to your stomach? Have you vomited?" Observation.	0 no nausea and no vomiting 1 mild nausea with no vomiting 2 3 4 intermittent nausea with dry heaves 5 6 7 constant nausea, frequent dry heaves, and vomiting
Tremor. Arms extended and fingers spread apart. Observation.	0 no tremor 1 not visible, but can be felt fingertip to fingertip 2 3 4 moderate, with patient's arms extended 5 6 7 severe, even with arms not extended
Paroxysmal sweats. Observation.	0 no sweat visible 1 barely perceptible sweating, palms moist 2 3 4 beads of sweat obvious on forehead 5 6 7 drenching sweats

Anxiety. Ask "Do you feel nervous?" Observation.	0 no anxiety, at ease
	1 mild anxious
	2 3 4 moderately anxious, or guarded, so anxiety is inferred
	5 6 7 equivalent to acute panic states as seen in severe delirium or acute schizophrenic reactions
Agitation. Observation.	0 normal activity
	1 somewhat more than normal activity
	2 3 4 moderately fidgety and restless
	5 6 7 paces back and forth during most of the interview, or constantly thrashes about
Tactile disturbances. Ask "Do you feel nervous?" Observation.	0 none
	1 very mild itching, pins and needles, burning or numbness
	2 mild itching, pins and needles, burning or numbness
	3 moderate itching, pins and needles, burning or numbness
	4 moderately severe hallucinations
	5 severe hallucinations
	6 extremely severe hallucinations
	7 continuous hallucinations

(*Continued on following page*)

BOX 5-2   CLINICAL INSTITUTE WITHDRAWAL ASSESSMENT SCALE (*continued*)

Symptoms and Assessment	Scores
Auditory disturbances. Ask "Are you more aware of sounds around you? Are they harsh? Do they frighten you? Are you hearing anything that is disturbing to you? Are you hearing things you know are not there?" Observation.	0 not present 1 very mild harshness or ability to frighten 2 mild harshness or ability to frighten 3 moderate harshness or ability to frighten 4 moderately severe hallucinations 5 severe hallucinations 6 extremely severe hallucinations 7 continuous hallucinations
Visual disturbances. Ask "Does the light appear to be too bright? Is its color different? Does it hurt your eyes? Are you seeing anything that is disturbing to you? Are you seeing things you know are not there?" Observation.	1 very mild sensitivity 2 mild sensitivity 3 moderate sensitivity 4 moderately severe hallucinations 5 severe hallucinations 6 extremely severe hallucinations 7 continuous hallucinations

Headache.	0 not present
Ask "Does your head feel different? Does it feel like there is a band	1 very mild
around your head?" Do not rate for dizziness or light-headedness.	2 mild
Otherwise, rate severity.	3 moderate
	4 moderately severe
	5 severe
	6 very severe
	7 extremely severe
Orientation and clouded sensorium.	0 oriented and can do serial additions
Ask "What day is this? Where are you? Who am I?"	1 cannot do serial additions or is uncertain about date
	2 disoriented for date by no more than 2 calendar days
	3 disoriented for date by more than 2 calendar days
	4 disoriented for place and/or person

Reprinted with permission from Sullivan, J. T., Sykora, K., Schneiderman, J., Naranjo, C. A., & Sellers, E. M. (1989). Assessment of alcohol withdrawal: The revised clinical institute withdrawal assessment for alcohol scale (CIWA-Ar). *British Journal of Addiction, 84*(11), 1353–1357. https://doi.org/10.1111/j.1360-0443.1989.tb00737.x

COLLECTING OBJECTIVE DATA

Equipment Needed

- Pencil and paper
- SBIRT

- CAGE Questionnaire and AUDIT Questionnaire. Both available at https://www.drugabuse.gov/nidamed-medical-health -professionals/tool-resources-your-practice/screening-assessment -drug-testing-resources/chart-evidence-based-screening-tools- adults

- Clinical Institute Withdrawal Assessment Scale
- Glasgow Coma Scale (GCS)
- Saint Louis University Mental Status (SLUMS) Examination Tool
- Primary Care Posttraumatic Stress Disorder Screen for *DSM-5* (PC-PTSD-5)
- Quick Inventory of Depressive Symptomatology (Self-Report)
- SAD PERSONS Suicide Risk Assessment

Physical Assessment

Perform an assessment of mental status by observing the client and asking questions. Much of this information may have already been assessed during the initial interview and general survey. There are several parts of the examination, which include assessment of the client's level of consciousness, posture, gait, body movements, dress, grooming, hygiene, facial expressions, behavior and affect, speech, mood, feelings, expressions, thought processes, perceptions, and cognitive abilities.

ASSESSMENT PROCEDURE	NORMAL FINDINGS	ABNORMAL FINDINGS
Observe level of consciousness • Note response to calling the client's name. If the client does not respond, call the name louder. If necessary, shake the client gently. If the client still does not respond, apply a painful stimulus.	• Alert and awake with eyes open and looking at examiner; client responds appropriately.	• Lethargy: Opens eyes, answers questions, and falls back asleep. • Obtunded: Opens eyes to loud voice, responds slowly with confusion, seems unaware of environment. • Stupor: Awakens to vigorous shake or painful stimuli, but returns to unresponsive sleep.

ASSESSMENT PROCEDURE	NORMAL FINDINGS	ABNORMAL FINDINGS
		• Coma: Remains unresponsive to all stimuli; eyes stay closed. Client with lesions of the corticospinal tract draws hands up to chest (*decorticate* or abnormal flexor posture) when stimulated. Client with lesions of the diencephalon, midbrain, or pons extends arms and legs, arches neck, and rotates hands and arms internally (*decorticate* or abnormal extensor posture) when stimulated.
• Use the GCS (Box 5-3) for clients who are at high risk for rapid deterioration of the nervous system. • If there is concern regarding the client's memory, use the SLUMS Dementia/Alzheimer's Test Examination (Box 5-4) if time is limited and a quick measure is needed to evaluate cognitive function.	• GCS score of 15 indicates an optimal level of consciousness. • A score between 27 and 30 for clients with a high school education and a score of 20 to 30 for clients with less than a high school education is considered normal.	• GCS score of less than 15 indicates some impairment of consciousness. A score of 3, the lowest possible score, indicates deep coma. • A SLUMS score of 20 to 27 for a high school educated client, or 14 to 19 for a less than high school educated client, indicates that mental cognition is impaired and the client should be referred for further testing.

(Continued on following page)

ASSESSMENT PROCEDURE	NORMAL FINDINGS	ABNORMAL FINDINGS
Ask client if they have had any past traumatic events in their life. Examples include experiencing a serious accident, fire, physical or emotional assault, or abuse, earthquake, flood, war, someone killed or dying, someone seriously injured, or had a loved one die through homicide or suicide. If the client indicates past history of traumatic events, use Box 5-5 Primary Care PTSD Screen for *DSM-5* (PC-PTSD-5).	Denies traumatic events.	Has experienced a traumatic event and is now having nightmares, avoids thinking of event, is on guard and easily startles, feels detached from people, feels guilty, blames self or others for the trauma that occurred. If a client answers "yes" to any three of five questions about how the traumatic event(s) have affected them over the past month, this is evidence of PTSD.
Observe appearance and movement • Posture	• Relaxed, with shoulders back and both feet stable	• Tense, rigid, slumped, asymmetrical posture. Slumped posture is seen with depression or organic brain disease.
• Gait	• Smooth, coordinated movements; client alters position occasionally.	• Uncoordinated—staggering, shuffling, and stumbling
• Motor movements	• Same as above	• Jerky, uncoordinated; tremors, tics, fast or slow movements. Bizarre movements are seen with schizophrenia; tense, fidgety, and restless behavior in anxious clients.

ASSESSMENT PROCEDURE	NORMAL FINDINGS	ABNORMAL FINDINGS
• Dress	• Clothes fit and are appropriate for occasion and weather.	• Clothes extra large or small and inappropriate for occasion. Inappropriate dress is seen with depression, dementia, Alzheimer disease, and schizophrenia.
• Hygiene	• Skin clean, nails clean and trimmed	• Dirty, unshaven; dirty nails; foul odors. Poor hygiene is seen with depression, dementia, Alzheimer disease, and schizophrenia; meticulous, finicky grooming in obsessive-compulsive disorder.
• Facial expression	• Good eye contact, smiles/frowns appropriately	• Poor eye contact is seen in apathy or depression; mask-like expression in Parkinson disease; extreme anger or happiness in anxious clients.
• Speech	• Clear with moderate pace	• High pitched; monotonal; hoarse; very soft or weak. Slow, repetitive speech is present in depression or Parkinson disease; loud and rapid in manic phases; irregular, uncoordinated speech in multiple sclerosis; dysphonia in impairment of cranial nerve X; dysarthria in Parkinson or cerebellar disease; aphasia in lesions of dominant hemisphere.

(Continued on following page)

ASSESSMENT PROCEDURE	NORMAL FINDINGS	ABNORMAL FINDINGS
Observe **mood** by asking, "How are you feeling?" or "What are your plans for the future?" • Feelings (vary from joy to anger) • Expressions	• Responds appropriately to the topic discussed; expresses feelings appropriate to the situation. • Expresses good feelings about self, others, and life; verbalizes positive coping mechanisms (talking, support systems, counseling, exercise, etc.)	• Expresses feelings inappropriate to the situation (e.g., extreme anger or euphoria). • Expresses dissatisfaction with self, others, and life in general; verbalizes negative coping mechanisms (use of alcohol, drugs, etc.); prolonged negative feelings seen with depression; elation and high energy seen with manic phases; excessive worry seen in obsessive-compulsive disorders; eccentric moods not relevant to situation are seen in schizophrenia.
Use Box 5-6: Quick Inventory of Depressive Symptomatology (Self-Report) to determine if the client is at risk for depression and needs to be referred to a primary care health provider for further evaluation.	Inventory scores of 0–5 = No risk of depression.	Inventory scores of 6–10 = Mild 11–15 = Moderate 16–20 = Severe 21–27 = Very severe
Observe **thought process and perceptions** by stating, "Tell me your understanding of your current health situation."		

ASSESSMENT PROCEDURE	NORMAL FINDINGS	ABNORMAL FINDINGS
• Clarity and content	• Expresses full and free-flowing thoughts during interview.	• Expressed thoughts are jumbled, confusing, and not reality oriented. Repetition and expression of illogical thoughts are seen with schizophrenia; rapid flight of ideas with manic phases; irrational fears with phobias; delusions seen with psychotic disorders, delirium, and dementia; illusions seen with acute grief, stress reactions, schizophrenia, and delirium; hallucinations with organic brain disease or psychotic illness.
• Perceptions	• Follows directions accurately; perceptions realistic and consistent with yours and others.	• Is unable to follow-through with directives; perceptions unrealistic and inconsistent with yours and others.
• Judgment	• Answers to questions are based on sound rationale.	• Impaired judgment may be seen in organic brain syndrome, emotional disturbances, mental retardation, or schizophrenia.

(Continued on following page)

ASSESSMENT PROCEDURE	NORMAL FINDINGS	ABNORMAL FINDINGS
• Identify possibly destructive or suicidal tendencies in client's thought processes and perceptions by asking, "How do you feel about the future?" or "Have you ever had thoughts of hurting yourself or doing away with yourself?" or "How do others feel about you?"	• Verbalizes positive, healthy thoughts about the future and self.	• Clients who are suicidal may share past attempts of suicide, give plan for suicide, verbalize feelings of worthlessness about self, joke about death frequently. Clients who are depressed or feel hopeless are at higher risk for suicide. Clients who have depression early in life have an increased risk for dementia (Bowers, 2014).
• Use Box 5-7, the SAD PERSONS Suicide Risk Assessment Tool, to determine the risk factors the client may have that may put them at risk for suicide.	• No risk factors are present on the SAD PERSONS factors.	• Evaluate any risk factors on the SAD PERSONS guide. Suicide was the 10th leading cause of death in the United States for all ages and is four times more prevalent in men (Centers for Disease Control and Prevention [CDC], 2017). Firearms, followed by suffocation or choking, and poisoning were the three most used methods (CDC, 2020b).
Observe cognitive abilities		
• Orientation—Ask client name, hour, date, season, where they live now.	• Aware of self, others, place, time; has address	• Unable to express where they are, time, and who others are; does not follow instructions. Reduced level of orientation is seen with organic brain disorders.

ASSESSMENT PROCEDURE	NORMAL FINDINGS	ABNORMAL FINDINGS
• Length of concentration	• Listens to you and responds with full thoughts.	• Fidgets; does not listen attentively to you; expresses incomplete thoughts. Distraction and inability to focus are noted with anxiety, fatigue, attention deficit disorders, and altered states due to drug or alcohol intoxication.
• Memory—Ask client, "What did you eat today?" (recent) and "When is your birthday?" (past).	• Correctly answers questions about current day's activities; recalls significant past events.	• Unable to recall any recent events with delirium, dementia, depression, and anxiety; unable to recall past events with cerebral cortex disorders. Use Box 5-8: The 10 Signs and Symptoms of Alzheimer Disease to screen for signs of Alzheimer disease. Use Table 5-1: Identifying the Cause of Confusion: Dementia, Delirium, or Depression to differentiate between dementia, delirium, or depression.
• Abstract reasoning—Ask client to explain a proverb, for example, "A stitch in time saves nine."	• Explains proverb accurately.	• Unable to give abstract meaning of proverb with schizophrenia, mental retardation, delirium, or dementia.

(Continued on following page)

ASSESSMENT PROCEDURE	NORMAL FINDINGS	ABNORMAL FINDINGS
• Ability to make sound judgments—Ask client questions such as "Why did you come to the hospital?" or "What do you do when you have pain?"	• Answers to questions are based on sound rationale.	• Answers to questions are not based on sound rationale in organic brain syndrome, emotional disturbances, mental retardation, or schizophrenia.
• Ability to identify similarities—Ask client questions such as "How are birds and bees alike?"	• Identifies similarity.	• Unable to identify similarity with schizophrenia, mental retardation, delirium, or dementia.
• Sensory perception and coordination—Ask client to write name and draw the face of a clock or copy simple figures such as:	• Writes name, draws clock and/or simple figures.	• Does not write name or draw clock/figures accurately with mental retardation, dementia, or parietal lobe dysfunction.

BOX 5-3   GLASGOW COMA SCALE-P

(A) Glasgow Coma Scale

The GCS is useful for rating one's response to stimuli. The client who scores 10 or lower needs emergency attention. The client with a score of 7 or lower is generally considered to be in a coma.

		Score
Eye opening response	Spontaneous opening	4
	To verbal command	3
	To pain	2
	No response	1
Most appropriate verbal response	Oriented	5
	Confused	4
	Inappropriate words	3
	Incoherent	2
	No response	1
Most integral motor response (arm)	Obeys verbal commands	6
	Localizes pain	5
	Withdraws from pain	4
	Flexion (decorticate rigidity)	3
	Extension (decerebrate rigidity)	2
	No response	1
TOTAL SCORE		3–15

(B) Pupil Reactivity Score

Pupils Unreactive to Light	Pupil Reactivity Score
Both pupils	2
One pupil	1
Neither pupil	0

The GCS-P is calculated by subtracting the Pupil Reactivity Score (PRS) from the GCS total score:

GCS-P = GCS – PRS

Part A: From Teasdale, G., & Jennett, B. (1974). Assessment of coma and impaired consciousness: A practical scale. *The Lancet, 304*(7872), 81–84. https://doi.org/10.1016/S0140-6736(74)91639-0. Used with permission; Part B: Reprinted with permission from American Association of Neurological Surgeons. (2019). *What is the Glasgow Coma Scale pupils score?* https://www.glasgowcomascale.org/what-is-gcs-p/. For more on the use of the pupils score see the following article, which documents the research supporting the use of the pupils score: Brennan, P. M., Murray, G. D., & Teasdale, G. M. (2018). Simplifying the use of prognostic information in traumatic brain injury. Part 1: The GCS-Pupils score: An extended index of clinical severity. *Journal of Neurosurgery, 128*(6), 1612–1620. https://doi.org/10.3171/2017.12.JNS172780

BOX 5-4   SLUMS MENTAL STATUS EXAMINATION

Saint Louis University

Mental Status (SLUMS) Examination

Name _____   Age _____
                                Level of education _____

Is patient alert? _____

☐1 1. What day of the week is it?
☐1 2. What is the year?
☐1 3. What state are we in?
      4. Please remember these five objects. I will ask you what they are later.
           Apple   Pen   Tie   House   Car
☐3 5. You have $100 and you go to the store and buy a dozen apples for $3 and a tricycle for $20.
      How much did you spend?
      How much do you have left?
☐3 6. Please name as many animals as you can in 1 minute.
      ⓪ 0–5 animals   ① 5–10 animals   ② 10–15 animals   ③ 15+ animals
☐5 7. What were the five objects I asked you to remember? 1 point for each one correct.
      8. I am going to give you a series of numbers and I would like you to give them to me backward
☐2   For example, if I say 42, you would say 24.
      ⓪ 87   ① 649   ② 8,537
      9. This is a clock face. Please put in the hour markers and the time at 10 minutes
☐4   to 11 o'clock.
      ☐ Hour markers okay
      ☐ Time correct
☐2 10. Please place an X in the triangle.
      ☐ Which of the above figures is largest?
☐8 11. I am going to tell you a story. Please listen carefully because afterward I'm going to ask you some questions about
      it.
      Jill was a very successful stockbroker. She made a lot of money on the stock market. She then met Jack, a devastatingly
      handsome man. She married him and had three children. They lived in Chicago. She then stopped work and stayed at home
      to bring up her children. When they were teenagers, she went back to work. She and Jack lived happily ever after.
      ② What was the female's name?   ② What work did she do?
      ② When did she go back to work?   ② What state did she live in?

Scoring

High School Education		Less Than High School Education	
27–30	Normal	20–25	
21–26	MNCD*	20–24	
19–20	Dementia	14–19	

*Mild Neurocognitive Disorder

For further information on using the tool, visit http://www.elderguru.com/downloads/SLUMS_instructions.pdf.

BOX 5-5 PRIMARY CARE PTSD SCREEN FOR *DSM-5* (PC-PTSD-5)

Scale

Sometimes things happen to people that are unusually or especially frightening, horrible, or traumatic. For example:

- a serious accident or fire
- a physical or sexual assault or abuse
- an earthquake or flood
- a war
- seeing someone be killed or seriously injured
- having a loved one die through homicide or suicide

Have you ever experienced this kind of event?
YES/NO

If no, screen total = 0. Please stop here.

If yes, please answer the questions below.

In the past month, have you ...

1. Had nightmares about the event(s) or thought about the event(s) when you did not want to?
   YES/NO
2. Tried hard not to think about the event(s) or went out of your way to avoid situations that reminded you of the event(s)?
   YES/NO
3. Been constantly on guard, watchful, or easily startled?
   YES/NO

4. Felt numb or detached from people, activities, or your surroundings?
   YES/NO
5. Felt guilty or unable to stop blaming yourself or others for the event(s) or any problems the event(s) may have caused?
   YES/NO

Administration and Scoring

Preliminary results from validation studies suggest that a cut-point of 3 on the PC-PTSD-5 (e.g., respondent answers "yes" to any three of five questions about how the traumatic event(s) have affected them over the past month) is optimally sensitive to probable PTSD. Optimizing sensitivity minimizes false-negative screen results. Using a cut-point of 4 is considered optimally efficient. Optimizing efficiency balances false-positive and false-negative results. As additional research findings on the PC-PTSD-5 are published, updated recommendations for cut-point scores as well as psychometric data will be made available.

Citation

Prins, A., Bovin, M. J., Kimerling, R., Kaloupek, D. G., Marx, B. P., Pless Kaiser, A., & Schnurr, P. P. (2015). *Primary Care PTSD Screen for DSM-5 (PC-PTSD-5)* [Measurement instrument]. https://www.ptsd.va.gov/professional/assessment/screens/pc-ptsd.asp

---

BOX 5-6 QUICK INVENTORY OF DEPRESSIVE SYMPTOMATOLOGY (SELF-REPORT)

PLEASE CHECKMARK THE ONE RESPONSE TO EACH ITEM THAT IS MOST APPROPRIATE TO HOW YOU HAVE BEEN FEELING OVER THE PAST 7 DAYS.

1. **Falling asleep:**
   - ☐ 0 I never took longer than 30 minutes to fall asleep
   - ☐ 1 I took at least 30 minutes to fall asleep, less than half the time (3 days or less out of the past 7 days)
   - ☐ 2 I took at least 30 minutes to fall asleep, more than half the time (4 days or more out of the past 7 days)
   - ☐ 3 I took more than 60 minutes to fall asleep, more than half the time (4 days or more out of the past 7 days)

2. **Sleep during the night:**
   - ☐ 0 I didn't wake up at night
   - ☐ 1 I had a restless, light sleep, briefly waking up a few times each night
   - ☐ 2 I woke up at least once a night, but I got back to sleep easily
   - ☐ 3 I woke up more than once a night and stayed awake for 20 minutes or more, more than half the time (4 days or more out of the past 7 days)

3. **Waking up too early:**
   - ☐ 0 Most of the time, I woke up no more than 30 minutes before my scheduled time

   - ☐ 1 More than half the time (4 days or more out of the past 7 days), I woke up more than 30 minutes before my scheduled time
   - ☐ 2 I almost always woke up at least 1 hour or so before my scheduled time, but I got back to sleep eventually
   - ☐ 3 I woke up at least 1 hour before my scheduled time and couldn't get back to sleep

4. **Sleeping too much:**
   - ☐ 0 I slept no longer than 7 to 8 hours per night, without napping during the day
   - ☐ 1 I slept no longer than 10 hours in a 24-hour period including naps
   - ☐ 2 I slept no longer than 12 hours in a 24-hour period including naps
   - ☐ 3 I slept longer than 12 hours in a 24-hour period including naps

5. **Feeling sad:**
   - ☐ 0 I didn't feel sad
   - ☐ 1 I felt sad less than half the time (3 days or less out of the past 7 days)
   - ☐ 2 I felt sad more than half the time (4 days or more out of the past 7 days)
   - ☐ 3 I felt sad nearly all of the time

Please complete either 6 or 7 (not both)

6. **Decreased appetite:**
   - ☐ 0 There was no change in my usual appetite
   - ☐ 1 I ate somewhat less often or smaller amounts of food than usual
   - ☐ 2 I ate much less than usual and only by forcing myself to eat
   - ☐ 3 I rarely ate within a 24-hour period and only by really forcing myself to eat or when others persuaded me to eat

7. **Increased appetite:**
   - ☐ 0 There was no change in my usual appetite
   - ☐ 1 I felt a need to eat more frequently than usual
   - ☐ 2 I regularly ate more often and/or greater amounts of food than usual
   - ☐ 3 I felt driven to overeat both at mealtime and between meals

Please complete either 8 or 9 (not both)

8. **Decreased weight (within the last 14 days):**
   - ☐ 0 My weight has not changed
   - ☐ 1 I feel as if I've had a slight weight loss
   - ☐ 2 I've lost 2 lb (about 1 kg) or more
   - ☐ 3 I've lost 5 lb (about 2 kg) or more

9. **Increased weight (within the last 14 days):**
   - ☐ 0 My weight has not changed
   - ☐ 1 I feel as if I've had a slight weight gain
   - ☐ 2 I've gained 2 lb (about 1 kg) or more
   - ☐ 3 I've gained 5 lb (about 2 kg) or more

10. **Concentration/decision making:**
    - ☐ 0 There was no change in my usual ability to concentrate or make decisions
    - ☐ 1 I occasionally felt indecisive or found that my attention wandered
    - ☐ 2 Most of the time, I found it hard to focus or to make decisions
    - ☐ 3 I couldn't concentrate well enough to read or I couldn't make even minor decisions

(Continued on following page)

BOX 5-6 QUICK INVENTORY OF DEPRESSIVE SYMPTOMATOLOGY (SELF-REPORT) (*continued*)

11. Perception of myself:
- ☐ 0 I saw myself as equally worthwhile and deserving as other people
- ☐ 1 I put the blame on myself more than usual
- ☐ 2 For the most part, I believed that I caused problems for others
- ☐ 3 I thought almost constantly about major and minor defects in myself

12. Thoughts of my own death or suicide:
- ☐ 0 I didn't think of suicide or death
- ☐ 1 I felt that life was empty or wondered if it was worth living
- ☐ 2 I thought of suicide or death several times for several minutes over the past 7 days
- ☐ 3 I thought of suicide or death several times a day in some detail, or I made specific plans for suicide or actually tried to take my life

13. General interest:
- ☐ 0 There was no change from usual in how interested I was in other people or activities
- ☐ 1 I noticed that I was less interested in other people or activities
- ☐ 2 I found I had interest in only one or two of the activities I used to do
- ☐ 3 I had virtually no interest in the activities I used to do

14. Energy level:
- ☐ 0 There was no change in my usual level of energy
- ☐ 1 I got tired more easily than usual
- ☐ 2 I had to make a big effort to start or finish my usual daily activities (e.g., shopping, homework, cooking, or going to work)
- ☐ 3 I really couldn't carry out most of my usual daily activities because I just didn't have the energy

15. Feeling more sluggish than usual:
- ☐ 0 I thought, spoke, and moved at my usual pace
- ☐ 1 I found that my thinking was more sluggish than usual or my voice sounded dull or flat
- ☐ 2 It took me several seconds to respond to most questions and I was sure my thinking was more sluggish than usual
- ☐ 3 I was often unable to respond to questions without forcing myself

16. Feeling restless (agitated, not relaxed, fidgety):
☐ 0 I didn't feel restless
☐ 1 I was often fidgety, wringing my hands, or needed to change my sitting position
☐ 2 I had sudden urges to move about and was quite restless
☐ 3 At times, I was unable to stay seated and needed to pace around

Quick Inventory of Depressive Symptomatology (Score Sheet)

Note: This Section Is to be Completed by the Study Personnel Only.

_____ Enter the highest score on any one of the four sleep items (1–4)
_____ Item 5
_____ Enter the highest score on any one of the appetite/weight items (6–9)
_____ Item 10
_____ Item 11
_____ Item 12
_____ Item 13
_____ Item 14
_____ Enter the highest score on either of the two psychomotor items (15 and 16)
_____ Total score (range: 0–27)

Interpretation of scores

0–5 = No risk of depression

6–10 = Mild

11–15 = Moderate

16–20 = Severe

21–27 = Very severe

Reprinted with permission from Rush, A. J., Trivedi, M. H., Ibrahim, H. M., Carmody, T. J., Arnow, B., Klein, D. N., Markowitze, J. C., Ninan, P. T., Kornstein, S., Manber, R., Thase, M. E., Kocsis, J. H., & Keller, M. B. (2003). The 16-Item Quick Inventory of Depressive Symptomatology (QIDS), clinician rating (QIDS-C), and self-report (QIDS-SR): A psychometric evaluation in patients with chronic major depression. *Biological Psychiatry, 54*(5), 573–583. https://doi.org/10.1016/S0006-3223(02)01866-8. © UT Southwestern Medical Center, Dallas, Texas.

BOX 5-7 SAD PERSONS SUICIDE RISK ASSESSMENT TOOL

This box can be used to assess the likelihood of a suicide attempt. Consider risk factors within the context of the clinical presentation. Campbell (2004) recommends that scoring not be used, but the examiner should look at the risk factors and respond accordingly.

Risk Factors
- **S**ex
- **A**ge
- **D**epression
- **P**revious attempt
- **E**thanol abuse
- **R**ational thinking loss
- **S**ocial supports lacking
- **O**rganized plan
- **N**o spouse
- **S**ickness

Adapted from Patterson, W. M., Dohn, H. H., Bird J., & Patterson, G. A. (1983). Evaluation of suicidal patients: The SAD PERSONS scale. *Psychosomatics, 24*(4), 343–345, 348–349. https://doi.org/10.1016/S0033-3182(83)73213-5

BOX 5-8 THE 10 SIGNS AND SYMPTOMS OF ALZHEIMER DISEASE

1. Memory loss that disrupts daily life
2. Challenges in planning or solving problems
3. Difficulty completing familiar tasks
4. Confusion with time or place
5. Trouble understanding visual images or spatial relationships
6. New problems with words in speaking or writing
7. Misplacing things and losing the ability to retrace steps
8. Decreased or poor judgment
9. Withdrawal from work or social activities
10. Changes in mood or personality

Adapted with permission from Alzheimer's Association (2021). The 10 Signs and Symptoms of Alzheimer's. Available at https://www.alz.org/alzheimers-dementia/10_signs

TABLE 5-1   **Identifying the Cause of Confusion: Dementia, Delirium, or Depression**

	Dementia	Delirium	Depression
Duration	Chronic condition that does not resolve over time	Hours to weeks in duration	Can last weeks to months or years
Onset	Chronic onset	Acute onset	Often abrupt onset
Attention	Generally normal attention	Impaired/fluctuating attention	Distractible but minimal impairment of attention
Memory	Recent and remote memory impaired	Recent and immediate memory impaired	Islands of intact memory
Alertness	Generally normal alertness	Fluctuates between lethargic and hypervigilant	Alert
Thinking, judgment	May have word finding difficulties, judgment may be poor	Disorganized thinking, slow or accelerated	Thinking intact though with themes of helplessness or self-depreciation

Adapted with permission from NSW Agency for Clinical Innovation. (2020). *Care of Confused Hospitalised Older Persons. Principle 3: Assessment of older people with confusion.* https://www.aci.health.nsw.gov.au/chops/chops-key-principles/assessment-of-older-people-with-confusion

 PEDIATRIC VARIATIONS

Focus questions would include the following:
- How feelings/activities have changed over the past week
- Difficulty in concentrating with school tasks
- Decrease or increase in eating habits
- Difficulty with sleeping
- Social isolation
- Decreased self-esteem
- Extreme mood changes (happiness/sadness/acting out/temper tantrums)
- Feelings of fear, confusion
- Change in relationships with peers, family
- Use of drugs/alcohol

GERIATRIC VARIATIONS

- May seem confused in a new or acute care setting owing to slowed thought processes and slowed responses to questions; however, is oriented to person, time, and place
- Decreased ability to recall directions
- Slight decline in short-term memory
- Slowed reaction time
- Likes to reminisce and tends to wander from topic at hand
- May have hesitation with short-term memory
- Clients older than 80 years should be able to recall two to four words after a 5-minute time period.
- Use the GDS-5/15 Geriatric Depression Scale to screen older adults for depression.

 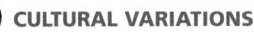 **CULTURAL VARIATIONS**

The stroke rate in most industrialized countries has been decreasing, but it remains high among African Americans (risk of first stroke is nearly twice as high as for whites, and African Americans have the highest death rate as a result of stroke in the United States) (CDC, 2020a). The CDC also noted that the Hispanic death rate from stroke is increasing, even though stroke deaths have declined for all racial/ethnic groups. The highest rate of stroke has continued to be in the Stroke Belt of the southeastern United States. Reasons for this high rate are thought to be larger proportion of rural areas (rural is associated with stroke prevalence), a higher proportion of African American residents (who have a higher stroke prevalence), higher prevalence of traditional stroke risk factors (and other cardiovascular risk factors), higher prevalence of inflammation and infection, and lower socioeconomic status (Howard & Howard, 2020).

Substance abuse, violence, human immunodeficiency virus (HIV) risk, depressive symptoms, and socioeconomic conditions are directly linked to health disparities among Latinas (Gonzalez-Guarda et al., 2012).

POSSIBLE COLLABORATIVE PROBLEMS—RISK FOR COMPLICATION

- Depression
- Suicide attempt
- Alcohol abuse
- Drug abuse

Teaching Tips for Selected Client Concerns

Client Concern: *Confusion associated with neurologic changes (aging, head injury, stroke, etc.)*

Inform client or caregiver of the purpose and benefits of community agencies that offer support. Refer client as necessary. Assist family in coping and explain how to communicate accurately using short sentences.

Client Concern: *Poor coping strategies associated with inadequate time to prepare for stressors from sudden crisis*

Teach client the use of appropriate stress-reducing measures (e.g., relaxation techniques, biofeedback, exercise, hobbies). Inform client of beneficial effects of decreasing coffee, sugar, and salt and maintaining adequate B and C vitamins in diet for adequate functioning of the endocrine and nervous systems. Refer client to community agencies and support groups as necessary.

Client Concern: *Poor memory*

Teach client memory-enhancing techniques.

Client Concern: *Opportunity to improve critical thinking skills*

Teach client critical thinking skills. Assist client to obtain resources to enhance critical thought processes.

 Client Concern: *Poor family coping ability associated with family crisis adjusting to poor infant/child development related to preterm infant*

Discuss social development of the child. Infant's "stranger anxiety" is normal. Teach parents ways to assist infant to warm up to strangers. Encourage verbalization, reassurance, and cuddling. Help parent assess child's readiness to begin school and to verbalize any school problems with child.

 Client Concern: *Poor coping strategies associated with inadequate social support*

Teach positive coping strategies to the child, such as relaxation and guided imagery. Identify family and friends that are supportive of the child and include them in identifying strategies to help improve self-esteem.

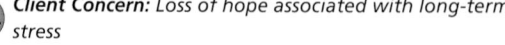 **Client Concern:** *Loss of hope associated with long-term stress*

Identify feelings of hopelessness, sadness, and pain. Encourage the child to discuss these feelings and develop strategies to use when these feelings are present.

Use play therapy for younger children to help identify these feelings and teach them resources and techniques to use when needed. Include parents/friends, especially for younger children, that will redirect the child's actions/thoughts when these feelings are exhibited.

References

Bowers, E. S. (2014). *8 Dementia risk factors*. http://www.everydayhealth.com/news/depression-risk-factor-dementia/

Brown, R., & Rounds, L. (1995). Conjoint screening questionnaires for alcohol and other drug abuse: Criterion validity in a primary care practice. *Wisconsin Medical Journal, 95*(3), 135–140. https://pubmed.ncbi.nlm.nih.gov/7778330/

Campbell, J.C. (2004). Danger Assessment. Retrieved from http://www.dangerassessment.org. A danger assessment questionnaire for women in a same sex relationship and (coming soon) a danger assessment questionnaire for immigrant women. http://www.dangerassessment.org

Centers for Disease Control and Prevention. (2017). *Leading causes of death reports, 1981–2018*. https://webappa.cdc.gov/sasweb/ncipc/leadcause.html

Centers for Disease Control and Prevention. (2020a). *Stroke facts*. https://www.cdc.gov/stroke/facts.htm

Centers for Disease Control and Prevention. (2020b). *Suicide and self-harm injury*. https://www.cdc.gov/nchs/fastats/suicide.htm

Ewing, J. A. (1984). Detecting alcoholism: The CAGE Questionnaire. *Journal of the American Medical Association, 252*(14), 1905–1907. https://doi.org/10.1001/jama.1984.03350140051025

Gonzalez-Guarda, R., McCabbe, F., Vermeesch, A., Cianelli, R., Florom-Smith, A., & Peragallo, N. (2012). Cultural phenomena and the syndemic factor: Substance abuse, violence, HIV, and depression among Hispanic women. *Annals of Anthropological Practice, 36*(2), 212–231. https://doi.org/10.1111/napa.12001

Howard, G., & Howard, V. (2020). Twenty years of progress toward understanding the Stroke Belt. *Stroke, 51*(3), 742–750. https://doi.org/10.1161/STROKEAHA.119.024155

National Institute on Drug Abuse. (2018). *Screening and assessment tools chart*. https://www.drugabuse.gov/nidamed-medical-health-professionals/tool-resources-your-practice/screening-assessment-drug-testing-resources/chart-evidence-based-screening-tools-adults

Substance Abuse and Mental Health Services Administration-Health Resources and Services Administration. (2011). *Screening, brief intervention, and referral to treatment (SBIRT)*. http://www.integration.samhsa.gov/clinical-practice/SBIRT

6 ASSESSING GENERAL HEALTH STATUS AND VITAL SIGNS

Structure and Function Overview

The general survey is the first part of the physical examination that begins the moment the nurse meets the client to obtain an overall impression about the client's general health status. The general survey includes observation of the client's physical development, body build, gender, apparent age as compared with reported age, skin condition and color, dress and hygiene, posture and gait, level of consciousness, behaviors, body movements, affect, facial expressions, speech patterns and clarity, and vital signs.

The client's vital signs, indicators of one's health, include temperature, pulse, respirations, and blood pressure. Pain for a time was considered to be the "fifth vital sign" but this designation was dropped because of the opioid crisis. For the body to function on a cellular level, a core body temperature between 35.5°C and 37.7°C (96°F and 99.9°F orally) must be maintained. Arterial or peripheral pulses are shock waves produced when the heart contracts and forcefully pumps blood out of the ventricles into the aorta. The body has many arterial pulse sites. One of them—the radial pulse—gives a good overall picture of the client's health status. The respiratory rate and character are additional clues to the client's overall health status. Blood pressure reflects the pressure exerted on the walls of the arteries. This pressure varies with the cardiac cycle, reaching a high point with systole and a low point with diastole. Therefore, blood pressure is a measurement of the pressure of the blood in the arteries when the ventricles are contracted (systolic blood pressure) and when the ventricles are relaxed (diastolic blood pressure). Blood pressure is expressed as the ratio of the systolic pressure over the diastolic pressure. *Cardiac output, distensibility of the arteries, blood volume, blood velocity, and blood viscosity (thickness)* all affect a client's blood pressure. The difference between systolic and diastolic pressure is termed the *pulse pressure.* Determine the pulse pressure after measuring the blood pressure because it reflects the stroke volume—the volume of blood ejected with each heartbeat. Finally, pain screening is essential for an overall impression of the client. See Chapter 7 for an in-depth Pain Assessment.

Nursing Assessment

COLLECTING SUBJECTIVE DATA

Name, address, current age, birth date, reason for seeking health care? Gender association? Major concern about current health? Current age, height, and weight? Recent weight change? High fevers? Change in pulse or heart rate? Usual blood pressure? Blood pressure last checked? Problem with hypertension or hypotension? Difficulty breathing? At rest?

With mild or strenuous exercise? Any pain? How does it feel (dull, sharp, aching, throbbing)? How does the area of pain look (shiny, bumpy, red, swollen, bruised)? Onset: when did it begin? Location: where is it? Does it radiate? Duration: how long does it last? Does it recur? Severity: how bad is it? Associated factors: what makes it better? What makes it worse? What other symptoms occur with it? See Chapter 7 for further assessment of pain. Over-the-counter and prescribed medications? Allergies? Family history of heart disease, diabetes, thyroid disease, lung disease, high blood pressure, cancer, or others? Educational background, employment? Disabilities, satisfaction with current life, frequency for seeking health care, use of tobacco products including cigarettes, chewing tobacco, snuff, or dip? Consumption of alcohol (amount, frequency, and type)? Use of illicit drugs (type and frequency)? Usual diet? Exercise (type and frequency)?

COLLECTING OBJECTIVE DATA

Equipment Needed

- Thermometer: tympanic thermometer, temporal artery thermometer, electronic oral and/or axillary thermometer, or rectal thermometer
- Protective, disposable covers for the type of thermometer used

- Aneroid or mercury sphygmomanometer or electronic blood pressure measuring equipment
- Stethoscope
- Watch with a second hand
- If available, use a mobile monitoring system, such as "DINAMAP," which can be taken room to room to perform multiple vital signs simultaneously. These devices often have a thermometer, electronic sphygmomanometer, oxygen saturation detector, and pulse monitor (Fig. 6-1)

Physical Assessment

When you meet the client, observe the client from head to toe to note any gross abnormalities in appearance or behavior. Assess vital signs (temperature, pulse, respirations, and blood pressure) to detect any severe deviations and to acquire baseline data. Then weigh the client and measure height with shoes and heavy clothing removed.

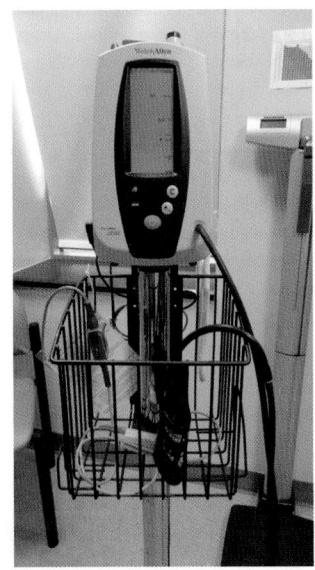

FIGURE 6-1 Mobile monitoring system.

GENERAL PHYSICAL SURVEY

PROCEDURE	NORMAL FINDINGS	ABNORMAL FINDINGS
Observe the following:		
• Physical development for age	• Appears to be stated chronologic age	• Appears older than age with evidence of hard manual labor, chronic illness, or alcoholism/smoking
• Dress	• Dressed for occasion	• Dress bizarre and inappropriate for occasion seen in mentally ill, grieving, depressed, or poor clients
• Posture and gait	• Erect posture. Gait is rhythmic, smooth, steady, and coordinated with arms swinging at side	• Curvatures of the spine (lordosis, scoliosis, or kyphosis) may indicate a musculoskeletal disorder. Stiff, rigid movements are common in arthritis or Parkinson disease. Slumped shoulders may signify depression. Clients with chronic obstructive pulmonary disease (COPD) tend to lean forward and brace themselves with their arms
• Body build	• A wide variety of body types fall within a normal range: from small amounts of fat and muscle to larger amounts of fat and developed muscle	• Lack of subcutaneous fat with prominent bones seen in the malnourished, abdominal ascites seen in starvation, abundant fatty tissue seen in obesity. Extreme weight loss is seen in anorexia nervosa (Abnormal Findings 6-1)

PROCEDURE	NORMAL FINDINGS	ABNORMAL FINDINGS
	• Body proportions are normal. Arm span (distance between fingertips with arms extended) is approximately equal. The distance from the head crown to the symphysis pubis is approximately equal to the distance from the symphysis pubis to the sole of the client's foot	• Decreased height and delayed puberty, with chubbiness, are seen in hypopituitary dwarfism (Abnormal Findings 6-1) • Skeletal malformations with a decrease in height are seen in achondroplastic dwarfism. In gigantism, there is increased height and weight with delayed sexual development (Abnormal Findings 6-1) • Overgrowth of bones in the face, head, hands, and feet with normal height is seen in hyperpituitarism (acromegaly) (Abnormal Findings 6-1) • Arm span is greater than height, and pubis to sole measurement exceeds pubis to crown measurement in Marfan syndrome (Abnormal Findings 6-1) • Excessive body fat that is evenly distributed is referred to as exogenous obesity. Central body weight gain with excessive cervical obesity (buffalo hump), also referred to as endogenous obesity, is seen in Cushing syndrome (Abnormal Findings 6-1)

(Continued on following page)

GENERAL PHYSICAL SURVEY

PROCEDURE	NORMAL FINDINGS	ABNORMAL FINDINGS
• Gender and sexual development	• Appropriate for age and gender	• Delayed or advanced puberty for stated age; male client with female characteristics, and female client with male characteristics
• Skin color and condition	• Varies from light to dark skinned. Color is even without obvious lesions: light to dark beige pink in light-skinned client; light tan to dark brown or olive in dark-skinned clients. Underlying red tones from good circulation give a liveliness or healthy glow to all shades of skin color	• Extreme pallor, flushed, yellow skin in light-skinned client; loss of red tones and ashen gray cyanosis in dark-skinned client
Monitor temperature with electronic thermometers. They may be used for tympanic, oral, rectal, axillary, or continuous temperatures depending on the model and type of probe used. See Table 6-1 for best route to take a temperature.	Body temperature is usually lowest in early AM and highest in late PM: 35.5°C–37.7°C (96°F–99.9°F)	Temperatures below 36.7°C (98°F) represent hypothermia and can be a result of prolonged exposure to cold, hypoglycemia, hypothyroidism, starvation, neurologic dysfunction, or shock

PROCEDURE	NORMAL FINDINGS	ABNORMAL FINDINGS
	Several factors may cause normal variations in the core body temperature. Body temperature is lowest early in the morning (4–6 AM) and highest late in the evening (8 PM to midnight). Strenuous exercise, stress, and ovulation may elevate temperature to 38.3°C (101°F). Hot fluids, smoking, and gum chewing may elevate temperature, whereas cold fluids may lower it	Temperatures above 38.3°C (100.9°F) represent hyperthermia and can indicate bacterial, viral, or fungal infections an inflammatory process; malignancies; trauma; or various blood, endocrine, and immune disorders
Tympanic. Tympanic membrane thermometers are gentle and noninvasive. Place the probe very gently at the opening of the ear canal for 2–3 seconds until the temperature appears in the digital display (Fig. 6-2)	Normal tympanic temperature range is 36.7°C–38.3°C (98°F–100.9°F). The tympanic membrane temperature is normally about 0.8°C (1.4°F) higher than the normal oral temperature	Tympanic temperature is under 36.7°C (98°F) or over 38.3°C (100.9°F)

(*Continued on following page*)

GENERAL PHYSICAL SURVEY

PROCEDURE	NORMAL FINDINGS	ABNORMAL FINDINGS
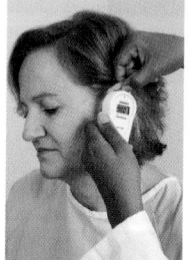 **FIGURE 6-2** Taking a tympanic temperature.		
Oral. Use an electronic thermometer with a disposable protective probe cover. Place the thermometer under the client's tongue to the right or left of the frenulum deep in the posterior sublingual pocket. Ask the client to close their lips around probe. Hold the probe until you hear a beep. Remove the probe and dispose of its cover by pressing the release button	Oral temperature is between 35.9°C and 37.5°C (96.6°F and 99.5°F)	Oral temperature is below 35.9°C (96.6°F) or over 37.5°C (99.5°F)

PROCEDURE	NORMAL FINDINGS	ABNORMAL FINDINGS
Electronic thermometers give a digital reading in 15–30 seconds if not quicker		
Rectal. Lubricate clean thermometer with water-soluble lubricant and insert 2.5–5.08 cm (1–2 in.) into rectum for 3 minutes. *Note: Use this method only when other routes are not practical (e.g., client cannot cooperate, is comatose, cannot close mouth, or tympanic thermometer is unavailable). Never force thermometer into rectum and never use a rectal thermometer for clients with severe coagulation disorders, recent rectal, anal, vaginal or prostate surgeries, diarrhea, hemorrhoids, colitis, or fecal impaction*	The rectal temperature is between 0.4°C and 0.5°C (0.7°F and 1°F) higher than the normal oral temperature. Normal rectal temperature range is 36.3°C–37.9°C (97.4°F–100.3°F)	Rectal temperature below 36.3°C (97.4°F) or above 37.9°C (100.3°F)
Axillary. Insert thermometer under axilla with arm down and across chest for 5–10 minutes	Normal axillary temperature range is 35.4°C–37°C (95.6°F–98.5°F). The axillary temperature is 0.5°C (1°F) lower than the oral temperature	Axillary temperature is below 35.4°C (95.6°F) or above 37°C (98.5°F)

(Continued on following page)

GENERAL PHYSICAL SURVEY

PROCEDURE	NORMAL FINDINGS	ABNORMAL FINDINGS
Temporal arterial. *Note: Temporal arterial temperature is measured by the thermometer reading the infrared heat waves released by the temporal artery through the skin.* Remove the protective cap and place the thermometer over the client's forehead. While holding and pressing the scan button, gently stroke the thermometer across the client's forehead over the temporal artery to a point directly behind the ear. You will hear beeping and a red light will blink to indicate a measurement is taking place. Release the scan button and remove the thermometer from the forehead. Read the temperature on display *Note: Temporal artery temperature measurement takes approximately 6 seconds*	The temporal artery temperature is approximately 0.4°C (0.8°F) higher than oral (Exegen Corporation, 2018). Normal temporal artery temperature range is 36.3°C–37.9°C (97.4°F–100.3°F)	Temporal artery temperature is below 36.3°C (97.4°F) or above 37.9°C (100.3°F)

PROCEDURE	NORMAL FINDINGS	ABNORMAL FINDINGS
Monitor for pulse		
Palpate radial pulse for rhythm and rate. Use the pads of your two middle fingers and lightly palpate the radial artery on the lateral aspect of the client's wrist (Fig. 6-3). Count the number of beats you feel for 30 seconds if the pulse rhythm is regular. Multiply by 2 to get the rate (or count for 15 seconds and multiply by 4). If the rhythm is irregular, count for a full minute. Then, verify by taking an apical pulse as well *Note: Perform cardiac auscultation of the apical pulse if the client exhibits any abnormal findings*	60–100 beats/min is normal for adults. Tachycardia may be normal in clients who have just finished strenuous exercise. Bradycardia may be normal in well-conditioned athletes 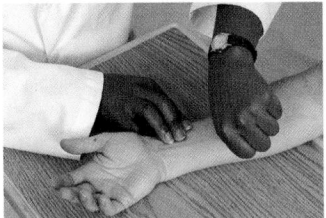 **FIGURE 6-3** Taking the radial pulse rate.	*Tachycardia* (>100 beats/min) may occur with fever, certain medications, stress, and other abnormal states, such as cardiac dysrhythmias *Bradycardia* (<60 beats/min) may be seen with sitting or standing for long periods causing blood to pool, decreasing pulse rate, with heart block or dropped beats
Palpate arterial elasticity	Artery feels straight, resilient, and springy	Artery feels rigid

(Continued on following page)

GENERAL PHYSICAL SURVEY

PROCEDURE	NORMAL FINDINGS	ABNORMAL FINDINGS
Palpate apical pulse. Auscultate heart sounds for 1 minute with stethoscope for the following:		
• Rate	• 60–100 beats/min	• > 100 beats/min equals tachycardia; <60 beats/min equals bradycardia
• Rhythm	• Regular	• Irregular; pulse deficit (difference between apical and radial pulses) may indicate atrial fibrillation, atrial flutter, premature ventricular contractions, and various degrees of heart block
Monitor respirations 1 full minute for the rate, rhythm, and depth (see Table 6-2). Observe the client's chest rise and fall with each breath. Count respirations for 30 seconds and multiply by 2. If you place the client's arm across the chest while palpating the pulse, you can also count respirations. Do this by keeping your fingers on the client's pulse even after you have finished taking it		

PROCEDURE	NORMAL FINDINGS	ABNORMAL FINDINGS
• Rate	• 12–20 breaths/min	• Fewer than 12 breaths/min or >20 breaths/min
• Rhythm	• Rhythm is regular	• Irregular (if irregular, count for 1 full minute)
• Depth	• Equal bilateral chest expansion of 2.5–5.08 cm (1–2 in.)	• Unequal, shallow, or extremely deep chest expansion, labored or gasping breaths
Measure oxygen saturation (amount of hemoglobin filed with oxygen). Use finger of extremity with palpable pulse and capillary refill. Remove nail polish of finger to be used and place pulse oximeter on finger (Fig. 6-4)	SpO_2 92%–99% 85%–89% may be acceptable in clients with chronic diseases such as emphysema	SpO_2 <92% (**hypoxia**) unless with chronic COPD and >99% which is **hyperoxemia**

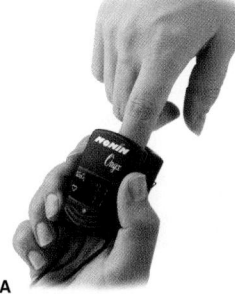
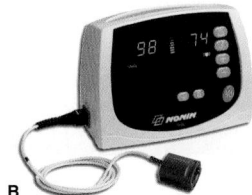

FIGURE 6-4 Measuring blood oxygenation with pulse oximetry reduces the need for invasive procedures, such as drawing blood for analysis of O_2 levels. **A.** Self-contained digital fingertip pulse oximeter, which incorporates the sensor and display into one unit. **B.** Tabletop model with sensor attached. Memory permits tracking heart rate and O_2 saturation over time. (Reprinted with permission from Honan, L. [2019]. *Focus on adult health* [2nd ed., Fig. 8-12]. Wolters Kluwer.)

(Continued on following page)

GENERAL PHYSICAL SURVEY

PROCEDURE	NORMAL FINDINGS	ABNORMAL FINDINGS
Measure blood pressure on dominant arm first. Take blood pressure in both arms when recording it for the first time. Take subsequent readings in arm with highest measurement. *Note: Advise client to avoid nicotine, caffeine, food, and alcohol consumption for 30 minutes prior to measurement (Skerrett, 2020) to avoid elevating the blood pressure reading. In addition, monitor these seven factors to prevent an inaccurate blood pressure reading:* *1. Client has a full bladder* *2. Client's back is unsupported* *3. Client's feet are unsupported* *4. Client's legs are crossed* *5. Sphygmomanometer cuff is over clothing* *6. Client's arm is unsupported* *7. Client is talking or hasn't had at least 3 minutes of quiet time prior to the measurement* (Source: American Medical Association, 2014)	Systolic pressure is <120 mmHg Diastolic pressure is <80 mmHg; varies with individuals. A pressure difference of 10 mmHg between arms is normal. Varies throughout the day due to external influences, including time of day, caffeine or nicotine intake, exercise, emotions, pain, temperature, and with body and arm positions. Usually slightly higher in a client who is standing due to compensation for the effects of gravity and slightly lower in a reclining client because of decreased resistance	Higher or lower than normal systolic and diastolic readings. Table 6-3 provides the latest blood pressure classifications (ACC et al., 2017). More than a 10 mmHg pressure difference between arms may indicate coarctation of the aorta or cardiac disease

PROCEDURE	NORMAL FINDINGS	ABNORMAL FINDINGS
Assess the pulse pressure, which is the difference between the systolic and diastolic blood pressure levels. Record findings in mmHg. For example, if the blood pressure was 120/80 mmHg, then the pulse pressure would be 120 minus 80, or 40 mmHg	Pulse pressure is 30–50 mmHg	Pulse pressure lower than 30 mmHg or higher than 50 mmHg may indicate cardiovascular disease
If the client takes antihypertensive medications or has a history of fainting or dizziness, **assess for possible orthostatic hypotension** by measuring the blood pressure and pulse with the client in a standing or sitting position after measuring the blood pressure with the client in a supine position	A drop of <20 mmHg from recorded sitting position	A drop of 20 mmHg or more from the recorded sitting blood pressure may indicate orthostatic (postural) hypotension. Pulse will increase to accommodate the drop in blood pressure. Orthostatic hypotension may be related to a decreased baroreceptor sensitivity, fluid volume deficit (e.g., dehydration), or certain medications (i.e., diuretics, antihypertensives). Symptoms of orthostatic hypotension include dizziness, light-headedness, and falling. Further evaluation and referral to the client's primary care provider are necessary
Observe comfort level Ask the client if they have any pain	Client assumes a relatively relaxed posture without excessive position shifting. Facial expression is alert and pleasant No subjective report of pain	Facial expression indicates discomfort (grimacing, frowning). Client may brace or hold a body part that is painful. Breathing pattern indicates distress (e.g., shortness of breath, shallow, rapid breathing). Explore any subjective report of pain. Refer to Chapter 7 for further assessment of pain

ABNORMAL FINDINGS **6-1** **Deviations Related to Physical Development, Body Build, and Fat Distribution**

DWARFISM
These images show the associated decreased height and skeletal malformations

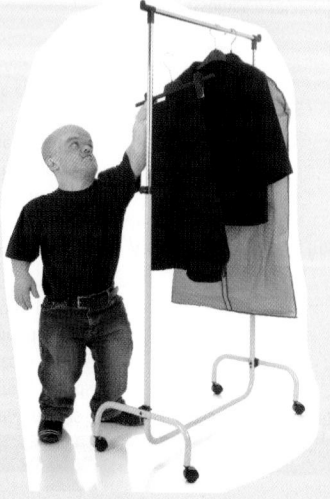

GIGANTISM
Note the disparity in height between the affected person and a person of the same age

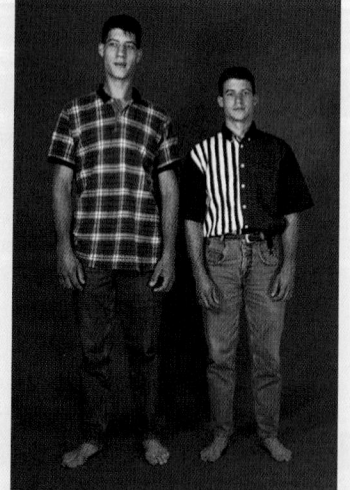

ACROMEGALY
The affected client shows the characteristic overgrowth of bones in the face, head, and hands

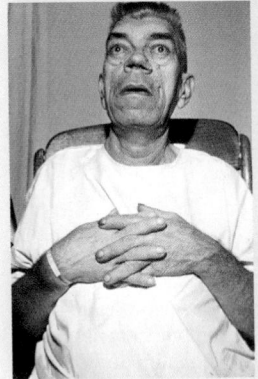

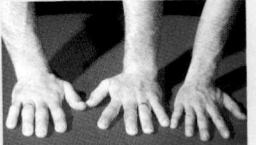

ANOREXIA NERVOSA
The client shows the emaciated appearance that follows self-starvation and accompanying extreme weight loss

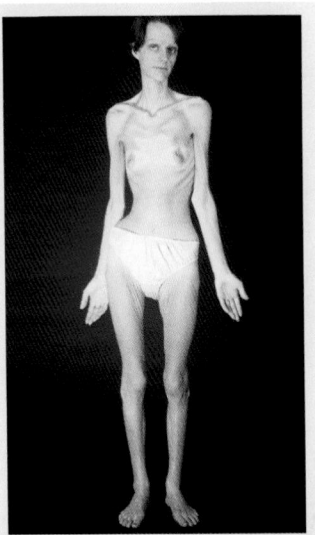

ABNORMAL FINDINGS

OBESITY

Obesity is a complex disease that involves an excessive amount of body fat. It increases the risk of diseases and health problems such as heart disease, diabetes, and high blood pressure (Mayo Clinic, 2020)

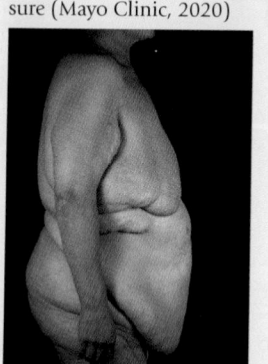

MARFAN SYNDROME

The elongated fingers are characteristic of this condition

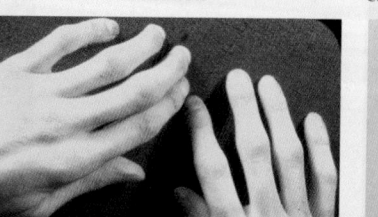

CUSHING SYNDROME

The affected client reflects the centralized weight gain

TABLE 6-1   Choosing the Correct Route to Measure Body Temperature

Route/Range	Client Type	Advantage	Disadvantage
Temporal 36.3°C–37.9°C (97.4°F–100.3°F)	All clients unless sweating profusely	Easy and quick to obtain	Sweating can interfere with accurate reading.
Tympanic 36.7°C–38.3°C (98.0°F–100.9°F)	All clients except with ear infection or ear pain	Easy and quick to obtain	There is no research to support the accuracy of this method (Mayo Clinic, 2018). Only one size of thermometer is available, and it is very difficult to use in children under 3 years of age.
Rectal 36.3°C–37.9°C (97.4°F–100.3°F)	Adults who require a very accurate core temperature	Most indicative of core body temperature (when compared to other routes)	Cannot be used with clients who have had rectal surgery, abscesses, diarrhea, low white blood cell count, or cardiac disease. Cannot be used in newborns. Use caution because there is a higher risk of exposure to body fluids.
Oral 35.9°C–37.5°C (96.6°F–99.5°F)	Older children and adults who are awake, cooperative, alert, and oriented. **Do not use if client has just consumed very cold or very warm food or drink.**	Easy and accurate	Cannot be used if client has had oral surgery, if the client is a smoker, or if the client is a mouth breather. Accuracy will be altered if client has just consumed very cold or hot foods.
Axillary 35.4°C–37.0°C (95.6°F–98.5°F)	Infants, young children, and anyone with an altered immune system, because this technique is noninvasive	Easy to take	Takes a very long time while nurse holds thermometer under client's arm. Not as accurate as oral or rectal.

TABLE 6-2   Types of Respirations

	Description	Pattern
Normal	12–20 breaths/min and regular	∿∿∿
Apnea	Absence of respiration	————
Bradypnea	Slow, shallow respiration	⌒‿⌒
Tachypnea	> 20 breaths/min and regular	∿∿∿∿∿
Hyperventilation	Increased rate and increased depth	∧∧∧∧∧
Hypoventilation	Decreased rate and decreased depth	———⌒———
Cheyne-Stokes	Periods of apnea and hyperventilation	∧∧___∧∧
Kussmaul	Very deep with normal rhythm	∧∧∧∧∧

TABLE 6-3   Changes in Blood Pressure Classification

Blood pressure categories in the new guidelines are:
- Normal: <120/80 mmHg;
- Elevated: Systolic between 120 and 129 and diastolic <80;
- Stage 1: Systolic between 130 and 139 or diastolic between 80 and 89;
- Stage 2: Systolic at least 140 or diastolic at least 90 mmHg;
- Hypertensive crisis: Systolic over 180 and/or diastolic over 120, with patients needing prompt changes in medication if there are no other indications of problems, or immediate hospitalization if there are signs of organ damage.

The guidelines eliminate the category of prehypertension, categorizing patients as having either Elevated (120–129 and <80) or Stage 1 hypertension (130–139 or 80–89). Although previous guidelines classified 140/90 mmHg as Stage 1 hypertension, this level is classified as Stage 2 hypertension under the new guidelines. In addition, the guidelines stress the importance of using proper technique to measure blood pressure; recommend use of home blood pressure monitoring using validated devices; and highlight the value of appropriate training of health care providers to reveal "white-coat hypertension."

PEDIATRIC VARIATIONS

Equipment Needed for Child

- Tape measure
- Growth charts for specific age comparisons (see the Centers for Disease Control and Prevention [CDC] and the World Health Organization [WHO] growth charts for children aged 0–2 years and from 2 years and older at https://www.cdc.gov/growthcharts/index.htm [CDC, 2010])
- Thermometer
- Stethoscope

Subjective Data: Pediatric Focus Questions

- Inquire about child's development milestones (see Appendix 5)
- Inquire about immunizations (see CDC [2020] recommended immunization schedules at https://cdc.gov/vaccines/schedules/index.html)
- Inquire about parent–child relationships (see Appendix 4)

Objective Data: Pediatric Assessment Techniques

PROCEDURE	NORMAL VARIATIONS
Observe **physical level of development** and compare with chronologic age *Note: When taking vital signs in infants, measure the respiratory and pulse rates first, as taking a temperature (especially a rectal temperature) may cause the infant to cry, which will alter the pulse and respiratory rates*	See Appendix 5
Monitor temperature. In infants <6 months old, use axillary, tympanic, or rectal measurements. In infants and children >6 months old, use temporal, tympanic, axillary, rectal, or oral measurements	Temperature fluctuates markedly in infants and young children

(Continued on following page)

PROCEDURE	NORMAL VARIATIONS
Temporal arterial. May be used in healthy infants <90 days old. Contraindicated in infants <90 days old who have illness, fever, etc. May be used in infants and children >90 days old with or without fever, illness, etc. *Note: The measurement technique is the same as for the adult client*	<38°C (100.4°F)
Rectal. The rectal temperature is considered the most accurate and should be used in children <4 years of age (American Academy of Pediatrics [AAP]); however, other clinical guidelines discourage rectal temperatures due to safety and practical issues, as well as physical and psychological discomfort (Barbi et al., 2017). Examples of these circumstances include a child who is critically ill, an uncooperative child, a child who is unconscious or at risk for seizures. Rectal measurement is contraindicated for premature infants, children with a medical history of gastrointestinal (GI) bleed, or other GI abnormalities (cancer, etc.)	<38°C (100.4°F) Rectal temperature measures higher in infants and children versus other routes. Rectal temperature may also measure higher in the late afternoon/evening and/or after playing/vigorous activity
Procedure. Position child prone, supine, or side lying (may use parent's lap). Insert lubricated thermometer no > 2.5 cm (1 in.) into rectum. For children <6 months of age, insert thermometer only 0.63–1.2 cm (1/4–1/2 in.). Never force thermometer into rectum against resistance	
Tympanic. Recommended for newborns, infants, toddlers through adolescence. Contraindicated in critically ill children younger than 7 years. Procedure: instruct child/parent on securing child's head to prevent movement while measuring temperature. Pull pinna down and back and proceed with the same measurement technique as is used for the adult client	<38°C (100.4°F)
Axillary. When taking axillary temperature, place tip of thermometer into axilla and hold arm down close to the body *Note: Measurement technique is the same as for the adult client*	<37.2°C (99°F)

PROCEDURE	NORMAL VARIATIONS

Oral. Starting at approximately 4 years, oral thermometers may be used in children; however, this will depend on the cooperation of the child. Instruct child to place probe under tongue and avoid biting on the probe. When using an electronic probe, cover it with a disposable probe cover to prevent breaking the probe or causing injury

Note: Measurement technique is the same as for the adult client

<37.8°C (100°F)

Monitor pulse. Take apical (not radial) pulse in children younger than 2 years (Fig. 6-5). Count pulse for 1 full minute

Awake and resting pulse rates vary with the age of the child: 1 week to 3 months, 100–160; 3 months to 2 years, 80–150; 2–10 years, 70–110; 10 years to adult, 55–90

Athletic adolescents tend to have lower pulse rates

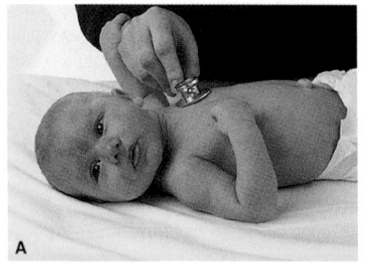 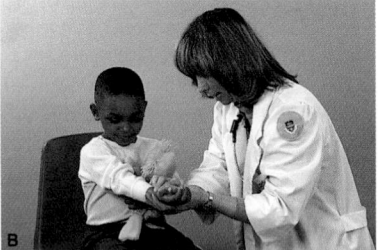

FIGURE 6-5 **(A)** Auscultating apical pulse rate in child <2 years. **(B)** Measuring radial pulse in child older than 2 years. (Photo by B. Proud.)

(Continued on following page)

PROCEDURE	NORMAL VARIATIONS
Monitor respirations by observing abdominal movement in infants and younger children	Respiratory rates: birth to 6 months, 30–50; 6 months to 2 years, 20–30; 3–10 years, 20–28; 10–18 years, 12–20
Monitor blood pressure. Blood pressure is not routinely performed on children younger than 3 years. Recommend annual screening beginning at 3 years of age and as indicated for high-risk children. Width of cuff should cover two thirds of upper arm or be 20% greater than diameter of the extremity. Length of bladder should encircle without overlapping. Take blood pressure while child is calm and quiet. For infants and children younger than 3 years, use an electronic DINAMAP that is designed to interpret blood pressure according to size and weight of young children	Blood pressure rates: *Systolic:* 1–7 years, age in years + 90; 8–18 years, (2 × age in years) + 90; *Diastolic:* 1–5 years, 56; 6–18 years, age in years + 52
• Measure height, weight, and head circumference and plot on growth chart • Height *Children younger than 24 months:* Measure length from vertex of head to heel in recumbent position *Children older than 24 months:* Measure standing height in bare feet	See normal height ranges at https://cdc.gov/growthcharts/clinical_charts.htm (CDC, 2017)
• Weight: For infants and young children up to 3 years old, use infant or platform balance scale. Weigh child with only clean diaper on. At approximately 3 years, or once child is able to stand, the upright scale may be used	At 1 year of age, the child's weight is usually three times the birth weight; see https://cdc.gov/growthcharts/clinical_charts.htm (CDC, 2017)

PROCEDURE	NORMAL VARIATIONS
• Head circumference *Children younger than 24 months:* Measure slightly above eyebrows, pinna of ears over occipital prominence of skull (see Fig. 6-6) 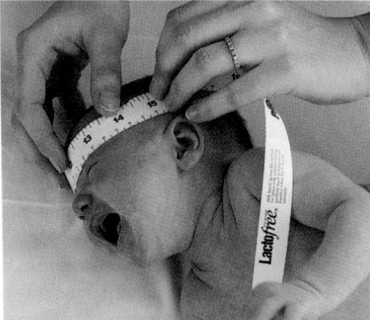 **FIGURE 6-6** Measuring the circumference of an infant's head. (Photo by B. Proud.)	• Plot head circumference on standard growth chart. Head circumference measurement should fall between the 5th and 95th percentiles and should be comparable with the child's height and weight percentiles. Those >95% may indicate macrocephaly. Those under the 5th percentile may indicate microcephaly. Increased head circumference in children older than 3 years may indicate separation of cranial sutures due to increased intracranial pressure

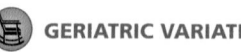 **GERIATRIC VARIATIONS**

- Dress may be heavier because of a decrease in body metabolism and a loss of subcutaneous fat.
- Osteoporotic thinning and collapse of the vertebrae secondary to bone loss may result in kyphosis.
- In older men, gait may be wider based with arms held outward.
- Older women tend to have a narrow base and may waddle to compensate for a decreased sense of balance.
- Mobility may be decreased, and gait may be rigid.
- Steps in gait may shorten with decreased speed and arm swing.
- Temperature may range from 35°C to 36.3°C (95°F–97.5°F). Therefore, the older client may not have an obviously elevated temperature with an infection or be considered hypothermic below 35.5°C (96°F). Normal body temperature values for all routes in older adults are consistently lower than values reported in younger populations (Harvard Medical School, 2020).

- Arteries are more rigid, hard, and bent.
- More rigid, arteriosclerotic arteries account for higher systolic blood pressure.
- Systolic pressure over 130 mmHg but diastolic pressure under 80 mmHg is called isolated systolic hypertension (Sheps, 2020).
- Systolic murmurs may be present.
- Widening of the pulse pressure is seen with aging due to less elastic peripheral arteries.

CULTURAL VARIATIONS

- Blood pressure percentiles of prepubertal children in nonindustrialized countries may fall well below Western percentiles.
- Asians and Native Americans have fewer sweat glands and, so, less obvious body odor than Whites and Black Africans.

POSSIBLE COLLABORATIVE PROBLEMS—RISK OF

- Hyperthermia
- Hypothermia
- Hypertension
- Hypotension
- Infection
- Dysrhythmia
- Dyspnea

Teaching Tips for Selected Client Concerns and Collaborative Problems

Client Concern: Opportunity to improve client health behaviors: Expresses desire to learn more about health promotion. Teach client self-assessment procedures (e.g., breast self-examination, testicular self-examination) and the importance of regular medical checkups. Refer to community wellness resources and support groups as they relate to client.

Collaborative Problem: Potential complication—hypertension

Explain the relationships between body weight, diet, exercise, stress, and blood pressure. Explain the possible effects of a low-fat, low-cholesterol diet along with vigorous exercise in reducing the atherosclerotic process. Explain the methods of preparing food low in sodium and fat, and high in potassium. Teach clients who drink alcohol to limit their intake. (See Tables 6-2 and 6-3 for follow-up and referral.)

Client Concern: Poor ambulation ability associated with deconditioning (inability to climb stairs) after illness

Teach client to increase muscle conditioning slowly. Refer to physician for physical therapy if necessary.

 Client Concern: Risk for poor thermoregulation associated with febrile illness

Instruct parents on proper method to assess temperature and detect fever. Teach proper method of giving tepid sponge baths and using antipyretics to reduce fever. Teach parents to avoid aspirin or aspirin products in children. Explain the use of quiet play and increasing fluids during this time. Teach parents to monitor for dehydration by assessing oral mucous membranes as needed.

Instruct parent to notify physician in case of high fever.

 Client Concern: Risk for infectious disease associated with loss of passive immunity of placenta (age 6–12 months)

Instruct parents to clothe infant well to decrease exposure to others with illnesses. Encourage use of good handwashing techniques for parents and children. Encourage parents to comply with the CDC recommendations on children's immunizations throughout childhood.

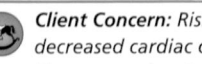 **Client Concern:** *Risk for poor growth and development associated with inadequate nutrition*

Instruct parents on adequate nutrient intake for developmental age of child. Refer to dietitian if necessary. Educate parents on the recommended dietary intake of the child for the appropriate age and changes to expect as the child gets older. Identify and discuss cultural beliefs related to dietary intake of the child and strategies to meet child's dietary needs. Teach parents normal eating behaviors of children, such as toddlers grazing with finger foods, etc. Identify community resources, as appropriate (early intervention, WIC, etc.) to assist the family in providing additional financial resources to support the family in purchasing healthy meals.

 Collaborative Problem: *Potential Complication—Postural Hypotension*

Identify postural hypotension in the older adult (difference of 20 mmHg systolic blood pressure and 10 mmHg diastolic blood pressure from a lying to a standing position). Instruct client to reduce risk of falls by moving from a lying to a sitting position slowly, then standing for 2 to 3 minutes before proceeding.

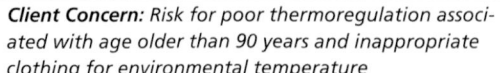 **Client Concern:** *Risk for hypothermia associated with decreased cardiac output and decreased subcutaneous tissue secondary to aging processes*

Encourage good heating in homes and added clothing in cold weather. Teach family to observe for signs of hypothermia, including facial edema, pallor, clouding of vision, decreased blood pressure, and decreased heart rate. Refer to community agencies that may provide shelter, clothing, and food when needed.

Client Concern: *Risk for poor thermoregulation associated with age older than 90 years and inappropriate clothing for environmental temperature*

Discuss with client decreasing ability to sense environmental temperature extremes with aging and effects of decreased efficiency of circulation to maintain body temperature. Teach client to seek assistance in determining adequate/appropriate clothing to match environment.

References

ACC/AHA/AAPA/ABC/ACPM/AGS/APhA/ASH/ASPC/NM/PCNA. (2017). 2017 Guideline for the prevention, detection, evaluation, and management of high blood pressure in adults: A report of the American College of Cardiology/American Heart Association Task Force on Clinical Practice Guidelines. *Journal of American College of Cardiology*, 71, e127–e248. https://www.acc.org/latest-in-cardiology/ten-points-to-remember/2017/11/09/11/41/2017-guideline-for-high-blood-pressure-in-adults

American Medical Association. (2014). *How a doctor quickly improved patients' blood pressure readings.* https://www.ama-assn.org/delivering-care/hypertension/how-doctor-quickly-improved-patients-blood-pressure-readings

Barbi, E., Marzuillo, P., Neri, E., Naviglio, S., & Krauss, B. S. (2017). Fever in children: Pearls and pitfalls. *Children (Basel)*, 4(9), 81. https://doi.org/10.3390/children4090081

Centers for Disease Control and Prevention. (2010). *Growth charts.* https://www.cdc.gov/growthcharts/index.htm

Centers for Disease Control and Prevention. (2017). *Clinical growth charts.* https://cdc.gov/growthcharts/clinical_charts.htm

Centers for Disease Control and Prevention. (2020). *Immunization schedules.* https://cdc.gov/vaccines/schedules/index.html

Exegen Corporation. (2018). Exegen temporalscanner calibration choices. https://www.exergen.com/wp-content/uploads/2018/05/Exergen-TemporalScanner-Calibration-Choices-873071.pdf

Harvard Medical School. (2020). *When is body temperature too low?* https://www.health.harvard.edu/staying-healthy/when-is-body-temperature-too-low#:~:text=Older%20adults%20often%20have%20an,about%201%C2%B0F%20lower

Mayo Clinic. (2020). Obesity: https://www.mayoclinic.org/diseases-conditions/obesity/symptoms-causes/syc-20375742

Sheps, S. (2020). *Isolated systolic hypertension: A health concern?* https://www.mayoclinic.org/diseases-conditions/high-blood-pressure/expert-answers/hypertension/faq-20058527#:~:text=Isolated%20systolic%20hypertension%20happens%20when,people%20older%20than%20age%2065

Skerrett, P. (2020). *Different blood pressure in right and left arms could signal trouble.* https://www.health.harvard.edu/blog/different-blood-pressure-in-right-and-left-arms-could-signal-trouble-201202014174

7 ASSESSING PAIN

Conceptual Foundations

The International Association for the Study of Pain (IASP) defined *pain* as "an unpleasant sensory and emotional experience, which we primarily associate with tissue damage or describe in terms of such damage" (IASP, 2017, p. 1). The definition of pain often emphasized in nursing is the one by Margo McCaffrey from 1968: "Pain is whatever the experiencing person says it is, existing whenever he says it does" (Pasero, 2018, front piece). It is important to remember this definition when assessing and treating pain.

The undertreatment of pain became a serious issue in the late 1990s. The Joint Commission designated "pain" as the "fifth vital sign" in 2001, but by 2004, this designation no longer appeared in the Standards for Accreditation (Baker, 2017; see Joint Commission, 2019, for Joint Commission Pain Standards) due to the opioid crisis.

The overtreatment of pain—resulting in overdoses of prescription pain relievers, heroin, and other opioids such as fentanyl—has been called the *opioid crisis*. The National Institute on Drug Abuse (2019) reported in 2018 a daily U.S. death rate of 128 persons due to opioid overdoses and a tremendous financial yearly burden from health care costs, lost productivity, treatment of addictions, and criminal justice expenses. This opioid crisis complicates pain assessment and treatment. Health care workers must collaborate to effectively assess and treat pain.

PATHOPHYSIOLOGY OF PAIN

The pathophysiologic phenomena of pain are associated with the central and the peripheral nervous systems. The source of pain stimulates the peripheral nerve endings (nociceptors), which transmit the sensations to the central nervous system. They are sensory receptors that detect signals from damaged tissue and to chemicals released from the damaged tissue. Nociceptors are sensitive to intense mechanical stimulation, temperature, or noxious stimuli (chemical, thermal, or mechanical). Nociceptors are distributed in the body, in the skin, subcutaneous tissue, skeletal muscle, joints, peritoneal surfaces, pleural membranes, dura mater, and blood vessel walls. Note that they are not located in the parenchyma of visceral organs. Physiologic processes involved in pain perception (or nociception) include transduction, transmission, perception, and modulation (see Fig. 7-1). These processes serve as means for the stimuli to be sent to various parts of the spinal cord and to the brain, where they are perceived and can be responded to. The modulation process, which changes or inhibits transmission, is poorly understood but affects the level of pain perceived.

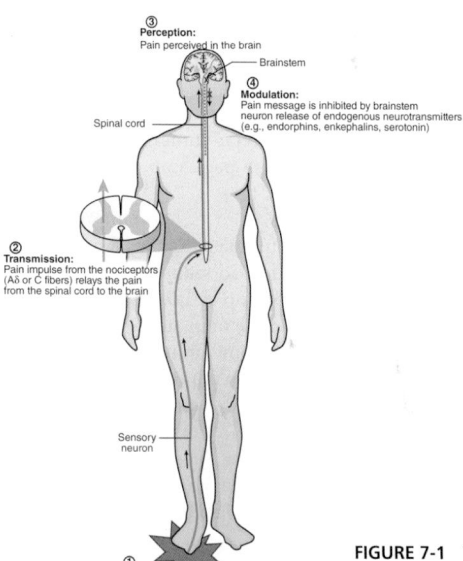

FIGURE 7-1 Transduction, transmission, perception, and modulation of pain.

PHYSIOLOGIC RESPONSES TO PAIN

Pain elicits a stress response in the human body, triggering the sympathetic nervous system, resulting in physiologic responses such as the following:

- Anxiety, fear, hopelessness, sleeplessness, and thoughts of suicide
- Focus on pain, reports of pain, cries and moans, and frowns and facial grimaces
- Decrease in cognitive function, mental confusion, altered temperament, high somatization, and dilated pupils
- Increased heart rate and peripheral, systemic, and coronary vascular resistance
- Increased respiratory rate and sputum retention, resulting in infection and atelectasis
- Decreased gastric and intestinal motility
- Decreased urinary output, resulting in urinary retention, fluid overload, and depression of all immune responses
- Increased antidiuretic hormone, epinephrine, norepinephrine, aldosterone, and glucagon; decreased insulin and testosterone
- Hyperglycemia, glucose intolerance, insulin resistance, and protein catabolism
- Muscle spasm, resulting in impaired muscle function and immobility and perspiration

CLASSIFICATION OF PAIN

Pain has many different classifications. Common categories of pain include the following:

- **Acute pain:** usually associated with an injury with a recent onset and duration of less than 6 months and usually lasts less than a month
- **Chronic nonmalignant pain:** usually associated with a specific cause or injury and is described as a constant pain that persists for more than 6 months
- **Cancer pain:** often due to the compression of peripheral nerves or meninges or from the damage to these structures following surgery, chemotherapy, radiation, or tumor growth and infiltration

Pain is also described as transient pain, tissue injury pain (surgical pain, trauma-related pain, burn pain, or iatrogenic pain as a result of an intervention), and chronic neuropathic pain.

Pain is also viewed in terms of its location, as follows:

- **Cutaneous pain** (skin or subcutaneous tissue)
- **Visceral pain** (abdominal cavity, thorax, cranium)
- **Deep somatic pain** (ligaments, tendons, bones, blood vessels, nerves)

Pain location can also be described as to whether or not it is perceived at the site of the pain stimuli, as follows:

- **Radiating** (perceived both at the source and extending to other tissues)
- **Referred** (perceived in body areas away from the pain source; see Fig. 7-2)
- **Phantom pain** (perceived in nerves left by a missing, amputated, or paralyzed body part)
  Other descriptions of pain include the following:
- **Neuropathic pain** causes an abnormal processing of pain messages and results from past damage to peripheral or central nerves due to sustained neurochemical levels
- **Intractable pain** is defined by its high resistance to pain relief

ASPECTS AND MANIFESTATIONS OF PAIN

There are many aspects that influence the way pain is manifested. The physiologic aspects of pain result from a client's physical response to a painful stimulus. For example, a client feels a pin pricking the skin of a finger through the nervous system; the sensation is interpreted by the brain, and the person pulls their hand away from the painful stimulus. Although they

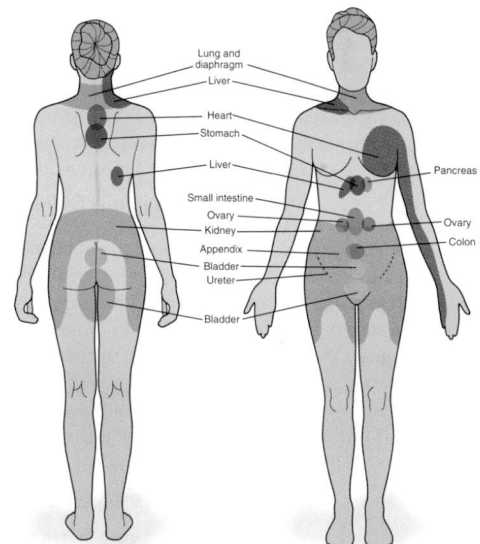

FIGURE 7-2 Areas of referred pain. *Left:* Posterior view. *Right:* Anterior view.

are physiologic in nature, the level of severity, the quality of the perceived pain, and the location where the pain is perceived to be are described as sensory aspects of the pain. For example, although a pin prick is usually felt at the site of the prick, other pain, such as severe chest pain felt in the back rather than in the chest, can be felt in a location other than the location of the actual pain stimulus; this is called *referred pain*. The quality of the perceived pain may vary and be felt, for example, as superficial or deep, shooting, sharp, electric, itchy, tingling, achy, cramping, or throbbing. When pain is perceived, the person responds with behaviors, both verbal and nonverbal. For example, for a pin prick, the person might say "ouch" and pull the hand away. Another aspect of pain relates to the cultural and social contexts of the client, which can affect the person's beliefs about the pain, its cause, and its purpose. For example, in some cultures, childbirth is expected to produce almost unbearable pain, and the woman in labor sobs and thrashes about and seems unable to help the nurse through the labor. Finally, the client's spiritual beliefs can affect their perceived pain sensations and responses. For example, persons who believe physical suffering to be offered up to God will expect pain and respond with resignation to it, not attempting to relieve it as much as someone would if not sharing a similar belief.

Nursing Assessment

COLLECTING SUBJECTIVE DATA

There are few objective findings on which the assessment of pain can rely. Pain is a subjective phenomenon, and thus, the main assessment lies in the client's reporting. The client's description of pain is quoted. The exact words used to describe the experience of pain are used to help in the diagnosis and management. The pain and its onset, duration, causes, and alleviating and aggravating factors are assessed. Then the quality, intensity, and effects of pain on the physical, psychosocial, and spiritual aspects are questioned. Past experience with pain in addition to past and current therapies are explored.

Preparing the Client

In preparation for the interview, clients are seated in a quiet, comfortable, and calm environment with minimal interruption. Explain to the client that the interview will entail questions to clarify the picture of the pain experienced in order to develop the plan of care.

Pain Assessment Tools

There are many assessment tools, some of which are specific to special types of pain. The main issues in choosing the tool are its reliability and its validity. Moreover, the tool must be clear and, therefore, easily understood by the client and require little effort from the client and the nurse.

Select one or more pain assessment tools appropriate for the client. There are many pain assessment scales, such as the following:

- Visual Analog Scale (VAS)
- Numeric Rating Scale (NRS) (Box 7-1)
- Numeric Pain Intensity Scale (NPIS)
- Behavioral Pain Scale (BPS) (Box 7-2)
- Pain Assessment in Advanced Dementia (PAINAD)
- Verbal Descriptor Scale

BOX 7-1 NUMERIC RATING SCALE (NRS)

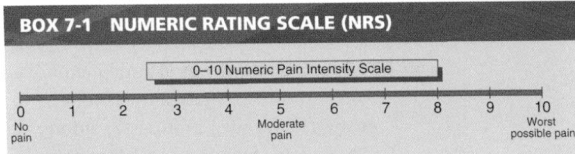

(Reprinted from *Acute pain management: Operative or medical procedures and trauma.* Clinical Practice Guideline No. 1. AHCPR Publication No. 92-0032; February 1992; with permission.)

BOX 7-2 BEHAVIORAL PAIN SCALE (BPS)

Item	Description	Score
Facial expression	Relaxed	1
	Partially tightened (e.g., brow lowering)	2
	Fully tightened (e.g., eyelid closing)	3
	Grimacing	4
Upper limbs	No movement	1
	Partially bent	2
	Fully bent with finger flexion	3
	Permanently retracted	4
Compliance with ventilation	Tolerating movement	1
	Coughing but tolerating ventilation for most of the time	2
	Fighting ventilator	3
	Unable to control ventilation	4

Reprinted with permission from Payen, J., Bru, O., Bosson, J., Lagrasta, A., Novel, E., Deschaux, L., & Jacquot, C. (2001). Assessing pain in critically ill sedated patients by using a behavioral pain scale. *Critical Care Medicine, 29*(12), 2258–2263. https://doi.org/10.1097/00003246-200112000-00004

- Faces Pain Scale (FPS), Faces Pain Scale – Revised (FPS-R), including the Wong-Baker FACES Scale (Box 7-3)
- Simple Descriptive Pain Intensity Scale
- Graphic Rating Scale
- Verbal Rating Scale
- McCaffrey Initial Pain Assessment Tool (see Box 7-4)

All of these and other scales can be found online. Most of these scales have been shown to be reliable measures of client pain. The three most popular scales are the NRS (Box 7-1), the Verbal Descriptor Scale, and the FPS (Box 7-3), although VASs are often mentioned as very simple. The NRS has been shown to be the best for older adults with no cognitive impairment and the FPS-R for cognitively impaired adults (Flaherty, 2012).

The Baker and Wong FACES Pain Scale (Wong-Baker FACES Foundations, 2015) is used for adults and especially for children to assess pain. See Box 7-3.

The BPS (Payen et al., 2001) has been used to assess pain in persons unable to verbally express their level of pain. As noted in the third category, the original intent was for ventilated clients. See Box 7-2.

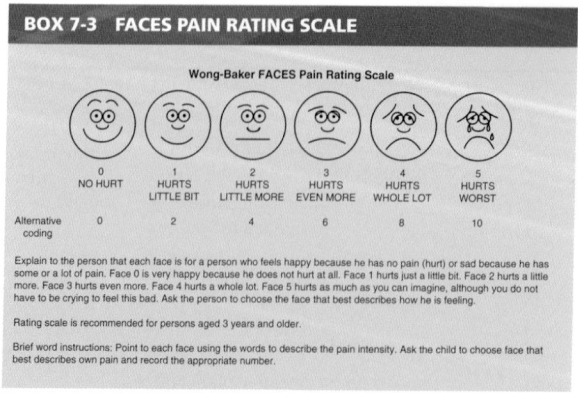

BOX 7-3 FACES PAIN RATING SCALE

Wong-Baker FACES Pain Rating Scale

| 0 NO HURT | 1 HURTS LITTLE BIT | 2 HURTS LITTLE MORE | 3 HURTS EVEN MORE | 4 HURTS WHOLE LOT | 5 HURTS WORST |

| Alternative coding | 0 | 2 | 4 | 6 | 8 | 10 |

Explain to the person that each face is for a person who feels happy because he has no pain (hurt) or sad because he has some or a lot of pain. Face 0 is very happy because he does not hurt at all. Face 1 hurts just a little bit. Face 2 hurts a little more. Face 3 hurts even more. Face 4 hurts a whole lot. Face 5 hurts as much as you can imagine, although you do not have to be crying to feel this bad. Ask the person to choose the face that best describes how he is feeling.

Rating scale is recommended for persons aged 3 years and older.

Brief word instructions: Point to each face using the words to describe the pain intensity. Ask the child to choose face that best describes own pain and record the appropriate number.

Used with permission from Wong-Baker FACES Foundation. (2015). *Wong-Baker FACES™ Pain Rating Scale*. Retrieved September 2017 with permission from http://www.WongBakerFACES.org

Effective pain assessment tools suitable for the client's initial assessment are the McCaffrey Initial Pain Assessment Tool (see Box 7-4) (McCaffery & Pasero, 1999) and the Brief Pain Inventory (Short Form)

BOX 7-4 MCCAFFERY INITIAL PAIN ASSESSMENT TOOL

McCaffery Initial Pain Assessment Tool

Patient's Name _____ Age _____ Date _____
Diagnosis _____ Physician _____ Room _____
Nurse _____

1. LOCATION: Patient or nurse marks drawing.

2. INTENSITY: Patient rates the pain. Scale used _____
   Present:
   Worst pain gets:
   Best pain gets:
   Acceptable level of pain:

3. QUALITY: (Use patient's own words, e.g., prick, ache, burn, throb, pull sharp) _____

4. ONSET, DURATION, VARIATIONS, RHYTHMS: _____

5. MANNER OF EXPRESSING PAIN? _____

6. WHAT RELIEVES THE PAIN? _____

7. WHAT CAUSES OR INCREASES THE PAIN? _____

8. EFFECTS OF PAIN: (Note decreased function, decreased quality of life.)
   Accompanying symptoms (e.g., nausea)
   Sleep
   Appetite
   Physical activity
   Relationship with others (e.g., irritability)
   Emotions (e.g., anger, suicidal, crying)
   Concentration
   Other

9. OTHER COMMENTS:
10. PLAN:

May be duplicated for use in clinical practice. From McCaffery M., & Pasero, C. (1999). *Pain: Clinical manual* (p. 60.). Copyright ©1999, Mosby, Inc.

PRESENT HEALTH CONCERNS

QUESTION	RATIONALE
Are you experiencing pain now or have you in the past 24 hours?	This helps establish the presence or absence of perceived pain.
Where is the pain located?	The location of pain helps identify the underlying cause.
Does it radiate or spread?	Radiating or spreading pain helps identify the source. For example, chest pain radiating to the left arm is most probably of cardiac origin, while pain that is pricking and spreading in the chest muscle area is probably musculoskeletal in origin.
Are there any other concurrent symptoms accompanying the pain?	Accompanying symptoms also help identify the possible source. For example, right lower quadrant pain associated with nausea, vomiting, and the inability to stand up straight is possibly associated with appendicitis.
When did the pain start?	The onset of pain is an essential indicator for the severity of the situation and suggests a source.
What were you doing when the pain first started?	This helps identify the precipitating factors and what might have exacerbated the pain.
Is the pain continuous or intermittent?	The pain pattern helps identify the nature of the pain and may assist in identifying the source.
If intermittent pain, how often do the episodes occur and for how long do they last?	Understanding the course of the pain provides a pattern that may help determine the source.

QUESTION	RATIONALE
Describe the pain in your own words.	Clients are quoted so that terms used to describe their pain may indicate the type and source. The most common terms used are throbbing, shooting, stabbing, sharp, cramping, gnawing, hot/burning, aching, heavy, tender, splitting, tiring/exhausting, sickening, fearful, and punishing.
What factors relieve your pain?	Relieving factors help determine the source and the plan of care.
What factors increase your pain?	Identifying factors that increase pain helps determine the source and helps in planning to avoid aggravating factors.
Are you on any therapy to manage your pain?	This question establishes any current treatment modalities and their effect on the pain. This helps in planning the future plan of care.
Is there anything you would like to add?	An open-ended question allows the client to mention anything that has been missed or the issues that were not fully addressed by the above questions.

PERSONAL HEALTH HISTORY

QUESTION	RATIONALE
Have you had any previous experience with pain?	Past experiences of pain may shed light on the previous history of the client in addition to possible positive or negative expectations of pain therapies.

(Continued on following page)

FAMILY HISTORY

QUESTION	RATIONALE
Does anyone in your family experience pain?	This helps assess the possible family-related perceptions or any past experiences with persons in pain.
How does pain affect your family?	This helps assess how much the pain is interfering with the client's family relations.

LIFESTYLE AND HEALTH PRACTICES

QUESTION	RATIONALE
What are your concerns about pain?	Identifying the client's fears and worries helps in prioritizing the plan of care and providing adequate psychological support.
How does your pain interfere with the following? • General activity • Mood/emotions • Concentration • Physical ability • Work • Relations with other people • Sleep • Appetite • Enjoyment of life	These are the main lifestyle factors that pain interferes with. The more the pain interferes with the client's ability to function in their daily activities, the more it will reflect on the client's psychological status and thus the quality of life.

COLLECTING OBJECTIVE DATA

Physical Assessment

Objective data for pain are collected by observing the client's movement and responses to touch or descriptions of the pain experience. Many of the pain assessment tools incorporate a section to evaluate the objective responses to pain. Key points to remember during a physical examination for pain include the following:

- Choose an assessment tool that is reliable and valid to the client's culture.
- Explain to the client the purpose of rating the intensity of pain.

- Ensure the client's privacy and confidentiality.
- Respect the client's behavior toward pain and the terms used to express it.
- Understand that different cultures express pain differently and maintain different pain thresholds and expectations.

Note: Refer to Chapter 2, Performing Physical Assessment Skills and Techniques, appropriate to affected body area. Body system assessments will include techniques for assessing pain (e.g., palpating the abdomen for tenderness or palpating the joints for tenderness or pain).

GENERAL OBSERVATION		
ASSESSMENT PROCEDURE	**NORMAL FINDINGS**	**ABNORMAL FINDINGS**
• Observe posture.	• Posture is upright when the client appears to be comfortable, attentive, and without excessive changes in position and posture.	• Client appears to be slumped with the shoulders not straight (indicates being disturbed/uncomfortable). Client is inattentive and agitated. Client might be guarding affected area and have breathing patterns reflecting distress.

(Continued on following page)

GENERAL OBSERVATION (*continued*)		
ASSESSMENT PROCEDURE	**NORMAL FINDINGS**	**ABNORMAL FINDINGS**
• Observe facial expression.	• Client smiles with appropriate facial expressions and maintains adequate eye contact.	• Client's facial expressions indicate distress and discomfort, including frowning, moans, cries, and grimacing. Eye contact is not maintained, indicating discomfort.
• Inspect joints and muscles.	• Joints appear normal (no edema); muscles appear relaxed.	• Edema of a joint may indicate injury or arthritis. Pain may result in muscle tension.
• Observe skin for scars, lesions, rashes, changes, or discoloration.	• No inconsistency, wounds, or bruising are noted.	• Bruising, wounds, or edema may be the result of injuries or infections, which may cause pain.
VITAL SIGNS		
PROCEDURE	**NORMAL FINDINGS**	**ABNORMAL FINDINGS**
• Measure heart rate.	• Heart rate ranges from 60 to 100 beats/min.	• Increased heart rate may indicate discomfort or pain.
• Measure respiratory rate.	• Respiratory rate ranges from 12 to 20 beats/min.	• Respiratory rate may be increased, and breathing may be irregular and shallow.
• Measure blood pressure.	• Blood pressure ranges from 100 to 130 mmHg (systolic) and 60 to 80 mmHg (diastolic).	• Increased blood pressure often occurs in severe pain.

PEDIATRIC VARIATIONS

It is hard to evaluate pain in neonates and infants. Behaviors that indicate pain are used to assess their pain.

A pain assessment tool that serves well for the client's initial assessment is the Initial Pain Assessment for Pediatric Use Only (About Kids Health, 2009).

 GERIATRIC VARIATIONS

Older people often suffer from pain related to chronic disorders, which is often undertreated. Untreated pain can lead to anxiety, depression, isolation, functional decline, and confusion. Aggressive or combative behaviors in the demented elderly may be the result of untreated pain.

 CULTURAL VARIATIONS

Pain is a universal human experience, but how people respond to it varies with the meaning placed on pain and the response to pain that is expected in the culture in which the person is raised. There are certain patterns of pain expression that vary across cultures. Pain can have several meanings between different cultures that lead to these difference response patterns. The most important factor is this: DO NOT STEREOTYPE! Even though there are tendencies for people from a particular cultural background to exhibit certain characteristics, many people of that culture will not. The nurse must assess what the person says about pain and how the person perceives pain.

POSSIBLE COLLABORATIVE PROBLEMS—RISK OF

Angina	Endocarditis
Decreased cardiac output	Peripheral vascular insufficiency
Paralytic ileus/small bowel obstruction	Osteoarthritis
Sickling crisis	Joint dislocation
Peripheral nerve compression	Pathologic fractures
Corneal ulceration	Renal calculi

Teaching Tips for Selected Client Concerns

Client Concern: Opportunity to improve spirituality associated with coping with prolonged physical pain

- Encourage the client to request interactions with spiritual leaders and to request forgiveness from family, friends, and others.
- Encourage the client to express reverence and awe and to participate in religious activities.
- Encourage the client to spend time outdoors and to display creative energy (e.g., writing, drawing, poetry).

Client Concern: Opportunity to improve comfort level

- Teach the client to identify comfortable positions.
- Teach the client to identify uncomfortable postures and to attempt to minimize their occurrences.

References

About Kids Health. (2009). Tools for measuring pain. https://www.aboutkidshealth.ca/Article?contentid=2994&language=English

Baker, D. (2017). *The Joint Commission's pain standards: Origins and evolution.* https://www.jointcommission.org/assets/1/6/Pain_Std_History_Web_Version_05122017.pdf

Flaherty, E. (2012). Pain assessment for older adults. *Try This: Best Practices in Nursing Care for Older Adults,* (7). http://catch-on.org/wp-content/uploads/2016/12/issue-7.pdf

Joint Commission. (2019). *Pain management standards for accredited organizations.* https://www.jointcommission.org/topics/pain_management_standards_hospital.aspx

McCaffery, M., & Pasero, C. (1999). *Pain: Clinical manual* (2nd ed.). Mosby.

National Institute on Drug Abuse. (2019). *Opioid overdose crisis.* https://www.drugabuse.gov/drugs-abuse/opioids/opioid-overdose-crisis

Pasero, C. (2018). In memoriam: Margo McCaffrey. *American Journal of Nursing, 118*(3), 3–17. https://doi.org/10.1097/01.NAJ.0000530929.65995.42

Payen, J., Bru, O., Bosson, J., Lagrasta, A., Novel, E., Deschaux, L., & Jacquot, C. (2001). Assessing pain in critically ill sedated patients by using a behavioral pain scale. *Critical Care Medicine, 29*(12), 2258–2263. https://doi.org/10.1097/00003246-200112000-00004

ASSESSING FOR VIOLENCE

Conceptual Foundations

Family violence (also called domestic violence) has been defined by the U.S. Department of Justice Office on Violence against Women (FindLaw, 2018, p. 1) as "a pattern of abusive behavior in any relationship that is used by one partner to gain or maintain control over another intimate partner." Family violence in U.S. sources tends to divide domestic violence from child abuse and elder abuse, but definitions from other countries, such as that of Australia, are broader and more readily focus on all family members (see Australian Law Reform Commission, 2010). A wheel representing this power and control model showing the relationship of physical abuse to other forms of abuse (developed by the Duluth Model Organization, 2017) can be found at https://www.theduluthmodel.org/wheels/. Family violence includes intimate partner violence (IPV), child abuse, and elder mistreatment and also affects people of all ages, sexes, religions, ethnicities, and socioeconomic levels.

IPV includes a range of behaviors, including physical abuse, emotional abuse, economic abuse, psychological abuse, and sexual assault. The Child Abuse Prevention and Treatment Act (CAPTA) defines *child abuse* as "any recent act or failure to act on the part of a parent or caretaker, which results in death, serious physical or emotional harm, sexual abuse, or exploitation, or an act or failure to act which presents an imminent risk of serious harm" (Public Law 104-235, §111; 42 U.S.C. 510g, 2003; and the CAPTA Reauthorization Act of 2010 [P.L. 111-320]). Elder mistreatment includes physical abuse, neglect, exploitation, abandonment, or prejudicial attitudes that decrease the quality of life and are demeaning to those older than 65 years.

TYPES OF FAMILY VIOLENCE

- **Physical abuse:** Pushing, shoving, slapping, kicking, choking, punching, burning; methods of restraint including holding, tying; attacks with household items (lamps, radios, ashtrays, irons, etc., or knives, guns)
- **Psychological abuse:** Constant use of insults or criticism, blaming the victim for things that are not the victim's faults, threats to hurt children or pets, isolation from supporters (family, friends, or coworkers), deprivation, humiliation, and intimidation
- **Economic abuse:** Preventing the victim from getting or keeping a job, controlling money and limiting access to funds, and controlling knowledge of family finances
- **Sexual abuse:** Forcing the victim to perform sexual acts against their will, pursuing sexual activity after the victim has said no, using violence during sex, and using weapons vaginally, orally, or anally

Nursing Assessment

Assessment for family violence mostly consists of the collection of adequate subjective data followed by a physical assessment. Before screening, discuss any legal, mandatory reporting requirements or other limits to confidentiality. Convey a concerned and nonjudgmental attitude. Show appropriate empathy.

To assess for the presence of family violence effectively, first examine your feelings, beliefs, and biases regarding violence.

No one under any circumstances should be physically, sexually, or emotionally abused. It is imperative that you become active in interrupting or ending cycles of violence. Be aware of "red flags" that may indicate the presence of family violence.

Because abuse, especially IPV, damages individuals, children, communities, and the social fabric of society, some government and professional organizations have recommended universal screening of all women for IPV as opposed to women in specific settings or with symptoms indicating abuse (O'Doherty et al., 2015). However, O'Doherty et al. found that, although screening in health care settings does indeed identify women experiencing IPV, current evidence does not support screening all women. Rather, screening women who are pregnant or those with symptoms is more likely to uncover abuse.

The U.S. Preventive Services Task Force (2019), in its final recommendation statement on IPV, recommended that clinicians screen women of childbearing age for IPV, such as domestic violence, and provide or refer women who screen positive to intervention services; however, the task force concluded that evidence is insufficient to recommend screening older or vulnerable adults for IPV.

Many organizations still recommend universal screening at initial and annual health care visits for a history of current and past abuse, regardless of the presence or absence of abuse indicators. Screen at each health care visit if there is a history of abuse. Screen all pregnant women at least once per trimester and once postpartum (Committee on Health Care for Underserved Women of American College of Obstetricians & Gynecologists, 2012, reaffirmed 2019). Screen mothers during well-child visits to the pediatrician. Also screen for abuse if the client is in a new relationship or if there are signs or symptoms indicating the presence of abuse.

COLLECTING SUBJECTIVE DATA

Creating a safe and confidential environment is essential when collecting subjective data from a client who has experienced family violence. Establish a trusting rapport and patiently listen. Use simple, direct questions with a relaxed and calm approach. If clients share the fact that they have experienced violence, do not ask them if they want to press charges, as this decision would require an attorney and is not part of assessing the client. For any client over the age of 3 years, ask screening questions in a secure, private setting with no one else present in the room. Do not screen if there are any safety concerns for you or the client. Prior to screening, discuss any legal, mandatory reporting requirements or other limits to confidentiality. Convey a concerned and nonjudgmental attitude. Show appropriate empathy and compassion (Fig. 8-1).

◎ CLINICAL TIP
There are four general areas to assess to determine the presence of family violence: physical abuse, psychological abuse, economic abuse, and sexual abuse. With physical abuse, it is important to remember that the abuse may start at any time during a relationship. The abuse may not be part of the presenting problem for which the client is being seen but may be the cause of the presenting problem.

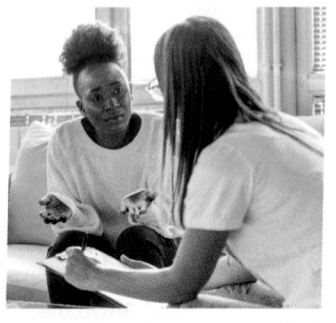

FIGURE 8-1 The nurse allows the woman to talk freely about her experience.

ASSESSMENT PROCEDURE	NORMAL FINDINGS	ABNORMAL FINDINGS (INDICATORS OF VIOLENCE OR POTENTIAL VIOLENCE)
Review past health history and physical examination records	No indicators of abuse are present	Documentation of past assaults. Unexplained injuries, symptoms of pain, nausea and vomiting, or choking. Repeated visits to emergency department. Signs and symptoms of anxiety. Use of sedatives or tranquilizers
		Injuries during pregnancy. History of drug or alcohol abuse, depression, and/or suicide attempts

ASSESSMENT PROCEDURE	NORMAL FINDINGS	ABNORMAL FINDINGS (INDICATORS OF VIOLENCE OR POTENTIAL VIOLENCE)
If partner/parent/caregiver is present at the visit, observe client's interactions with partner	Client is not afraid of partner. Client answers questions independently. Partner appears supportive	Partner criticizes client about appearance, feelings, and/or actions and is not sensitive to client's needs. Partner refuses to leave client's presence and speaks for client. Client is anxious and afraid of partner; is submissive to negative comments from partner. See Figure 8-1
Perform the rest of the examination without the partner, parent, or caregiver present		
Ask all clients: • Has anyone in your home ever hurt you? • Do you feel unsafe in your home? • Are you afraid of anyone in your home? • Has anyone made you do anything you did not want to do? • Has anyone ever touched you without your permission? • Has anyone ever threatened you?	Client answers no to all questions	"Yes" to any of the questions indicates abuse

(Continued on following page)

ASSESSMENT PROCEDURE	NORMAL FINDINGS	ABNORMAL FINDINGS (INDICATORS OF VIOLENCE OR POTENTIAL VIOLENCE)
For IPV, begin the screening by telling the woman that it is important to screen all women routinely for IPV because it affects so many women and men in our society. Ask the client to fill out or help the client fill out the Abuse Assessment. Tell the client "Because violence is common in many people's lives, I routinely ask all clients to complete the following questions or I can ask you these questions" (Assessment Screen in Box 8-1) **◎ CLINICAL TIP** Sometimes, no matter how carefully you prepare the client and ask the questions, she may not disclose abuse	Client answers "no" to all three questions (see Box 8-1). If the client replies "no" to screening questions and is not being abused, it is important for the client to know that you are available if she ever experiences abuse in the future Make statements that build trust such as: If your situation ever changes, please call me to talk about it. I am happy to hear that you are not being abused. If that should ever change, this is a safe place to talk	"Yes" to any of the questions strongly indicates initial disclosure of abuse. You should do the following: • Acknowledge the abuse and her courage • Use supportive statements such as "I'm sorry this is happening to you. This is not your fault. You are not responsible for his behavior. You are not alone. You don't deserve to be treated this way. Help is available to you" • Acknowledge her autonomy and right to self-determination • Reiterate confidentiality of disclosure

COLLECTING OBJECTIVE DATA

Equipment Needed

- All equipment for a complete head-to-toe physical examination

- Safe and secure private screening area (do not screen in an area that poses any safety concerns for the client or yourself)
  - Abuse Assessment Screen (Box 8-1)
  - Self-Assessment: Danger Assessment (Box 8-2)

BOX 8-1 ABUSE ASSESSMENT SCREEN

1. WITHIN THE LAST YEAR, have you been hit, slapped, kicked, or otherwise physically hurt by someone?   YES   NO
   If YES, by whom? _____
   Total number of times _____

2. SINCE YOU HAVE BEEN PREGNANT, have you been hit, slapped, kicked, or otherwise physically hurt by someone?   YES   NO
   If YES, by whom? _____
   Total number of times _____

MARK THE AREA OF INJURY ON THE BODY MAP. SCORE EACH INCIDENT ACCORDING TO THE FOLLOWING SCALE:
   SCORE
   1 = Threats of abuse including use of a weapon _____
   2 = Slapping, pushing: no injuries and/or lasting pain _____
   3 = Punching, kicking, bruises, cuts, and/or continuing pain _____
   4 = Beating up, severe contusions, burns, broken bones _____
   5 = Head injury, internal injury, permanent injury _____
   6 = Use of weapon; wound from weapon _____
   If any of the descriptions for the higher number apply, use the higher number.

3. WITHIN THE LAST YEAR, has anyone forced you to have sexual activities?   YES   NO
   If YES, by whom? _____
   Total number of times _____

Developed by the Nursing Research Consortium on Violence and Abuse. Readers are encouraged to reproduce and use this assessment tool. Reprinted with permission.

BOX 8-2 SELF-ASSESSMENT: DANGER ASSESSMENT

Several risk factors have been associated with increased risk of homicides (murders) of women and men in violent relationships. We cannot predict what will happen in your case, but we would like you to be aware of the danger of homicide in situations of abuse and for you to see how many of the risk factors apply to your situation.

Using the calendar, please mark the approximate dates during the past year when you were abused by your partner or ex-partner. Write on that date how bad the incident was according to the following scale:

1. Slapping, pushing; no injuries and/or lasting pain
2. Punching, kicking; bruises, cuts, and/or continuing pain
3. "Beating up"; severe contusions, burns, broken bones
4. Threat to use weapon; head injury, internal injury, permanent injury
5. Use of weapon; wounds from weapon

(If any of the descriptions for the higher number apply, use the higher number.)

Mark Yes or No for each of the following. ("He" refers to your husband, partner, ex-husband, ex-partner, or whoever is currently physically hurting you.)

1. Has the physical violence increased in severity or frequency over the past year?
2. Does he own a gun?
3. Have you left him after living together during the past year?
   a. (If you have *never* lived with him, check here:_____)
4. Is he unemployed?
5. Has he ever used a weapon against you or threatened you with a lethal weapon? (If yes, was the weapon a gun?)
6. Does he threaten to kill you?
7. Has he avoided being arrested for domestic violence?
8. Do you have a child that is not his?
9. Has he ever forced you to have sex when you did not wish to do so?
10. Does he ever try to choke you?
11. Does he use illegal drugs? By drugs, I mean "uppers" or amphetamines, speed, angel dust, cocaine, "crack," street drugs, or mixtures
12. Is he an alcoholic or problem drinker?
13. Does he control most or all of your daily activities? For instance, does he tell you who you can be friends with, when you can see your family, how much money you can use, or when you can take the car? (If he tries, but you do not let him, check here: _____)
14. Is he violently and constantly jealous of you? (For instance, does he say "If I can't have you, no one can"?)

15. Have you ever been beaten by him while you were pregnant? (If you have never been pregnant by him, check here: _____)
16. Have you ever threatened or tried to commit suicide?
17. Has he ever threatened or tried to commit suicide?
18. Does he threaten to harm your children?
19. Do you believe he is capable of killing you?

20. Does he follow or spy on you, leave threatening notes or messages on your answering machine, destroy your property, or call you when you don't want him to?
Total "Yes" Answers _____

Thank you. Please talk to your nurse, advocate, or counselor about what the danger assessment means in terms of your situation.

Campbell, J. C. (2004). Self-assessment: Danger assessment. In J. Humphreys & J. Campbell (Eds.), *Family violence and nursing practice*. Lippincott Williams & Wilkins.

Physical Assessment

During examination of a client who you suspect or know has been abused, it is essential to provide privacy for the client and keep your hands warm to promote the client's comfort during the examination. Also, remain nonjudgmental regarding client's habits, lifestyle, and any revelations about abuse. At the same time, educate and inform about risks and possibilities for assistance.

ASSESSMENT PROCEDURE	NORMAL FINDINGS	ABNORMAL FINDINGS
Perform a general survey. Observe general appearance and body build	Client appears to be stated age and well developed	Abused children may appear younger than stated age due to developmental delays or malnourishment. Older clients may appear thin and frail due to malnourishment

(Continued on following page)

ASSESSMENT PROCEDURE	NORMAL FINDINGS	ABNORMAL FINDINGS
Note dress and hygiene	Client is well-groomed and dressed appropriately for season and occasion	Poor hygiene and soiled clothing may indicate neglect. Long sleeves and pants in warm weather may be an attempt to cover bruising or other injuries. Victims of sexual abuse may dress provocatively
Assess the following: • Mental status	• Client is coherent and relaxed. A child shows proper developmental level for age	• Client is anxious, depressed, suicidal, withdrawn, or has difficulty concentrating. Client has poor eye contact or soft, passive speech. Client is unable to recall recent or past events. Child does not meet developmental expectations
• Vital signs	• Vital signs are within normal limits	• Hypertension may be seen in victims of abuse
• Skin	• Skin is clean, dry, and free of lesions or bruises. Skin fragility increases with age; bruising may occur with pressure and may mimic bruising associated with abuse. Be careful to distinguish between normal and abnormal findings	• Client has scars, bruises, burns, welts, or swelling on face, breasts, arms, chest, abdomen, or genitalia

ASSESSMENT PROCEDURE	NORMAL FINDINGS	ABNORMAL FINDINGS
• Head and neck	• Head and neck are free of injuries	• Client has hair missing in clumps, subdural hematomas, or rope marks or finger/hand strangulation marks on neck
• Eyes	• Eyes are free of injury	• Client has bruising or swelling around eyes, unilateral ptosis of upper eyelids (due to repeated blows causing nerve damage to eyelids), or a subconjunctival hemorrhage
• Ears	• Ears are clean and free of injuries	• Client has external or internal ear injuries
• Abdomen	• Abdomen is free of bruises and other injuries and is nontender	• Client has bruising in various stages of healing. Assessment reveals intra-abdominal injuries. A pregnant client has received blows to abdomen
• Genitalia and rectal area	• Client is free of injury	• Client has irritation, tenderness, bruising, bleeding, or swelling of genitals or rectal area. Discharge, redness, or lacerations may indicate abuse in young children. Hemorrhoids are unusual in children and may be caused by sexual abuse. Extreme apprehension during examination may indicate physical or sexual abuse

(Continued on following page)

ASSESSMENT PROCEDURE	NORMAL FINDINGS	ABNORMAL FINDINGS
• Musculoskeletal system	• Client shows full range of motion and has no evidence of injuries	• Dislocation of shoulder; old or new fractures of face, arms, or ribs; and poor range of motion of joints are indicators of abuse
• Neurologic system	• Client demonstrates normal neurologic function	• Tremors, hyperactive reflexes, and decreased sensations to areas of old injuries secondary to neurologic damage

Further Assessment for Positive IPV Findings

If screening for IPV is positive, ask the client to fill out a danger assessment questionnaire (Box 8-2)	Client has a safety plan to prevent further abuse and injury	If the client says she prefers to return home, ask her if it is safe for her to do so and have her respond to the questions in Box 8-3. Provide the client with contact information for shelters and groups. Encourage her to call with any concerns
If screening for IPV is positive and the client's answers on the danger assessment questionnaire indicate a high probability for serious violence, ask the client if she has a safety plan and where she would like to go when she leaves your agency (Box 8-3) Be sure to schedule a follow-up appointment and/or refer the client as appropriate		

BOX 8-3 ASSESSING A SAFETY PLAN

Ask the client: Do you:
- Have a packed bag ready? Keep it hidden but make it easy to grab quickly?
- Tell your neighbors about your abuse and ask them to call the police when they hear a disturbance?
- Have a code word to use with your kids, family, and friends so they will know to call the police and get you help?
- Know where you are going to go, if you ever have to leave?
- Remove weapons from the home?
- Have the following gathered:
  - Cash?
  - Social Security cards/numbers for you and your children?
  - Birth certificates for you and your children?
  - Driver's license?
  - Rent and utility receipts?
  - Bank account numbers?
  - Insurance policies and numbers?
  - Marriage license?
  - Jewelry?
  - Important phone numbers?
  - Copy of protection order?

Ask children: Do you:
- Know a safe place to go?
- Know who is safe to tell you are unsafe?
- Know how and when to call 911? Know how to make a collect call? Inform children that it is their job to keep themselves safe; they should not interject themselves into adult conflict.

If the client is planning to leave:
- Remind the client that this is a dangerous time that requires awareness and planning
- Review where the client is planning to go, shelter options, and the need to be around others to curtail violence
- Review the client's right to possessions and list of possessions to take

🐴 PEDIATRIC VARIATIONS

The Centers for Disease Control and Prevention (CDC, 2020b) has reported that one in seven children in the United States has experienced child abuse or neglect in the last year. In 2018, nearly 1,770 children died of abuse or neglect.

The following points are important to keep in mind when assessing for abuse in children:

- For any client older than 3 years, ask any screening questions in a secure, private setting with no one else present in the room.
- Receive any information the child may disclose to you in an interested, calm, and accepting manner. Avoid showing surprise or distaste.
- Do not coerce the child to answer questions by offering rewards.
- Establish the child's level of understanding by asking simple questions (name, how to spell name, age, birth date, how many eyes do you have, etc.). Then formulate questions the child can comprehend.

- The majority of children disclose to questions specific to the person suspected of abuse or related to the type of abuse (Hegar et al., 2000).
- Use multiple-choice or open-ended questions and avoid "yes or no" questions.
- The less information you supply in your questions and the more information the child gives in answering the questions, the higher the credibility of the collected data.
- Realize that there are significant behavioral consequences for children who are abused. Once these children reach adolescence and adulthood, they are likely to indulge in sexual and other risk-taking behaviors, juvenile delinquency and adult criminality, alcohol and other drug abuse, and are likely to be perpetrators or victims of abuse as adults (Castro et al., 2019; Office of Women's Health, 2019). However, these and other authors raise questions about the association between witnessing domestic violence and becoming an abusive adult.

See Figure 8-2 for examples of physical child abuse.

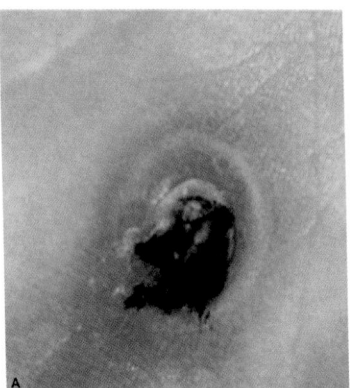
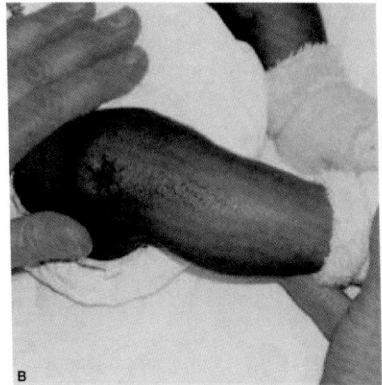
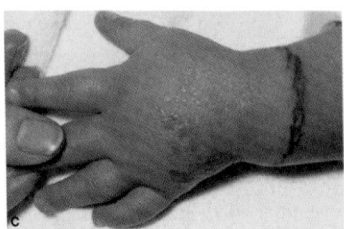
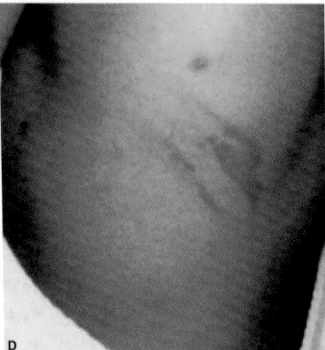

FIGURE 8-2 Examples of physical child abuse. Physical injuries may have distinctive outlines that indicate the instrument of abuse. (**A**) Cigarette burn on child's foot. (**B**) Imprint from a radiator cover. (**C**) Rope burn from being tied to crib rail. (**D**) Imprint from a looped electrical cord. (Reprinted with permission from Hatfield, N. T., & Kincheloe, C. [2018]. *Introductory maternity and pediatric nursing* (4th ed., Fig. 33-2). Wolters Kluwer.)

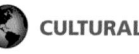 **GERIATRIC VARIATIONS**

- Elder abuse includes physical abuse, sexual abuse, emotional abuse, neglect (passive or active), willful deprivation, abandonment, confinement, and financial abuse or exploitation and is reported to be experienced by 1 in 10 persons aged 60 years and older in the United States (CDC, 2020a; National Council on Aging [NCOA], n.d.). The NCOA reported that 90% of abusers are family members, often adult children or spouses.
- The medical consequences of elder abuse include (1) inability of the frail older adult to handle the trauma; (2) inability to get food or medication because of neglect; (3) inability to pay for food or medication because of financial abuse; and (4) inability to deal with illness/malnutrition/problems because of depression associated with abuse.
- Statistics of economic abuse are difficult to find due to underreporting by abused elders.
- Start out by asking the older adult client to tell you about a typical day in their life. Be alert for indicators placing the older client at a high risk for abuse or neglect. Then ask the following ("Yes" to any of the questions indicates abuse):
  - Has anyone ever made you sign papers that you did not understand?
  - Are you alone often?
  - Has anyone refused to help you when you needed help?
  - Has anyone ever refused to give you or let you take your medications?
  - Has anyone ever taken your medications from you? Explain.

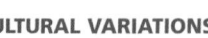 **CULTURAL VARIATIONS**

Conducting a cultural assessment using assessment guidelines is necessary before attempting to understand family violence. Although studies show some cultural variation, the rates seem to vary with poverty level and two extremes of living congestion; high rates exist in highly congested inner cities and also in very underpopulated rural areas (Maguire-Jack et al., 2015).

POSSIBLE COLLABORATIVE PROBLEMS—RISK OF

- Bone fractures
- Concussion
- Subdural hematoma
- Subconjunctival hemorrhage
- Intra-abdominal injury
- Depression
- Suicide
- Death

Teaching Tips for Selected *Client Concerns*

Client Concern: Risk for poor family relationships associated with indications of family violence

Teach the family about the availability of safe community resources.

Avoid giving the family print resources that may be accessed by the partner, who may respond in a violent manner to this information. Direct the client to online Internet resources as available.

Client Concern: Lack of safe environment associated with history of spousal abuse episodes

Teach the client that they are a victim and that no one deserves to be treated with violence in any situation or circumstance.

Teach the client ways to become empowered through healthy lifestyle practices including exercise, diet, and adequate rest and sleep.

Provide the client with contact details for a victim assistance program.

 Client Concern: Risk for low self-esteem associated with feelings of guilt and feeling responsible for being a victim

Explain to children that they are not responsible for the abusive behavior of the offender. Assess social and interpersonal relationships and identify a person that the child can depend on or call for support. Notify social services to assess family situation. Assess need for counseling for self-esteem.

 Client Concern: Lack of social interaction associated with feelings of embarrassment regarding family violence

Identify high-risk relationships and encourage family and social support for the client. Teach the client problem-solving skills and strategies to avoid social isolation. Explain to the client that they are not responsible for the violence and encourage the client to discuss concerns they may have to work through conflicting feelings.

 Client Concern: Lack of control of personal situation and life associated with abusive significant other who manipulates control of all family relationships and finances

Teach the older client about the hazards of myths (e.g., teach that this is not the client's fault and that they have a right to feel safe).

Give the client simple choices to make them feel empowered.

Teach problem-solving and decision-making skills to empower the older client.

References

American College of Obstetricians & Gynecologists. (2012/2019). *Committee opinion: Intimate partner violence.* https://www.acog.org/Clinical-Guidance-and-Publications/Committee-Opinions/Committee-on-Health-Care-for-Underserved-Women/Intimate-Partner-Violence

Australian Law Reform Commission. (2010). *Definition of family violence.* http://www.alrc.gov.au/publications/family-violence-and-commonwealth-laws%E2%80%94social-security-law/definition-family-violence

Castro, A., Ibáñez, J., Maté, B., Esteban, J., & Barrada, J. (2019). Childhood sexual abuse, sexual behavior, and revictimization in adolescence and youth: A mini review. *Frontiers in Psychology.* https://doi.org/10.3389/fpsyg.2019.02018

Centers for Disease Control and Prevention. (2020a). *Elder abuse.* https://www.cdc.gov/violenceprevention/elderabuse/index.html

Centers for Disease Control and Prevention. (2020b). *Preventing child abuse & neglect.* https://www.cdc.gov/violenceprevention/childabuseandneglect/fastfact.html

FindLaw. (2018). *What is the definition of domestic violence?* https://www.findlaw.com/family/domestic-violence/what-is-domestic-violence.html

Hegar, A., Emans, S., & Muram, D. (2000). *Evaluation of the sexually abused child: A medical textbook and photographic atlas.* Oxford University Press.

Maguire-Jack, K., Lanier, P., Johnson-Motoyama, M., Welch, H., & Dineen, M. (2015). Geographic variation in racial disparities in child maltreatment: The influence of county poverty and population density. *Child Abuse and Neglect, 47,* 1–13. https://doi.org/10.1016/j.chiabu.2015.05.020

National Council on Aging. (n.d.). *Elder abuse facts.* https://www.ncoa.org/public-policy-action/elder-justice/elder-abuse-facts/

O'Doherty, L., Hegarty, K., Ramsay, J., Ramsay, J., Davidson, L., Feder, G., & Taft, A. (2015). Screening women for intimate partner violence in healthcare settings. *Cochrane Database Systematic Review, 22*(7), CD007007. https://doi.org/10.1002/14651858.CD007007.pub3

Office of Women's Health. (2019). *Effects of domestic violence on children.* https://www.womenshealth.gov/relationships-and-safety/domestic-violence/effects-domestic-violence-children

The Duluth Model. (2017). *What is the Duluth model?* https://www.theduluthmodel.org/what-is-the-duluth-model/

U.S. Preventive Services Task Force. (2019, July). *Final recommendation statement: Intimate partner violence, elder abuse, and abuse of vulnerable adults: Screening.* https://www.uspreventiveservicestaskforce.org/Page/Document/RecommendationStatementFinal/intimate-partner-violence-and-abuse-of-elderly-and-vulnerable-adults-screening1

9 ASSESSING NUTRITIONAL STATUS

Structure and Function Overview

Nutrition is the "process by which substances in *food* are transformed into body tissues and provide *energy* for the full range of physical and mental activities that make up human life (Carpenter, 2016, p. 1). Adequate nutrition requires that essential nutrients—including carbohydrates, proteins, fats, vitamins, minerals, and water—be ingested in appropriate amounts.

Optimal nutritional status results in more energy to meet activity demands, higher levels of immunity, and faster healing. When nutrition is not optimal, undernutrition (malnutrition) or overnutrition (overweight or obesity) occurs, both of which are associated with many diseases and disorders.

Hydration status also affects health and is assessed with nutrition. Many people do not drink enough fluids, which puts them at risk for chronic mild dehydration. Overhydration is rare in healthy individuals and is only assessed in clients who are at risk for fluid retention, such as those with kidney, liver, and cardiac diseases in which the fluid dynamic mechanisms are impaired.

Nutritional and hydration assessment helps identify the client's overall health status and need for health promotion. It identifies risk factors for obesity, dietary deficits (malnutrition and undernutrition), dehydration, food allergies, food intolerances, and food contamination.

The most beneficial nutritional status requires a balance of nutrient intake to meet daily metabolic demands. Metabolic demands vary based on developmental level, lifestyle, and other energy demands. Optimal nutrition is often thought to be a balance of calories and exercise, but metabolic demands require a variety of nutrients and not just a focus on calories.

Dietary guidelines for Americans include:

1. Follow a healthy eating pattern across the lifespan
2. Focus on variety, nutrient density, and amount
3. Limit calories from added sugars and saturated fats and reduce sodium
4. Shift to healthier foods and beverage choices
5. Support healthy eating patterns for all

(U.S. Department of Health and Human Services [UHHS] and U.S. Department of Agriculture [USDA], 2015, Executive Summary, p. 1). (See the full report of the 2020–2025 *Dietary Guidelines for Americans* at https://www.dietaryguidelines.gov/sites/default/files/2020-12/Dietary_Guidelines_for_Americans_2020-2025.pdf.)

Nursing Assessment

COLLECTING SUBJECTIVE DATA

Describe appetite and daily food intake. Special diet? Number of meals and snacks per day? Do you consider your diet to be healthy? Any food preferences, intolerances, and allergies? Who shops and prepares food in your household? How is food stored? Number of meals eaten out weekly? Describe what you have eaten over the last 24 hours (see Box 9-1). Use of special health foods, vitamins, or other supplements? Explain. Amount and type of daily fluid intake? Usual daily activities? Unintended weight loss or gain in the past 6 months? Use Box 9-2 to assess nutritional health and Box 9-3 to assess feeding in dementia.

COLLECTING OBJECTIVE DATA

Equipment

- Balance beam scale with height attachment or digital scale and height measuring device
- Metric measuring tape
- Marking pencil
- Skinfold calipers

Physical Assessment

Assessment of the client's nutritional status consists of an overall inspection of muscle mass, distribution of fat, and skeleton. It is important to determine whether abnormalities found during assessment of the skin, thyroid, mouth, lungs, abdomen, and nervous system are related to alterations in nutrition.

BOX 9-1 CLIENT'S 24-HOUR DIET RECALL

Patient's name: _____

Date taken: _____

Pregnant: ☐ yes ☐ no   Nursing: ☐ yes ☐ no

Taking nutritional supplements: ☐ yes ☐ no

Amount of money spent on food last month: _____

Check which food record: ☐ entry ☐ exit

Activity level: ☐ <30 minutes ☐ 30–60 minutes ☐ >60 minutes

Meal type:
1 = Morning
2 = Mid-morning
3 = Noon
4 = Afternoon
5 = Evening
6 = Late evening

Serving abbreviations:
Tablespoon — T
Teaspoon — t
Cup — c
Pound — lb
Ounce — oz
Slice — sl

What did the patient eat and drink in the last 24 hours? (be thorough)

Describe in detail foods and beverages consumed. List one food/drink per line.

	Amount eaten	Meal type

Number of lessons taught since last record:

Individual _____   Group _____   Other _____

Insert state EEO here

(Courtesy of Gail Mooney Hanula, PhD)

BOX 9-2 DETERMINE YOUR NUTRITIONAL HEALTH NUTRITIONAL RISK ASSESSMENT

The Nutrition Screening Initiative (NSI), developed by the American Academy of Family Physicians and the American Dietetic Association to promote the integration of nutrition screening and intervention into health care for older adults (Texas Department of Aging and Disability Services, 2010), identified the following warning signs and created a checklist based on these warning signs:

The Warning Signs of Poor Nutrition:
- Disease
- Eating poorly
- Tooth loss/mouth pain
- Economic hardship
- Reduced social contact
- Multiple medicines
- Involuntary weight loss/gain
- Needs assistance in self-care
- Elder years above age 80

The following checklist based on these warning signs may be used to find out if your client is at nutritional risk. Read the following statements. Circle the number in the "yes" column for those that apply to the client. For each "yes" answer, score the number in the box. Total the nutrition score.

	YES
Illness or condition that made client change the kind and/or amount of food eaten	2
Eats fewer than two meals per day	3
Eats few fruits or vegetables, or milk products	2
Has three or more drinks of beer, liquor, or wine almost every day	2
Tooth or mouth problems that make it hard to eat	2
Does not always have enough money to buy the food needed	4
Eats alone most of the time	1
Takes three or more different prescribed or over-the-counter drugs a day	1
Without wanting to, has lost or gained 10 lb in the past 6 months	2
Not physically able to shop, cook, and/or feed self	2

TOTAL
Total the nutritional score.
0–2 Good. Recheck the score in 6 months.

3–5 Moderate nutritional risk. See what can be done to improve eating habits and lifestyle. Recheck score in 3 months.
6 or more High nutritional risk. Consult with physician, dietician, or other qualified health or social service professional.

Note: Remember that warning signs suggest risk but do not represent diagnosis of any condition.
Reprinted from Texas Department of Aging and Disability Services. (2010). *DETERMINE your Nutritional Health: Nutrition Screening Initiative (NSI)*. https://hhs.texas.gov/sites/default/files/documents/doing-business-with-hhs/providers/health/nra.pdf

---

BOX 9-3   EDINBURGH FEEDING EVALUATION IN DEMENTIA QUESTIONNAIRE (EDFED-Q)

Score answers to questions 1–10: never (0), sometimes (1), often (2)

1. Does the patient require close supervision while feeding?
2. Does the patient require physical help with feeding?
3. Is there spillage while feeding?
4. Does the patient tend to leave food on the plate at the end of the meal?
5. Does the patient ever refuse to eat?
6. Does the patient turn their head away while being fed?
7. Does the patient refuse to open their mouth?
8. Does the patient spit out their food?
9. Does the patient leave their mouth open allowing food to drop out?
10. Does the patient refuse to swallow?

Total Score:
(Total scores range from 0 to 20, with 20 being the most serious. Scores can be used to track change)

11. Indicate appropriate level of assistance required by patient: supportive educative, partly compensatory, wholly compensatory

Used with permission from Watson, R., & Deary, I. J. (1997). A longitudinal study of feeding difficulty and nursing intervention in elderly patients with dementia. *Journal of Advanced Nursing, 26*(1), 25–32. https://doi.org/10.1046/j.1365-2648.1997.1997026025.x

General Inspection

ASSESSMENT PROCEDURE	NORMAL FINDINGS	ABNORMAL FINDINGS
Observe body build in addition to muscle mass and fat distribution	A wide variety of body types fall within a normal range—from fat and muscle. In general, the normal body is proportional	
Note tone	Firm, developed	Flaccid, wasted, underdeveloped
Note strength with voluntary movement	Strength equal bilaterally	Weak, sluggish, or unequal
Note body fat for distribution over waist, thighs, and triceps	Equal distribution; some fat under skin	Lack of fat under skin, increased bony prominences, emaciated, cachexic, abundant fatty tissue seen in obesity, abdominal ascites (due to fluid shift in protein)
Posture	Erect, no malformations, smooth and coordinated gait	Poor posture, difficulty walking, bowlegged, knock knees
Energy level	Energetic	Fatigued, irritable
Observe skin for color and texture	Pink, smooth	Pale, rough, dry, flaky, petechiae

ASSESSMENT PROCEDURE	NORMAL FINDINGS	ABNORMAL FINDINGS
Observe skin turgor. Pinch a small fold of skin, observing elasticity, and watch how quickly the skin returns to its original position	There is no tenting; skin returns to original position	Tenting can indicate fluid loss but is also present in malnutrition and loss of collagen in older adults. This finding must be correlated with other hydration findings
Observe for pitting edema (observable swelling of body tissues due to fluid accumulation that occurs when pressure is applied to the swollen area and indentation of the tissues occurs and or persists)	No edema is present	Pitting edema is a sign of fluid retention, especially in cardiac and renal diseases
Observe nails for color and texture	Nails firm; skin under nails pink	Pale, brittle, opaque, spoon shaped, ridged
Observe hair for texture	Lustrous and shiny	Brittle, dry
Observe lips for color and texture	Pink, smooth, moist	Swollen, puffy, lesions, fissures at corners of mouth
Observe tongue's condition and furrows	Tongue is moist, plump with central sulcus, and no additional furrows	Tongue is dry with visible papillae and several longitudinal furrows, suggesting loss of normal third-space fluid and dehydration
Observe teeth for position and condition	Straight with no cavities	Missing, malpositioned, cavities

(Continued on following page)

ASSESSMENT PROCEDURE	NORMAL FINDINGS	ABNORMAL FINDINGS
Observe gums for condition and color	Smooth, firm, pink	Inflamed, spongy, swollen, red, bleed easily
Observe neck veins with client in the supine position, then with the head elevated above 45 degrees	Neck veins are softly visible in supine position. With head elevated above 45 degrees, the neck veins flatten or are slightly visible but soft	Flat veins in supine client may indicate dehydration. Visible firm neck veins indicate distension, possibly resulting from fluid retention and heart disease
Observe eye position and surrounding coloration	Eyes not sunken, no dark circles appear under eyes	Sunken eyes—especially with deep, dark circles—indicate dehydration or malnutrition
Take blood pressure with the client in lying, sitting, and standing positions. Palpate the radial pulse. Count the client's respirations. Take the client's temperature	There are no orthostatic changes; blood pressure and pulse rate remain within normal range for client's activity level and status	Blood pressure registers lower than usual and/or drops >20 mmHg from lying to standing position, thereby indicating fluid volume deficit, especially if the pulse rate is also elevated. Radial pulse rate +1 and thready denotes dehydration. Elevated pulse rate and blood pressure indicate overhydration
Measure pulse	Normal heart rate for age	Tachycardia, hypertension, irregular pulse

Anthropometric Measurements

ASSESSMENT PROCEDURE	NORMAL FINDINGS	ABNORMAL FINDINGS
Measure height using the L-shaped measuring attachment on the balance scale. Instruct the client to stand shoeless on the balance scale platform with heels together and back straight and to look straight ahead. Raise the attachment above the client's head. Then lower it to the top of the client's head *Note: When you do not have access to a measuring attachment on a scale, have the client stand shoeless with their back and heels against the wall. Balance a straight, level object (ruler) atop the client's head—parallel to the floor—and mark the object's position on the wall. Measure the distance between the mark and the floor. If the client cannot stand, measure the arm span to estimate height. Have the client stretch one arm straight out sideways. Measure from the tip of one middle finger to the tip of the nose. Multiply by 2 and record the arm span height*	Compare findings for normal adult height and weight Height is within range for age and ethnic and genetic heritage. Children are usually within the range of parents' heights	Extreme shortness seen with achondroplastic dwarfism and Turner syndrome. Extreme heights are seen with Marfan syndrome, gigantism, and with excessive secretion of growth hormone

(Continued on following page)

ASSESSMENT PROCEDURE	NORMAL FINDINGS	ABNORMAL FINDINGS
Measure weight. Level the balance beam scale at zero before weighing the client. Do this by moving the weights on the scale to zero and adjusting the knob by turning it until the balance beam is level. Ask the client to remove shoes and heavy outer clothing and to stand on the scale. Adjust the weights to the right and left until the balance beam is level again. Record weight (2.2 lb = 1 kg) *Note: If you are weighing a client at home, you may have to use an electronic scale with an automatically adjusting true zero*	Desirable weights for men and women are listed in the body mass index (BMI) table (see Table 9-1)	Weight does not fall within range of desirable weights for women and men. Excessive weight increases one's risks for additional health problems
Determine ideal body weight (IBW) and percentage of IBW. Use this formula to calculate the client's IBW: *Female:* 100 lb for 5 ft + 5 lb for each inch over 5 ft + 10% for small or large frame	Body weight is within 10% of ideal range	A current weight that is 80%–90% of IBW indicates a lean client and possibly mild malnutrition. Weight that is 70%–80% indicates moderate malnutrition; <70% may indicate severe malnutrition possibly from systemic disease, eating disorders,

ASSESSMENT PROCEDURE	NORMAL FINDINGS	ABNORMAL FINDINGS
Male: 106 lb for 5 ft + 6 lb for each inch over 5 ft $\pm$ 10% for small or large frame Calculate the client's percentage of IBW by the following formula: $$\frac{\text{Actual weight}}{\text{IBW}} \times 100 = \%\text{IBW}$$		cancer therapies, and other problems. Weight exceeding 10% of the IBW range is considered overweight; weight exceeding 20% of IBW is considered obesity
Measure BMI Though a number of methods are available to evaluate weight status, the most commonly used screening method is the BMI (Weight-control Information Network, 2012) BMI is calculated based on height and weight, regardless of gender. It is a practical measure for estimating total body fat and is calculated as weight in kilograms divided by the square height in meters	BMI is between 18.5 and 24.9	BMI <18.5 is considered underweight. BMI between 25.0 and 29.9 is considered overweight and increases risk for health problems. A BMI of 30 or greater is considered obese and places the client at a much higher risk for type 2 diabetes, cardiovascular disease, osteoarthritis, and sleep apnea
Determine waist circumference Waist circumference is the most common measurement used to determine the extent of abdominal visceral fat in relation to body fat Waist circumference can be used either alone as a predictor of health risk or in conjunction with waist-to-hip ratio	*Females:* ≤35 in. (88 cm) *Males:* ≤40 in. (102 cm) These findings are associated with reduced disease risk	*Females:* >35 in. (88 cm) *Males:* >40 in. (102 cm) These findings are associated with disorders such as diabetes, hypertension, hyperlipidemia, and cardiovascular disease. See Table 9-2

(Continued on following page)

ASSESSMENT PROCEDURE	NORMAL FINDINGS	ABNORMAL FINDINGS
Measure mid-arm circumference (MAC) MAC evaluates skeletal muscle mass and fat stores Have the client fully extend and dangle the nondominant arm freely next to the body. Locate the arm's midpoint (halfway between the top of the acromion process and the olecranon process). Mark the midpoint and measure the MAC (Fig. 9-1), holding the tape measure firmly around, but not pinching, the arm Record the measurement in centimeters. Refer to Table 9-3 to compare with the standard reference. For example, record both the MAC and the standard reference number. "MAC = 25 cm; 88% of standard. Standard = 28.5" (25/28.5 = 88%)	Compare the client's current MAC to prior measurements and compare to the standard MAC measurements for the client's age and sex listed in Table 9-3. Standard reference is 29.3 cm for men and 28.5 cm for women	Measurements <90% of the standard reference are in the category of moderately malnourished. Less than 60% of the standard reference indicates severe malnourishment. See Table 9-3

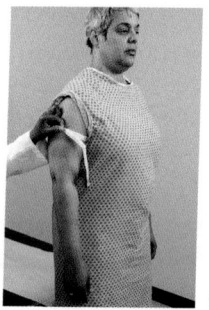

FIGURE 9-1 Measuring mid-arm circumference.

ASSESSMENT PROCEDURE	NORMAL FINDINGS	ABNORMAL FINDINGS
Measure triceps skinfold thickness (TSF). Take the TSF measurement to evaluate the degree of subcutaneous fat stores. Instruct the client to stand and hang the nondominant arm freely. Grasp the skinfold and subcutaneous fat between the thumb and forefinger midway between the acromion process and the tip of the elbow. Pull the skin away from the muscle (ask client to flex arm: if you feel a contraction with this maneuver, you still have the muscle) and apply the calipers (Fig. 9-2). Repeat three times and average the three measurements. Record the measurements in millimeters. Refer to Table 9-4 to compare with the standard reference. For example: Record both the TSF and the standard reference number: "TSF = 15 mm; 91% of standard. Standard = 16.5" (15/16.5 = 91%)	Compare the client's current measurement with past measurements and with the standard TSF measurements for the client's gender listed in Table 9-4. Standard reference is 13.5 mm for men and 16.5 mm for women	Measurements <90% of the standard reference indicate a loss of fat stores and place the client in the moderately malnourished category. See Table 9-4. Less than 60% of the standard reference indicates severe malnourishment. Measurements >130% of the standard indicate obesity

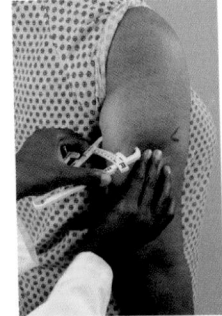

FIGURE 9-2 Measuring triceps skinfold thickness.

(Continued on following page)

ASSESSMENT PROCEDURE	NORMAL FINDINGS	ABNORMAL FINDINGS
Calculate mid-arm muscle circumference (MAMC). (See Table 9-5.) To determine skeletal muscle reserves or the amount of lean body mass and evaluate malnourishment in clients, calculate the MAMC. MAMC is derived from MAC and TSF by the following formula: MAMC (cm) = MAC (cm) − (0.314 × TSF)	Compare the client's current MAMC with past measurements and with the data for MAMCs for the client's age and gender listed in Table 9-5. Standard reference is 25.3 cm for men and 23.2 cm for women	The MAMC decreases to the lower percentiles with malnutrition and in obesity if TSF is high. If the MAMC is in a lower percentile and the TSF is in a higher percentile, the client may benefit from muscle-building exercises that increase muscle mass and decrease fat See Table 9-5 Malnutrition: • Mild—MAMC of 90%–99% • Moderate—MAMC 60%–90% • Severe—MAMC <60% as seen in protein-calorie malnutrition

ASSESSMENT PROCEDURE	NORMAL FINDINGS	ABNORMAL FINDINGS
Assessing Hydration		
Measure intake and output (I&O) in inpatient settings Measure all fluids taken in by oral and parenteral routes, through irrigation tubes, as medications in solution, and through tube feedings Measure all fluid output (urine, stool, drainage from tubes, perspiration). Calculate insensible loss at 800–1,000 mL daily, and add to total output	I&O are closely balanced over 72 hours when insensible loss is included *Note: Fluid is normally retained during acute stress, illness, trauma, and surgery. Expect diuresis to occur in most clients in 48–72 hours*	Imbalances in either direction suggest impaired organ function and fluid overload or inability to compensate for losses, resulting in dehydration
Weigh clients at risk for hydration changes daily	Weight is stable or changes <2–3 lb over 1–5 days	Weight gains or losses of 6–10 lb in 1 week or less indicate a major fluid shift. A change of 2.2 lb (1 kg) is equal to a loss or gain of 1 L of fluid

TABLE 9-1 Body Mass Index (BMI) and Corresponding Body Weight Categories for Children and Adults

Body Weight Category	Children and Adolescents (Ages 2–19 Years) (BMI-for-Age Percentile Range)	Adults (BMI) kg/m^2
Underweight	<5th percentile	<18.5
Normal weight	5th to <85th percentile	18.5–24.9
Overweight	85th to <95th percentile	25.0–29.9
Obese	≥95th percentile	30.0 and greater

Reprinted from U.S. Department of Health and Human Services and U.S. Department of Agriculture. (2015). *2015–2020 dietary guidelines for Americans* (8th ed.). http://health.gov/dietaryguidelines/2015/guidelines/

TABLE 9-2 Disease Risk for Type 2 Diabetes, Hypertension, and Cardiovascular Diseases Relative to Body Mass index (BMI) and Waist Circumference

BMI	Waist Size Women: 88.9 cm (35 in.) Men: 101.6 cm (40 in.)	Waist Size Women: >88.9 cm (35 in.) Men: >101.6 cm (40 in.)
25–29.9	Increased	High
30–34.9	High	Very high
35–39.9	Very high	Very high
40 and above	Extremely high	Extremely high

From National Heart, Lung, and Blood Institute. (n.d.). *Assessing your weight and health risk.* https://www.nhlbi.nih.gov/health/educational/lose_wt/risk.htm

TABLE 9-3 Mid-Arm Circumference (MAC) Standard Reference

Adult MAC (cm)	Standard Reference	60% of Standard Reference—Moderately Malnourished	Severely Malnourished
Men	29.3	26.3	17.6
Women	28.5	25.7	17.1

TABLE 9-4 Triceps Skinfold Thickness (TSF) Standard Reference

Adult TSF (mm)	Standard Reference	90% of Standard Reference—Moderately Malnourished	60% of Standard Reference—Severely Malnourished
Men	12.5	11.3	7.5
Women	16.5	14.9	9.9

TABLE 9-5 Mid-Arm Muscle Circumference (MAMC) Standard Reference

Adult MAMC (cm)	Standard Reference	90% of Standard Reference—Moderately Malnourished	60% of Standard Reference—Severely Malnourished
Men	25.3	22.8	15.2
Women	23.2	20.9	13.9

Dietary Assessment

Assess client's dietary requirements and intake by asking client to keep a 3-day diary of food and fluid intake. You may also use Box 9-2.

ASSESSMENT PROCEDURE	NORMAL FINDINGS	ABNORMAL FINDINGS
Estimate client's daily caloric requirements. See Table 9-6 for estimated daily calorie needs. Compare intake with USDA-recommended food guidelines (Fig. 9-3)	Meets caloric requirements	Consumes more or less than caloric requirements for age, height, body build, and weight. Consumes more or less than recommended

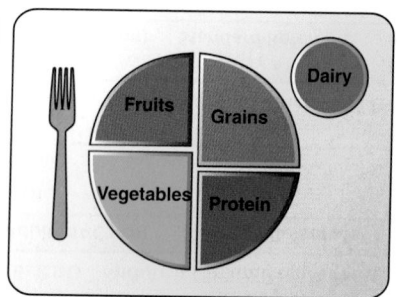

FIGURE 9-3 MyPlate/MyWins. See U.S. Department of Agriculture food guidelines and further explanation of the newest guidelines at https://www.cnpp.usda.gov/dietary-guidelines

TABLE 9-6 Estimated Calorie Needs per Day, by Age, Sex, and Physical Activity Level

	Males				Females[d]		
Age	Sedentary[a]	Moderately Active[b]	Active[c]	Age	Sedentary[a]	Moderately Active[b]	Active[c]
2	1,000	1,000	1,000	2	1,000	1,000	1,000
3	1,000	1,400	1,400	3	1,000	1,200	1,400
4	1,200	1,400	1,600	4	1,200	1,400	1,400
5	1,200	1,400	1,600	5	1,200	1,400	1,600
6	1,400	1,600	1,800	6	1,200	1,400	1,600
7	1,400	1,600	1,800	7	1,200	1,600	1,800
8	1,400	1,600	2,000	8	1,400	1,600	1,800
9	1,600	1,800	2,000	9	1,400	1,600	1,800
10	1,600	1,800	2,200	10	1,400	1,800	2,000
11	1,800	2,000	2,200	11	1,600	1,800	2,000
12	1,800	2,200	2,400	12	1,600	2,000	2,200

(*Continued on following page*)

TABLE 9-6 Estimated Calorie Needs per Day, by Age, Sex, and Physical Activity Level (*continued*)

Males				Females[d]		
Age	Sedentary[a]	Moderately Active[b]	Active[c]	Age	Sedentary[a]	Moderately Active[b]	Active[c]
13	2,000	2,200	2,600	13	1,600	2,000	2,200
14	2,000	2,400	2,800	14	1,800	2,000	2,400
15	2,200	2,600	3,000	15	1,800	2,000	2,400
16	2,400	2,800	3,200	16	1,800	2,000	2,400
17	2,400	2,800	3,200	17	1,800	2,000	2,400
18	2,400	2,800	3,200	18	1,800	2,000	2,400
19–20	2,600	2,800	3,000	19–20	2,000	2,200	2,400
21–25	2,400	2,800	3,000	21–25	2,000	2,200	2,400
26–30	2,400	2,600	3,000	26–30	1,800	2,000	2,400
31–35	2,400	2,600	3,000	31–35	1,800	2,000	2,200
36–40	2,400	2,600	2,800	36–40	1,800	2,000	2,200
41–45	2,200	2,600	2,800	41–45	1,800	2,000	2,200

46–50	2,200	2,400	2,800	46–50	1,800	2,000	2,200
51–55	2,200	2,400	2,800	51–55	1,600	1,800	2,200
56–60	2,200	2,400	2,600	56–60	1,600	1,800	2,200
61–65	2,000	2,400	2,600	61–65	1,600	1,800	2,000
66–70	2,000	2,200	2,600	66–70	1,600	1,800	2,000
71–75	2,000	2,200	2,600	71–75	1,600	1,800	2,000
76 and up	2,000	2,200	2,400	76 and up	1,600	1,800	2,000

[a]Sedentary means a lifestyle that includes only the physical activity of independent living.

[b]Moderately active means a lifestyle that includes physical activity equivalent to walking about 1.5–3 miles/day at 3–4 mph, in addition to the activities of independent living.

[c]Active means a lifestyle that includes physical activity equivalent to walking > 3 miles/day at 3–4 mph, in addition to the activities of independent living.

[d]Estimates for females do not include women who are pregnant or breastfeeding.

From Institute of Medicine. (2002). *Dietary reference intakes for energy, carbohydrate, fiber, fat, fatty acids, cholesterol, protein, and amino acids.* The National Academies Press.

Reprinted from U.S. Department of Health and Human Services and U.S. Department of Agriculture. (2015). *2015–2020 dietary guidelines for Americans* (8th ed.). http://health.gov/dietaryguidelines/2015/guidelines/

🐎 PEDIATRIC VARIATIONS

Physiologic Growth Patterns

- Growth is most rapid during the first year of life.
- Birth weight doubles at age 4 to 6 months and triples by 1 year.
- Length increases 50% the first year of life.
- Teeth erupt at first year of life.
- Growth decreases from ages 1 to 6 years, but biting, chewing, and swallowing abilities increase.
- Muscle mass and bone density increase from ages 1 to 6 years.
- There is a latent uneven period of growth from ages 1 to 12 years.
- Permanent teeth erupt at ages 6 to 12 years.
- School-age children tolerate larger, less frequent meals.
- Nutritional needs increase during growth spurts (ages 10–15 years for girls and ages 12–19 years for boys).

Dietary Requirements

- Allow 1,000 calories plus 100 more per each year of age (e.g., a 5-year-old needs 1,500 calories/day).
- Children need three milks, two meats, four fruits or vegetables, and four grains per day.
- Adolescents need four milks, two meats, four fruits or vegetables, and four grains per day.
- The American Academy of Pediatrics (2012) recommends exclusive breastfeeding for about 6 months, followed by breastfeeding as complementary foods are added into the infant's diet, with continuation of breastfeeding for 1 year or longer as mutually desired by mother and infant. Exclusive breastfeeding is sufficient for optimal growth and development for approximately the first 6 months. Solid foods should not be introduced before age 6 months. When they are introduced, solid foods should be iron enriched.

Physical Assessment

- Infants: Obtain weight, length, and head circumference. Identify type of feeding and iron source.
- Children and adolescents: Weigh child and obtain height. Identify adequacy of meals and snacks and sources of iron, calories, and protein.

GERIATRIC VARIATIONS

- Older clients may have atrophy on dorsum of hands even with good nutrition.
- Assess for poor-fitting dentures and decreased ability to taste.
- Body weight may decrease with aging because of a loss of muscle or lean body tissue.
- Older adults tend to consume less food and eat more irregularly as they age. This tends to increase with social isolation.
- Older adults have decreased peristalsis and nerve sensation, which may lead to constipation. Encourage fluids and dietary bulk to avoid laxative abuse.
- Caloric requirements decrease in response to a decreased basal metabolic rate, decreased activity, and change in body composition. A 10% decrease in calories is recommended for people aged 51 to 75 years and a 20% to 25% decrease in calories for people older than 75 years.
- A decrease in mobility and vision may impair the ability to purchase and prepare food. Sensory taste losses may lead to anorexia.

- Fifty percent of older adults are thought to be economically deprived. This factor may affect their nutrition if meat and milk are omitted from the diet to save money.
- Dietary recall may be difficult for older adults.
- Skinfold measurements are often inaccurate owing to changes in subcutaneous fat.

 CULTURAL VARIATIONS

- Great variations may be seen in nutritional preferences, eating habits, and patterns of various groups.
- Foods, beverages, and medications are classified as hot/cold by many Asians and Hispanics (e.g., yin/yang by Chinese); it is very important to these clients to seek a balanced consumption based on these theories.
- Many people, especially of non–northern European descent, have some degree of lactose intolerance.[1]

---

[1]Clients with lactose intolerance may be able to consume yogurt, buttermilk, fermented cheese, and acidophilus milk, or they may use products such as chewable tablets or liquid drops to act in place of the lactose enzyme.

- Classifications of "food" and "nonfood" items vary in cultures.
- Cultural or religious dietary rules or laws are of great importance to some groups (e.g., Orthodox Jews).
- Some groups may have diseases precipitated by certain foods or medications (e.g., glucose-6-phosphate dehydrogenase [G-6-PD] deficiency, lactose deficiency).
- Some cultural food preferences are contraindicated in specific disease states (e.g., Japanese client with hypertension who consumes high-sodium soy sauce).

Teaching Tips for Selected Client Concerns

Client Concern: Opportunity for learning about ways to improve nutrition and metabolism

- Encourage proper oral hygiene.
- Teach nutritional guidelines.
- Eat a variety of foods.
- Balance the food you eat with physical activity—maintain or improve your weight. All adults should get at least 30 minutes of moderate physical activity most or all days of the week. Regular physical activity is important for a healthy body,
enhancing psychological well-being, and preventing premature death (Healthy People, 2020 [2013]).
- Choose a diet with more dark green and orange vegetables, legumes, fruits, whole grains, and low-fat milk and milk products.
- Choose a diet with less total fats.
- Choose a diet with less added sugar and calories.
- Choose a diet with less salt and sodium.
- If you drink alcoholic beverages, do so in moderation. According to Healthy People, 2020 (2013), alcohol as well as illegal drug use is linked to violence, injury, and HIV infection. Indicators set forth by Healthy People, 2020 (2013) include increasing the proportion of adolescents not using alcohol or any illicit drugs and reducing the proportion of adults using any illicit drug during the past 30 days.
- Teach client how to get the most for their food dollar, how to read food labels, and ways to maintain nutrients in foods.
- Buy frozen vegetables and ripe fresh produce when available.
- Encourage safe food storage and preparation to retain nutritional value and prevent foodborne illnesses.
- Prepare low-fat foods—suggest substituting applesauce or yogurt for butter when baking. Use bouillon or tomato juice instead of oil for sautéing. For added flavor, use herbs and spices to replace some or all of the fat.

- Suggest using the online dietary and physical activity assessment tool *SuperTracker* to help plan, analyze, and track dietary choices and physical activity at www.choosemyplate.gov.

Client Concern: Obesity

Provide client with information on social support groups. Teach client self-assessment and rewarding techniques when proper nutrition is followed. Teach client how to calculate caloric intake and caloric expenditure and how to explore forms of exercise that meet client's needs. Assist client to replace frequent unhealthy snacking with nutritious snacks. Teach dietary guidelines and food choices for Americans recommended by the U.S. Department of Agriculture (2020–2025), Center for Nutrition Policy and Promotion (April, 2012).

 ### *Client Concern: Risk for developing obesity*

Teach parents to avoid overfeeding infants. Encourage proper formula dilution. Teach avoidance of empty caloric foods. Discourage use of food for rewarding behavior. Teach parents that childhood obesity has been shown to increase the risk of developing cardiovascular disease, prediabetes/diabetes, bone and joint disorders, sleep apnea, and social/psychological problems such as decreased self-esteem. Encourage healthy lifestyle practices such as eating and exercising daily to lower the risk of childhood obesity and developing the related chronic diseases.

The Dietary Guidelines for Americans (2020–2025) recommend that children aged 6 to 17 years get at least 60 minutes of physical activity each day. Furthermore, parents should limit inactive forms of play, such as television viewing and computer gaming.

 ### *Client Concern: Inadequate nutritional intake*

- Teach parents to avoid restricting normal intake of fat. Teach that low-fat diets are dangerous to growing infants because fat is essential to metabolism of some vitamins and other substances and to hormone production associated with growth and development. Educate parents regarding the nutritional daily guidelines for girls and boys for each age. The recommended daily intake of calories, protein, fruits, vegetables, grains, and dairy products varies according to age and size.

- Encourage parent and child to discuss with health care provider alternative nutritional guidelines, considering the client's age and any conditions the client has.

References

American Academy of Pediatrics. (2012). *AAP reaffirms breastfeeding guidelines*. https://www.aap.org/en-us/about-the-aap/aap-press-room/pages/AAPReaffirms- Breastfeeding-Guidelines.aspx

Carpenter, K. (2016). *Human nutrition*. http://www.britannica.com/ science/human-nutrition

Healthy People. (2020). *Nutrition and weight status*. https://www.healthypeople.gov/2020/topics-objectives/topic/nutrition-and-weight-status/objectives

Texas Department of Aging and Disability Services. (2010). *DETERMINE your Nutritional Health: Nutrition Screening Initiative (NSI)*. https://hhs.texas.gov/sites/default/files/documents/doing-business-with-hhs/providers/health/nra.pdf

U.S. Department of Agriculture (USDA). *Dietary guidelines for Americans 2020-2025*. https://www.dietaryguidelines.gov/sites/default/files/2020-12/Dietary_Guidelines_for_Americans_2020-2025.pdf

U.S. Department of Health and Human Services and U.S. Department of Agriculture. (2015). *2015–2020 dietary guidelines for Americans* (8th ed.). http://health.gov/dietaryguidelines/2015/guidelines/

Weight-Control Information Network. (2012). https://newsinhealth.nih.gov/2012/05/weight-control-information-network

Nursing Assessment of Physical Systems

10 ⟩ ASSESSING SKIN, HAIR, AND NAILS

Structure and Function Overview

SKIN

The skin is composed of three layers: the epidermis, dermis, and subcutaneous tissue (Fig. 10-1). The skin is a physical barrier that protects the underlying tissues and structures and plays a vital role in temperature maintenance, fluid and electrolyte balance, absorption, excretion, sensation, immunity, vitamin D synthesis, and individual identity related to appearance. The **sebaceous glands** are attached to hair follicles over most of the body, excluding the soles and palms, and secrete an oily substance called *sebum* that waterproofs the hair and skin.

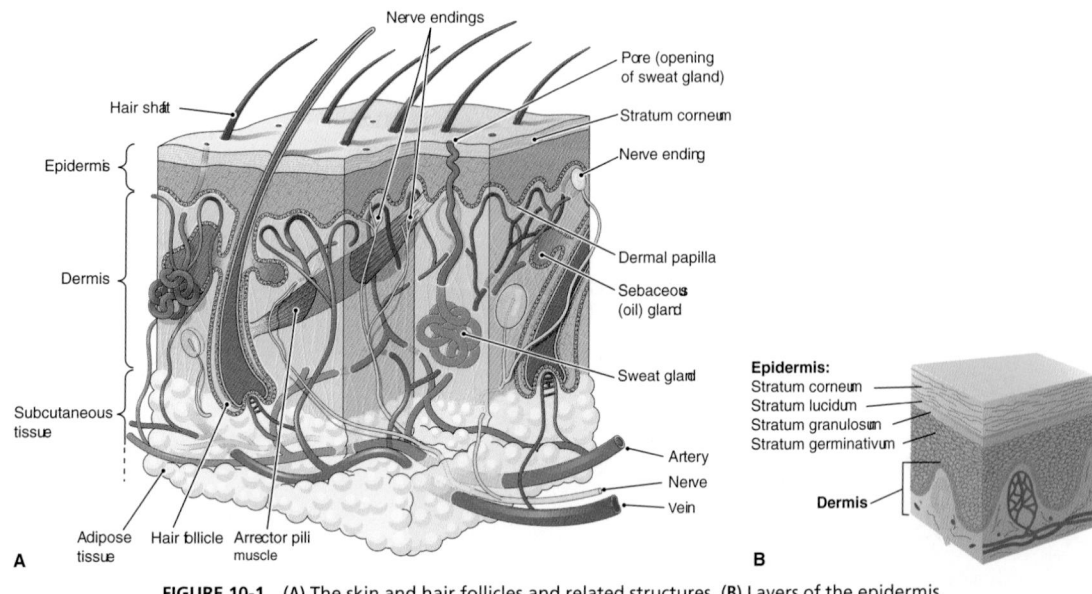

FIGURE 10-1 (A) The skin and hair follicles and related structures. (B) Layers of the epidermis.

There are two types of **sweat glands.** The **eccrine glands,** located over the entire skin, secrete sweat and affect thermoregulation by evaporation of sweat from the skin surface. The **apocrine glands,** associated with hair follicles in the axillae, perineum, and areolae of the breasts, are small and nonfunctional until puberty, when they secrete a milky sweat.

HAIR

Hair consists of layers of keratinized cells found over much of the body, except for the lips, nipples, soles of the feet, palms of the hands, labia minora, and penis. There are two types of hair. **Vellus hair (peach fuzz)** is short, pale, and fine over much of the body and provides thermoregulation by wicking sweat away from the body. **Terminal hair** (particularly scalp and eyebrows) is longer, generally darker, and coarser than vellus hair, and provides insulation and allows for self-expression. Nasal hair, auditory canal hair, eyelashes, and eyebrows filter dust and other airborne debris. Puberty initiates the growth of additional terminal hair in both sexes on the axillae, perineum, and legs. Hair color varies and is determined by the type and amount of pigment (melanin and pheomelanin) production.

NAILS

The nails, located on the distal phalanges of fingers and toes, are hard, transparent plates of keratinized epidermal cells that grow from a root underneath the skinfold called the *cuticle* (Fig. 10-2). The **nail body** extends over the entire nail bed and has a pink tinge as a result of blood vessels underneath. The **lunula** is a crescent-shaped area located at the base of the nail. It is the visible aspect of the nail matrix. The nails protect the distal ends of the fingers and toes, enhance precise movement of the digits, and allow for an extended precision grip.

Nursing Assessment

COLLECTING SUBJECTIVE DATA

Interview Questions

Skin rashes, lesions, itching, dryness, oiliness, bruising, tingling, numbness, stretch marks, skin tags, dark patches, or skin infections (location; onset; precipitating factors: stress, weather, drugs, exposure to allergens)? Methods of relief (e.g., medications, lotions, soaks)? Changes in skin color, lesions, bruising

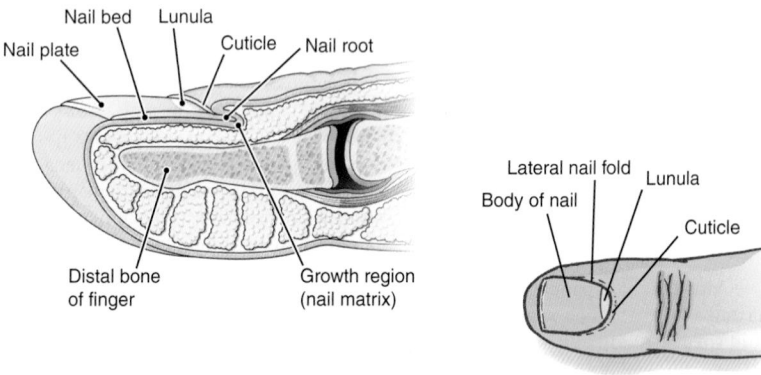

FIGURE 10-2 The nail and related structures.

(onset, type of change)? Scalp lesions, itching, infections? Excessive or insufficient sweating or uncontrolled body odors? History of skin disorders (acne, dermatitis, cancer, ulcers, others)? Viruses (chicken pox, measles)? Sunburns or other burns? Surgical excision of skin lesions? Tattoos (if yes, what type: traumatic, caused by debris embedded in skin, as after a motorcycle accident; amateur, placed by nonprofessionals using India ink with a pin; professional, applied by a professional or skilled tattoo artist; medical, used to delineate a landmark for radiation; or cosmetic, used for permanent eyeliner, lipstick, hair, blush, or

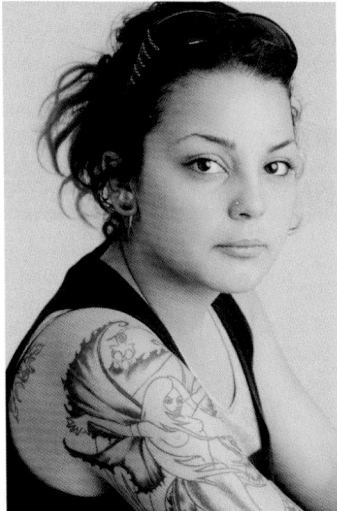

FIGURE 10-3 Tattoos and piercings. (Reprinted with permission from Hatfield, N. T., & Kincheloe, C. [2018]. *Introductory maternity and pediatric nursing* [4th ed., Fig. 27-5]. Wolters-Kluwer.)

eyebrows? (Rarely seen today in humans are tattoos used for identification such as concentration camp numbers.) Body piercings? (See Fig. 10-3.) Describe. Changes in texture, condition, and amount of hair? Changes in condition of nails and cuticles? Nail breaking, splitting? Cuticle inflammation? Artificial nails? Changes in body odor? Skin, hair, and nail care habits; bathing patterns; soaps and lotions used? Shampoo, hair spray, coloring, nail enamels used? Amount of sun/tanning exposure (types of oils and lotions used)? Exposure to chemicals? Knowledge of warning sign for skin cancer (see http://www.skincancer.org/skin-cancer-information/melanoma/melanoma-warning-signs-and-images/do-you-know-your-abcdes#panel1-4) and skin self-inspection?

Risk Factors

Risk for skin cancer related to repeated, intermittent sun exposure with sunburn beginning at early age; use of tanning booths; medical therapies (PUVA and radiation); genetic susceptibility; fair skin and light eyes and hair; immunosuppression; human papillomavirus (HPV); chemical exposure (tar, coal, arsenic, paraffin, some oils); age; actinic keratosis or change in mole; long-term skin irritation.

COLLECTING OBJECTIVE DATA

Equipment Needed

- Adequate lighting (natural daylight is the best) or examination light
- Comfortable room temperature
- Gloves
- Penlight
- Magnifying glass
- Centimeter ruler
- Mirror for client's self-examination of skin
- Wood light
- Examination gown or drape
- Braden Scale to measure pressure sore risks
- Pressure Ulcer Scale for Healing (PUSH) tool to measure pressure injury healing

Physical Assessment

Review Figures 10-1 and 10-2 for a diagram of the skin and related structures and the nails. Expose the body part to be inspected by asking the client to remove clothing, jewelry, nail polish, makeup, wigs, toupees, or hairpieces and to put on a gown. Cleanse skin as needed. Provide privacy, comfortable temperature, and good lighting for skin inspection.

SKIN INSPECTION AND PALPATION

ASSESSMENT PROCEDURE	NORMAL FINDINGS	ABNORMAL FINDINGS
Inspect the skin for the following:		
• Generalized color	• *In white skin:* Light to dark pink • *In dark skin:* Light to dark brown, olive	• *In white skin:* Extreme pallor, flushed, bluish (cyanosis). • *In dark skin:* Loss of red tones in pallor; ashen gray in cyanosis.
Note: *Keep in mind that the amount of pigment in the skin accounts for the intensity of color as well as hue. Table 10-1 describes the six skin types.*	A generalized loss of pigmentation is seen in albinism.	Bluish-colored palms, soles, lips, nails, and earlobes are seen with cyanosis. Cyanosis is seen in vasoconstriction, myocardial infarction, or pulmonary insufficiency. Pallor is seen in arterial insufficiency and anemia.

ASSESSMENT PROCEDURE	NORMAL FINDINGS	ABNORMAL FINDINGS
• Color variations in patches on the body	• *In white skin:* Sun-tanned areas, white patches (vitiligo) • **Pale or light-skinned clients have darker pigment around nipples, lips, and genitalia.** • *In dark skin:* Lighter colored palms, soles, nail beds, and lips; black/blue area over lower lumbar area (Mongolian spot); freckle-like pigmentation of nail beds and sclerae	• *In white skin:* Generalized pale yellow to pumpkin color (jaundice) • *In dark skin:* Yellow color may appear in sclerae, oral mucous membranes, hard and soft palates, palms, and soles. Increased pigmented areas; decreased pigmented areas; reddened, warm areas (erythema); black and blue marks (ecchymosis); tiny red spots (petechiae). Jaundice is often seen in liver or gallbladder disease, hemolysis, or anemia. • Rashes, such as the reddish (in light-skinned people) or darkened (in dark-skinned people) • Erythema (skin redness and warmth) is seen in inflammation, allergic reactions, or trauma. ⊚ **CLINICAL TIP** **Erythema in the dark-skinned client may be difficult to see. However, the affected skin feels swollen and warmer than the surrounding skin.**

(Continued on following page)

ASSESSMENT PROCEDURE	NORMAL FINDINGS	ABNORMAL FINDINGS
Note any odors emanating from the skin.	Slight or no odor of perspiration, depending on activity.	A strong odor of perspiration or foul odor may indicate disorder of sweat glands or infected tissues. Poor hygiene practices may indicate a need for client teaching or assistance with activities of daily living.
Palpate skin for the following:		Rough, thick, dry skin is seen in hypothyroidism.
• Texture	• Smooth, soft	• Extremely cool or warm, wet, oily. Cold skin is seen in shock, hypotension, and arterial insufficiency. Very warm skin is seen in fever and hyperthyroidism.
• Temperature and moisture: Feel with back of hand.	• Warm, dry	• Pinched-up skin takes 30 seconds or longer to return to original position. Turgor is decreased in dehydration.
• Turgor: Pinched-up skin on sternum or under clavicle.	• Pinched-up skin returns immediately to original position.	• Swollen, shallow to deep pitting, ascites. Generalized edema is seen in congestive heart failure or kidney disease. Unilateral, localized edema is seen in peripheral vascular problems such as venous stasis, obstruction, or lymphedema.
• Edema: Press firmly for 5–10 seconds over tibia and ankle.	• No swelling, pitting, or edema	• Skin breakdown: See Assessment Guide 10-1 for staging of any pressure injury detected. See the PUSH tool (Box 10-1) to document the degree of skin breakdown and to measure pressure injury healing over time.

ASSESSMENT PROCEDURE	NORMAL FINDINGS	ABNORMAL FINDINGS
• Skin integrity: Pay special attention to pressure point areas. Use Braden Scale (Box 10-2) to determine the client's risk for skin breakdown.	• Skin intact, no reddened areas	• Primary lesions arise from normal skin owing to disease or irritation (see Abnormal Findings 10-1). Secondary lesions arise from changes in primary lesions (see Abnormal Findings 10-2). Vascular lesions may be seen with increased venous pressure, aging, liver disease, or pregnancy (see Abnormal Findings 10-3). Skin cancer can manifest as either primary or secondary lesions.
• If a skin lesion is detected, inspect and palpate for size, location, mobility, consistency, and pattern (circular, clustered, or straight-lined).	• Silver-pink stretch marks (striae), moles (nevi), freckles, birthmarks. See Box 10-3 for common skin variations	

TABLE 10-1 **Six Skin Types**

Type	Description	Color	Tanning Behavior	von Luschan Scale
I	Very light, "Celtic" type		Often burns, occasionally tans	1–5
II	Light, or light-skinned European		Usually burns, sometimes tans	6–10
III	Light intermediate, or dark-skinned European		Rarely burns, usually tans	11–15
IV	Dark intermediate, also "Mediterranean" or "olive skin"		Rarely burns, often tans	16–21
V	Dark or "brown" type		Naturally brown skin, sometimes darkens	22–28
VI	Very dark, or "black" type		Naturally black-brown skin	29–36

Adapted with permission from Weller, R., Hunter, J., Mann, M. W. (2015). *Clinical dermatology* (5th ed.). Blackwell Publishing.

BOX 10-1 PUSH TOOL TO MEASURE PRESSURE INJURY HEALING

PUSH Tool 3.0

Patient's Name _____   Patient ID#_____

Ulcer Location_____   Date_____

Directions: Observe and measure the pressure injury. Categorize the ulcer with respect to surface area, exudate, and the type of wound tissue. Record a subscore for each of these ulcer characteristics. Add the subscores to obtain the total score. A comparison of total scores measured over time provides an indication of the improvement or deterioration in pressure injury healing.

	0	1	2	3	4	5	Subscore
Length × Width (in cm²)	0	<0.3	0.3–0.6	0.7–1.0	1.1–2.0	2.1–3.0	
		6	7	8	9	10	
		3.1–4.0	4.1–8.0	8.1–12.0	12.1–24.0	≥24.0	
Exudate Amount	0	1	2	3			Subscore
	None	Light	Moderate	Heavy			
Tissue Type	0	1	2	3	4		Subscore
	Closed	Epithelial Tissue	Granulation Tissue	Slough	Necrotic Tissue		
							Total score

Length × Width: Measure the greatest length (head to toe) and the greatest width (side to side) using a centimeter ruler. Multiply these two measurements (length × width) to obtain an estimate of surface area in square centimeters (cm^2). Caveat: Do not guess! Always use a centimeter ruler and always use the same method each time the ulcer is measured.

Exudate Amount: Estimate the amount of exudate (drainage) present after removal of the dressing and before applying any topical agent to the ulcer. Estimate the exudate (drainage) as none, light, moderate, or heavy.

Tissue Type: This refers to the types of tissue that are present in the wound (ulcer) bed. Score as a "4" if there is any necrotic tissue present. Score as a "3" if there is any amount of slough present and necrotic tissue is absent. Score as a "2" if the wound is clean and contains granulation tissue. A superficial wound that is re-epithelializing is scored as a "1." When the wound is closed, score as a "0."

4—Necrotic Tissue (Eschar): Black, brown, or tan tissue that adheres firmly to the wound bed or ulcer edges and may be either firmer or softer than surrounding skin.

3—Slough: Yellow or white tissue that adheres to the ulcer bed in strings or thick clumps, or is mucinous.

2—Granulation Tissue: Pink or beefy red tissue with a shiny, moist, granular appearance.

1—Epithelial Tissue: For superficial ulcers, new pink or shiny tissue (skin) that grows in from the edges or as islands on the ulcer surface.

0—Closed/Resurfaced: The wound is completely covered with epithelium (new skin).

Reprinted with permission from National Pressure Injury Advisory Panel. Available at https://npiap.com/

ASSESSMENT GUIDE 10-1   Identification of Pressure Injury Stage

Pressure Injury: A pressure injury is localized damage to the skin and/or underlying soft tissue, usually over a bony prominence or related to a medical or other device. The injury can present as intact skin or an open ulcer and may be painful. The injury occurs as a result of intense and/or prolonged pressure or pressure in combination with shear. The tolerance of soft tissue for pressure and shear may also be affected by microclimate, nutrition, perfusion, comorbidities, and condition of the soft tissue.

Stage 1 Pressure Injury: Nonblanchable erythema of intact skin. Intact skin with a localized area of nonblanchable erythema, which may appear differently in darkly pigmented skin. Presence of blanchable erythema or changes in sensation, temperature, or firmness may precede visual changes. Color changes do not include purple or maroon discoloration; these may indicate deep tissue pressure injury (DTPI).

Stage 2 Pressure Injury: Partial-thickness skin loss with exposed dermis. Partial-thickness loss of skin with exposed dermis. The wound bed is viable, pink or red, moist, and may also present as an intact or ruptured serum-filled blister. Adipose (fat) is not visible, and deeper tissues are not visible. Granulation tissue, slough, and eschar

are not present. These injuries commonly result from adverse microclimate and shear in the skin over the pelvis and shear in the heel. This stage should not be used to describe moisture-associated skin damage (MASD), including incontinence-associated dermatitis (IAD), intertriginous dermatitis (ITD), medical adhesive-related skin injury (MARSI), or traumatic wounds (skin tears, burns, abrasions).

Stage 3 Pressure Injury: Full-thickness skin loss. Full-thickness loss of skin, in which adipose (fat) is visible in the ulcer, and granulation tissue and epibole (rolled wound edges) are often present. Slough and/or eschar may be visible. The depth of tissue damage varies by anatomical location; areas of significant adiposity can develop deep wounds. Undermining and tunneling may occur. Fascia, muscle, tendon, ligament, cartilage, and/or bone are not exposed. If slough or eschar obscures the extent of tissue loss, this is an unstageable pressure injury.

Stage 4 Pressure Injury: Full-thickness skin and tissue loss. Full-thickness skin and tissue loss with exposed or directly palpable fascia, muscle, tendon, ligament, cartilage, or bone in the ulcer. Slough and/or eschar may be visible. Epibole (rolled edges), undermining, and/or tunneling often occur. Depth varies by anatomical location. If slough or eschar obscures the extent of tissue loss, this is an unstageable pressure injury.

Unstageable Pressure Injury: Obscured full-thickness skin and tissue loss. Full-thickness skin and tissue loss in which the extent of tissue damage within the ulcer cannot be confirmed because it is obscured by slough or eschar. If slough or eschar is removed, a Stage 3 or Stage 4 pressure injury will be revealed. Stable eschar (i.e., dry, adherent, intact without erythema or fluctuance) on the heel or ischemic limb should not be softened or removed.

DTPI: Persistent nonblanchable deep red, maroon, or purple discoloration. Intact or nonintact skin with localized area of persistent nonblanchable deep red, maroon, purple discoloration or epidermal separation reveals a dark wound bed or blood-filled blister. Pain and temperature change often precede skin color changes. Discoloration may appear differently in darkly pigmented skin. This injury results from intense and/or prolonged pressure and shear forces at the bone–muscle interface. The wound may evolve rapidly to reveal the actual extent of tissue injury or may resolve without tissue loss. If necrotic tissue, subcutaneous tissue, granulation tissue, fascia, muscle, or other underlying structures are visible, this indicates a full-thickness pressure injury (Unstageable, Stage 3, or Stage 4). Do not use DTPI to describe vascular, traumatic, neuropathic, or dermatologic conditions.

BOX 10-2 BRADEN SCALE FOR PREDICTING PRESSURE SORE RISK

Patient's Name _____ Evaluator's Name _____ Date of Assessment _____

Sensory Perception	1. Completely Limited	2. Very Limited	3. Slightly Limited	4. No Impairment
Ability to respond meaningfully to pressure-related discomfort.	Unresponsive (does not moan, flinch, or grasp) to painful stimuli, due to diminished level of consciousness or sedation OR Limited ability to feel pain over most of the body.	Responds only to painful stimuli. Cannot communicate discomfort, except by moaning or restlessness OR Has a sensory impairment that limits the ability to feel pain or discomfort over half of the body.	Responds to verbal commands, but cannot always communicate discomfort or the need to be turned OR Has some sensory impairment that limits the ability to feel pain or discomfort in one or two extremities.	Responds to verbal commands. Has no sensory deficit that would limit the ability to feel or voice pain or discomfort.
Moisture	**1. Constantly Moist**	**2. Very Moist**	**3. Occasionally Moist**	**4. Rarely Moist**
Degree to which skin is exposed to moisture.	Skin is kept moist almost constantly by perspiration, urine, etc. Dampness is detected every time the patient is moved or turned.	Skin is often, but not always moist. Linen must be changed at least once a shift.	Skin is occasionally moist, requiring an extra linen change approximately once a day.	Skin is usually dry. Linen only requires changing at routine intervals.

Friction and Shear	1. Problem	2. Potential Problem	3. No Apparent Problem
Ability to lift and move body without rubbing or tearing skin against surface	Requires moderate to maximum assistance in moving. Complete lifting without sliding against sheets is impossible. Frequently slides down in bed or chair, requiring frequent repositioning with maximum assistance. Spasticity, contractures, or agitation leads to almost constant friction.	Moves feebly or requires minimum assistance. During a move, the skin probably slides to some extent against sheets, chair, restraints, or other devices. Maintains relatively good position in chair or bed most of the time but occasionally slides down.	Moves in bed and independently and has sufficient muscle strength to lift up completely during move. Maintains position in bed or chair.

Reprinted with permission from Braden Scale for Predicting Pressure Sore Risk. © Barbara Braden and Nancy Bergstrom

Activity	1. Bedfast	2. Chairfast	3. Walks Occasionally	4. Walks Frequently
Degree of physical activity.	Confined to bed.	Ability to walk severely limited or nonexistent. Cannot bear own weight and/or must be assisted into a chair or a wheelchair.	Walks occasionally during day, but for very short distances, with or without assistance. Spends majority of each shift in bed or chair.	Walks outside the room at least twice a day and inside the room at least once every 2 hours during waking hours.

Mobility	1. Completely Immobile	2. Very Limited	3. Slightly Limited	4. No Limitation
Ability to change and control body position.	Does not make even slight changes in body or extremity position without assistance.	Makes occasional slight changes in body or extremity position but unable to make frequent or significant changes independently.	Makes frequent though slight changes in body or extremity position independently.	Makes major and frequent changes in position without assistance.

(Continued on following page)

BOX 10-3   COMMON VARIATIONS: SKIN VARIATIONS

Many skin assessment findings are considered normal variations in that they are not health- or life-threatening. For example, freckles are common variations in fair-skinned clients, whereas unspotted skin is considered the ideal. Scars and vitiligo, on the other hand, are not exactly normal findings because scars suggest a healed injury or surgical intervention and vitiligo may be related to a dysfunction of the immune system. However, they are common and usually insignificant. Common findings are pictured as follows:

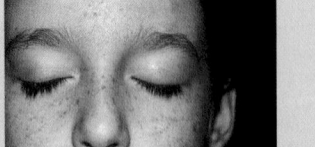

Freckles—Flat, small macules of pigment that appear following sun exposure.

Vitiligo depigmentation of the skin.

Striae (sometimes called *stretch marks*).

meal and generally only about half of any food offered. Protein intake includes only three servings of meat or dairy products per day. Occasionally will take a dietary supplement

OR

Receives less than optimum amount of liquid diet or tube feeding.

dairy products) per day. Occasionally will refuse a meal, but will usually take a supplement when offered

OR

Is on a tube feeding or total parenteral nutrition (TPN) regiment that probably meets most nutritional needs.

and dairy pro casionally eats between meals. Does not require supplementation.

Seborrheic keratosis, a warty or crusty pigmented lesion.

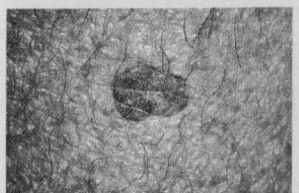

Scar.

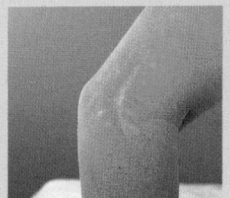

Mole (also called *nevus*), a flat or raised tan/brownish marking up to 6 mm wide.

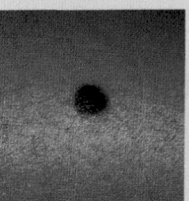

Cutaneous tag, raised papule with a depressed center.

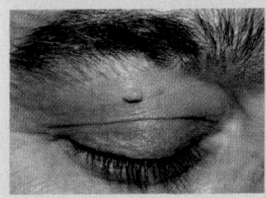

Cutaneous horn.

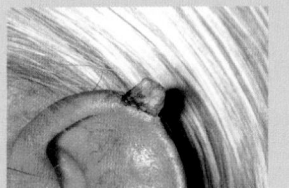

Cherry angiomas, small raised spots (1–5 mm wide) typically seen with aging.

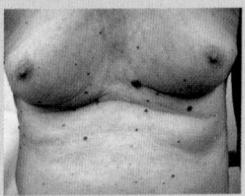

Photo credits: Used with permission from Goodheart, H., & Gonzalez, M. E. (2016). *Goodheart's photoguide to common pediatric and adult skin disorders* (4th ed.). Wolters Kluwer; Striae reprinted with permission from Craft, N., Fox, L. P., Goldsmith, L. A., Papier, A., Birnbaum, R., Mercurio, M. G., Miller, D., Rajendran, P., Rosenblum, M., Taylor, E., & Tumeh, P. C. (2010). *VisualDx: Essential adult dermatology.* Wolters Kluwer.

HAIR INSPECTION AND PALPATION

ASSESSMENT PROCEDURE	NORMAL FINDINGS	ABNORMAL FINDINGS
Inspect and palpate hair for the following: • Color	• Varies	• Patchy gray areas are seen in nutritional deficiencies. Copper-red hair in an African-American child may indicate severe malnutrition.
• Amount and distribution	• Varies	• Sudden loss of hair (alopecia) or increase in facial hair in females (hirsutism). Hirsutism is seen in Cushing syndrome; general hair loss seen in infections, nutritional deficiencies, hormonal disorders, some types of chemotherapy, or radiation therapy; patchy loss seen with scale infection and lupus erythematosus.
• Texture	• Fine to coarse, pliant	• Change in texture, brittle. Dull, dry hair is seen in hypothyroidism and malnutrition.
• Presence of parasites	• None	• Lice (body or head), eggs attached to hair shaft, usually accompanied by severe itching.

SCALP INSPECTION AND PALPATION

ASSESSMENT PROCEDURE	NORMAL FINDINGS	ABNORMAL FINDINGS
Inspect and palpate scalp for the following: • Symmetry	• Symmetrical	• Asymmetrical
• Texture	• Smooth, firm	• Bumpy, scaly, excoriated. Scaly, dry flakes are seen in dermatitis; gray scaly patches seen in fungal infections; dandruff seen with psoriasis.
• Lesions	• None	• Open or closed lesions

NAIL INSPECTION AND PALPATION

ASSESSMENT PROCEDURE	NORMAL FINDINGS	ABNORMAL FINDINGS
Inspect and palpate nails for the following: • Color	• Pink nail bed *In dark skin:* May have small or large pigmented deposits, streaks, freckles	• Pale or cyanotic nails are seen in hypoxia or anemia; yellow discoloration seen in fungal infections or psoriasis; splinter hemorrhages (vertical lines) seen in trauma; Beau lines (horizontal) seen in acute trauma; nail pitting seen in psoriasis (see Abnormal Findings 10-4).

(Continued on following page)

ASSESSMENT PROCEDURE	NORMAL FINDINGS	ABNORMAL FINDINGS
• Shape	Round nail with 160-degree nail base (see Fig. 10-4). 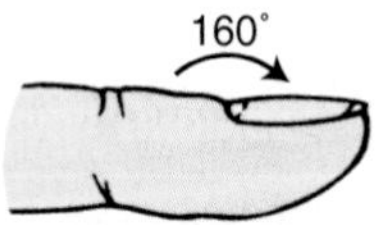 FIGURE 10-4 Normal angle.	• Clubbing: 180-degree or more nail base is seen with hypoxia. Spoon nails occur with iron deficiency anemia.
• Texture • Condition of nail bed	• Nail is round, hard, immobile. *In dark skin:* May be thick • Smooth, firm, and pink	• Thickened nails are seen with decreased circulation. • Paronychia (inflamed nail head) indicates infection (see Abnormal Findings 10-4). Onycholysis (detached nail plate from nail bed) indicates infection or trauma

| ABNORMAL FINDINGS | **10-1** | **Primary Skin Lesions** |

NONPALPABLE LESION
Macule: Flat and colored (e.g., freckle, petechia, ecchymoses)

PALPABLE LESIONS
Papule: Elevated and superficial (e.g., wart)

PALPABLE LESIONS WITH FLUID
Bulla, vesicle: Elevated and filled with fluid (e.g., blister)

Cyst: Encapsulated, filled with fluid or semi-solid mass (e.g., epidermoid cyst)

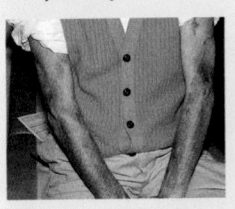 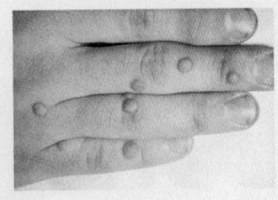 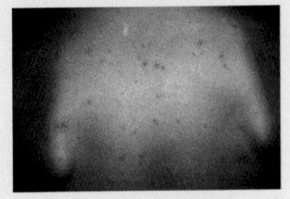 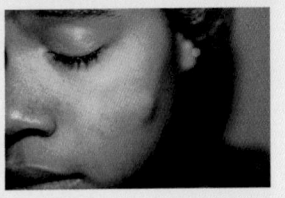

(*Continued on following page*)

ABNORMAL FINDINGS | 10-1 | Primary Skin Lesions (*continued*)

Nodule, tumor: Elevated and firm, has the dimension of depth (e.g., lipoma)

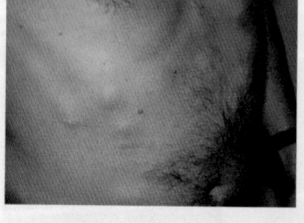

Wheal: Localized edema (e.g., insect bite)

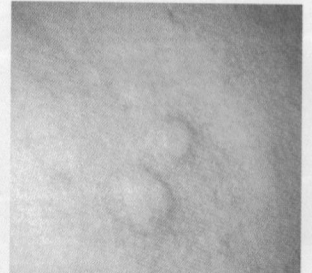

Pustule: Elevated and filled with pus (e.g., acne)

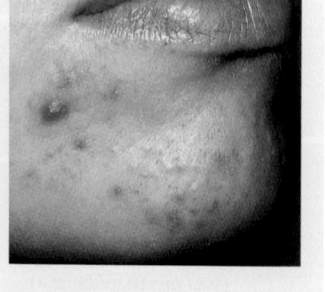

ABNORMAL FINDINGS 10-2 Secondary Skin Lesions (Changes in Primary Skin Lesions)

Ulcer: Skin surface loss, often bleeds

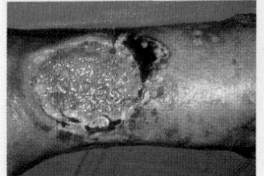

Atrophy: Thin, shiny, taut skin

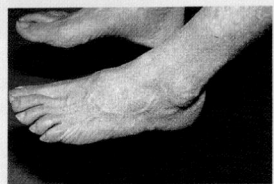

Crust: Dried pus or blood

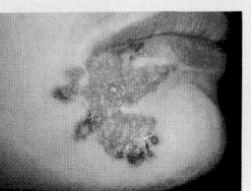

Lichenification: Thickened, roughened skin

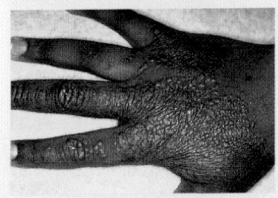

Scale: Thin, flaky skin

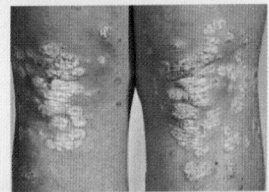

Keloid: Hypertrophied scar

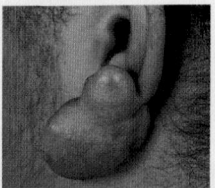

ABNORMAL FINDINGS　10-3　Vascular Lesions

Cherry angioma: Ruby red; flat or raised

Spider vein: Bluish; may have radiating legs; seen mostly on legs

Spider angioma: Bright red with radiating legs; pullulating seen on the center of lesion, or legs, or arms, and upper trunk; blanches when pressure is applied to the center.

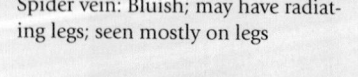

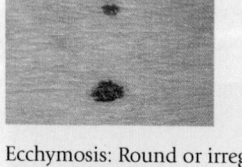

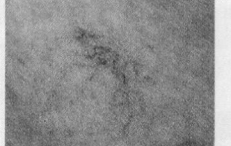

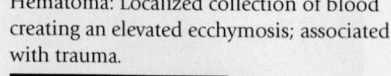

Ecchymosis: Round or irregular macular lesion; larger than petechia; color varies and changes black, yellow, and green.

Petechiae: Round red or purple macules

Hematoma: Localized collection of blood creating an elevated ecchymosis; associated with trauma.

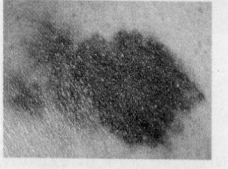

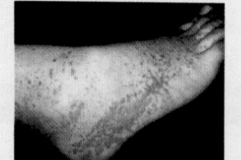

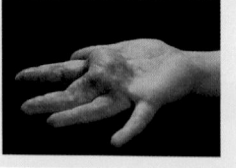

ABNORMAL FINDINGS   **10-4**   **Common Nail Disorders**

Many clients have nails with discoloration, lines, ridges, and spots and uncommon shapes that suggest an underlying disorder. Some examples are as follows:

LONGITUDINAL RIDGING
Parallel ridges running length wise. May be seen in the elderly and some young people with no known etiology.

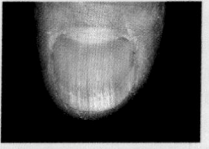

HALF-AND-HALF NAILS
Nails that are half white on the upper proximal half and pink on the distal half. May be seen in chronic renal disease.

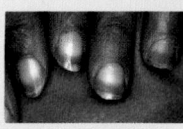

PITTING
Seen with psoriasis.

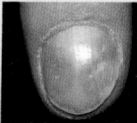

KOILONYCHIA
Spoon-shaped nails that may be seen with trauma to cuticles or nail folds or in iron deficiency anemia, endocrine or cardiac disease.

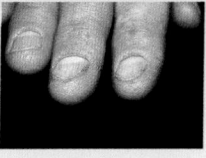

YELLOW NAIL SYNDROME
Yellow nails grow slow and are curved. May be seen in AIDS and respiratory syndromes.

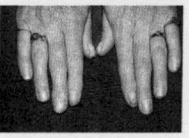

PARONYCHIA
Local infection.

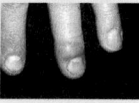

Photo credits: Half-and-half nails used with permission from Hall, B. J., & Hall, J. C. (2010). *Sauer's manual of skin diseases* (10th ed.). Lippincott Williams & Wilkins; All other photographs used with permission from Goodheart, H., & Gonzalez, M. E. (2016). *Goodheart's photoguide to common pediatric and adult skin disorders* (4th ed.). Wolters Kluwer.

ABNORMAL FINDINGS

PEDIATRIC VARIATIONS

Subjective Data: Interview Questions

Skin eruptions or rashes and relationship to any allergies (e.g., food, formula, type of diapers used, diaper creams, soaps, dust)? Bathing routines and soap used? Play injuries (cuts, abrasions, bruises)? Indicators of physical abuse (bruises)? Exposure to communicable diseases? Exposure to pets, stuffed animals? Eczema (onset, precipitating factors, treatment)? Acne (during adolescence; location: face, back, chest; onset; precipitating factors; treatment)? Excessive nail biting? Twirling of hair? History of communicable diseases?

Objective Data: Assessment Techniques

ASSESSMENT PROCEDURE	NORMAL FINDINGS	ABNORMAL FINDINGS
Inspect the following: • Skin color	• Infant's skin is lighter shade than parents'; Mongolian spot is a common hyperpigmentation variation in African Americans, Native Americans, Latin Americans, and Asians. Body piercing may be cultural or a fad. Excessive piercing or tattooing that is "homemade" may increase the risk for hepatitis B or HIV from infected needles.	• Yellow skin is seen in jaundice or with ingestion of too many yellow/orange vegetables in infants/toddlers. Bruising (purple, green, yellow) discoloration in the skin indicates injury to the skin tissue. If markings suggest imprint of hand/fingers, evaluate for physical abuse.
• Oiliness and acne	• Adolescents have increased sebaceous gland activity.	• Cystic acne, acne vulgaris

ASSESSMENT PROCEDURE	NORMAL FINDINGS	ABNORMAL FINDINGS
• Skin lesions	• None	• Crusted or ruptured vesicles are seen in impetigo. Pruritic macular–papular skin eruptions that become vesicular are seen in chicken pox. Pink to red macular–papular rash is seen in measles. Erythemic vesicular rash in linear formation may indicate contact dermatitis (poison ivy). Annular, raised erythemic lesion with central clearing indicates fungal infection
• Hand creases: Assess dermatoglyphics by inspecting flexion creases in palm **FIGURE 10-5** Normal creases.	• Three flexion creases present in palm (Fig. 10-5) **FIGURE 10-6** Simian creases seen in Down syndrome.	• More or fewer than three flexion creases with varied pattern in palm (e.g., one horizontal crease in palm [Simian crease]) (Fig. 10-6)

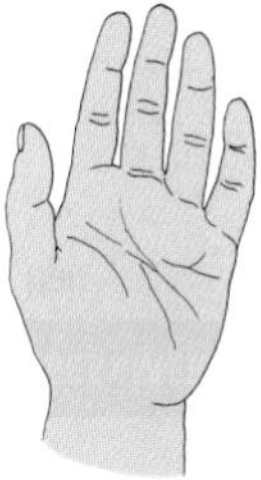

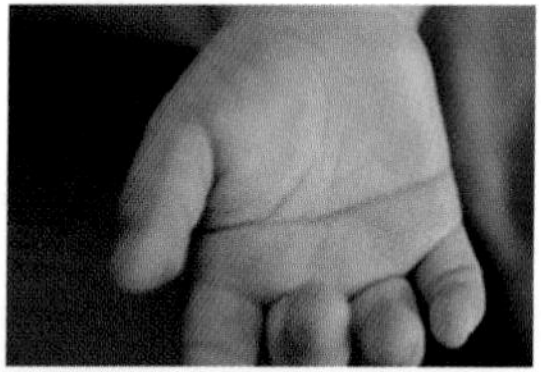

(Continued on following page)

ASSESSMENT PROCEDURE	NORMAL FINDINGS	ABNORMAL FINDINGS
• Hair	• Lustrous, strong, elastic, shiny. Scalp clean and dry. No scaling, flaking.	• Thick or flaky greasy yellow scales on scalp in young children, flakes in hair with yellow greasy scales on scalp, forehead eyebrows, and ears indicate seborrhea (cradle cap). Small white nits in hair shaft (resembles a piece of rice) are eggs of head lice, *Pediculosis capitis.* Adult lice are tiny, brown bugs found in hair shaft.

 GERIATRIC VARIATIONS

Skin

- Thinning epithelium
- Wrinkles, decreased turgor, and elasticity
- Dry, itchy skin due to decrease in activity of eccrine and sebaceous glands
- Seborrheic or senile keratosis (tan to black macular–papular lesions on neck, chest, or back)
- Senile lentigines ("liver spots" or "age spots"—flat brown maculae on hands, arms, neck, and face) (Fig. 10-7)
- Cherry angiomas (small, round, red elevated spots)

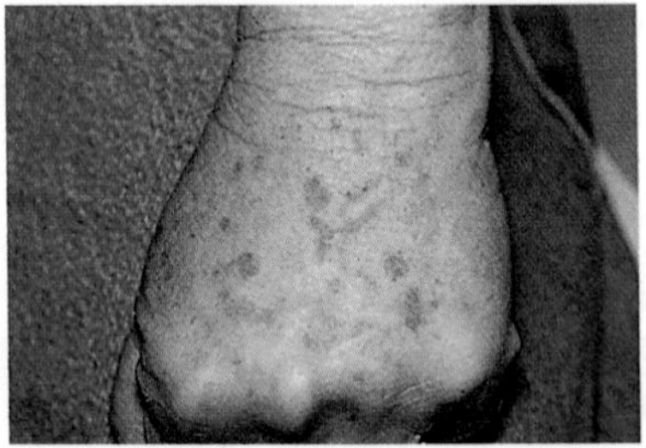

FIGURE 10-7 Senile lentigines are common on aging skin.

- Senile purpura (vivid purple patches)
- Acrochordons (soft, light-pink to brown skin tags)
- Prominent veins due to thinning epithelium

Hair

- Loss of pigment; fine, brittle texture
- Alopecia, especially in men; sparse body hair
- Coarse facial hair, especially in women
- Decreased axillary, pubic, and extremity hair

Nails

- Thickened, yellow, brittle nails
- Ingrown toenails

 CULTURAL VARIATIONS

- Infants and newborns of African American, Native American, or Asian descent often have Mongolian spots, a blue-black or purple macular area on buttocks and sacrum; sometimes this pattern appears on the abdomen, thighs, or upper extremities.
- Dark-skinned clients tend to have lighter colored palms, soles, nail beds, and lips. They may also have freckle-like pigmentation of nail beds and sclera. Nails may also be thick.

- Females of certain cultural groups shave or pluck pubic hair.
- Pallor is assessed in the dark-skinned client by observing the absence of underlying red tones. (Brown skin appears yellow brown; black skin appears ashen gray.)
- Erythema is detected by palpation of increased warmth of skin in dark-skinned clients.
- Cyanosis is detected in dark-skinned clients by observing the lips and tongue, which become ashen gray.
- Inspect for petechiae in the oral mucosa or conjunctiva of the dark-skinned client, because they are difficult to see in dark-pigmented areas; also observe the sclerae, hard palate, palms, and soles for jaundice.
- Social stigma toward some dermatologic disorders is widespread. Dermatologic diseases are found to affect quality of life in many cultures, especially of females (Ribeiro de Paula et al., 2014).
- Systemic lupus erythematosus (SLE) prevalence is higher in Asians, African Americans, Afro Caribbeans, Native Americans, and Hispanics in the United States, especially affecting African-American women, at three to four times the rate of White women (Maningding et al., 2020; Rodriguez, 2018).
- Butterfly rash (also called *Malar rash*) across the bridge of the nose and cheeks (Fig. 10-5) is characteristic of SLE.
- Presence of body piercing may be a fad or a cultural norm.

POSSIBLE COLLABORATIVE PROBLEMS—RISK OF

Skin infections
Skin rashes
Skin lesions
Burns
Graft rejection
Hemorrhage
Allergic reactions (skin)
Insect/animal bite

- Understand the link between sun exposure and skin cancer and the accumulating effects of sun exposure on developing cancers.
- Carry out routine skin self-assessment (Box 10-4) and seek professional advice as soon as possible if anything unusual is detected.

Teaching Tips for Selected Client Concerns

Client Concern: Opportunity to improve health associated with request to learn how to protect skin from sun damager

Teach the client that regular exercise improves circulation and oxygenation of skin.

Encourage protective clothing and boots when walking in wooded areas.

Teach client to:

- Reduce sun exposure.
- Always use sunscreen (solar protection factor [SPF] 15 or higher) when sun exposure is anticipated.
- Wear long-sleeved shirts and wide-brimmed hats.
- Avoid sunburns.
- Avoid intermittent tanning.

Client Concern: Poor care of skin, nail, and hair integrity associated with poor skin, hair, and nails hygiene, and/or excessive piercing/tattooing performed with "homemade" materials, or prolonged use of nail polish or artificial nails

Assess hair, nail, and skin care, and instruct the client on appropriate hygiene measures as necessary (e.g., use mild soap, lotion for dry skin; wash oily areas with warm soap and water three times a day).

Teach dangers of hepatitis B and HIV when using contaminated needles.

Caution the client about potential nail damage caused by nail polish and artificial nails.

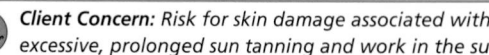 *Client Concern:* Risk for skin damage associated with excessive, prolonged sun tanning and work in the sun

BOX 10-4 SELF-ASSESSMENT: HOW TO EXAMINE YOUR OWN SKIN

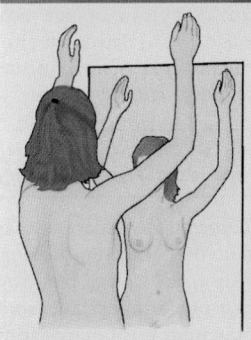 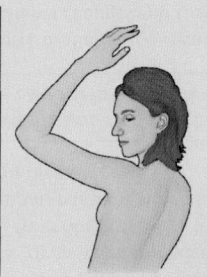 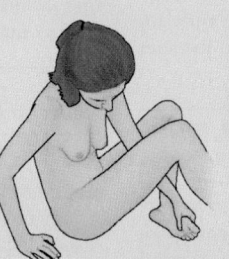 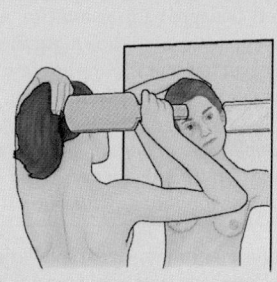 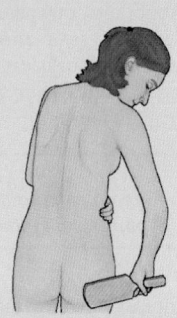

1. Examine the body front and back in the mirror, then the right and left sides, with the arms raised.

2. Bend the elbows, looking carefully at the forearms, back of the upper arms, and palms

3. Next, look at the back of the legs and feet, the spaces between the toes, and the soles of the feet,

4. Examine the back of the neck and the scalp with a handheld mirror. Part the hair to lift.

5. Finally, check the back and buttocks with a hand mirror.

Reprinted with permission from Jensen, S. (2019). *Nursing health assessment: A best practices approach* (3rd ed., Fig. 11.10). Wolters Kluwer Health

Caution the client against prolonged sun exposure or tanning lamp, and instruct that proper use of sunscreen agents can decrease the risk of skin pathologies. Teach the client to report a change in the size or appearance of a mole, nodule, pigmented area, new growth on the skin; to limit or avoid sun exposure between 10 AM and 4 PM, when the sun's ultraviolet rays are strongest; to use a sunscreen with an SPF of at least 15; to wear protective clothing and hats, or as recommended, Slip, Slop, Slap, and Wrap© (American Cancer Society, 2019). Slip on a shirt, slop on sunscreen, slap on a hat, wrap on sunglasses to protect eyes and sensitive skin around them.

Client Concern: *Risk for skin rash associated with lack of parental knowledge of diaper skin care for infant or child*

Inform parents of products available for treatment of rash and importance of frequent diaper changes and cleansing of skin with mild soap (e.g., Ivory or Dove). Teach parents to keep skin cool and dry, avoid restricting clothing, and allow air drying for 15 to 20 minutes several times a day.

 Client Concern: *Poor skin integrity associated with improper care of acne lesions*

Teach adolescents proper skin cleansing, using mild soaps such as Cetaphil soap on face, good hand washing, and avoid picking lesions. Stress the importance of adequate rest, moderate exercise, and a balanced diet. Encourage hydration and avoiding foods, soaps, and creams that irritate skin.

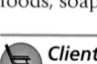 ***Client Concern:*** *Risk for poor skin integrity associated with prolonged immobility, decreased production of natural oils, and thinning skin in older adults*

Teach the client and family the benefits of turning of client, range-of-motion (ROM) exercises, massage, and cleaning of skin for reducing the risk of skin breakdown. Teach the family and client how to observe for reddened pressure areas. Encourage the use of lotions to replace skin oils. Massage skin with lotions. Instruct the client to decrease the frequency of baths and use a humidifier during the cold seasons. Explain the effects of proper nutrition and adequate fluids on skin integrity.

Client Concern: *Risk for foot infection associated with lack of knowledge of how to select proper-fitting shoes to avoid toe pressure and how to care for thickened, dried toenails due to decreased peripheral circulation*

Instruct the client to soak nails 15 minutes in warm water before cutting. Use good scissors and lighting. Explain importance of proper-fitting, breathable, supportive shoes. Refer to podiatrist as necessary. Ascertain whether shoes fit correctly.

References

American Cancer Society (ACS). (2019). *How do I protect myself from ultraviolet (UV) rays?* https://www.cancer.org/healthy/be-safe-in-sun/uv-protection.html

Maningding, E., Dall'Era, M., Trupin, L., Murphy, L., & Yazdany, J. (2020). Racial and ethnic differences in the prevalence and time to onset of manifestations of systemic lupus erythematosus: The California Lupus Surveillance Project. *Arthritis Care Research, 72*(5), 622–629. https://doi.org/10.1002/acr.23887

Ribeiro de Paula, H., Haddad, A., Alves Weiss, M., Moreira Dini, G., & Masako Ferreira, L. (2014). Translation, cultural adaptation, and validation of the American Skindex-29 quality of life index. *Annals of Brazilian Dermatology, 89*(4), 600–607. https://doi.org/10.1590/abd1806-4841.20142453

Rodriguez, T. (2018). *Addressing racial disparities in systemic lupus erythematosus treatment*. https://www.rheumatologyadvisor.com/home/topics/systemic-lupus-erythematosus/addressing-racial-disparities-in-systemic-lupus-erythematosus-treatment/#:~:text=SLE%20develops%20in%20African%20American%20women%2C%20for%20example%2C,individuals%2C%20are%20also%20at%20increased%20risk%20for%20SLE

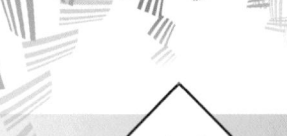

11   ASSESSING HEAD AND NECK

Structure and Function Overview

HEAD

The framework of the head is the skull, which can be divided into two subsections, the cranium and the face (Fig. 11-1). The cranium has eight bones that protect the brain and the major sensory organs: frontal (1), parietal (2), temporal (2), occipital (1), ethmoid (1), and sphenoid (1). In adults, these bones are joined together by immovable sutures: the sagittal, coronal, squamosal, and lambdoid sutures. The face has 14 bones: maxilla (2), zygomatic (cheek) (2), inferior conchae (2), nasal (2), lacrimal (2), palatine (2), vomer (1), and mandible (jaw) (1). The mandible is the only movable facial joint and joins the cranium at the temporal bone forming the temporomandibular joint (TMJ). Other important structures in the head are the temporal artery, the parotid glands, and the submandibular glands.

NECK

The structure of the neck is composed of muscles, ligaments, and the cervical vertebrae. Contained within the neck are the hyoid bone, several major blood vessels, the larynx, the trachea, and the thyroid gland (Fig. 11-2).

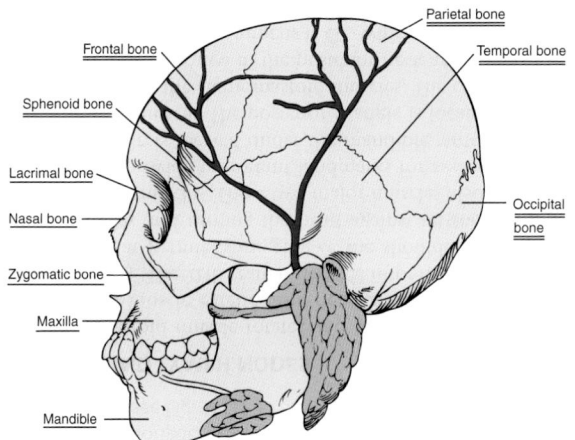

FIGURE 11-1 Bones and sutures of the skull (face and cranium).

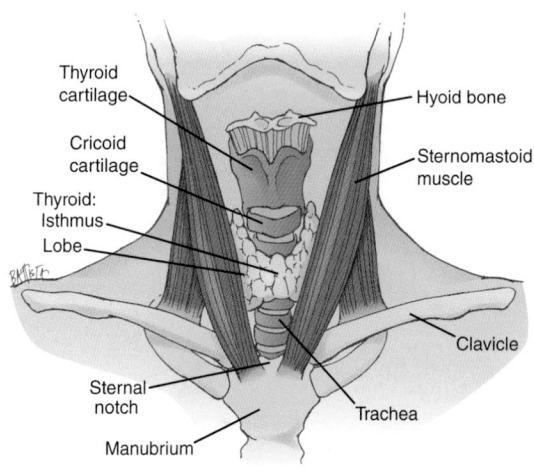

FIGURE 11-2 Structures of the neck.

The thyroid gland is the largest endocrine gland in the body. The first upper tracheal ring, called the *cricoid cartilage*, has a small notch in it. The thyroid cartilage (Adam's apple) is larger and located just above the cricoid cartilage. The hyoid bone, which is attached to the tongue, lies above the thyroid cartilage and under the mandible (see Fig. 11-2).

MUSCLES AND LYMPH NODES

The sternomastoid muscle rotates and flexes the head, whereas the trapezius muscle extends the head and moves the shoulders (Fig. 11-3). The 11th cranial nerve is responsible for muscle movement that permits shrugging of the shoulders by the trapezius muscles and turning the head against resistance by the sternomastoid muscles. These two major muscles also form two triangles that provide important landmarks for assessment. The anterior triangle is located under the mandible, anterior to the sternomastoid muscle. The posterior triangle is located between the trapezius and the sternomastoid muscles. The cervical vertebrae (C1–C7) are located in the posterior neck and support the cranium. The vertebra prominens is C7, which can easily be palpated when the neck is flexed. Using C7 as a landmark will help you locate other vertebrae. In addition, several lymph nodes are located in the head and the neck (see Fig. 11-8).

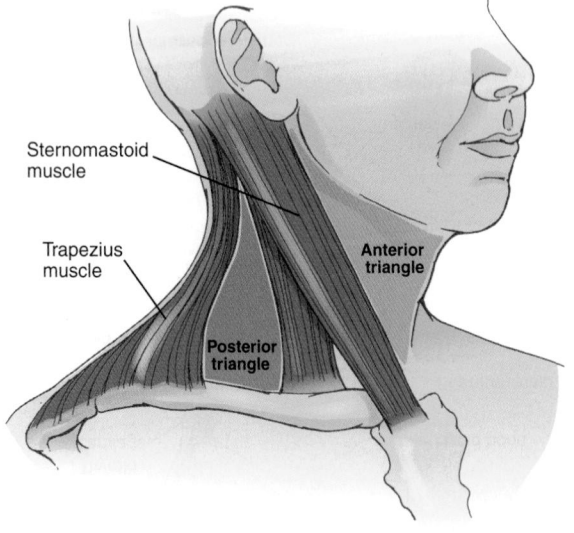

FIGURE 11-3 Neck muscles and landmarks.

Nursing Assessment

COLLECTING SUBJECTIVE DATA

Interview Questions

Lumps (onset, location, size, texture)? Limited movement of neck? Describe. Facial pain/neck pain/headaches (location, onset, duration, precipitating factors, relief)? Do you find that you have headaches when you take certain medications? See Box 11-1 for kinds and characteristics of headaches. Have the client complete the Headache Impact Test at www.bash.org.uk/wp-content/uploads/2012/07/English.pdf and share the results. Muscle tension, vertebral joint dysfunction, limited mobility of head and neck? Prior head or face injuries? Difficulty concentrating, organizing your thoughts, or remembering? Changes in behavior? Experiencing dizziness, lightheadedness, spinning sensation, blurred vision, or loss of consciousness? History of hypothyroidism or hyperthyroidism (see Box 11-2)? Prior neck injuries (date, related to work, recreation, treatment)? Prior radiation therapy to head or neck? Prior thyroid surgery? Family history of head/neck cancer, migraines? Head and neck self-care: posture, use of helmet, seat belts, tobacco products? Use of tobacco, caffeine, or alcohol? Type of work and recreation in relation to impact on posture and possible head and neck injuries? Any protective gear used when riding a horse, bicycle, or other open sports vehicle (e.g., helmet)?

One short tool with instructions for use is the HELPS screening instrument: https://www.nashia.org/resources-list/cdxvc5lcq3q3ycesazm0wfyg9umxye. There are also screening tools specific for mild concussions and military personnel.

Risk Factors

For head injury: age (newborn to 4 years old), high-risk sports, lack of protective devices (e.g., seat belts, helmet), violence, falls (especially after age 65), excessive alcohol ingestion. For thyroid disease: radiation to upper body, family history. For lymphatic enlargement: immunosuppression, chronic disease, malnutrition.

COLLECTING OBJECTIVE DATA

Equipment Needed

- Clean gloves
- Small cup of water for client during thyroid examination
- Stethoscope

BOX 11-1 TYPES AND CHARACTERISTICS OF HEADACHES

Sinus Headache

Character: Deep, constant, throbbing pain; pressure-like pain in one specific area of the face or the head (e.g., behind the eyes); face tender to the touch

Onset and precipitating factors: Occurs with or after a cold or acute sinusitis or acute febrile illness with purulent discharge from nose

Location: May occur in one area of the face or along the eyebrow ridge and below the cheek bone (see figure below)

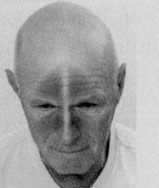

Sinus
headache

Duration: Lasts until associated condition is improved
Severity: May be moderately severe; not debilitating

Pattern: Pain worsens with sudden movements of the head, bending forward, lying down, in the morning (due to mucus collecting and draining all night), or with sudden temperature changes (going from warm room to cold)

Associated factors: Associated with other symptoms of sinusitis, such as nasal drainage and congestion, fever, and foul-smelling breath. Sinus headaches may be confused with tension headaches and migraines. Key points about sinus headaches noted by Hutchinson (2016) are as follows:

- Migraine is commonly misdiagnosed as sinus headache.
- Self-diagnosed sinus headache is nearly always migraine (90% of the time).
- Migraine is commonly associated with forehead and facial pressure over the sinuses, nasal congestion, and runny nose.
- In the absence of fever, pus from your nose, alteration in smell or foul-smelling breath, you likely have a migraine headache.
- Your diagnosis needs health practitioner confirmation for accuracy and best treatment.

Cluster Headache

Character: Stabbing pain; may be accompanied by tearing, eyelid drooping, reddened eye, or runny nose

Onset and precipitating factors: Has a sudden onset; may be precipitated by ingesting alcohol
Location: Localized in the eye and orbit and radiating to the facial and temporal regions

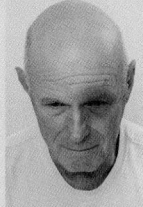

Cluster

Duration: Typically occurs in the late evening or night

Severity: Intense
Pattern: Movement or walking back and forth may relieve the discomfort
Associated factors: Occurs more in young males

Tension Headache

Character: Dull, tight, diffuse

Onset and precipitating factors: No prodromal stage, may occur with stress, anxiety, or depression
Location: Usually located in the frontal, temporal, or occipital region

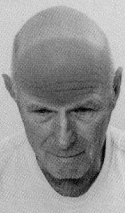

Tension

Duration: Lasts for days, months, or years
Severity: Aching
Pattern: Symptomatic relief may be obtained by local heat, massage, analgesics, antidepressants, and muscle relaxants
Associated factors: Affects women more often than men

Migraine Headache

Character: Accompanied by nausea, vomiting, and sensitivity to noise or light

(Continued on following page)

BOX 11-1 TYPES AND CHARACTERISTICS OF HEADACHES (*continued*)

Onset and precipitating factors: May have prodromal stage (visual disturbances, vertigo, tinnitus, numbness, or tingling of fingers or toes); may be precipitated by emotional disturbances, anxiety, or ingestion of alcohol, cheese, chocolate, or other foods and substances to which the client is sensitive

Location: Located around eyes, temples, cheeks, or forehead; may affect only one side of the face

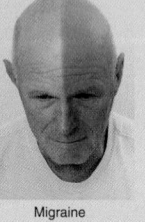
Migraine

Duration: Lasts up to 3 days
Severity: Throbbing, severe
Pattern: Rest may bring relief
Associated factors: Occurs more often in women

Tumor-Related Headache

Character: Aching, steady; neurologic and mental symptoms and nausea and vomiting may develop
Onset and precipitating factors: No prodromal stage; may be aggravated by coughing, sneezing, or sudden movements of the head
Location: Varies with location of tumor
Duration: Commonly occurs in the morning and lasts for several hours
Severity: Variable in intensity
Pattern: Usually subsides later in the day

Source: Hutchinson, S. (2016). *Sinus headaches.* https://www.americanmigrainefoundation.org/living-with-migraines/types-of-headachemigraine/sinus-headaches/; University of Maryland. (2019). *Headaches.* https://www.umms.org/ummc/health-services/neurology/services/headache-migraine; University of Maryland. (2016). *Migraine headache.* http://www.umm.edu/health/medical/altmed/condition/migraine-headache; University of Maryland. (2016). *Sinus headache.* https://americanmigrainefoundation.org/resource-library/sinus-headaches/; University of Maryland. (2016). *Tension headache.* http://www.umm.edu/health/medical/ency/articles/tension-headache

BOX 11-2 SIGNS AND SYMPTOMS OF ALTERED THYROID FUNCTION

Hypothyroidism

Signs and symptoms of hypothyroidism are often nonspecific and include (Skugor, 2014):

- Sleepiness
- Cold intolerance
- Weight gain (especially unintentional)
- Muscle aches
- Fatigue
- Menstrual irregularities
- Pale, dry skin
- Thin, brittle hair or nails
- Bradycardia
- Constipation
- Edema (especially periorbital)
- Difficulty with concentration and memory
- Slowing of relaxation phase of tendon reflexes
- May have higher diastolic blood pressure
- Most serious form of hypothyroidism is myxedema

Hyperthyroidism (Thyrotoxicosis)

Signs and symptoms of hyperthyroidism (Skugor, 2014) include:

Symptoms
  Nervousness
  Fatigue
  Weakness
  Palpitations
  Heat intolerance
  Excessive sweating
  Dyspnea
  Diarrhea
  Insomnia
  Poor concentration
  Oligomenorrhea

Signs
  Weight loss
  Hair loss
  Tachycardia
  Proximal myopathy
  Warm, moist skin
  Hyperkinesis
  Stare, lid lag, lid retraction, and exophthalmos (with Graves disease)
  Emotional liability
  Hyperactive reflexes
  Thyroid enlargement (in most cases)

Physical Assessment

See Figures 11-1 to 11-3 for a review of the anatomy of the head and the neck.

Ask the client to remove any hats, hairpieces, wigs, hair ornaments, pins, rubber bands, jewelry, and head or neck scarves. Ask client to put on a gown if they are wearing clothing that covers the neck. Explain what you are doing through the examination to decrease client anxiety.

SCALP, FACE, AND NECK INSPECTION AND PALPATION

ASSESSMENT PROCEDURE	NORMAL FINDINGS	ABNORMAL FINDINGS
Inspect and palpate the **scalp** for the following:		
• Size	• Varies, especially in accord with ethnicity. Usually, the head is symmetric, round, erect, and in midline, and appropriately related to body size (normocephalic)	• Extremely large or small. Scalp is thick in acromegaly (Box 11-3) (increase in growth hormones); large, acorn shaped in Paget disease
• Shape	• Symmetrical and round. May vary, especially in accord with ethnicity	• Asymmetrical
• Consistency	• Hard and smooth	• Bumpy or soft. Lumps or lesions are seen in cancer and trauma

ASSESSMENT PROCEDURE	NORMAL FINDINGS	ABNORMAL FINDINGS
Observe the **face** for the following: • Symmetry **The nasolabial folds and palpebral fissures are ideal places to check facial features for symmetry.** ◎ **CLINICAL TIP:** **If drooping of one side of the face is noted, assess for other signs of stroke using Box 11-4, Recognizing Symptoms of Stroke.**	• The face is symmetrical, with a round, oval, elongated, or square appearance. No abnormal movements noted.	• Asymmetrical. Face is asymmetrical (drooping, weakness, or paralysis) with parotid gland enlargement or Bell palsy (see Box 11-3), mask-like face in Parkinson disease. Asymmetric orofacial movements may be from organic disease or neurologic problem; refer client for follow-up. Drooping, weakness, or paralysis on one side of the face may occur with stroke (cerebrovascular accident [CVA]). See Box 11-3. "Sunken" face with depressed eyes and hollow cheeks is typical of cachexia (emaciation or wasting). Pale, swollen face may result from nephritic syndrome

(Continued on following page)

SCALP, FACE, AND NECK INSPECTION AND PALPATION (*continued*)		
ASSESSMENT PROCEDURE	**NORMAL FINDINGS**	**ABNORMAL FINDINGS**
• Facial features	• Features vary.	• Distorted features: mask-like face in Parkinson disease; tightened, hard face in scleroderma; sunken, hollow face in cachexia; swollen face in nephrotic syndrome; moon shape with red cheeks, facial hair in Cushing syndrome
Observe the **neck** for the following:		
• Appearance	• Symmetrical neck with head centered. No bulging masses or swollen enlarged lymph nodes	• Asymmetrical head position, masses, or scars present. Swelling is seen in cancer, enlarged thyroid, or inflamed lymph nodes
• Movement	Smooth, controlled movements; range of motion (ROM) from upright position: • Flexion = 45 degrees • Extension = 55 degrees • Lateral abduction = 40 degrees • Rotation = 70 degrees	• Rigid, jerky movements; ROM less than normal values; pain on movement. Limited ROM, stiffness, and rigidity are seen with muscle spasms, inflammation, meningitis, cervical arthritis

ASSESSMENT PROCEDURE	NORMAL FINDINGS	ABNORMAL FINDINGS
		Notify primary care provider and seek emergency care if client has stiff neck along with fever, headache, nausea, vomiting, photophobia, and/or confusion, which are indicative of meningococcal meningitis or meningococcal septicemia (Centers for Disease Control and Prevention [CDC], 2017).
		SAFETY TIP If symptoms of meningococcal illness are present, seek immediate emergency care.
		See Chapter 21 to test for signs of meningeal irritation, Brudzinski sign, and Kernig sign.
Palpate the temporal artery, located between the top of the ear and the eye (Fig. 11-4).	Temporal artery elastic and nontender	Temporal artery is hard, thick, and tender with inflammation as seen with temporal arteritis (inflammation of the temporal arteries that may lead to blindness). This condition requires urgent attention

(Continued on following page)

SCALP, FACE, AND NECK INSPECTION AND PALPATION (*continued*)

ASSESSMENT PROCEDURE	NORMAL FINDINGS	ABNORMAL FINDINGS
Palpate the TMJ by placing your index finger over the front of each ear as you ask the client to open mouth (Fig. 11-5)	No swelling, tenderness, or crepitation with movement. Mouth opens and closes fully (3–6 cm between upper and lower teeth). Lower jaw moves laterally 1–2 cm in each direction	Limited ROM, swelling, tenderness, or crepitation may indicate TMJ syndrome

⊚ **CLINICAL TIP**
When assessing TMJ syndrome, be sure to explore the client's history of headaches, if any.

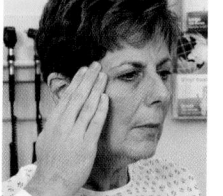

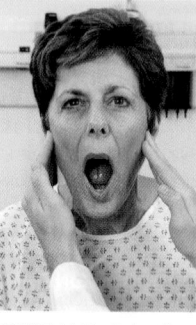

FIGURE 11-4 Palpating the temporal artery.

FIGURE 11-5 Palpating.

BOX 11-3 ABNORMALITIES OF THE HEAD AND NECK

Acromegaly

Acromegaly is characterized by enlargement of the feet, hands (A), and facial features (nose, ears) (B).

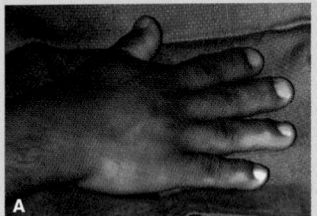

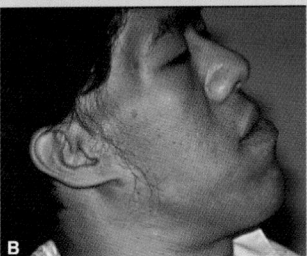

Bell Palsy

Bell palsy usually begins suddenly and reaches a peak within 48 hours. Symptoms may include twitching, weakness, paralysis, drooping eyelid or corner of the mouth, drooling, dry eye, dry mouth, decreased ability to taste, eye tearing, and facial distortion. One-sided facial paralysis is characteristic (National Institute of Neurological Disorders and Stroke [NINDS], 2015).

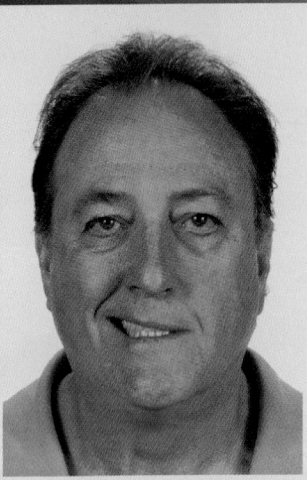

(Continued on following page)

BOX 11-3 ABNORMALITIES OF THE HEAD AND NECK (*continued*)

Hypothyroidism/Myxedema
Myxedema (severe hypothyroidism) is characterized by a dull, puffy face; edema around the eyes; and dry, coarse, and sparse hair.

Hair dry, coarse, sparse

Lateral eyebrows thin

Periorbital edema

Puffy dull face with dry skin

Hyperthyroidism
Exophthalmos is seen in hyperthyroidism.

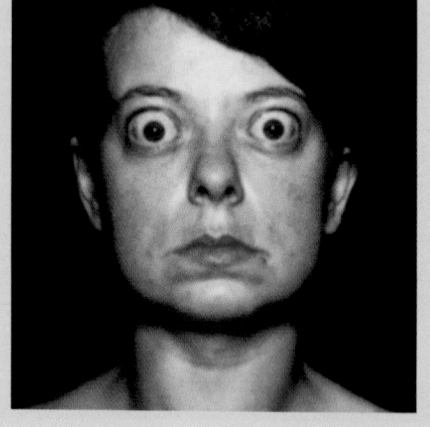

Photo credits: Reprinted with permission from Acromegaly from DeLong, L., & Burkhart, N. (2012). *General and oral pathology for the dental hygienist* (2nd ed.). Wolters Kluwer Heath; Hypothyroidism/myxedema reprinted with permission from Bickley, L. S., & Szilagyi, P. (2003). *Bates' guide to physical examination and history taking* (8th ed.). Lippincott Williams & Wilkins.

BOX 11-4   RECOGNIZING SYMPTOMS OF STROKE

Recognize the signs of stroke and ACT F.A.S.T.:
  Face drooping
  Arm weakness
  Speech difficulties
  Time to call: Time loss is brain loss

Other Symptoms of Stroke Beyond F.A.S.T. (American Stroke Association, 2018)

- Sudden NUMBNESS or weakness of face, arm, or leg, especially on one side of the body
- Sudden CONFUSION, trouble speaking or understanding speech
- Sudden TROUBLE SEEING in one or both eyes
- Sudden TROUBLE WALKING, dizziness, loss of balance or coordination
- Sudden SEVERE HEADACHE with no known cause

Symptoms of Stroke in the Posterior Circulation

- Vertigo, feels like the room is spinning
- Imbalance
- One-sided arm or leg weakness
- Slurred speech or dysarthria
- Double vision or other vision problems
- A headache
- Nausea and/or vomiting

If these symptoms are present, call for emergency care immediately.

Text adapted with permission from American Stroke Association (2018).

(Continued on following page)

BOX 11-4   RECOGNIZING SYMPTOMS OF STROKE (*continued*)

Learn to Recognize the Signs of a Stroke

Act 'F.A.S.T'

Stroke symptoms are unique because they come on suddenly, without warning.
The National Stroke Association suggests using the term "F.A.S.T" to help you recognize common
stroke symptoms.

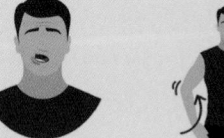 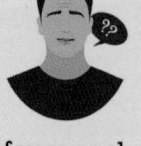 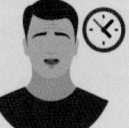

F for face
If you notice a droop or
uneven smile on a person's
face, this is a warning sign.

A for arms
Arm numbness or weakness
can be a warning sign. You
can ask the person to raise
their arms if you are unsure.
It's a warning sign if the arm
drops down or isn't steady.

S for speech
difficulty
Ask the person to repeat
something. Slurred speech
can indicate that the
person is having a stroke.

T for time
Act fast if someone is
experiencing stroke
symptoms.

Call 911 if you feel or see these signs happening to someone.

TRACHEA, THYROID, AND LYMPH NODE PALPATION

Palpate the trachea first, followed by observing and then palpating of the thyroid gland using the guidelines described below. After palpating the thyroid gland, palpate the cervical lymph nodes.

ASSESSMENT PROCEDURE	NORMAL FINDINGS	ABNORMAL FINDINGS
Palpate the **trachea** for position and landmarks (tracheal rings, cricoid, and thyroid cartilage) (see Fig. 11-2 for location)	Midline position; symmetrical; landmarks identifiable	Asymmetrical position deviates from the midline with tumor, enlarged thyroid, aortic aneurysm, pneumothorax, atelectasis, or fibrosis
Observe the movement of the thyroid cartilage. Ask the client to swallow a small sip of water	The thyroid cartilage and the cricoid cartilage move upward symmetrically as the client swallows	Asymmetric movement or generalized enlargement of the thyroid gland is considered abnormal
Palpate the thyroid by standing behind the client and asking them to lower the chin to the chest and turn the neck slightly to the right. This will relax client's neck muscles. Place your thumbs on the nape of the client's neck with your other fingers on either side of the trachea below the cricoid cartilage		

(Continued on following page)

TRACHEA, THYROID, AND LYMPH NODE PALPATION (*continued*)

ASSESSMENT PROCEDURE	NORMAL FINDINGS	ABNORMAL FINDINGS
Use your left fingers to push the trachea to the right. Then use your right fingers to feel deeply in front of the sternomastoid muscle (Fig. 11-6). Repeat on the opposite side. You may offer the client a sip of water to assist with swallowing Note the position, landmarks, and characteristics as you palpate	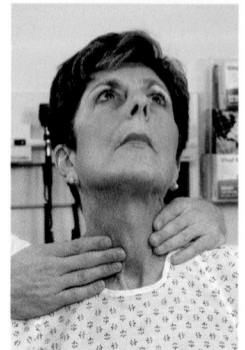 **FIGURE 11-6** Palpating the thyroid.	
• Position	• Usually not palpable. However, isthmus may be palpated in midline. Ability to see or palpate the thyroid varies considerably with client's thyroid size and body build	• Deviates from the midline if obscured by masses or growths

ASSESSMENT PROCEDURE	NORMAL FINDINGS	ABNORMAL FINDINGS
• Characteristics, landmarks	• Glandular thyroid tissue may be felt rising underneath your fingers. Lobes should feel smooth, rubbery, firm, nontender, and free of nodules. The right lobe is often 25% larger than the left lobe	• Enlarged lobes, irregular consistency, tender on palpation. Diffuse enlargement is seen in hyperthyroidism, Graves disease (Box 11-3), or endemic goiter; rapid enlargement of a single nodule suggests malignancy Diffuse enlargement of the thyroid gland
Auscultate the thyroid only if you find an enlarged thyroid gland during inspection or palpation. Place the bell of the stethoscope over the lateral lobes of the thyroid gland (Fig. 11-7). Ask the client to hold their breath (to obscure any tracheal breath sounds while you auscultate)	No bruits are auscultated 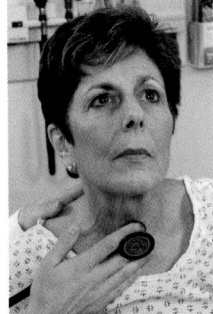	A soft, blowing, swishing sound auscultated over the thyroid lobes is often heard in hyperthyroidism because of an increase in blood flow through the thyroid arteries

FIGURE 11-7 Auscultating for bruits over the thyroid gland.

(Continued on following page)

TRACHEA, THYROID, AND LYMPH NODE PALPATION (*continued*)

ASSESSMENT PROCEDURE	NORMAL FINDINGS	ABNORMAL FINDINGS

Palpate the **cervical lymph nodes** (Fig. 11-8 for location) for the following:

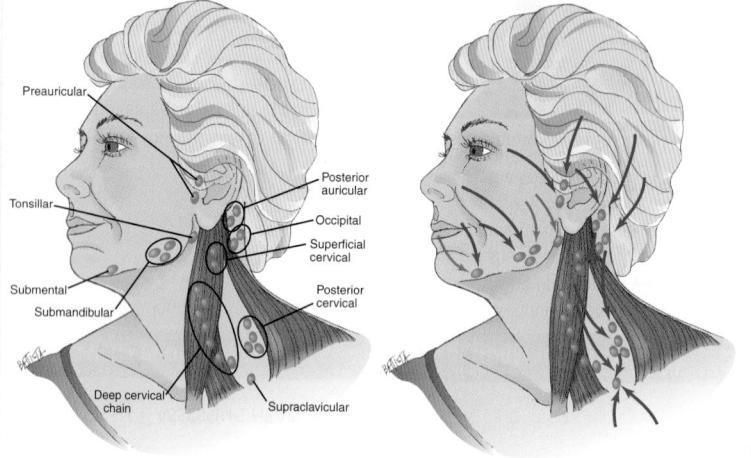

FIGURE 11-8 *Left:* Lymph nodes in the neck. *Right:* Direction of lymph flow. Note: Lymph nodes (represented by green dots) that are covered by hair may be palpated in the scalp under the hair.

ASSESSMENT PROCEDURE	NORMAL FINDINGS	ABNORMAL FINDINGS
• Size and shape	• Cervical lymph nodes are usually not palpable. If palpable, they should be 1 cm or less and round	• Enlarged nodes with irregular borders. Enlarged nodes >1 cm are seen in acute or chronic infection, autoimmune disorders, or metastatic disease; hard, fixed, enlarged, unilateral nodes seen in metastasis; tender, enlarged nodes seen in acute infections; enlarged occipital nodes seen in HIV infection
• Delineation	• Discrete	• Confluent
• Mobility	• Mobile	• Fixed to tissue
• Consistency	• Soft	• Hard, firm
• Tenderness	• Nontender	• Client verbalizes pain on palpation

 CULTURAL VARIATIONS

Hair varies widely genetically. For example, in the United States, African Americans often have tightly curled, short hair to which they apply oil to combat dryness; Whites have a variety of hair shapes, including straight to tightly curled and from nearly white to nearly black in color; and Asian Americans generally have very straight, silky black hair (Andrews et al., 2020). The timing of gray hair varies by cultural group (Andrews et al., 2020). Whites gray faster than other groups, followed by African Americans, and then Asians (who may not develop gray hair until their 80s or 90s).

A few cultural factors can occasionally contribute to head injuries, such as the use of poorly maintained automobiles or bicycles, lack of use of protective gear, inadequate and unsafe housing, and unsafe celebratory practices (such as shooting guns to welcome the new year) (CDC, 2019).

 PEDIATRIC VARIATIONS

ASSESSMENT PROCEDURE	NORMAL FINDINGS	ABNORMAL FINDINGS
Observe **head shape, size, and symmetry**	Normocephalic and symmetrical, features appropriate for size. Head may have odd shape due to molding during birth	Uneven molding, asymmetrical masses, enlarged head. Hydrocephalus is seen with increased cerebrospinal fluid. Microcephaly is a head circumference that is less than normal
Observe **head control**	Holds head erect in midline by 4 months; moves head up and down, side to side	Resistance to movement (head lag after 6 months seen with cerebral injury)
Palpate **skull and fontanelles** very gently when infant is quiet in sitting position	Smooth, fused, except for fontanelles. Immediately following birth, edema crossing suture lines is normal (caput succedaneum). Edema not crossing the suture line indicates cephalohematoma	Ecchymotic areas on scalp; loss of hair in spots; posterior fontanelle (triangular) open after 2 months of age, anterior fontanelle open after 12–18 months of age. Bulging fontanelle is seen in increased intracranial pressure; depressed fontanelles seen in dehydration or malnutrition; delayed fusion of fontanelles seen with hydrocephalus, Down syndrome, hypothyroidism, or rickets; third fontanel seen in Down syndrome; limited ROM seen in torticollis (wryneck)
Palpate the **neck** for lymph nodes	Moderate number of small (>3 mm), shotty, firm lymph nodes in child (age 3–12 years)	Diffuse large lymph nodes, asymmetrical placement. Enlarging supraclavicular lymph nodes are seen with Hodgkin disease

GERIATRIC VARIATIONS

- Lower face may shrink and the mouth may be drawn inward as a result of resorption of mandibular bone.
- Bones of face and nose are more angular in appearance.
- Facial wrinkles are prominent because subcutaneous fat decreases with age.
- Muscle atrophy and loss of fat cause shortening of neck.
- Strength of the pulsation of the temporal artery may be decreased.
- Cervical curvature may increase because of kyphosis of the spine.
- Fat may accumulate around the cervical vertebrae (especially in women) and is referred to as a "Dowager hump."
- Decreased flexion, extension, lateral bending, and rotation of the neck due to arthritis.
- Thyroid may feel more nodular or irregular because of fibrotic changes and may be felt lower in neck because of age-related structural changes.

POSSIBLE COLLABORATIVE PROBLEMS—RISK OF

- Lymphedema
- Hypercalcemia
- Hypocalcemia

Teaching Tips for Selected Client Concerns

Client Concern: *Risk for head and neck injury associated with poor posture*

Teach correct posture and body mechanics for sitting, lifting, and pushing.

Client Concern: *Risk for head or neck injury associated with not wearing protective devices (e.g., head gear during contact sports, seat belts, eye goggles)*

Teach risk reduction tips:

- Use safe driving techniques.
- Wear protective gear such as helmets and seat belts, especially when riding a bicycle or motorcycle.
- Avoid violent or potentially violent environments when possible.
- Modify one's residence to prevent falls.
- Avoid dangerous contact sports likely to cause brain injury; wear protective equipment when engaging in such activity.

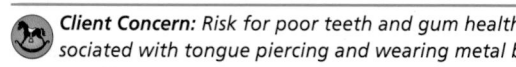 **Client Concern:** *Risk for injury to infant associated with open fontanelles*

Teach parents normal development of fontanelles and how to protect infants from pressure and injury.

Client Concern: *Risk for poor health habits associated with a lack of knowledge on the effects of smokeless tobacco*

Teach that "dipping snuff" increases the risk of cancer (oral, tongue, cheek, gum, esophageal, and pancreatic), leukoplakia, receding gums, bone loss around roots of teeth, tooth loss, stained teeth, and bad breath; is associated with nicotine addiction, heart disease, and hypertension; increases risk of heart attack and stroke and of early delivery and stillbirth in pregnant women (American Cancer Society, 2015). Furthermore, it is *not* a healthy substitute for smoking cigarettes.

Client Concern: *Risk for poor teeth and gum health associated with tongue piercing and wearing metal balls in mouth*

Teach risks of teeth chipping with tongue piercing. Explain that there is high risk of contacting hepatitis B virus and HIV when contaminated needles are used.

References

American Cancer Society (ACS). (2015). *Health risks of smokeless tobacco*. http://www.cancer.org/cancer/cancercauses/tobaccocancer/smokeless-tobacco

American Stroke Association. (2018). *Learn more stroke warning signs and symptoms*. https://www.stroke.org/en/about-stroke/stroke-symptoms/learn-more-stroke-warning-signs-and-symptoms

Andrews, M., Boyle, J., & Collins, J. (2020). *Transcultural concepts in nursing care* (8th ed.). Wolters Kluwer.

Centers for Disease Control & Prevention (CDC). (2017). *Meningococcal disease*. https://www.cdc.gov/meningococcal/about/symptoms.html

Centers for Disease Control and Prevention. (2019). *Traumatic brain injury & concussion: TBI: Get the facts*. https://www.cdc.gov/traumaticbraininjury/get_the_facts.html

Hutchinson, S. (2016). *Sinus headaches*. https://www.americanmigrainefoundation.org/living-with-migraines/types-of-headachemigraine/sinus-headaches/

National Institute of Neurological Disorders & Stroke (NINDS). (2015). *Bell's palsy face sheet*. http://www.ninds.nih.gov/disorders/bells/detail_bells.htm#281243050

Skugor, M. (2014). *Hypothyroidism and hyperthyroidism*. http://www.clevelandclinicmeded.com/medicalpubs/diseasemanagement/endocrinology/hypothyroidism-and-hyperthyroidism/Default.htm

ASSESSING EYES

Structure and Function Overview

EXTERNAL STRUCTURES OF THE EYE

The *eyelids* (upper and lower) are two movable structures composed of skin and two types of muscle—striated and smooth (Fig. 12-1). The palpebral conjunctiva lines the inside of the eyelids, and the bulbar conjunctiva covers most of the anterior eye, merging with the cornea at the limbus.

The *lacrimal apparatus* consists of glands and ducts that serve to lubricate the eye (Fig. 12-2). The *lacrimal gland*, located in the upper outer corner of the orbital cavity just above the eye, is responsible for tear production. Tears are channeled into the *nasolacrimal sac*, through the *nasolacrimal duct*. They drain into the nasal meatus.

The *extraocular muscles* are the six muscles attached to the outer surface of each eyeball (Fig. 12-3), which control six different directions of eye movement. Four rectus muscles are responsible for straight movement, and two oblique muscles are responsible for diagonal movement. Each muscle coordinates with a muscle in the opposite eye. This allows for parallel movement of the eyes and thus the binocular vision characteristic of humans.

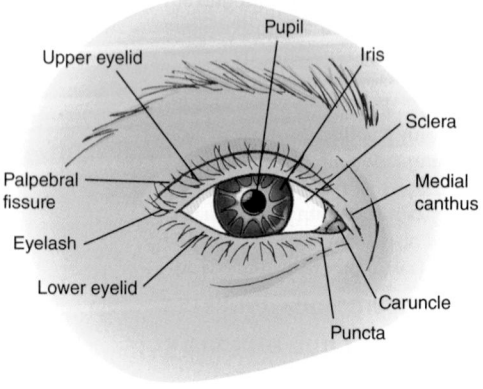

FIGURE 12-1 External structures of the eye.

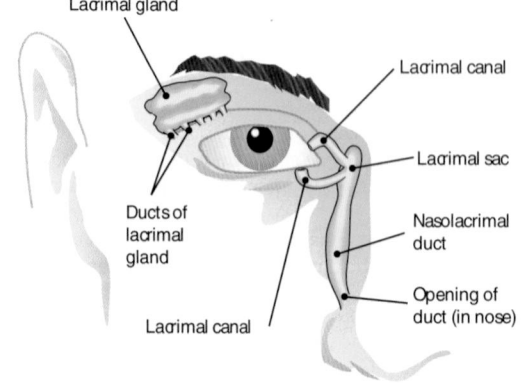

FIGURE 12-2 The lacrimal apparatus consists of tear (lacrimal) glands and ducts.

INTERNAL STRUCTURES OF THE EYE

The eyeball is composed of three separate coats or layers (Fig. 12-4). The outermost layer consists of the *sclera* and *cornea*.

The *iris* is a circular disc of muscle that contains pigments that determine eye color. The central aperture of the iris is called the *pupil*.

The *lens* is a biconvex, transparent, avascular, encapsulated structure located immediately posterior to the iris.

The innermost layer, the *retina*, extends only to the ciliary body anteriorly and consists of numerous layers of nerve cells, including the cells commonly called *rods* and *cones*.

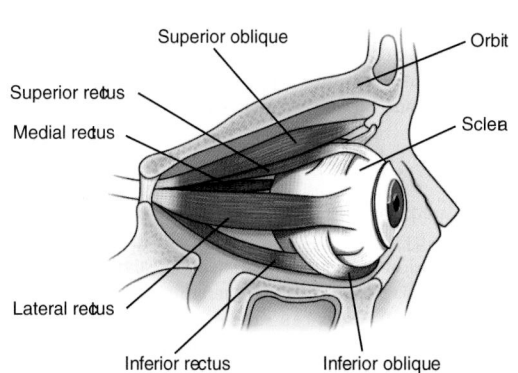

FIGURE 12-3 Extraocular muscles control the direction of eye movement.

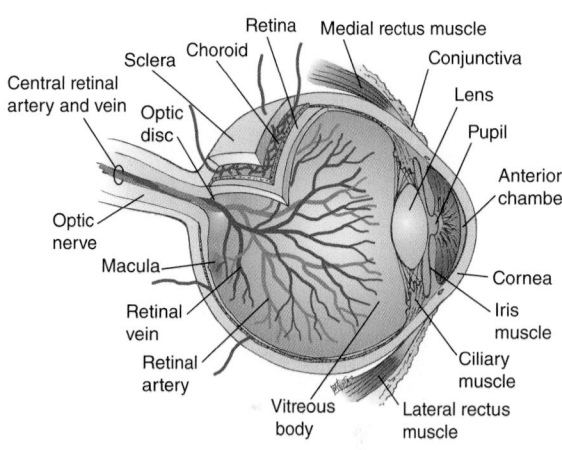

FIGURE 12-4 Anatomy of the eye.

The *optic disc* is a cream-colored circular area located on the retina toward the medial or nasal side of the eye (Fig. 12-5). A small circular area that appears slightly depressed is referred to as the *physiologic cup*.

The *retinal vessels* can be readily viewed with the aid of an ophthalmoscope. Four sets of *arterioles* and *venules* travel through the optic disc, bifurcate, and extend to the periphery of the fundus. Vessels are dark red and grow progressively narrower as they extend out to the peripheral areas. A retinal depression known as the *fovea centralis* is located adjacent to the optic disc in the temporal section of the fundus (see Fig. 12-5). This area is surrounded by the macula, which appears darker than the rest of the fundus.

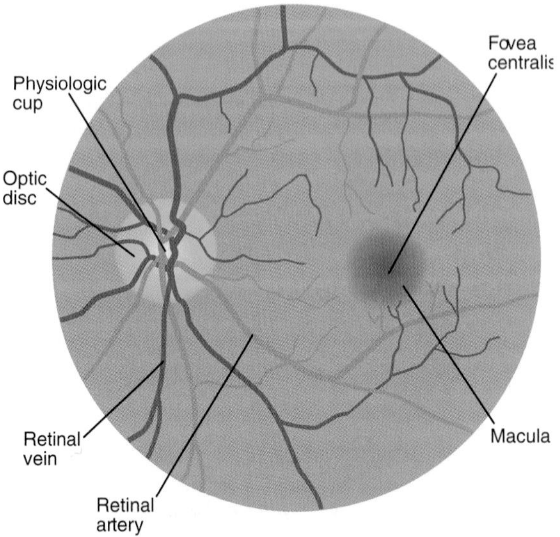

VISION

A **visual field** refers to what a person sees with one eye. The visual field of each eye can be divided into four quadrants: upper temporal, lower temporal, upper nasal, and lower nasal.

Visual perception occurs as light rays strike the retina, where they are transformed into nerve impulses, conducted to the brain through the optic nerve, and interpreted. In the eye, light must

FIGURE 12-5 Normal ocular fundus.

pass through transparent media (cornea, aqueous humor, lens, and vitreous body) before reaching the retina.

Visual Reflexes

The **pupillary light reflex** causes pupils to constrict when exposed to bright light. This can be seen as a *direct reflex*, in which constriction occurs in the eye exposed to the light, or as an *indirect or consensual reflex*, in which exposure to light in one eye results in constriction of the pupil in the opposite eye.

Accommodation is a functional reflex allowing the eyes to focus on near objects. This is accomplished through movement of the ciliary muscles, causing an increase in the curvature of the lens, which is not visible. However, convergence of the eyes and constriction of the pupils can be seen.

Nursing Assessment

COLLECTING SUBJECTIVE DATA

Interview Questions

Recent changes in vision? Spots? Floaters? Blind spots? Halos? Rings? Difficulty with night vision? Double vision? Blurred vision? Strabismus? Macular degeneration? Use of Amsler grid? Eye pain? Redness or swelling? Eye discharge? Excessive watering or tearing? History of prior eye surgery? Trauma? Use of corrective glasses or contact lenses? Date of last eye examination with ophthalmologist? Tested for glaucoma? Eye care habits? (Use of sunglasses? Safety glasses? Work around chemicals, sparks, smokes, fumes, or dust?) Have visual changes affected work or ability to care for self? Typical 24-hour dietary recall? Use of vitamins or supplements (lutein, zeaxanthin, zinc, vitamin C, vitamin E, zinc, and beta-carotene supplements)? Use of medications that may affect vision such as corticosteroids, lovastatin, pyridostigmine, quinidine, risperidone, and rifampin?

Teach clients to have regular eye examinations—if healthy, at 65 years of age, at least every year or 2. If client has diabetes or has other risk factors or takes such medications as corticosteroids, encourage them to talk with their health care provider to determine eye examination schedule; protect eyes if exposed to ionizing radiation sources (x-rays or radiation therapy); avoid smoking or stop smoking; avoid excessive alcohol intake; maintain healthy weight, exercise most days, and develop a plan to lose weight if overweight; eat well-rounded diet with a variety of colorful fruits and vegetables for vitamins, antioxidants, and other nutrients;

ask health care provider about antioxidant supplements that have been shown to prevent cataracts; use eye protective equipment if necessary to prevent eye injuries; and seek medical care for prolonged or unusual eye inflammation or for any eye injury.

Risk Factors

Risk for glaucoma related to diabetes mellitus, myopia, age older than 60 years, hypothyroidism, eye injury or prolonged inflammation, prolonged steroid drop use, ethnic origin (African American, Mexican American, Asian American), or family history of glaucoma. Risk for cataracts related to increasing age, ultraviolet light exposure, excessive sunlight exposure, diabetes mellitus, hypertension, smoking, alcohol use, diet low in antioxidant vitamins, obesity, previous eye surgery, injury, prolonged inflammation, prolonged corticosteroid medication use in any form, exposure to ionizing radiation (e.g., x-rays), and family history. The American Academy of Ophthalmology (AAO, 2020a) suggests that **people who have diabetes mellitus or are at risk for glaucoma** have complete eye examinations according to the schedules found in Table 12-1.

The AAO (2015) recommends clients younger than 40 years who have no risk factors for glaucoma should have a complete eye examination every 5 to 10 years, including tests for glaucoma. The AAO suggests more frequent routine eye examinations with increasing age.

COLLECTING OBJECTIVE DATA

Equipment Needed

- Eye chart (Snellen, E Chart, or handheld Rosenbaum)
- Near-vision chart or newsprint
- Amsler grid
- Cover card or occluder
- Penlight
- Ophthalmoscope (see Assessment Guide 12-1)
- Ruler
- Disposable gloves for eye drainage/exudates to prevent infection spread

TABLE 12-1   Recommended Frequency of Comprehensive Medical Eye Examinations

Age	Frequency
Asymptomatic clients:	
Under 40 years	Every 5–10 years
40–54 years	Every 2–4 years
55–64 years	Every 1–3 years
65 years and older	Every 1–2 years
Clients at risk for glaucoma (such as African Americans and Hispanics): increase frequency (frequency not specified)	
Clients with diabetes mellitus:	
Diabetes mellitus type 1:	
Onset at any age	5 years after onset and yearly thereafter
Diabetes mellitus type 2:	
Diagnosis	Examination at diagnosis and yearly thereafter
Women with diabetes mellitus type 1 or type 2	
Prior to pregnancy conception	First baseline examination
First trimester of pregnancy	Examination early in first trimester and interval thereafter determined by findings

Women who develop gestational diabetes do not seem to be at risk for diabetic retinopathy during pregnancy.
Source: American Academy of Ophthalmology. (2020). *Comprehensive adult medical eye evaluation PPP 2020.* https://www.aao.org/preferred-practice-pattern/comprehensive-adult-medical-eye-evaluation-ppp

ASSESSMENT GUIDE 12-1 Using the Ophthalmoscope

The examiner can rotate the lenses that are labeled with a negative or positive number. Red numbers indicate a negative diopter and are used for myopic (nearsighted) clients. Black numbers indicate a positive diopter and are used for hyperopic (farsighted) clients. The zero lens is used if neither the examiner nor the client has a refractive error.

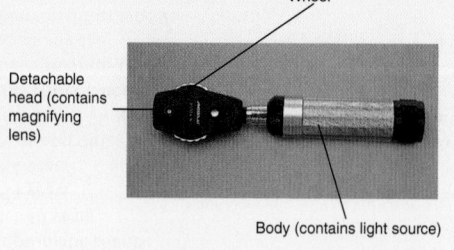

Wheel

Detachable head (contains magnifying lens)

Body (contains light source)

Ophthalmoscope
1. Turn ophthalmoscope on and select the aperture with the large, round beam of white light.
2. Ask the client to remove glasses. Remove your glasses. Contact lenses can be left in the eyes of the client or examiner.
3. Ask the client to fix gaze on an object that is straight ahead and slightly upward.
4. Darken the room to allow pupils to dilate.
5. Hold the ophthalmoscope in your right hand with your index finger on the lens wheel and place the instrument to your right eye (braced between the eyebrow and the nose). Examine the client's right eye. Use your left hand and left eye to examine the client's left eye.
6. Begin about 25.4–38.1 cm (10–15 in.) from the client at a 15-degree angle to the client's side.
7. Keep focused on the red reflex as you move in closer and then rotate the diopter setting to see the optic disc.

Physical Assessment

Review Figures 12-1 to 12-5 for diagrams of the anatomy of the internal and external eye structures. Make sure the client is seated comfortably in a well-lighted room that can be darkened for the ophthalmic examination. First, visual acuity, visual fields for peripheral vision, corneal light perception, eye alignment, extraocular muscle strength, and cranial nerve function are tested. Next, the external eye structures are assessed. Finally, the ophthalmic examination of internal eye structures is performed.

TESTING VISION		
ASSESSMENT PROCEDURE	**NORMAL FINDINGS**	**ABNORMAL FINDINGS**
Check **visual acuity** (have client wear contacts or glasses unless they are reading glasses, which will blur distant vision):		
• Test **distance visual acuity** with Snellen chart 609.6 cm (20 ft) from client (Fig. 12-6). Position client 20 ft from the Snellen or E chart and ask the client to read each line, starting at the top, until they cannot decipher the letters or their direction. Document the results by recording the number of feet the client is from the chart on the top and recording the smallest line of numbers the client can read on the bottom.	• 20/20 OD (oculus dexter) and OS (oculus sinister) with no hesitation, frowning, or squinting.	• Any letters missed on 20/20 line or above; client reads chart by leaning forward, with head tilted or squinting. *Myopia,* impaired far vision, occurs when second number is larger than first number (e.g., 20/40).

(Continued on following page)

TESTING VISION (continued)		
ASSESSMENT PROCEDURE	**NORMAL FINDINGS**	**ABNORMAL FINDINGS**
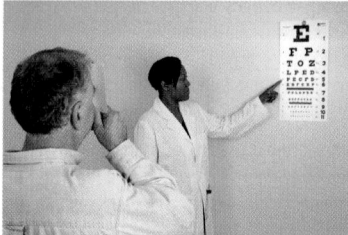 **FIGURE 12-6** Checking distance vision. • Test **near visual acuity** with newspaper ~35.6 cm (14 in.) from client's head.	• Client reads print at 35.6 cm (14 in.) without difficulty.	• Client reads print by holding it closer or farther away than 35.6 cm (14 in.). *Presbyopia,* impaired near vision, is seen when client moves reading material farther away to read owing to decreased accommodation of lenses.

ASSESSMENT PROCEDURE	NORMAL FINDINGS	ABNORMAL FINDINGS
• Test **vision for signs of macular degeneration or retinal changes with Amsler chart** posted at eye level with client wearing their glasses, using bottom portion to view chart if they wear bifocals. Ask client to stand 30.5–35.6 cm (12–14 in.) away from covering one eye. They should look at the center dot. Clients over the age of 45 years or with a family history of retinal problems, such as macular degeneration, should have eyes checked periodically.	• No distortions, graying, blurring, or blank spots seen by client. No changes from prior baseline with Amsler chart as noted previously by primary health care provider.	• Mark areas of distortion, graying, blurring, or blank spots seen by client on their chart and notify the primary care provider. If client has already developed a baseline with distortions that their primary care provider is aware of, then report any changes from their baseline to their primary care provider.
• Check **peripheral vision** (Fig. 12-7): Face client at a distance of 61.0–91.4 cm (2–3 ft); client and examiner look directly ahead and cover eye directly opposite each other. Extend your arm and bring in one to two fingers and ask client if they see one or two fingers. Repeat this in all four visual fields (inferior, superior, nasal, and temporal).	• Client and examiner report seeing object at the same time as it approaches from the periphery. 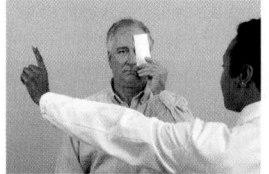	• With reduced peripheral vision, client does not report seeing object at the same time as the examiner.

FIGURE 12-7 Checking peripheral vision.

(Continued on following page)

TESTING EXTRAOCULAR MUSCLE FUNCTION

ASSESSMENT PROCEDURE	NORMAL FINDINGS	ABNORMAL FINDINGS
• Test **corneal light reflex to assess parallel alignment of the eyes.** Ask client to look straight ahead. Then hold a penlight ~12 in. from the client's face. Shine the light toward the bridge of the nose while the client stares straight ahead. Note the light reflected on the corneas.	• Reflections of light noted at same location on both eyes, which indicates parallel alignment.	• Light reflections noted at different areas on both eyes occur with deviation in alignment of eyes due to muscle weakness or paralysis (see Abnormal Findings 12-1) • *Strabismus* is constant malalignment of eyes. • *Tropia* is a specific type of misalignment; *esotropia* is an inward turn of the eye, and *exotropia* is an outward turn of the eye.
• Test for **abnormal eye movement using cover/uncover test** (Fig. 12-8). This test detects deviation in alignment or strength and slight deviations in eye movement by interrupting the fusion reflex that normally keeps the eyes parallel. Ask client to look straight ahead, covering one eye with a cover card, and observe uncovered eye for movement. Now remove the cover card and observe the previously covered eye for any movement. Repeat the test on the opposite eye.	• Uncovered eye does not move when opposite eye is covered. • Covered eye does not move as cover is removed.	• Uncovered eye moves to focus when the opposite eye is covered. Covered eye moves to focus when cover is removed. These findings are seen with eye muscle weakness and deviation in alignment of eyes. • *Phoria* is a term used to describe misalignment that occurs only when fusion reflex is blocked (see Abnormal Findings 12-1).

ASSESSMENT PROCEDURE	NORMAL FINDINGS	ABNORMAL FINDINGS

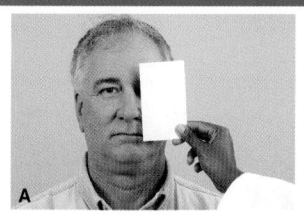 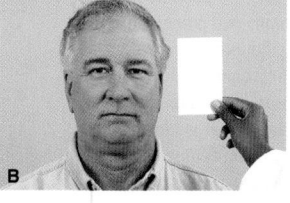

FIGURE 12-8 Performing the cover/uncover test. **A.** Cover one eye with cover card, and observe uncovered eye for movement. **B.** Remove the cover card and observe the previously covered eye for any movement. Repeat on opposite eye.

• Test **extraocular movements by performing the position test** (Fig. 12-9): Ask client to focus on an object that you are holding. Instruct the client to follow its movement through the *six cardinal fields of gaze*. Observe the client's eye movements.

• Both eyes move in a smooth, coordinated manner in all directions.

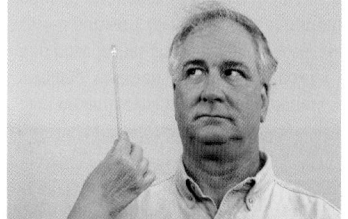

FIGURE 12-9 Checking extraocular movements.

• Nystagmus (oscillating, shaking eye movements) is seen with inner ear disorders, multiple sclerosis, brain lesions, or narcotics use. A couple of beats of nystagmus at extreme lateral gaze is considered normal.
• Failure to follow object with one or both eyes indicates muscle weakness or cranial nerve dysfunction.

(Continued on following page)

INSPECTING EXTERNAL EYE STRUCTURES		
ASSESSMENT PROCEDURE	**NORMAL FINDINGS**	**ABNORMAL FINDINGS**
Inspect **eyelids and lashes** (see Fig. 12-1) for the following: • Position and appearance	• Skin on both eyelids is without redness, swelling, or lesions. Lid margins moist and pink; lashes short, evenly spaced, and curled outward; lower margins at bottom edge of iris; upper lid margin should be between the upper margin of the iris and the upper margin of the pupil. No white sclera is seen above or below the iris. Palpebral fissures may be horizontal • The upper and lower lids close easily and meet completely when closed • The lower eyelid is upright with no inward or outward turning. Eyelashes are evenly distributed and curve outward along the lid margins	Crusting, scales; lashes absent or curled inward; edema or xanthelasma present; itching; ulcerative lesions; asymmetry of lids; weak muscles. See Abnormal Findings 12-1 for illustrations of the following: • *Ectropion:* Lower lids turn outward • *Chalazion:* Inflammation of meibomian glands • *Hordeolum:* Stye or inflammation of glands in lid • *Entropion:* Lower lids turn inward • *Blepharitis:* Waxy, white scales (seborrheic) or inflammation of hair follicles (*Staphylococcus*) • *Ptosis:* Drooping of lids; seen with oculomotor nerve damage, myasthenia gravis. Protrusion of eyeballs with retracted lids seen with hyperthyroidism

ASSESSMENT PROCEDURE	NORMAL FINDINGS	ABNORMAL FINDINGS
• Blinking	• Blinking symmetrical, involuntary, at ~15 blinks/min	• Asymmetrical blink, incomplete closure, rapid blinking
• Inspect **bulbar conjunctiva** and **sclera** for clarity and appearance by asking the client to keep the head still while looking up, down, and to either side. An object may be moved up, down, and to either side to guide the client's eye movements (Fig. 12-10)	• Bulbar conjunctiva is clear, moist, smooth, and transparent, with visible tiny blood vessels. Sclera is smooth and white, with no lesions, foreign bodies, or exudates.	• Lesions, nodules, discharge, crusting, or foreign body present. Marked redness of the conjunctiva is seen with conjunctivitis (see Abnormal Findings 12-2). Sclera with petechiae; marked jaundice

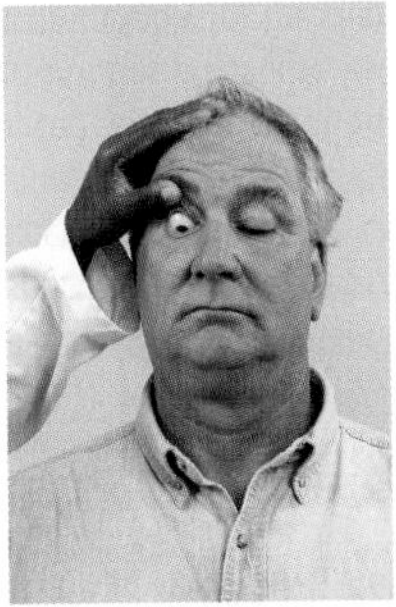

FIGURE 12-10 Inspecting the conjunctiva.

(Continued on following page)

INSPECTING EXTERNAL EYE STRUCTURES (*continued*)

ASSESSMENT PROCEDURE	NORMAL FINDINGS	ABNORMAL FINDINGS
Inspection of the **palpebral conjunctiva** should be performed only if the client voices pain or "something in the eye." It is best that an experienced advanced practitioner or eye specialist perform this procedure, as it may be stressful and uncomfortable for the client		
• Wear gloves to inspect the palpebral conjunctiva of the lower eyelid by placing thumbs bilaterally at the level of the lower bony orbital rim and gently pulling down to expose the palpebral conjunctiva. Avoid putting pressure on the eye. Ask the client to look up as you observe the exposed areas	• The lower and upper palpebral conjunctivae are clear and free of swelling or lesions	• Cyanosis of the lower lid suggests a heart or lung disorder
• Evert the upper eyelid. Ask the client to look down with their eyes slightly open. Gently grasp the client's upper eyelashes and pull the lid downward. Place a cotton-tipped applicator ~1 cm above the eyelid margin and push down with the applicator while still holding the eyelashes	• Palpebral conjunctiva is free of swelling, foreign bodies, or trauma	• A foreign body or lesion may cause irritation, burning, pain, and/or swelling of the upper eyelid

ASSESSMENT PROCEDURE	NORMAL FINDINGS	ABNORMAL FINDINGS
• Hold the eyelashes against the upper ridge of the bony orbit just below the eyebrow, to maintain the everted position of the eyelid. Examine palpebral conjunctiva for swelling, foreign bodies, or trauma. Return the eyelid to normal by moving the lashes forward and asking the client to look up and blink. The eyelid should return to normal		
⊙ **CLINICAL TIP** When palpating, always begin with the eye that is not red or infected to avoid transmission of infection from one eye to the other.		
• Inspect **cornea and lens** (using oblique lighting) for appearance. Cataracts are the leading cause of blindness. More than 24.4 million Americans aged 40 years and older have cataracts, and by age 75, half of Americans develop cataracts (AAO, 2020b).	• Transparent, smooth, moist	• Lesions, opacities, irregular light reflections, or foreign body present. Rough or dry cornea is seen with trauma or allergic responses

(Continued on following page)

INSPECTING EXTERNAL EYE STRUCTURES (*continued*)

ASSESSMENT PROCEDURE	NORMAL FINDINGS	ABNORMAL FINDINGS
Inspect **iris and pupil** for the following: • Shape	• Round and flat	• Irregular. Miosis is constricted, fixed pupils; mydriasis is excessive dilatation of the pupil (see Abnormal Findings 12-3)
• Color (iris)	• Uniform color. Brown is the most common color, but green, hazel, or blue may also be seen. • Pupil, round with regular border, centered in the iris	• Inconsistent color
• Equality	• Equal in size (3–5 mm) • An inequality in pupil size of <0.5 mm occurs in 20% of clients. This condition, called *anisocoria*, is normal	• Unequal; if the difference in pupil size (anisocoria) changes throughout pupillary response tests, the inequality of size is abnormal (see Abnormal Findings 12-3)
Test **pupillary reaction to light** by performing the following tests. Use a pupillary gauge to measure the constricted pupil. Document the pupil's eye at rest as the top (or first) number and the size of the constricted pupil as the bottom (or second) number (i.e., OS [left eye] **3/2;** OD [right eye] **3/1**)	Bilateral constriction of pupils to light.	

ASSESSMENT PROCEDURE	NORMAL FINDINGS	ABNORMAL FINDINGS
Check **direct pupil response** by asking the client to look straight ahead and approaching each eye from the client's side with a penlight (Fig. 12-11). Observe the pupillary reaction	• Illuminated pupil constricts 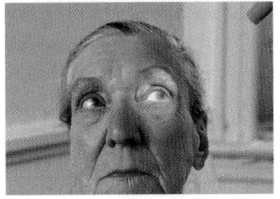 FIGURE 12-11 Observe the pupils with a penlight or similar device, test pupillary reaction to light (Photo by B. Proud).	• Illuminated pupil fails to constrict
Check **consensual pupil response** by asking the client to look straight ahead and approaching each eye from the client's side with a penlight. Observe the pupillary reaction in the opposite eye	• Pupil opposite the one illuminated constricts simultaneously	• Monocular blindness can be detected when light directed to the blind eye results in no response in either pupil. When light is directed into the unaffected eye, both pupils constrict
Check **accommodation** (Fig. 12-12): Ask client to stare at an object 91.4–122 cm (3–4 ft) away, and move object in toward client's nose	• Pupils converge and constrict as object moves in toward the nose; pupil responses are uniform	• Pupils do not converge or constrict. Pupil responses are unequal
Inspect **lens** for clarity.	• Clear	• Cloudy; opacities are seen with cataracts

(Continued on following page)

INSPECTING EXTERNAL EYE STRUCTURES (*continued*)

ASSESSMENT PROCEDURE	NORMAL FINDINGS	ABNORMAL FINDINGS
Inspect and palpate **lacrimal apparatus** (Fig. 12-13) for the following: 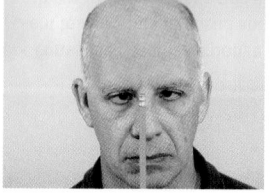 **FIGURE 12-12** Checking accommodation of pupils.	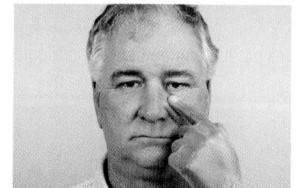 **FIGURE 12-13** Palpating the lacrimal apparatus.	
• Appearance	Puncta (small elevations on the nasal side of the upper and lower lids), mucosa pink	Puncta markedly reddened and edematous with infection, blockage, or inflammation
• Response to pressure applied at nasal side of lower orbital rim	No tenderness or discharge noted when pressure is applied	Fluid or purulent discharge expressed with pain on palpation with duct blockage Excessive tearing may indicate a nasolacrimal sac obstruction

OPHTHALMIC EXAMINATION OF INTERNAL EYE STRUCTURES		
ASSESSMENT PROCEDURE	**NORMAL FINDINGS**	**ABNORMAL FINDINGS**
Use the ophthalmoscope to view internal eye structures (see Assessment Guide 12-1: Guidelines for Using Ophthalmoscope). **Hold the ophthalmoscope in your right hand, to your right eye, to inspect the client's right eye. Hold the ophthalmoscope in your left hand, to your left eye, to inspect the client's left eye.**		
• Inspect **red reflex** for shape and color (Fig. 12-14) 	• Red reflex is round, bright, with red-orange glow	• Red reflex has decreased color or abnormal shape; dark spots are seen with cataracts • Nuclear cataracts appear gray when seen with a flashlight; they appear as a black spot against the red reflex when seen through an ophthalmoscope

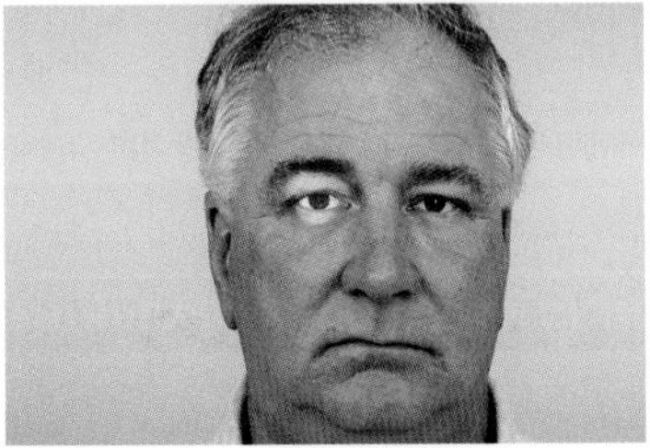

FIGURE 12-14 Inspecting the red reflex.

(Continued on following page)

OPHTHALMIC EXAMINATION OF INTERNAL EYE STRUCTURES

ASSESSMENT PROCEDURE	NORMAL FINDINGS	ABNORMAL FINDINGS
Inspect **optic disc** (see Fig. 12-15) for the following: • Shape **FIGURE 12-15** Normal ocular fundus (also called the *optic disc*).	• Round or slightly oval disc with sharply defined margins (Fig. 12-15)	• Irregularly shaped disc, blurred margins. A swollen disc with blurred margins is papilledema and is seen with hypertension or increased intracranial pressure (see Abnormal Findings 12-4). Optic atrophy is a white-colored disc without vessels and is seen with the death of optic nerves
• Color • Size	• Creamy pink (lighter than retina) • Approximately 1.5 mm size, symmetrical in both eyes	• Pallor of entire disc or one section • Size of disc not equal in both eyes

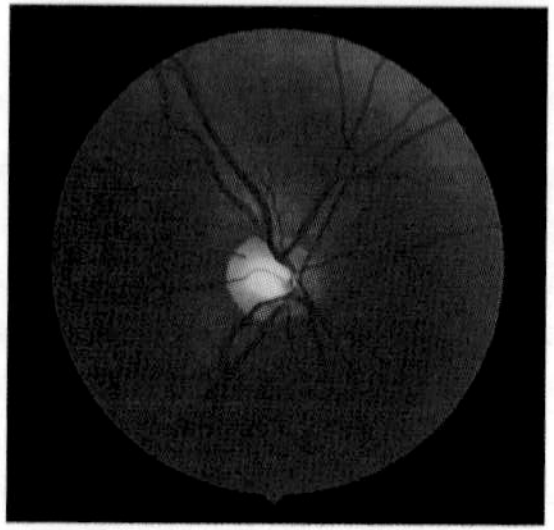

ASSESSMENT PROCEDURE	NORMAL FINDINGS	ABNORMAL FINDINGS
• Physiologic cup *Note: The diameter of the optic disc (DD) is used as the standard of measure for the location and size of other structures seen in the ocular fundus. Document the position of the structure as it relates to clock number (i.e., lesion at 2:00, 1 DD in size, 2 DD from optic disc)*	• Small area is noted as paler than disc located just temporal of center of disc; occupies $^4/_{10}$–$^5/_{10}$ of the diameter of the disc	• Cup location and size are not symmetrical in both eyes; cup occupies $>^5/_{10}$ diameter of the disc • Enlarged physiologic cup seen in glaucoma (see Abnormal Findings 12-4)
• Inspect **the retinal vessels.** Remain in the same position as described previously. Inspect the sets of retinal vessels by following them out to the periphery of each section of the eye. **Note:** • number of sets of arterioles and venules • color and diameter of the arterioles • arteriovenous (AV) ratio	• Four sets of arterioles and venules pass through the optic disc. Arterioles are bright red and narrow as they move away from the optic disc. Arterioles have a light reflex that appears as a thin, white line in the center of the arteriole. Venules are darker red and larger than arterioles and narrow as they move away from the optic disc. The ratio of arteriole diameter to vein diameter (AV ratio) is 2:3 or 4:5	• Changes in the blood supply to the retina may be observed in constricted arterioles, dilated veins, or absence of major vessels • Initially, hypertension may cause a widening of the arterioles' light reflex and the arterioles take on a copper color. With long-standing hypertension, arteriole walls thicken and appear opaque or silver

(Continued on following page)

OPHTHALMIC EXAMINATION OF INTERNAL EYE STRUCTURES (*continued*)

ASSESSMENT PROCEDURE	NORMAL FINDINGS	ABNORMAL FINDINGS
• Inspect AV crossings	• Veins pass underneath the arteriole and are seen right up to the column of blood on either side of the arteriole (the arteriole wall itself is normally transparent)	• Arterial nicking, tapering, and banking are abnormal AV crossings caused by hypertension or arteriosclerosis
• Inspect **retinal background**. Remain in the same position described previously and search the retinal background from the disc to the macula, noting the color and the presence of any lesions	• General background appears consistent in texture. The red-orange color of the background is lighter near the optic disc	• Cotton-wool patches (soft exudates) and hard exudates from diabetes and hypertension appear as light-colored spots on the retinal background. Hemorrhages and microaneurysms appear as red spots and streaks on the retinal background (see Abnormal Findings 12-4)
• Inspect **fovea (sharpest area of vision) and macula**. Remain in the same position described previously. Shine the light beam toward the side of the eye or ask the client to look directly into the light. Observe the fovea and the macula that surround it	• The macula is the darker area, one disc diameter in size, located to the temporal side of the optic disc. Within this area is a star-like light reflex called the fovea	• Excessive clumped pigment appears with detached retinas or retinal injuries. Macular degeneration may be due to hemorrhages, exudates, or cysts (see Abnormal Findings 12-4)

ASSESSMENT PROCEDURE	NORMAL FINDINGS	ABNORMAL FINDINGS
• Inspect **anterior chamber.** Remain in the same position and rotate the lens wheel slowly to +10, +12, or higher to inspect the anterior chamber of the eye	• The anterior chamber is transparent	• *Hyphema* occurs when injury causes red blood cells to collect in the lower half of the anterior chamber. *Hypopyon* usually results from an inflammatory response in which white blood cells accumulate in the anterior chamber and produce cloudiness in front of the iris
ASSESSING EYE TRAUMA		
With eye trauma accompanied by eye pain, discomfort, or feeling that something is in the eye, observe for: • Foreign body that remains after gentle washing • Perforated globe • Blood in eye	• No foreign body is observed • Eye globe intact with no indication of blood in eye	• Refer the client to an eye doctor immediately if a foreign body cannot be removed with gentle washing, there is perforation of globe, blood in eye, and/or client has impaired vision (Mayo Clinic, 2020)
With a blunt eye trauma, observe for: • Lid swollen shut • Blood in anterior chamber • White/hazy cornea • Irregularly shaped fixed, dilated, or constricted pupil	• No swelling of lid • No blood in anterior chamber • Cornea clear • Pupils equal and reactive to light	Refer client to eye doctor immediately if eye is swollen, blood is observed in anterior chamber, cornea is hazy, or pupils are irregularly shaped, fixed, dilated, or constricted

ABNORMAL FINDINGS 12-1 Extraocular Muscle Function

CORNEAL LIGHT REFLEX TEST ABNORMALITIES

Strabismus (or Tropia)

A constant malalignment of the eye axis, strabismus is defined according to the direction toward which the eye drifts and may cause amblyopia.

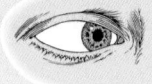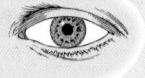

Esotropia (eye turns inward)

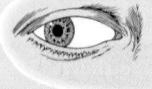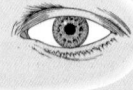

Exotropia (eye turns outward)

COVER/UNCOVER TEST ABNORMALITIES

Phoria (Mild Weakness)

Noticeable only with the cover test, phoria is less likely to cause amblyopia than strabismus. **Esophoria is an inward drift and exophoria an outward drift of the eye.**

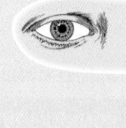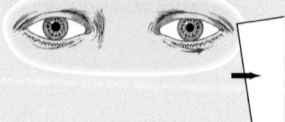

The uncovered eye is weaker; when the stronger eye is covered, the weaker eye moves to refocus.

Once the eye is uncovered, it will quickly move back to re-establish fixation.

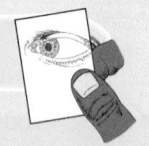

When the weaker eye is covered, it will drift to a relaxed position.

ABNORMAL FINDINGS | 12-2 | **External Eye Examination: Deviations from Normal**

ECTROPION

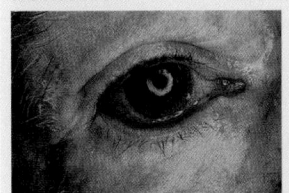

CHALAZION

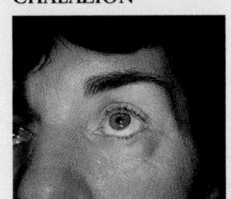

HORDEOLUM (stye)

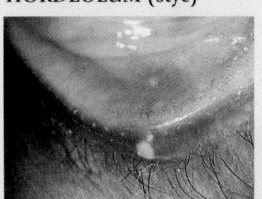

ENTROPION

BLEPHARITIS

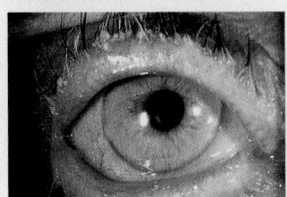

PTOSIS

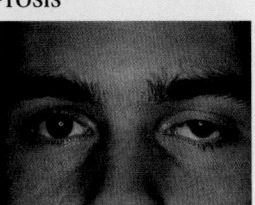

(*Continued on following page*)

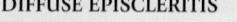

ABNORMAL FINDINGS **12-2** **External Eye Examination: Deviations from Normal (*continued*)**

CONJUNCTIVITIS

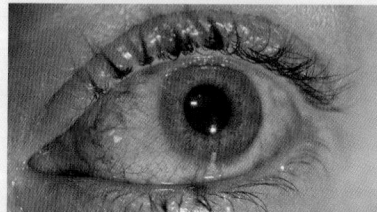

CATARACTS

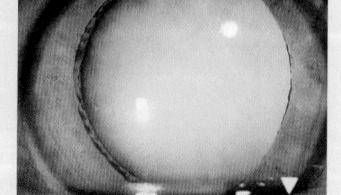

DIFFUSE EPISCLERITIS

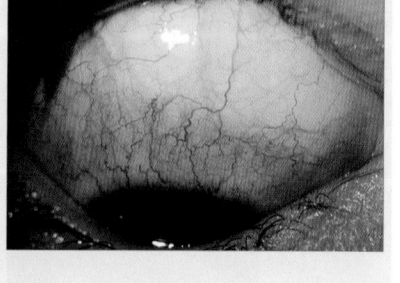

ABNORMAL FINDINGS **12-3** **Pupil and Iris Abnormalities**

IRREGULARLY SHAPED IRIS

An irregularly shaped iris causes a shallow anterior chamber, which may increase the risk for narrow-angle (closed-angle) glaucoma.

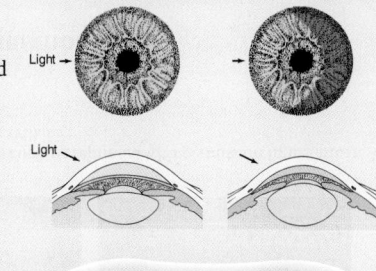

ABNORMALITIES OF THE PUPILS

Miosis

Also known as *pinpoint pupils*, miosis is characterized by constricted and fixed pupils—possibly a result of narcotic drugs or brain damage.

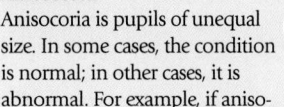

Anisocoria

Anisocoria is pupils of unequal size. In some cases, the condition is normal; in other cases, it is abnormal. For example, if aniso-

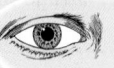 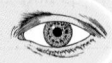

coria is greater in bright light compared with dim light, the cause may be trauma, tonic pupil (caused by impaired parasympathetic nerve supply to iris), and oculomotor nerve paralysis. If anisocoria is greater in dim light compared with bright light, the cause may be Horner syndrome (caused by paralysis of the cervical sympathetic nerves and characterized by ptosis, sunken eyeball, flushing of the affected side of the face, and narrowing of the palpebral fissure).

Mydriasis

Dilated and fixed pupils, typically resulting from central nervous system injury, circulatory collapse, or deep anesthesia.

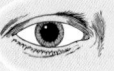 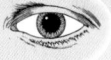

| ABNORMAL FINDINGS | 12-4 | **Ophthalmoscope Examination: Deviations from Normal** |

PAPILLEDEMA **GLAUCOMATOUS CUPPING** **COTTON-WOOL PATCHES** **RETINAL HEMORRHAGE**

Photo credits: Glaucomatous cupping reprinted with permission from Tasman, W., & Jaeger, E. (Eds.) (2001). *The Wills Eye Hospital atlas of clinical ophthalmology* (2nd ed.). Lippincott Williams & Wilkins.

PEDIATRIC VARIATIONS

Explain procedure to decrease child's fear when room is darkened.

Assess cranial nerves III and IV (oculomotor and abducens) by evaluating extraocular muscle function in children by assessing the six cardinal positions of gaze. Test young children by having them follow a toy or an interesting object.

In older children, evaluate eye muscle strength by performing the Hirschberg test and the cover/uncover test.

ASSESSMENT PROCEDURE	NORMAL FINDINGS	ABNORMAL FINDINGS
Inspect **placement of light** on cornea (Hirschberg test)	• Light falls symmetrically within each pupil. *Note: Pseudostrabismus is considered normal in young children. The pupils will appear at the inner canthus due to the epicanthic fold*	• Asymmetrical location of light reflection on pupil signals strabismus. The absence of the red reflex may indicate the presence of cataracts
Measure **inner canthal distance**	• Average distance 3 cm (1.2 in.)	• Wide-set eyes, upward slant, and thick epicanthal folds may suggest Down syndrome
Assess **palpebral slant**	• Outer canthus aligns with tips of pinna (except in Asian children) (Fig. 12-16)	• Presence of upward slant in non-Asians • Upper lid that lies above iris ("setting-sun" sign) suggests hydrocephalus • Black and white speckling of iris (Brushfield spots) seen in Down syndrome

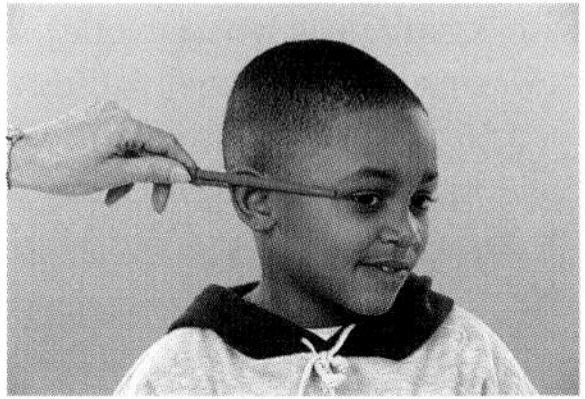

FIGURE 12-16 Outer canthus is in alignment with the tip of the pinna (Photo by B. Proud).

(Continued on following page)

ASSESSMENT PROCEDURE	NORMAL FINDINGS	ABNORMAL FINDINGS
• Observe **placement of lids** • Inspect iris • Inspect **lacrimal apparatus** • Perform **visual acuity tests.** Use E chart for preschoolers	• With eye open, lids lie between the upper iris and the pupil • Color varies from brown to green to blue • Lacrimal meatus not present until 3 months of age • Children can differentiate colors by the age of 5 years	• A one-line difference indicates visual impairment and should be referred; may be due to congenital defects, chronic disease, or refractive errors

 OLDER ADULT VARIATIONS

Vision examination reveals the following:
- Presbyopia (decreased near vision due to decreased elasticity of lens) common in clients older than 45 years
- Poorer night vision and decreased tolerance to glare
- Decreased peripheral vision
- Difficulty in differentiating blues from greens

External eye examination reveals the following:
- Dry eyes due to decreased tear production
- Drooping eyelids (senile ptosis)
- Entropion and ectropion common in the older adult

- Conjunctiva thins and becomes yellowish
- Clouding of lens (cataracts)
- Xanthelasma, raised yellow plaques, most often near the inner canthus, are a normal variation associated with increasing age and high lipid levels
- Yellowish nodules on bulbar conjunctiva (pinguecula), common and harmless
- White ring around iris (arcus senilis)—does not affect vision
- Slowed pupillary response and slowed accommodation

Ophthalmic examination reveals the following:
- Pale, narrowed arterioles

CULTURAL VARIATIONS

- Asians and members of some other groups may have common variation of epicanthal folds or narrowed palpebral fissures.
- Dark-skinned clients may have sclera with yellow or pigmented freckles.
- Non-Hispanic Whites have lower rates of diabetic retinopathy and glaucoma, but higher rates of age-related macular degeneration (AMD) than do African Americans and Hispanics. Hispanics have higher rates of cataracts, but all three groups have a relatively high rate compared with other eye diseases. Glaucoma is much more prevalent in African Americans than in the other groups (Charlson et al., 2015).
- Visual acuity varies by population areas worldwide and by ethnic group in the United States. Myopia (mild and moderate) and high myopia are increasing in prevalence, especially in Asian countries (Holden et al., 2016).
- Racial disparities exist in refractive error correction in the United States, where 50.6% had corrections to 20/40 or better. However, inadequate correction was greater in Mexican Americans and non-Hispanic Blacks than in non-Hispanic Whites in all age groups, especially in those under 20 years of age, and was related to low income, lower education level, and lack of health insurance (Ou, 2018).
- **The eyes of African Americans protrude slightly more than those of Whites, and those of Hispanics protrude less. Eyes of African Americans of both sexes may have eyes protruding beyond 21 mm. A difference of more than 2 mm between the two eyes is abnormal** (Miller et al., 2016; Weaver et al., 2010).
- Optic discs are larger in African Americans, which is thought to be associated with the higher rate of glaucoma in this group (Swanson, 2014).

POSSIBLE COLLABORATIVE PROBLEMS—RISK OF

Visual changes	Glaucoma
Eye infections	Impaired functioning of lacrimal apparatus
Cataracts	Corneal abrasions

Teaching Tips for Selected Client Concerns

Client Concern: Poor management of eye care associated with a lack of knowledge of recommended eye examinations

Teach clients that a comprehensive eye examination every 2 years is recommended for healthy clients without risk factors between 18 and 60 years of age; annually for aged 61 years and older (American Optometric Association [AOA], 2020b). Clients at risk for eye problems should be examined annually or as recommended by their physician. Clients at risk include those:

- With diabetes, hypertension, or a family history of ocular disease (e.g., glaucoma, macular degeneration)
- Working in occupations that are highly demanding visually or hazardous to the eyes
- Taking prescription or nonprescription drugs with ocular side effects
- Wearing contact lenses
- Who have had eye surgery
- With other health concerns or conditions

See Table 12-1 for guidelines for clients with risk factors.

Client Concern: *Risk for spread of infection associated with a lack of knowledge of eye infection care*

Instruct client on proper administration of eye drops and ointments. Discuss proper cleansing from inner to outer canthus and changing of cleansing cloth to prevent cross contamination

Client Concern: *Opportunity to enhance knowledge of eye care during the growing years*

Teach parents the schedule found in Table 12-2 for eye examinations.

TABLE 12-2 **Recommended Eye Examination Frequency for the Pediatric Patient**

	Examination Interval	
Patient Age	**Asymptomatic/ Low Risk**	**At Risk**
Birth through 2 years	At 6–12 months of age	At 6–12 months of age or as recommended
3–5 years	At least once between 3 and 5 years of age	At least once between 3 and 5 years of age or as recommended
6–18 years	Before first grade and annually thereafter	Before first grade and annually, or as recommended, thereafter

Reprinted with permission from American Optometric Association. *Comprehensive eye examinations.* https://www.aoa.org/healthy-eyes/caring-for-your-eyes/eye-exams. © 2021 American Optometric Association.

Children considered at risk for the development of eye and vision problems may need additional testing or more frequent re-evaluation. Factors placing an infant, toddler, or child at significant risk for visual impairment include (AOA, 2020b) the following:

- Prematurity, low birth weight, oxygen deficiency at birth, grade III or IV intraventricular hemorrhage
- Family history of retinoblastoma, congenital cataracts, or metabolic or genetic disease
- Infection of mother during pregnancy (e.g., rubella, toxoplasmosis, venereal disease, herpes, cytomegalovirus, or AIDS)
- Difficult or assisted labor, which may be associated with fetal distress or low Apgar scores
- High refractive error
- Strabismus
- Anisometropia
- Known or suspected central nervous system dysfunction evidenced by developmental delays

 Client Concern: *Risk for eye dryness associated with decreased tear production secondary to the aging process*

Instruct client on the use of artificial tears as necessary.

 Client Concern: *Risk for falling associated with impaired vision secondary to the aging process*

Explore visual aids for independent living to assist client with visual loss (magnifying glasses, audio tapes, CDs, large-print books, special glasses for viewing television, large-numbered phones, large-print checks, cane).

Encourage further evaluation, if necessary. Instruct family to keep furniture in same place and to provide better lighting. Provide the following eye care guidelines: adults aged 65 years or older with no risk factors should have an ophthalmologic eye examination every 1 to 2 years. To promote this goal, the National Eye Care Project is a nationwide outreach program sponsored by the AAO as a public service. It is designed to help the disadvantaged elderly obtain medical eye care. The toll-free phone number is 1-800-222-EYES. To be eligible, a person must be a U.S. citizen or legal resident, age 65 years or older, who does not have access to an ophthalmologist whom they may have seen in the past.

Instruct clients to wear sunglasses and hats in the sun. This is important because even on bright cloudy days, ultraviolet light can penetrate clouds. Squinting does not eliminate ultraviolet light entering the eye.

Explain that adults with diabetes mellitus should have an ophthalmologic eye examination at the time of diagnosis and yearly thereafter. Abnormal findings may require more frequent examinations.

Following are eye disorders commonly seen in older clients. Discuss symptoms of each with the client.

- Presbyopia (difficulty reading printed material)
- Floaters (moving specks or clouded vision)
- Cataracts (painless blurring of vision, glare or light sensitivity, poor night vision, double vision in one eye, needing brighter light to read, fading or yellowing of colors)
- Glaucoma (symptoms of glaucoma are not noticeable until damage has already occurred. Early diagnosis and treatment are keys to preventing blindness). Tonometry is used to measure pressure within the eye. Normal eye pressures range from 10 to 21 mmHg. Eye pressures greater than 22 mmHg increases one's risk for developing glaucoma. However, people with normal eye pressure may develop **glaucoma** (AOA, 2020a).
- Macular degeneration (words on a page look blurred in the center; straight lines look distorted, especially toward the center; a dark or empty area appears in the center of vision; colors look dim). Refer the client to the Macular Degeneration Partnership website http://www.amd.org/living-with-amd/resources-and-tools/31-amsler-grid.html to download the Amsler grid with directions to use to test for any visual changes.

References

American Academy of Ophthalmology. (2015). *Frequency of ocular examinations - 2015.* https://www.aao.org/clinical-statement/frequency-of-ocular-examinations

American Academy of Ophthalmology. (2020a). *Comprehensive adult medical eye evaluation PPP 2020.* https://www.aao.org/preferred-practice-pattern/comprehensive-adult-medical-eye-evaluation-ppp

American Academy of Ophthalmology. (2020b). *Eye health statistics.* https://www.aao.org/newsroom/eye-health-statistics

American Academy of Ophthalmology. (2021). *Have AMD? Save your sight with an Amsler grid.* https://www.aao.org/eye-health/tips-prevention/facts-about-amsler-grid-daily-vision-test

American Optometric Association. (2016). *Comprehensive eye exams.* https://www.aoa.org/healthy-eyes/caring-for-your-eyes/eye-exams?sso=y

American Optometric Association. (2020a). *Glaucoma.* https://www.aoa.org/patients-and-public/eye-and-vision-problems/glossary-of-eye-and-vision-conditions/glaucoma

American Optometric Association. (2020b). *Recommended eye examination frequency for pediatric patients and adults.* https://idaho.aoa.org/

patients-and-public/caring-for-your-vision/comprehensive-eye-and-vision-examination/recommended-examination-frequency-for-pediatric-patients-and-adults

Charlson, E., Sankar, P., Miller-Ellis, E., Regina, M., Fertig, R., Salinas, J., Pistilli M., Salowe, R. J., Rhodes, A. L., Merritt, W. T., 3rd., Chua, M., Trachtman, B. T., Gudiseva, H. V., Collins, D. W., Chavali, V. R., Nichols, C., Henderer, J., Ying, G. S., Varma, R., … O'Brien, J. M. (2015). The primary open-angle African American glaucoma genetics study. *Ophthalmology, 122*(4), 711–720. https://doi.org/10.1016/j.ophtha.2014.11.015

Holden, B., Fricke, T., Wilson, D., Jong, M., Naidoo, K., Sankaridurg, P., Wong, T. Y., Naduvilath, T. J., & Resnikoff, S. (2016). Global prevalence of myopia and high myopia and temporal *trends* from 2000 through 2050. *Ophthalmology, 123*(5), 1036–1042. https://doi.org/10.1016/j.ophtha.2016.01.006

Miller, N., Subramanian, P., & Patel, V. (2016). Walsh & Hoyt's clinical neuro-ophthalmology: The essentials (Vol. 3). Wolters Kluwer, Lippincott Williams & Wilkins.

Ou, Y. (2018). *Glaucoma in the African American and Hispanic communities.* https://www.brightfocus.org/glaucoma/article/glaucoma-african-american-and-hispanic-communities

Swanson, M. (2014). *The changing and challenging epidemiology of glaucoma.* http://www.reviewofoptometry.com/content/c/49437/dnnprintmode/true/?skinsrc=%;5Bl%;5Dskins/ro2009/pageprint&containersrc=%;5Bl%;5Dcontainers/ro2009/simple

Weaver, A., Loftis, K., Tan, J. C., Duma, S. M., & Stitzel, J. D. (2010). CT based three-dimensional measurement of orbit and eye anthropometry. *Investigative Ophthalmology & Visual Science, 51*(10), 4892–4897. https://pubmed.ncbi.nlm.nih.gov/20463322/

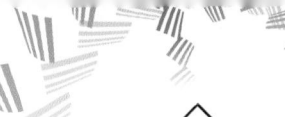

13 ASSESSING EARS

Structure and Function Overview

EXTERNAL STRUCTURES OF THE EAR

The external ear is composed of the auricle or pinna (Fig. 13-1B) and the external auditory canal (Fig. 13-1A). Modified sweat glands in the external ear canal secrete *cerumen*, a wax-like substance that keeps the tympanic membrane (TM) soft and has bacteriostatic properties, a defense against foreign bodies. The TM or eardrum, a translucent, pearly gray, concave membrane, seen in Figure 13-1C, serves as a partition stretched across the inner end of the auditory canal, separating it from the middle ear.

The middle ear (a small, air-filled chamber in the temporal bone) contains three auditory ossicles: the malleus, the incus, and the stapes. These tiny bones are responsible for transmitting sound waves from the eardrum to the inner ear through the oval window. Air pressure is equalized on both sides of the TM by means of the *eustachian tube*, which connects the middle ear to the nasopharynx. The distinct landmarks of the TM (Fig. 13-1C) include the following:

- Handle and short process of the malleus
- Umbo, the base of the malleus
- Cone of light reflection of the otoscope light due to the concave membrane

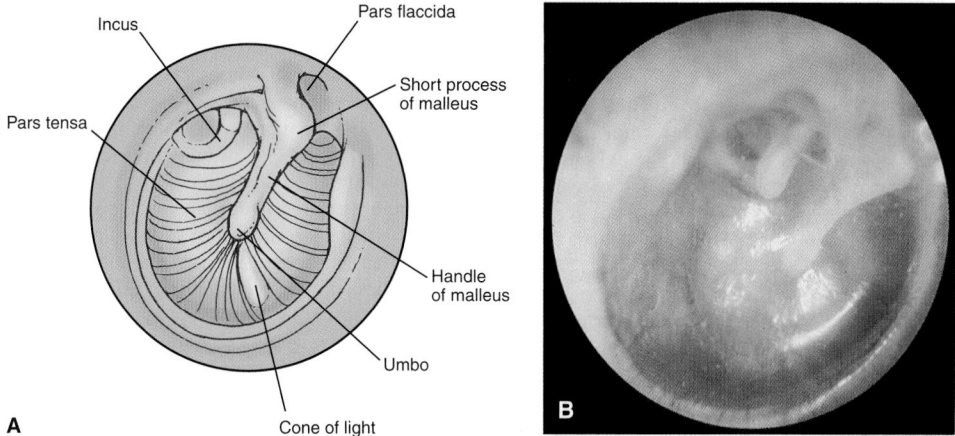

FIGURE 13-1 Structures in the outer, middle, and inner divisions. **(A)** Landmarks of Right Tympanic Membrane. **(B)** Normal Otoscopic view of Right Tmpanic Membrane.

- Pars flaccid, top portion of the membrane that appears to be less taut
- Pars tensa, the bottom of the membrane that appears to be taut

The middle ear is separated from the inner ear (Fig. 13-1A) by a bony partition containing two openings, the round and oval windows. The inner ear, or labyrinth, is fluid filled and is made up of the bony labyrinth and an inner membranous labyrinth. The bony labyrinth has three parts: the cochlea, the vestibule, and the semicircular canals.

HEARING

The ears serve as sensory organs for hearing. Sound vibrations traveling through air are collected by and funneled through the external ear and cause the eardrum to vibrate. Sound waves are then transmitted through auditory ossicles as the vibration of the eardrum causes the malleus, the incus, and then the stapes to vibrate. As the stapes vibrates at the oval window, the sound waves are passed to the fluid in the inner ear. The movement of this fluid stimulates the hair cells of the spiral organ of Corti and initiates the nerve impulses that travel to the brain by way of the acoustic nerve.

Sounds waves are transmitted through:

- The external and middle ear. This is referred to as **conductive hearing.** Conductive hearing loss is related to dysfunction of the external or middle ear (e.g., impacted earwax, otitis media, foreign object, perforated eardrum, middle ear drainage, otosclerosis).
- The inner ear. This is referred to as **sensorineural hearing** (or perceptive hearing). Sensorineural hearing loss is related to dysfunction of the inner ear (i.e., organ of Corti, cranial nerve VIII, temporal lobe of the brain).

- the skull bones, which serve to augment usual sound waves through air, bone, and, finally, fluid. This pathway is less efficient than the conductive or sensorineural pathway.

Nursing Assessment

COLLECTING SUBJECTIVE DATA

Collecting subjective data consists of asking the client focus questions and assessing for risk factors.

Interview Questions

Recent changes in hearing? All or some sounds affected? History of otosclerosis? Excessive earwax? Method of wax removal? Ear drainage? Type? Pain that occurs when manipulating, or wiggling, the pinna (may suggest otitis externa [swimmer's ear])? Middle or inner ear pain? Occurrence? Relief? Associated factors such as sore throat, sinus infection, or gum/teeth problems? Ringing or cracking in ears (tinnitus)? Dizziness, feeling of being unbalanced or spinning (vertigo)? Loss of high-frequency sounds? History of prior ear surgery? Trauma? Ear infections? Swimmer's ear? Sudden deafness? Use of ototoxic medications? Prolonged exposure to loud noises? Use of protective hearing devices? Method used for cleaning ears? Use of hearing aids? Last hearing examination?

Risk Factors

Risk for hearing loss related to genetic predisposition, congenital anomalies, otitis media, fluid in inner ear, loud noises (especially prolonged exposure or short exposure to >110 dB), ototoxic medications, aging (presbycusis), trauma to eardrum, otosclerosis, viral inner ear infections, impacted cerumen, hypoxia during birth, or neonatal jaundice.

COLLECTING OBJECTIVE DATA

Equipment Needed

- Otoscope with good batteries (pneumatic bulb device for young children) (Assessment Guide 13-1)
- Tuning fork (512 and 1,024 Hz)

Physical Assessment

Review Figures 13-1 and 13-2 for the anatomy of the external, middle, and inner ear.

Make sure the client is seated comfortably in such a way that you can easily visualize both ears. First examine the external ear, then examine the ear canal and TM with the otoscope, and finally assess hearing function.

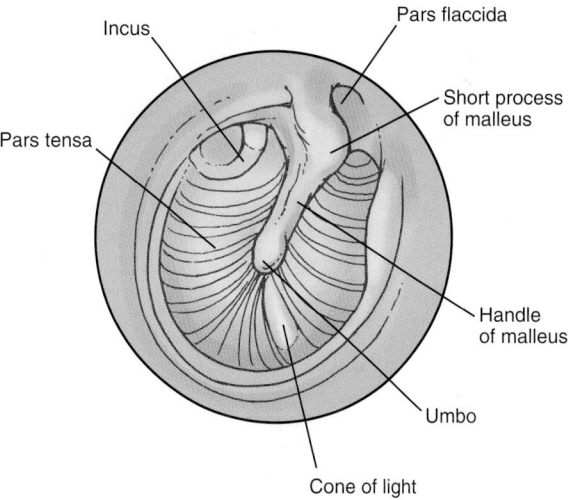

FIGURE 13-2 Right tympanic membrane.

ASSESSMENT GUIDE 13-1   Using an Otoscope to Inspect the External Canal and the Tympanic Membrane

1. Ask clients to sit comfortably with the back straight and the head tilted slightly away from you toward their opposite shoulder.
2. Choose the largest speculum that fits comfortably into the ear canal (usually 5 mm in the adult) and attach it to the otoscope. Hold otoscope in your dominant hand and turn the otoscope light "on."
3. Use thumb and fingers of your opposite hand to grasp client's auricle firmly but gently. Pull out, up, and back to straighten the external auditory canal. Do not alter this position during the examination.
4. Grasp the otoscope handle between your thumb and fingers. Hold otoscope up or down, whichever is comfortable for you. If you hold the otoscope down, steady your hand holding the otoscope against the client's head or face.
5. Insert the speculum gently down and forward into the ear canal (~1.27 cm [0.5 in.]). Be careful not to touch the inner portion of the sensitive canal wall.
6. Position your eye against the lens.

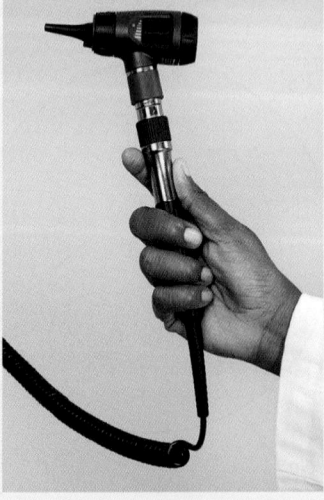

Otoscope

ASSESSMENT PROCEDURE	NORMAL FINDINGS	ABNORMAL FINDINGS
Inspect **external ear** (Fig. 13-3) for the following: 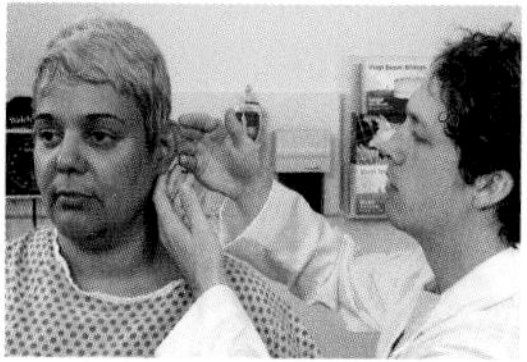 FIGURE 13-3 Inspecting the external ear.		
• Size and shape	• Ears of equal size and similar appearance	• Ears of unequal size or configuration (<4 cm or >10 cm)
• Position	• Alignment of pinna with corner of eye and within 10-degree angle of vertical position	• Pinna positioned below a line from corner of eye, or unequal alignment. Malaligned or low-set ears are seen with chromosomal defects or genitourinary disorders.
• Lesions and discolorations	• Skin smooth and without nodules; pink color	• Erythema, edema, nodules, or areas of discoloration. Postauricular cysts are seen with blocked sebaceous glands; ulcerated crusted nodules may be malignant; pale blue color seen in frostbite.

(Continued on following page)

ASSESSMENT PROCEDURE	NORMAL FINDINGS	ABNORMAL FINDINGS
Palpate **external ear** (see Fig. 13-1)	Nontender auricle, **tragus**	Painful auricle or tragus associated with otitis externa or post-auricular cyst. Tenderness behind ear is associated with otitis media.
Palpate **mastoid process** for the following: • Tenderness • Temperature • Edema	• No tenderness or pain when palpated • Warm • Mastoid process easily palpated	• Pain on palpation of mastoid process with mastoiditis • Erythema • Actual process difficult to palpate; ear displaced outward owing to edema
Inspect **auditory canal** using otoscope (see Assessment Guide 13-1) for the following: • Cerumen	• *Color:* Black, dark red, gray, or brown • *Consistency:* Waxy, flaky, soft, or hard • *Odor:* None	• Impacted cerumen (obstructs visualization of membrane); bloody purulent discharge is seen in otitis media with perforated eardrum; foul-smelling discharge associated with otitis externa or impacted foreign body (see Abnormal Findings 13-1).

ASSESSMENT PROCEDURE	NORMAL FINDINGS	ABNORMAL FINDINGS
• Appearance	• Canal walls pink and uniform with TM visible	• Lesions, foreign body, erythema, or edema present in canal. Red, swollen canals are seen with otitis media; polyps or nonmalignant nodular swellings can block the view of the eardrum (see Abnormal Findings 13-1).
• Tenderness	• Little or no discomfort on manipulation of pinna; inner two-thirds of canal very tender if touched with speculum	• Moderate-to-severe pain when pinna is moved or otoscope speculum is inserted
The entire TM may not be visible at one glance. Rotate the otoscope around to view images. The images can be "piecemealed" together to fully assess the TM. Use the largest speculum that the canal will allow. Once inserted into the ear canal, the otoscope may need to be positioned slightly anterior to see the TM.		

(Continued on following page)

ASSESSMENT PROCEDURE	NORMAL FINDINGS	ABNORMAL FINDINGS
Inspect **TM**, using otoscope (see Assessment Guide 13-1), for the following:		
• Color	• Pearly gray, shiny, translucent, with no bulging or retraction	• Dull appearance: Blue (blood) or pink/red (inflammation). Red, bulging TM is seen with acute otitis media (see Abnormal Findings 13-2); yellow, bulging TM seen with serous otitis media; blue or dark color seen in trauma when there is blood behind the TM.
• Consistency	• Intact; may show movement when swallowing	• Perforations, scarring, or immobility. White spots are seen with scarring of the TM (see Abnormal Findings 13-2).
• Landmarks (see Fig. 13-1)	• Cone of light, umbo, handle of malleus, and short process of malleus easily visualized	• Retracted TM accentuates landmarks; bulging TM partially occludes landmarks. Prominent landmarks indicate TM retraction due to negative pressure from obstructed eustachian tube, whereas obscured landmarks indicate thickened TM due to chronic otitis media.

ASSESSMENT PROCEDURE	NORMAL FINDINGS	ABNORMAL FINDINGS
Perform **the whisper test** (or whispered voice test) by asking the client to gently occlude the ear not being tested and rub the tragus with a finger in a circular motion. Start with testing the better hearing ear and then the poorer one. With your head 2 feet behind the client (so that the client cannot see your lips move), whisper a two-syllable word such as "popcorn" or "football." Ask the client to repeat it back to you. If the response is incorrect the first time, whisper the word one more time.	• Able to correctly repeat the two-syllable word as whispered. Identifying three of six whispered words is considered passing the test.	• Unable to repeat the two-syllable word after two tries indicates hearing loss and requires follow-up testing by an audiologist.

(Continued on following page)

ASSESSMENT PROCEDURE	NORMAL FINDINGS	ABNORMAL FINDINGS
Perform **Weber test** (Fig. 13-4A) if the client reports diminished or lost hearing in one ear. This tests conduction of sound waves through bone to help distinguish between conductive hearing (sound waves transmitted by the external and middle ear) and sensorineural hearing (sound waves transmitted by the inner ear). Strike a tuning fork softly with the back of your hand and place it at the center of the client's head or forehead. Centering is the important part. Ask whether the client hears the sound better in one ear or the same in both ears.	Vibrations are heard equally well in both ears. No lateralization of sound to either ear.	• With *conductive hearing loss*, the client reports lateralization of sound to the poor ear—that is, the client "hears" the sounds in the poor ear. The good ear is distracted by background noise and conducted air, which the poor ear has trouble hearing. Thus, the poor ear receives most of the sound conducted by bone vibration. With *sensorineural hearing loss*, the client reports **lateralization** of sound to the good ear. This is because of limited perception of the sound due to nerve damage in the bad ear, making sound seems louder in the unaffected ear.

ASSESSMENT PROCEDURE	NORMAL FINDINGS	ABNORMAL FINDINGS
◎ **CLINICAL TIP** Hold the tuning fork by the handle and do not touch the tines.	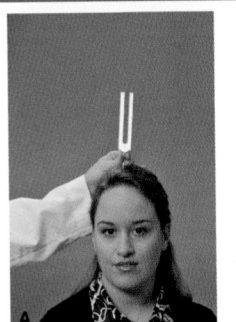	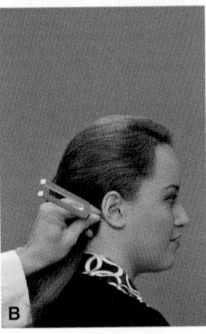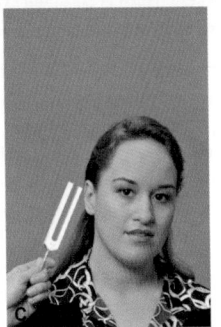

FIGURE 13-4 Using a tuning fork to assess auditory function. **(A)** Weber test. **(B)** Rinne test: Bone conduction. **(C)** Rinne test: Air conduction. (Reprinted with permission from Jensen, S. [2015]. *Nursing health assessment* [2nd ed.]. Wolters Kluwer.)

(Continued on following page)

ASSESSMENT PROCEDURE	NORMAL FINDINGS	ABNORMAL FINDINGS
Perform the **Rinne test** (Fig. 13-4B and C). The Rinne test compares air and bone conduction (AC and BC, respectively) sounds. Strike a tuning fork and place the base of the fork on the client's mastoid process. (Ask the client to tell you when the sound is no longer heard.) Move the prongs of the tuning fork to the front of the external auditory canal. Ask the client to tell you if the sound is audible after the fork is moved.	AC sound is normally heard longer than BC sound (AC > BC).	Although AC > BC in normal hearing, the Rinne test is used to determine the cause of the hearing loss (conductive or sensorineural) once it is determined that there is a hearing loss. If the cause is sensorineural, the finding will also be AC>BC. With *conductive hearing loss*, BC sound is heard longer than or equally as long as AC sound (BC ≥ AC). *Conductive hearing loss*: Sound is not conducted through the outer ear canal to the eardrum and ossicles of the middle ear. Causes include fluid in middle ear, middle ear infection (otitis media), allergies (serous otitis media), eustachian tube dysfunction, perforated eardrum, benign tumors, impacted cerumen, infection in the ear canal (external otitis), or the presence of a foreign body (American Speech-Language-Hearing Association [ASHA], 2020a). *Sensorineural hearing loss:* AC > BC. Sensorineural hearing loss occurs with damage to the inner ear (cochlea), or to nerve pathways between the inner ear and brain. This is the most common type of permanent hearing loss. Causes include ototoxic drugs, genetic hearing loss, aging, head trauma, malformation of the inner ear, and loud noise exposure (ASHA, 2020b).

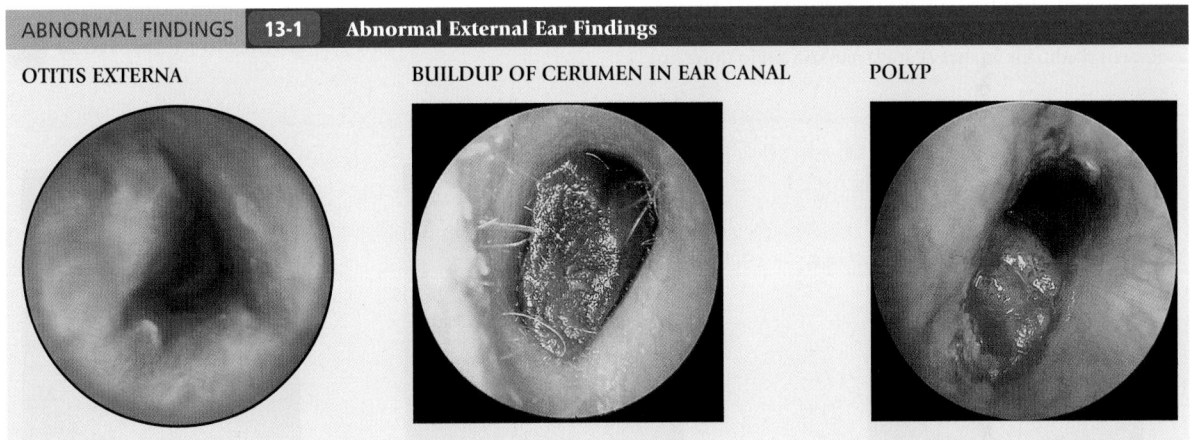

ABNORMAL FINDINGS   13-1   **Abnormal External Ear Findings**

OTITIS EXTERNA

BUILDUP OF CERUMEN IN EAR CANAL

POLYP

Photo credits: Otitis externa, reprinted with permission from Bickley, L. S. (2002). *Bates' guide to physical examination and history taking* (8th ed.). Lippincott Williams & Wilkins.

ABNORMAL FINDINGS	13-2	Abnormal Tympanic Membrane Findings

ACUTE OTITIS MEDIA

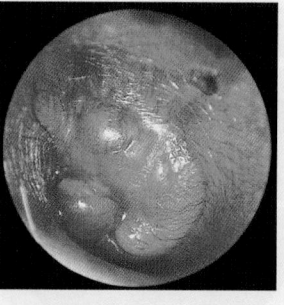

PERFORATED TYMPANIC MEMBRANE

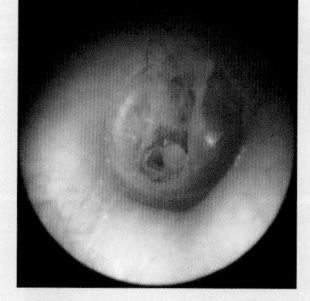

SCARRED TYMPANIC MEMBRANE

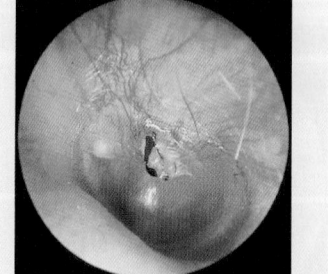

PEDIATRIC VARIATIONS

- Impacted cerumen in the canal may impede visual examination of TM. Careful removal of wax with a curette may be performed.

- Irrigation of the external ear may also be attempted to remove cerumen with warm water. Never use hot or cold water.
- Scarring may be visible in children with a history of tympanostomy tubes.

- The TM should appear pink, shiny, and translucent, allowing visualization of the bony landmarks. If child has been crying, then the TM may appear red.
- Assess the TM for mobility by compressing a pneumatic insufflator bulb with a small puff of air. The healthy membrane should be mobile. Immobility of the TM may be caused by fluid or pus accumulation behind the TM, perforation of the TM, scarring, or the presence of tympanostomy tubes.

ASSESSMENT PROCEDURE	NORMAL FINDINGS	ABNORMAL FINDINGS
Observe for **placement and alignment of pinna**.	Pinna slightly crosses the horizontal line (Fig. 13-5A), extends slightly forward from skull symmetrically.	Pinna falls below horizontal line (Fig. 13-5B); low ears with vertical alignment > 10-degree angle suggest mental retardation or congenital syndrome; abnormal shape indicates renal pathology.
Observe **inner canal**.		
Note: For otoscope examination of infants and young children, restraint may be necessary to accomplish a safe, effective assessment (Fig. 13-6). In infants and young children, perform the otoscope examination last in the assessment because this part of the examination is often distressing to children in this age group.		
Child younger than 3 years.		
Restrain; pull pinna downward and backward.		

(Continued on following page)

ASSESSMENT PROCEDURE	NORMAL FINDINGS	ABNORMAL FINDINGS

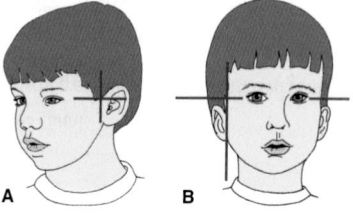

FIGURE 13-5 Placement and alignment of pinna in children. (**A**) Normal. (**B**) Low-set ears with alignment greater than 10-degree angle.

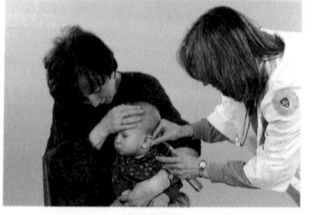

FIGURE 13-6 Infant being restrained in the upright position (Photo by B. Proud.)

Children older than 3 years. Pull pinna upward and backward.		
Inspect TM using otoscope with pneumatic device.	TM moves with introduction of air.	TM does not move with introduction of air.

GERIATRIC VARIATIONS

- Elongated lobule with linear wrinkles.
- Tuft of wire-like hair may be present at entrance of ear canal.
- More cerumen buildup; drier, harder cerumen due to rigid cilia in ear canal.
- Perception of consonants (Z, T, F, G) and high-frequency sounds (S, Sh, Ph, K) decreases.
- Dull, retracted TM—may be cloudy with more prominent landmarks owing to normal aging process.
- Diminished hearing acuity (presbycusis). More than 30% of people over age 65 have some type of hearing loss; 14% of people between 45 and 64 years of age have hearing loss. Most age-related hearing loss cannot be corrected, but some can, and the functional status caused by the loss needs to be addressed. McCabe (2019) recommends hearing screening for older adults.
- Older client may refuse to wear hearing aid due to a bad past experience or feelings of embarrassment. Improved, more discreet hearing aids are now available.

 CULTURAL VARIATIONS

- Consistency and color of earwax varies. Dry, gray, flaky earwax is usual in northern Asians and Native Americans. Wetter, light honey to orange to dark brown wax is most common in tropical areas of Asia, Africa, and the Americas and in African Americans and Whites (Molnar, 2016).
- Dry earwax has been associated with lower apocrine gland secretion/sweat production and, thus, less body odor, and lower rates of breast cancer.
- Race and ethnicity have been found to be associated with hearing thresholds wherein Blacks had the best hearing followed by Hispanics and Whites (and darker-skinned Hispanics better than lighter-skinned Hispanics even though study of skin color itself did not show significant differences; Lin et al., 2012).

POSSIBLE COLLABORATIVE PROBLEMS—RISK OF

- Otitis media: acute, chronic, serous otitis externa
- Perforated TM
- Hearing impairment

Teaching Tips for Selected Client Concerns

Client Concern: *Risk for loss of hearing associated with working in loud, noisy environment*

Teach client to:

- Wear a protective hearing device when in an environment with loud noises (e.g., loud music, loud engines, aircraft, explosives, or firearms).
- Avoid sound exposure louder than a washing machine. Avoid noises that are very loud, very close, or last too long.
- Avoid listening to extremely loud music for long periods of time.
- Have hearing checked periodically, and if there is hearing loss, obtain and use hearing aids.
- Recognize hearing loss using the self-assessment tool in Box 13-1 to determine the need to seek medical evaluation if hearing loss is suspected.

Client Concern: *Risk for injury associated with decreased auditory perception*

Teach safety measures (e.g., burglar alarms, lights on telephone and alarms, phone designed for hearing impaired). Explore availability of resources for hearing aids, and refer client to reading materials or sign language learning if appropriate. Encourage client to ask others to repeat what is not heard.

Client Concern: *Opportunity to promote ear care associated with client's request to learn safe ear care*

Avoid the use of instruments to remove wax from ears due to chance of impacting it further. See professional for earwax removal.

Teach client to cleanse outer ears with damp cloth and to *never insert anything into ear canal, including cotton-tipped swabs, pens, hairpins, and so on. Instruct to never use an "ear candle" to remove earwax. These are ineffective and may cause burns, obstruction of the ear canal, or perforation of the TM. Irrigation devices should only be used by health care professionals* (American Family Physician, 2017). Encourage use of sunscreen on external ear. Teach client to shake head to remove water in ear and to dry ear after swimming to prevent swimmer's ear.

BOX 13-1   TEN WAYS TO RECOGNIZE HEARING LOSS

The following questions will help you determine whether you need to have your hearing evaluated by a medical professional:

Do you have a problem hearing over the telephone?	Yes ☐	No ☐
Do you have trouble following the conversation when two or more people are talking at the same time?	Yes ☐	No ☐
Do people complain that you turn the TV volume up too high?	Yes ☐	No ☐
Do you have to strain to understand conversation?	Yes ☐	No ☐
Do you have trouble hearing in a noisy background?	Yes ☐	No ☐
Do you find yourself asking people to repeat themselves?	Yes ☐	No ☐
Do many people you talk to seem to mumble (or not speak clearly)?	Yes ☐	No ☐
Do you misunderstand what others are saying and respond inappropriately?	Yes ☐	No ☐
Do you have trouble understanding the speech of women and children?	Yes ☐	No ☐
Do people get annoyed because you misunderstand what they say?	Yes ☐	No ☐

If you answered "yes" to three or more of these questions, you may want to see an otolaryngologist (an ear, nose, and throat specialist) or an audiologist for a hearing evaluation.

The material on this page is for general information only and is not intended for diagnostic or treatment purposes. A doctor or other health care professional must be consulted for diagnostic information and advice regarding treatment.

Excerpt from NIH Publication No. 01-4913

For more information, contact the **NIDCD Information Clearinghouse**.

The NIDCD Information Clearinghouse is a service of the National Institute on Deafness and Other Communication Disorders (NIDCD), National Institutes of Health (NIH), and U.S. Department of Health and Human Services (HHS).

Client Concern: *Risk for Injury related to attempts to insert foreign objects in ear*

Teach parents and child (as appropriate for age) about dangers of insertion of foreign objects in ear. Teach parents to avoid toys with small, removable parts. Also, teach parents to avoid putting infant to bed with bottle filled with formula, juices, or sugar water, because this can settle in the oral pharynx and provide medium for bacterial growth and cause middle ear infections. Encourage yearly ear screening with physical examination during growing years.

Client Concern: *Opportunity to enhance child ear care associated with request from parent as to how to care for child's ears and hearing health*

- Immunize children against childhood diseases, including measles, meningitis, rubella, and mumps.
- Be immunized against rubella before pregnancy if a woman is of child-bearing age.
- If pregnant, get screening for syphilis and other sexually transmitted infections (STIs), adequate antenatal and prenatal care, and diagnosis and treatment for a baby born with jaundice.
- Avoid the use of ototoxic drugs unless prescribed by a qualified health care worker and properly monitored for correct dosage.
- If you have a newborn, avoid feeding from bottle while infant is lying on back.
- Have newborn infant screened for hearing.
- Get treatment for ear infections as soon as they are noticed; follow up with health care provider after symptoms seem to be gone to make sure there is no fluid left in the ear.
- Get treatment for tonsil and adenoid infections and inflammation.
- Keep child home from day care if possible when there is an outbreak of ear infections.
- Teach child to avoid putting foreign bodies in ears.

Client Concern: *Loss of hearing associated with aging process*

Advise caregivers and family to speak clearly, and allow client to see your lips. Speak within distance of 91.4 to 122 cm (3–6 ft).

References

American Family Physician. (2017). Practice guidelines: Cerumen impaction: An updated guideline from the AAO-HNSF. *American Family Physician, 96*(4), 263–264. https://www.aafp.org/afp/2017/0815/p263.html

American Speech-Language-Hearing Association. (2020a). *Conductive hearing loss.* https://www.asha.org/public/hearing/conductive-hearing-loss/

American Speech-Language-Hearing Association. (2020b). *Sensorineural hearing loss.* https://www.asha.org/public/hearing/sensorineural-hearing-loss/#:~:text=Sensorineural%20hearing%20loss%2C%20or%20SNHL,type%20of%20permanent%20hearing%20loss

Lin, F. R., Maas, P., Chien, W., Carey, J. P., Ferrucci, L., & Thorpe, R. (2012). Association of skin color, race/ethnicity, and hearing loss among adults in the USA. *Journal of the Association for Research in Otolaryngology, 13*(1), 109–117.

McCabe, D. (2019). *Hearing screening in older adults.* https://hign.org/consultgeri/try-this-series/hearing-screening-older-adults

Molnar, S. (2016). *Human variation: Races, types, and ethnic groups.* Routledge.

14 ASSESSING MOUTH, THROAT, NOSE, AND SINUSES

Structure and Function Overview

The mouth or oral cavity is formed by the lips, cheeks, hard and soft palates, uvula, and the tongue and its muscles (Fig. 14-1).

Contained within the mouth are the tongue, teeth, gums, and openings of the salivary glands (parotid, submandibular, and sublingual). The gums (gingiva) are covered by mucous membrane and normally hold 32 permanent teeth in the adult (Fig. 14-2).

Three pairs of salivary glands secrete saliva (watery, serous fluid containing salts, mucus, and salivary amylase) into the mouth (Fig. 14-3): the parotid glands, the submandibular glands, and the sublingual glands.

The throat (pharynx), located behind the mouth and nose, serves as a muscular passage for food and air (see Fig. 14-4). The upper part of the throat is the nasopharynx. Below the nasopharynx lies the oropharynx, and below the oropharynx lies the laryngopharynx.

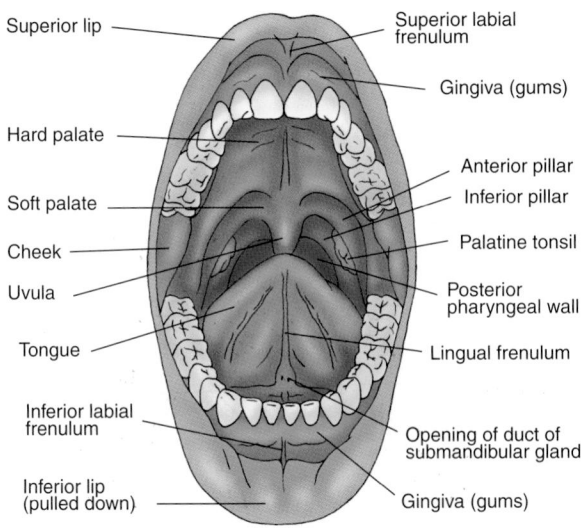

FIGURE 14-1 Structures of the mouth.

Superior lip
Superior labial frenulum
Gingiva (gums)
Hard palate
Anterior pillar
Inferior pillar
Soft palate
Palatine tonsil
Cheek
Uvula
Posterior pharyngeal wall
Tongue
Lingual frenulum
Inferior labial frenulum
Opening of duct of submandibular gland
Inferior lip (pulled down)
Gingiva (gums)

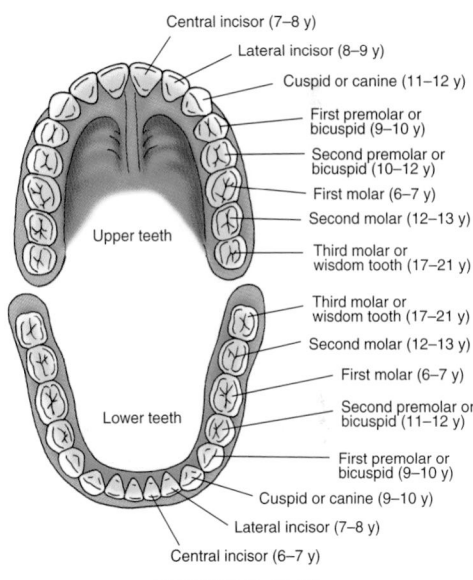

FIGURE 14-2 Teeth.

Central incisor (7–8 y)
Lateral incisor (8–9 y)
Cuspid or canine (11–12 y)
First premolar or bicuspid (9–10 y)
Second premolar or bicuspid (10–12 y)
First molar (6–7 y)
Second molar (12–13 y)
Third molar or wisdom tooth (17–21 y)
Upper teeth
Third molar or wisdom tooth (17–21 y)
Second molar (12–13 y)
First molar (6–7 y)
Second premolar or bicuspid (11–12 y)
First premolar or bicuspid (9–10 y)
Cuspid or canine (9–10 y)
Lateral incisor (7–8 y)
Central incisor (6–7 y)
Lower teeth

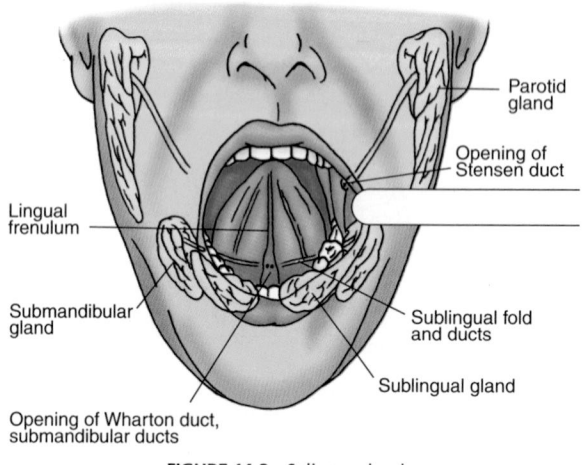

FIGURE 14-3 Salivary glands.

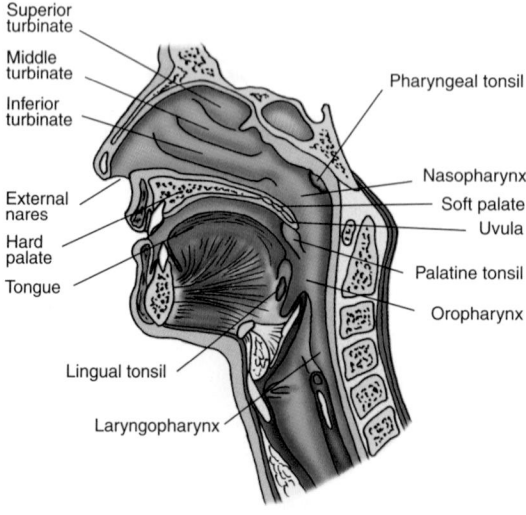

FIGURE 14-4 Nasal cavity and throat structures.

The nose is composed of bone and cartilage covered with skin and an internal nasal cavity, lined with mucous membrane. The **external nose** consists of a bridge (upper portion), tip, and two oval openings called **nares**. The **nasal cavity** (Fig. 14-4) is located between the roof of the mouth and the cranium separated into halves by the nasal septum. The front of the nasal **septum** contains Kiesselbach area, a rich supply of blood vessels.

The superior, middle, and inferior **turbinates (conchae)** are bony lobes that project from the nasal cavity, increasing the surface area that is exposed to incoming air (see Fig. 14-4). As the person inspires air, nasal hairs (vibrissae) filter large particles from the air. Ciliated mucosal cells then capture and propel debris toward the throat, where it is swallowed. A meatus underlies each turbinate and receives drainage from the **paranasal sinuses** and the **nasolacrimal duct.**

Four pairs of **paranasal sinuses** (frontal, maxillary, ethmoidal, and sphenoidal) are located in the skull. The paranasal sinuses are lined with ciliated mucous membrane that traps debris and propels it toward the outside. The **frontal sinuses** (above the eyes) and the **maxillary sinuses** (in the upper jaw) are accessible to the examiner, whereas the **ethmoidal and sphenoidal sinuses** are smaller, located deeper in the skull, and not accessible for direct examination.

Nursing Assessment

COLLECTING SUBJECTIVE DATA

Interview Questions

Prior dental issues? Dentures? Lip or oral lesions; cold sores? Redness or swelling (location, occurrence, relief)? Sore throat? Dysphagia? Hoarseness? History of mouth, nose, or throat cancer in family? Smoking history or use of smokeless tobacco? Excessive use of alcohol? Dental care practices: brushing, flossing, dental checkups? Teeth grinding? History of braces? Nosebleeds? Change in ability to smell? Nasal drainage and character of drainage? Seasonal or other allergies? Use of nose sprays or allergy medications? Difficulty breathing through nostrils? Sinus pain? Past sinus infections (frequency)? Past oral, nasal, or sinus surgery? Trauma? Headaches located in sinus areas? Postnasal drip?

Risk Factors

Risk for oropharyngeal cancer related to smoking or use of smokeless tobacco; family history; alcoholism or heavy alcohol use; working with wood, nickel refining, or textile fibers; infection with certain human papillomaviruses (HPVs); poor oral hygiene; poor diet/nutrition (low in fruits, vegetables, vitamin A deficiency); and chewing betel nuts containing a mild stimulant that is popular in Asia.

COLLECTING OBJECTIVE DATA

Equipment Needed

- Penlight
- Tongue blade
- 4- × 4-in. gauze pad
- Clean gloves
- Nasal speculum or short, wide-tipped speculum attached to head of otoscope (Assessment Guide 14-1)

Physical Assessment

Review Figures 14-1 to 14-4 for diagrams of the mouth, oropharynx, and nose.

ASSESSMENT GUIDE 14-1   Using Otoscope with Wide-Tipped Attachment

- Use nondominant hand to stabilize and gently tilt the client's head back.
- Insert the short, wide tip of the otoscope into the client's nostril without touching the sensitive nasal septum.
- Slowly direct the otoscope back and up.
- View the nasal mucosa, nasal septum, the inferior and middle turbinates, and the nasal passage (the narrow space between the septum and the turbinates).

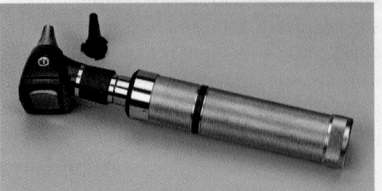

Otoscope with wide-tipped attachment.

ASSESSMENT PROCEDURE	NORMAL FINDINGS	ABNORMAL FINDINGS
Mouth		
Inspect **mouth** for symmetry and alignment while asking client to open and close mouth (Fig. 14-5).	Lips and surrounding tissue relatively symmetrical in net position and with smiling. No lesions, swelling, drooping.	Asymmetrical mouth may indicate neurologic condition (e.g., Bell palsy, stroke), tumors, infections, or dental abnormalities or poorly fitting dentures.
	Upper teeth resting on the top of lower teeth with upper incisors slightly overriding lower ones	Malocclusion of teeth, separation of individual teeth, or protrusion of upper or lower incisors
Wearing gloves, inspect and palpate **lips** for the following (Fig. 14-6): • Consistency, moisture, and color. Check for lesions or ulcers.	Lips are smooth and moist without lesions or swelling. • *In white skin*: Pink • *In dark skin:* May have bluish hue or freckle-like pigmentation	• Dry, cracked lips are seen with dehydration. Pallor around the lips (circumoral pallor) is seen in anemia and shock. Bluish (cyanotic) lips may result from cold or hypoxia. Reddish lips are seen in clients with ketoacidosis, carbon monoxide poisoning, and chronic obstructive pulmonary disease (COPD) with polycythemia. Swelling of the lips (edema) is common in local or systemic allergic or anaphylactic reactions. Lesions or ulcers of the lips are seen with viral infections. **Lip cancer** can occur

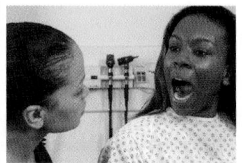

FIGURE 14-5   Inspecting the open mouth.

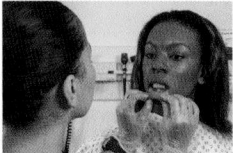

FIGURE 14-6   Palpating the lips.
• Moist, smooth with no lesions

(Continued on following page)

ASSESSMENT PROCEDURE	NORMAL FINDINGS	ABNORMAL FINDINGS
		anywhere but is most common on lower lip. Most lip cancers are squamous cell carcinomas. Cheilosis (cracking in the corners) seen in riboflavin deficiencies; broken vesicles with crusting in herpes simplex type I; scaly nodular lesions or ulcers occur with lip carcinoma (see Abnormal Findings 14-1).
Note: Ask client to remove any dentures or dental appliances before continuing examination.		
Wearing gloves, inspect and palpate **buccal mucosa** for the following (Fig. 14-7):		
• Color 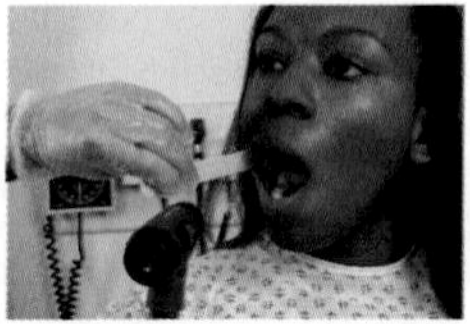 **FIGURE 14-7** Inspecting the buccal mucosa.	• Pink (increased pigmentation often noted in dark-skinned clients)	• Pale, cyanotic, or reddened mucosa

ASSESSMENT PROCEDURE	NORMAL FINDINGS	ABNORMAL FINDINGS
	• Smooth, moist, without lesions	• Ulcers, dry mucosa, bleeding, or white patches are present. Thick, elevated white patches (leukoplakia) that do not scrape off are precancerous; white, curdy patches that scrape off and bleed indicate thrush; red spots over red mucosa (Koplik spots) indicate measles. Canker sores (painful vesicles that erupt) are seen with allergies and stress (see Abnormal Findings 14-1).
• Landmarks	• Parotid duct (Stensen duct) openings are seen as small papillae located near upper second molar	• Elevated, markedly reddened area near upper second molar
Wearing gloves, retract client's lips to inspect and palpate **gums** for the following:		
• Color	• Pink	• Pale, markedly reddened. Swollen gums that bleed are seen with gingivitis; recessed red gums with tooth loss seen with periodontitis (see Abnormal Findings 14-1); bluish-black gum line present in lead poisoning.
• Consistency	• Moist, clearly defined margins	• Dry, edema, ulcers, bleeding, white patches, tenderness

(Continued on following page)

ASSESSMENT PROCEDURE	NORMAL FINDINGS	ABNORMAL FINDINGS
Wearing gloves, inspect and palpate **teeth** for the following: • Number (see Fig. 14-2) • Position and condition • Color	• 32 teeth • Stable fixation, smooth surfaces, and edges • Pearly white and shiny	• Missing teeth • Loose or broken teeth, jagged edges, dental caries • Darkened, brown, or chalky white discoloration. Teeth may be yellow brown in clients who use excessive coffee, tea, tobacco, or fluoride. Chalky white area is seen with beginning cavity.
Inspect protruded **tongue** for the following: • Color, symmetry, and texture	• Pink, moist, papillae present; symmetrical appearance; midline fissures present • *Common variations:* Fissured, geographic tongue (Fig. 14-8A)	• Dry; nodules, ulcers present; papillae or fissures absent; asymmetrical. Deep longitudinal fissures are seen in dehydration; *black hairy tongue* seen with conditions causing hyposalivation, heavy smoking, alcohol intake, use of antibiotics that inhibit

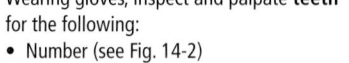

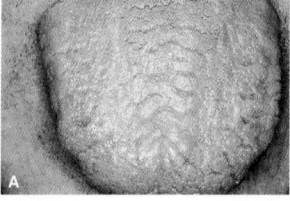

FIGURE 14-8 Normal tongue variations. (**A**) Fissured tongue. (**B**) Fordyce granules. (Part A: Courtesy of Dr. Michael Bennett. Part B: Reprinted with permission from Jensen, S. [2019]. Nursing health assessment: A best practices approach [3rd ed., Fig. 17-16]. Wolters Kluwer.)

ASSESSMENT PROCEDURE	NORMAL FINDINGS	ABNORMAL FINDINGS
	• Fordyce granules (ectopic sebaceous glands) are a common variation seen in the oral cavity. They are yellowish-white papular lesions scattered across the oral mucous membrane of the cheeks, tongue, or lips (Fig. 14-8B).	normal bacteria leading to fungus, use of mouthwashes; also seen with bismuth intake (Pepto-Bismol) (Exodontia.Info, 2019; Mayo Clinic, 2018); smooth, red, shiny tongue seen in niacin or vitamin B_{12} deficiency • Raised whitish feathery areas on sides of tongue that cannot be scraped off suggest hairy leukoplakias seen in HIV infection and AIDS. • See Abnormal Findings 14-1
• Movement • Color	• Smooth • Pink	• Jerky or unilateral movement • Markedly reddened; white patches; pale. • Smokers may have a yellow-brown coating on the tongue, which is not leukoplakia.
Inspect **ventral surface of the tongue and mouth floor** for the following: • Color, consistency, and lesions	• Smooth, shiny, pink, or slightly pale with visible veins and no lesions. • Slightly pale	• Markedly reddened, cyanotic, or extreme pallor, lesions

(Continued on following page)

ASSESSMENT PROCEDURE	NORMAL FINDINGS	ABNORMAL FINDINGS
• Landmarks	• Submandibular duct openings (Wharton ducts) are located on both sides of the frenulum. Tongue is free of lesions or increased redness; frenulum is centered (see Fig. 14-3).	• Lesions, ulcers, nodules, or hypertrophied duct openings are present on either side of the frenulum.
• Size	• Moderate size with papillae (little protuberances) present	• A smooth, reddish, shiny tongue without papillae indicative of niacin or vitamin B_{12} deficiencies, certain anemias, and antineoplastic therapy (Stanford Medicine, 2020; Abnormal Findings 14-1). • An enlarged tongue suggests hypothyroidism, acromegaly, or Down syndrome and angioneurotic edema of anaphylaxis. A very small tongue suggests malnutrition. An atrophied tongue or fasciculations point to cranial nerve (CN) (hypoglossal, CN 12) damage.
Inspect and palpate **sides of tongue** for color and lesions (Fig. 14-9).	Pink, smooth, moist; no lesions	White or reddened areas, ulcerations, or indurations present. Leukoplakia indicates precancerous lesions; may see canker sores (see Abnormal Findings 14-1).

ASSESSMENT PROCEDURE	NORMAL FINDINGS	ABNORMAL FINDINGS
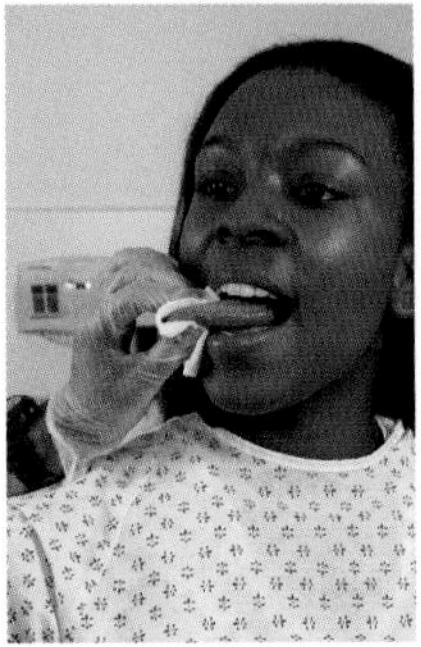 FIGURE 14-9 Inspecting sides of tongue.		
Inspect **hard and soft palates** (see Fig. 14-4) for the following:		
• Color	• *Hard palate:* Pale • *Soft palate:* Pink	• Extreme pallor, white patches, or markedly reddened areas

(Continued on following page)

ASSESSMENT PROCEDURE	NORMAL FINDINGS	ABNORMAL FINDINGS
• Consistency	*Hard palate:* Firm with irregular transverse rugae *Common variation:* Palatine torus (bony protuberance) on hard palate (Fig. 14-10) *Soft palate:* Spongy texture with symmetrical elevation or phonation 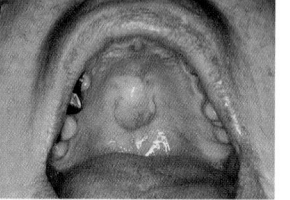 **FIGURE 14-10** Torus palatinus.	• Softened tissue over hard palate; lesions present; absence of elevation; soft palate asymmetrical elevation with phonation. Thick, white plaques are seen in *Candida* infection; deep, purple lesions may indicate Kaposi sarcoma (see Abnormal Findings 14-1).

ASSESSMENT PROCEDURE	NORMAL FINDINGS	ABNORMAL FINDINGS
Throat		
Inspect **oropharynx** (see Fig. 14-11) for the following: • Color • Landmarks 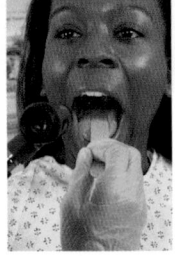 **FIGURE 14-11** Inspecting oropharynx.	 • Pink • Tonsillar pillars symmetrical; tonsils present (unless surgically removed) and without exudate; uvula at midline and rises on phonation	 • Markedly reddened with exudate seen in pharyngitis; yellow mucus seen with postnasal sinus drainage. • Enlarged tonsils (tonsils are red, enlarged, and covered with exudate in tonsillitis); see tonsillitis grading scale in Abnormal Findings 14-2; asymmetrical; uvula deviates from midline; edema, ulcers, lesions.
Nose		
Inspect and palpate the **external nose.** Note nasal color, shape, consistency, and tenderness.	Color same as the rest of the face; smooth and symmetrical structure; no tenderness.	Nasal tenderness on palpation accompanies a local infection.

(Continued on following page)

ASSESSMENT PROCEDURE	NORMAL FINDINGS	ABNORMAL FINDINGS
Check **patency of air flow through the nostrils** by occluding one nostril at a time and asking client to sniff.	Client is able to sniff through each nostril while other is occluded.	Client cannot sniff through a nostril that is occluded nor can they sniff or blow air through the nostrils. May be a sign of swelling, rhinitis, or an obstructing foreign object.
Inspect the **internal nose** using an otoscope with a short, wide-tipped attachment (or you can also use a nasal speculum and penlight) (Fig. 14-12). See Assessment Guide 14-1. 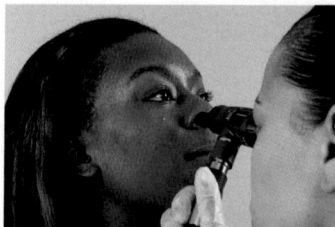 **FIGURE 14-12** Inspecting the internal nose.	Nasal mucosa dark pink, moist, and free of exudate. Nasal septum intact and free of ulcers or perforations. Turbinates dark pink, moist, and free of lesions (Fig. 14-13A). *Note: The superior turbinate will not be visible from this point of view.* A deviated septum may appear to be an overgrowth of tissue. This is a normal finding as long as breathing is not obstructed (Fig. 14-13B).	Nasal mucosa swollen and pale pink or bluish gray in clients with allergies. Nasal mucosa red and swollen with upper respiratory infection. Exudate seen with infections. Purulent nasal discharge seen with acute bacterial rhinosinusitis. Bleeding (epistaxis) or crusting may be noted on lower anterior part of nasal septum with local irritation. Ulcers of the nasal mucosa or a perforated septum may be seen with the use of cocaine, trauma, chronic infection, or chronic nose picking. Small, pale, round, firm overgrowths or masses on mucosa (polyps) seen in clients with chronic allergies (Fig. 14-14).

ASSESSMENT PROCEDURE	NORMAL FINDINGS	ABNORMAL FINDINGS

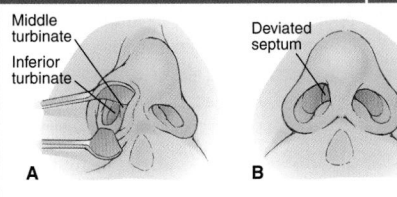

FIGURE 14-13 (A) Normal internal nose. **(B)** Deviated septum.

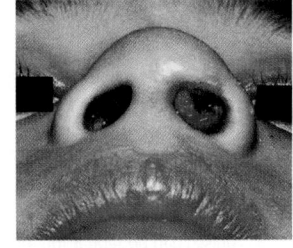

FIGURE 14-14 Nasal polyp.

Sinuses

Palpate the **sinuses.** When an infection is suspected, the nurse can examine the sinuses through palpation, percussion, and transillumination.

Palpate the **frontal sinuses** by using your thumbs to press up on the brow on each side of nose (Fig. 14-15A).

Frontal and maxillary sinuses are nontender to palpation, and no crepitus is evident.

Frontal or maxillary sinuses are tender to palpation in clients with allergies or acute bacterial rhinosinusitis. If the client has a large amount of exudate, you may feel crepitus upon palpation over the maxillary sinuses.

(Continued on following page)

ASSESSMENT PROCEDURE	NORMAL FINDINGS	ABNORMAL FINDINGS
Palpate the **maxillary sinuses** by pressing with thumbs up on the maxillary sinuses (Fig. 14-15B).	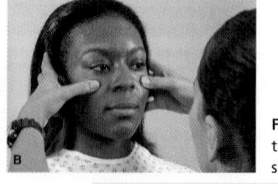 FIGURE 14-15 **(A)** Palpating frontal sinuses. **(B)** Palpating maxillary sinuses.	
Percuss the **sinuses.** Lightly tap (percuss) over the frontal sinuses and over the maxillary sinuses for tenderness.	The sinuses are not tender on percussion.	The frontal and maxillary sinuses are tender upon percussion in clients with allergies or sinus infection.
Transillumination		
Transilluminate the sinuses if sinus tenderness is present to detect the presence of fluid or pus. Transilluminate the frontal sinuses by holding light source snugly under the eyebrows in a dark room. Use other hand to shield the light. Repeat for other frontal sinus. Transilluminate the maxillary sinuses by holding light over maxillary sinus and asking the client to open their mouth. Repeat for the other side.	A red glow transilluminates the frontal sinuses. This indicates a normal, air-filled sinus. A red glow transilluminates the maxillary sinuses. The red glow will be seen on the hard palate.	Absence of a red glow usually indicates a sinus filled with fluid or pus. Absence of a red glow usually indicates a sinus filled with fluid, pus, or thick mucus (from chronic sinusitis).

ABNORMAL FINDINGS   **14-1**   **Mouth and Throat Abnormalities**

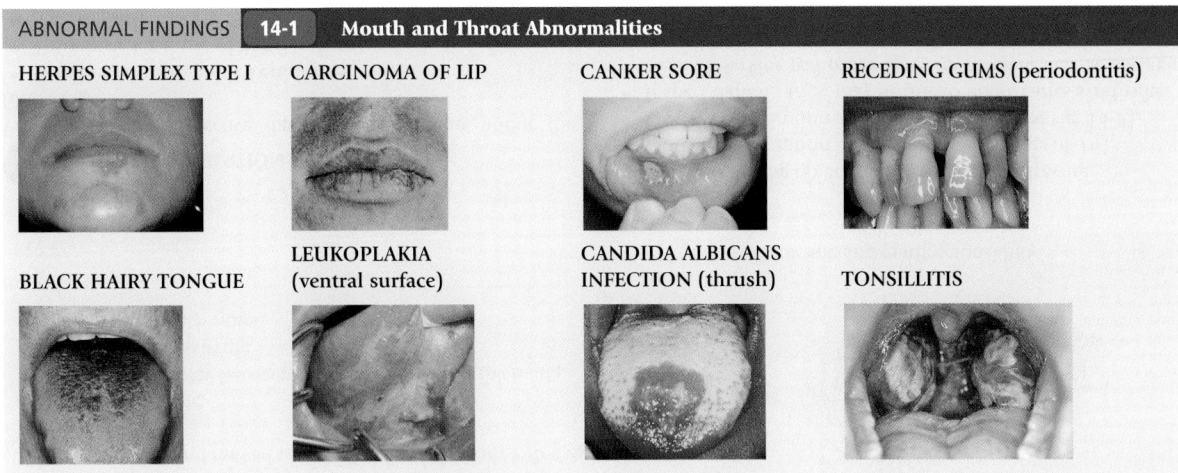

HERPES SIMPLEX TYPE I

CARCINOMA OF LIP

CANKER SORE

RECEDING GUMS (periodontitis)

BLACK HAIRY TONGUE

LEUKOPLAKIA (ventral surface)

CANDIDA ALBICANS INFECTION (thrush)

TONSILLITIS

Photo credits: Black hairy tongue, receding gums, courtesy of Dr. Michael Bennett.

ABNORMAL FINDINGS | **14-2** | **Detecting and Grading Tonsillitis**

In a client who has both tonsils and a sore throat, tonsillitis can be identified and ranked with a grading scale from 1 to 4 as follows:

- Tonsils are visible.
- Tonsils are midway between tonsillar pillars and the uvula.
- Tonsils touch the uvula.
- Tonsils touch each other.

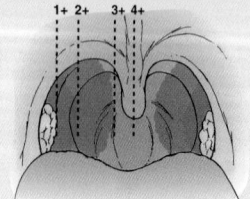

Detecting and grading tonsillitis

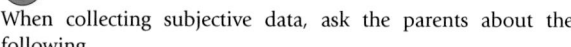 **PEDIATRIC VARIATIONS**

When collecting subjective data, ask the parents about the following.

- Number of teeth, time of eruptions
- Thumb sucking, use of pacifier (type)
- Sore throats
- Use of bottle
- Fluoridated water

When collecting objective data, note the following:

- Observe for eruption of deciduous teeth (Fig. 14-16).
- Observe for eruption of permanent teeth (see Fig. 14-2).
- Inspect dental caries; may be due to bottle caries syndrome.
- Note: *A sucking pad inside upper lip of infant may be apparent due to sucking friction.*
- Tonsils reach adult size by the age of 6 years and continue to grow. By the age of 10 to 12 years, they are twice the adult

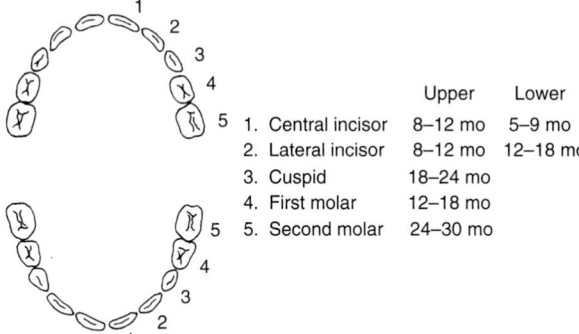

	Upper	Lower
1. Central incisor	8–12 mo	5–9 mo
2. Lateral incisor	8–12 mo	12–18 mo
3. Cuspid	18–24 mo	
4. First molar	12–18 mo	
5. Second molar	24–30 mo	

FIGURE 14-16 Timetable for eruption of deciduous teeth.

size. By the end of adolescence, they begin to atrophy back to normal adult size.

GERIATRIC VARIATIONS

- Worn teeth from prolonged use, abraded enamel, and yellowing teeth.
- Teeth may appear longer as the gums recede, become ischemic, and undergo fibrotic changes, which make the older client more susceptible to periodontal disease and tooth loss.
- Poor fitting dentures may cause facial asymmetry and poor eating habits.
- Oral mucosa is drier owing to decreased production of saliva.
- Tongue may be fissured and have varicose veins on ventral surface.
- Decreased taste sensations due to a decrease in number of taste buds.
- Decreased sense of smell due to progressive atrophy of olfactory bulbs.

CULTURAL VARIATIONS

- Dark-skinned clients:
  - May have lips with bluish hue or freckle-like pigmentation.
  - May have dark pigment or freckling on side or ventral surface of tongue and floor of mouth; hard and soft palate may also be darkly pigmented.
- Tori, both palatinus and mandibular, are normal variations in which there is a bony protuberance in the midline of the hard palate. Tori tend to occur more in Native Americans, Eskimos, Norwegians, and Thais (Cleveland Clinic, 2016).

- Physical variations related to the mouth, nose, and sinuses involve color differences and structures of the uvula, lip, palate, and teeth. Darker-skinned people often develop hyperpigmentation of the buccal mucosa by age 50 (10% of U.S. Whites and 90% of African Americans). Also, a benign leukoedema (grayish-white lesion) occurs on the buccal mucosa of 68% to 90% of African Americans and 43% of Whites (Andrews et al., 2020). This condition can be mistaken for oral thrush or other infection.
- Structure of the uvula varies, and a cleft or partial or completely split uvula is found in 10% of Native Americans and Asians. The highest incidence of cleft lip and palate is seen in Native Americans, followed by Asians, then Whites, and the lowest incidence is seen in African Americans. In addition to ethnicity, older age of the mother correlates with cleft lip and palate (Andrews et al., 2020).
- The number of teeth and their size vary widely. Many tooth variations have little clinical significance, but denser tooth enamel in African Americans makes their teeth less susceptible to dental caries. Periodontal disease is highest among Chinese (Chinese, 39.8%; Blacks, 32%; Whites, 26%; Weatherspoon et al., 2016). Poor oral hygiene increases the risk for periodontal disease. Loss of teeth due to periodontal disease is now highest among non-Hispanic Black adults living in the United States (Andrews et al., 2020).
- Oral diseases are prevalent in poorer populations in developed and developing countries, including dental caries, periodontal disease, tooth loss, oral mucosal and oropharyngeal lesions and cancers, HIV-related diseases, and trauma. The following poor living conditions contribute to developing oral disease: diet; nutrition; hygiene; the use of alcohol, tobacco, and tobacco-related products; and limited oral health care.
- Very high rates of oral cancer (five to six times higher than in the United States) are reported for South Asia, where tobacco mixed with betel nut, lime, spices, perfumes, and other substances are smoked, chewed, and used in South Asian rituals (Niaz et al., 2017).
- Sinusitis is widespread. However, the prevalence is higher in U.S. Whites and African Americans than in Hispanics (Sinuswars, 2012).

POSSIBLE COLLABORATIVE PROBLEMS—RISK OF

- Stomatitis
- Gingivitis
- Oral lesions
- Periodontal (gum) disease (periodontitis)
- Nosebleed

Teaching Tips for Selected Client Concerns and Collaborative Problems

Client Concern: *Unhealthy oral mucous membranes associated with poor oral hygiene practices*

Instruct client on proper brushing and flossing. (Client should brush teeth at least twice a day and floss once a day to remove plaque from under gum line and sides of teeth.)

Recommend a toothbrush with soft, rounded end or polished bristles, to be replaced every 3 to 4 months or sooner when frayed, in addition to an "American Dental Association—accepted" fluoride toothpaste and mouth rinse. Explain the role of fluoride in decreasing tooth decay. Refer to dentist for fluoride protection advice if client's water supply is not fluoridated. Explain the significance of a well-balanced diet in decreasing tooth decay and periodontal (gum) disease. Dry mouth can cause problems with oral health. Refer to dentist or physician for possible recommendation of artificial saliva or fluoride mouth rinse.

Encourage routine dental screenings, including a mouth and throat screening (American Cancer Society [ACS], 2018, 2019; National Cancer Institute, 2020). Regular screening, especially at routine dental examinations, is beneficial, especially for those who are at higher risk, such as those who use tobacco, drink alcohol frequently, have had previous oral cancers, or have had heavy sun exposure.

Collaborative Problem: *Risk for complication: Periodontal (gum) disease*

Teach client warning signs:
- Gums that bleed with brushing
- Red, swollen, tender gums or gums that pull away from teeth
- Pus between teeth and gums
- Loose or separating teeth
- Change in position of teeth or denture fit
- Persistent bad breath

Teach prevention:
- Brush twice daily with soft toothbrush and fluoride toothpaste, and floss every day
- Replace toothbrush every 3 to 4 months, or sooner if bristles are frayed
- Eat a balanced diet and limit between-meal snacks
- Schedule regular dental visits (Healthline Editorial Team, 2019).

***Collaborative Problem:** Risk for Complication: Oral cancer*

Teach client risk factors for oropharyngeal cancer as listed by the ACS (2019): tobacco use (and possibly secondhand smoke); alcohol consumption; frequent and heavy, prolonged sun exposure (cancer of the lip); HPV, especially with oral sex; Gender (men more than women); fair skin (lip); age (especially over 45); poor oral hygiene; poor diet/nutrition (low in fruits and vegetables); weakened immune system; marijuana use; and chewing betel nut and mixtures of betel nut (often used in South and Southeast Asia) (National Cancer Institute, n.d.).

Teach client warning signs of oral cancer:
- Sore in mouth that does not heal
- White scaly patches in mouth
- Swelling or lumps in mouth/in throat/on lips
- Numbness or pain in mouth/in throat/on lips
- Repeated bleeding in mouth
- Difficulty chewing, swallowing, speaking, or moving tongue or jaw
- Change in bite

Teach client to:
- Understand that there *is no safe tobacco use. Spit tobacco (chewing tobacco) leads to gum inflammation, tooth loss, and oral cancer. Cigar smoking leads to mouth, throat, and lung cancer* (Healthy People 2020, 2020).
- Avoid smoking cigarettes or using oral tobacco, or get assistance to stop if smoking or chewing currently.
- Avoid excessive alcohol use, especially if you smoke.
- Avoid chewing betel nuts.
- Avoid infection with HPV, which can be transmitted through oral sex or contact with others who are infected, or seek medical assistance if infection suspected.
- Avoid excessive sun exposure (or tanning booth exposure) to lips. Use adequate sunscreen if unable to avoid sun.
- Eat a diet that is rich in fruits, vegetables, and vitamin A and that is generally well rounded.
- Practice regular oral hygiene, using a soft toothbrush twice per day and dental floss at least once per day, and have routine dental care.
- If you have a weakened immune system, take extra precautions to avoid risks for oral cancer.
- Avoid smoking marijuana, especially if you have any of the other risk factors.

Collaborative Problem: Risk for Complication: Nosebleed

Instruct client to apply pressure for 5 minutes while breathing through mouth and leaning forward. Caution against blowing nose for several hours afterward. Refer a client who experiences frequent nosebleeds for further evaluation.

 Client Concern: Poor development of teeth and gums associated with lack of proper infant and child mouth care

Instruct parents not to put child to bed with a bottle filled with formula, milk, juices, or sugar water, because these liquids pool around teeth and promote decay. Use only water in bottles when putting child to bed, to prevent the so-called *baby bottle tooth decay.* Teach the importance of fluoride in drinking water and proper nutrition to prevent decay. Fluoride drops are recommended for infants, and fluoride tablets for children up to the age of 14 years if adequate fluoride is not in water. Refer child to dentist if thumb sucking continues when permanent teeth begin to erupt. Explain the benefits of using a small, cool spoon rubbed over gums or using teething rings during teething period. Instruct parents to start brushing the child's teeth with eruption of first tooth. Begin flossing when primary teeth have erupted (2–2 1/2 years). Teach parents to brush and floss child's teeth until child can be taught to do this alone (approximately at the age of 7 years for brushing and at the age of 10 years for flossing). Encourage a dental examination by a dentist when the child is between 6 and 12 months of age.

 Client Concern: Risk for oral injury associated with developmental age and play activities

In case of broken or knocked-out tooth, instruct parents to rinse the tooth in cool water (do not scrub it); when possible, insert back in socket and hold in place. If this cannot be done, put tooth in cup of milk or water, or wrap it in wet cloth and take the child to dentist at once for possible replacement. Recommend use of mouth guards to prevent injuries in contact sports.

 Client Concern: Risk for nose injury associated with insertion of foreign bodies into nasal cavity

Caution and give instructions to parents about child's interest in inserting objects into body openings such as the nose. Instruct on common objects to remove from child's reach.

Client Concern: *Explore food preferences with older client and use visual appeal of food to enhance appetite. Use of lemons may help restore the sense of smell and taste by fighting bacterial and viral infections, thus making the nasal passage clear. Mixing lemon juice and honey in a glass of water may help. Using fresher spices can increase flavor in food. Encourage client to stay hydrated. Artificial saliva products may also help in some cases. Encourage brightly colored vegetables like carrots, sweet potatoes, broccoli, and tomatoes. Also, if their diet allows, flavor food with a little butter, olive oil, cheese, nuts, or fresh herbs like sage, thyme, or rosemary. Poor nutrition associated with decreased appetite secondary to decreased senses of taste and smell secondary to aging, especially after age 60, nasal and sinus problems such as allergies, sinusitis or nasal polyps, and/or use of certain medications including beta-blockers and angiotensin-converting enzyme (ACE).*

◎ CLINICAL TIP
A loss of smell and taste may be an indication that the person is a carrier of COVID-19 and other viruses before any symptoms appear (Bienkov, 2020).

References

American Cancer Society. (2018). *Can oral cavity and oropharyngeal cancers be found early?* https://www.cancer.org/cancer/oral-cavity-and-oropharyngeal-cancer/detection-diagnosis-staging/detection.html

American Cancer Society. (2019). *Oral and oropharyngeal cancer: Screening.* https://www.cancer.net/cancer-types/oral-and-oropharyngeal-cancer/screening

Andrews, M., Boyle, J., & Collins, J. (2020). *Transcultural concepts in nursing care* (8th ed.). Wolters Kluwer.

Bienkov, A. (2020). *If you've lost your sense of smell or taste, you could be a 'hidden carrier' of the coronavirus.* https://www.businessinsider.com/coronavirus-symptoms-loss-of-smell-taste-covid-19-anosmia-hyposmia-2020-3

Cleveland Clinic. (2016). *Bony bumps in the mouth.* https://consultqd.clevelandclinic.org/bony-bumps-in-the-mouth/

Exodontia.Info. (2019). *Black hairy tongue. Lingua villosa nigra.* http://www
.exodontia.info/Black_Hairy_Tongue.html

Healthline Editorial Team. (2019). *Gum disease (gingivitis or periodontitis).* https://www.healthline.com/health/gingivitis#associated-health-conditions

Healthy People 2020. (2020). *Oral health.* https://www.healthypeople
.gov/2020/topics-objectives/topic/oral-health

Mayo Clinic. (2018). *Black hairy tongue.* https://www.mayoclinic.org/
diseases-conditions/black-hairy-tongue/symptoms-causes/syc-20356077

National Cancer Institute. (n.d.). *Betel quid with tobacco.* https://www
.cancer.gov/publications/dictionaries/cancer-terms/def/betel-quid-with-tobacco

National Cancer Institute. (2020). *Oral cavity, pharyngeal, and laryngeal cancer screening (PDQ®) Health professional version.* https://www.cancer.gov/
types/head-and-neck/hp/oral-screening-pdq

Niaz, K., Maqbool, F., Khan, F., Bahadar, H., Hassan, F., & Abdullahi, M.
(2017). Smokeless tobacco (*paan* and *gutkha*), consumption, prevalence, and contribution to oral cancer. *Epidemiological Health, 39,* e2017009. https://doi.org/10.4178/epih.e2017009

Sinuswars. (2012). *People that may be prone to developing sinusitis.* http://
www.sinuswars.com/archive/ProneToDevelopingSinusitis.asp

Stanford Medicine. (2020). *Technique of the tongue exam.* https://
stanfordmedicine25. stanford.edu/the25/tongue.html

Weatherspoon, D., Borrell, L., Johnson, C., Mujahid, M., Neighbors, H., &
Adar, S. (2016). Racial and ethnic differences in self-reported periodontal disease in the multi-ethnic study of atherosclerosis (MESA). *Oral Health and Preventive Dentistry, 14*(3), 249–257. https://doi
.org/10.3290/j.ohpd.a35614

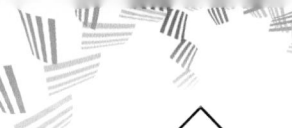

15 ASSESSING THORAX AND LUNGS

Structure and Function Overview

THORAX

The term *thorax* identifies the portion of the body extending from the base of the neck superiorly to the level of the diaphragm inferiorly. This thoracic cage is constructed of the sternum, 12 pairs of ribs, 12 thoracic vertebrae, muscles, and cartilage. The thorax consists of the anterior thoracic cage (Fig. 15-1) and the posterior thoracic cage (Fig. 15-2).

The sternum, or breastbone, lies in the center of the chest anteriorly and is divided into three parts: the manubrium, the body, and the xiphoid process. The clavicles (collar bones) extend from the manubrium to the acromion of the scapula. The manubrium connects laterally with the clavicles and the first two pairs of ribs. A U-shaped indentation located on the superior border of the manubrium is an important landmark known as the *suprasternal notch*. A few centimeters below the suprasternal notch, a bony ridge can be palpated at the point where the manubrium articulates with the body of the sternum. This landmark is referred to as the *sternal angle* (or angle of Louis).

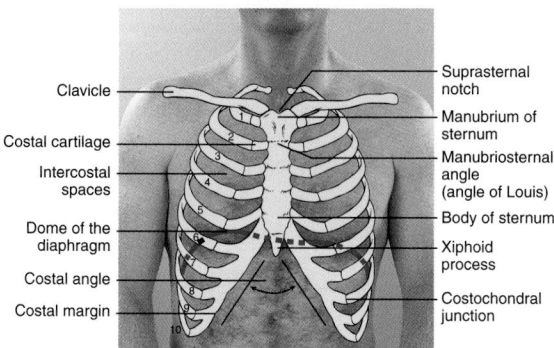

FIGURE 15-1 Anterior thoracic cage.

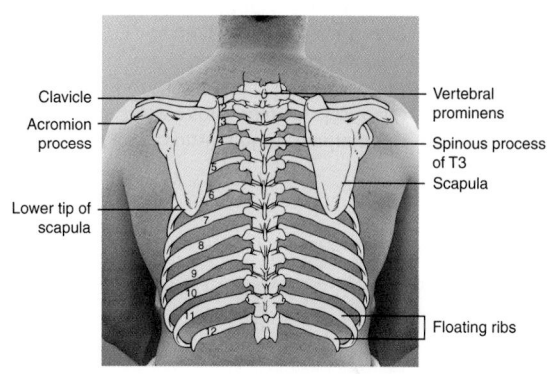

FIGURE 15-2 Posterior thoracic cage.

Ribs (7–10) connect to the cartilages of the pair lying superior to them rather than to the sternum (see Fig. 15-1). This configuration forms an angle between the right and left costal margins meeting at the level of the xiphoid process, referred to as the *costal angle.*

Each pair of ribs articulates with its respective thoracic vertebra. The spinous process of the seventh cervical vertebra (C7), also called

the *vertebra prominens,* can be easily felt with the client's neck flexed. The lower tip of each scapula is at the level of the seventh or eighth rib when the client's arms are at their side (see Fig. 15-2).

To describe a location around the circumference of the chest wall, imaginary lines running vertically on the chest wall are used. On the anterior chest, these lines are known as the *midsternal line* and the *right and left midclavicular lines* (Fig. 15-3A).

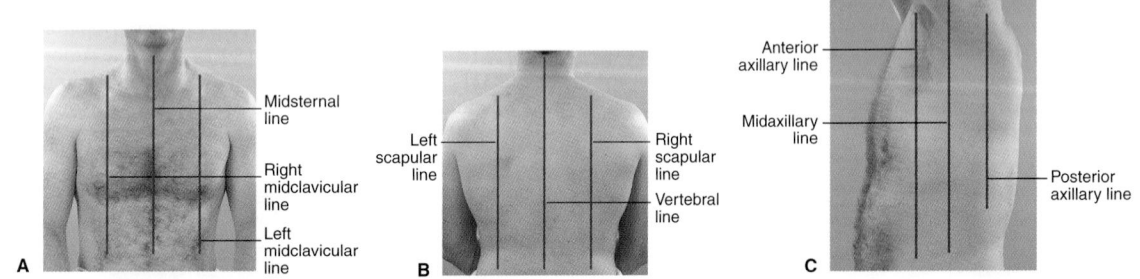

FIGURE 15-3 **(A)** Anterior vertical lines, imaginary landmarks. **(B)** Posterior vertical lines, imaginary landmarks. **(C)** Lateral vertical lines, imaginary landmarks.

The posterior thorax includes the vertebral (or spinal) line and the right and left scapular lines, which extend through the inferior angle of the scapulae when the arms are at the client's side (Fig. 15-3B).

The lateral aspect of the thorax is divided into three parallel lines. The *midaxillary line* runs from the apex of the axillae to the level of the 12th rib. The *anterior axillary line* extends from the anterior axillary fold along the anterolateral aspect of the thorax, whereas the *posterior axillary line* runs from the posterior axillary fold down the posterolateral aspect of the chest wall (Fig. 15-3C).

THORACIC CAVITY

The thoracic cavity consists of the mediastinum and the lungs.

The lungs are two cone-shaped, elastic structures suspended within the thoracic cavity. The *apex* of each lung extends slightly above the clavicle, whereas the *base* is at the level of the diaphragm. At the point of the midclavicular line on the anterior surface of the thorax, the lung extends to approximately the sixth rib. Laterally, lung tissue reaches the level of the eighth rib, and, posteriorly, the lung base is at about the tenth rib (Fig. 15-4).

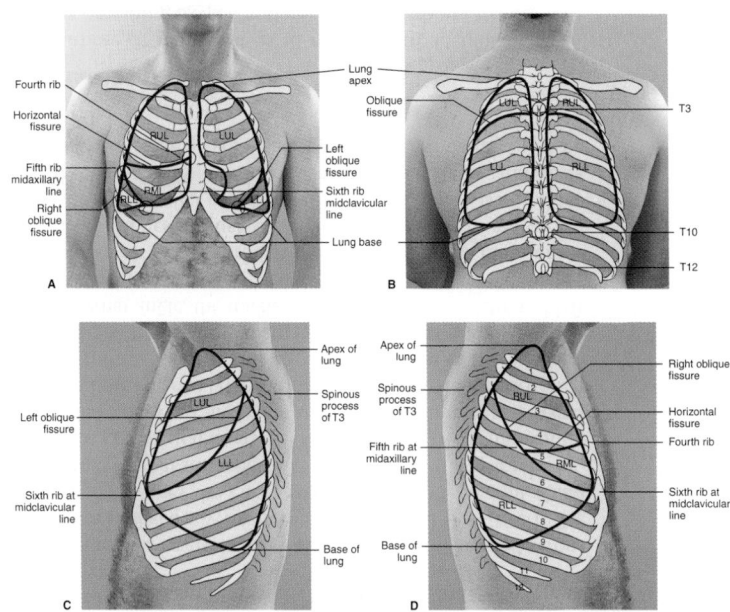

FIGURE 15-4 (**A**) Anterior view of lung position. (**B**) Posterior view of lung position. (**C**) Lateral view of left lung position. (**D**) Lateral view of right lung position. LLL, left lower lobe; LUL, left upper lobe; RLL, right lower lobe; RML, right middle lobe; RUL, right upper lobe.

The thoracic cavity is lined by a thin, double-layered serous membrane collectively referred to as the *pleura* (Fig. 15-5). The *parietal pleura* lines the chest cavity, whereas the *visceral pleura* covers the external surfaces of the lungs. The *pleural space* lies between the two pleural layers. In the healthy adult, the lubricating serous fluid between the layers allows movement of the visceral layer over the parietal layer during ventilation without friction.

The trachea lies anterior to the esophagus and is approximately 10 to 12 cm long in an adult (see Fig. 15-5). At the level of the sternal angle, the trachea bifurcates into the right and left main bronchi.

Inspired air travels through the trachea into the main bronchi and continues through the system as the bronchi repeatedly bifurcate into smaller passageways known as *bronchioles*. Eventually, the bronchioles terminate at the alveolar ducts, and air is channeled into the alveolar sacs, which contain the alveoli (see Fig. 15-5).

MECHANICS OF BREATHING

The purpose of respiration is to maintain an adequate oxygen level by providing oxygen and eliminating carbon dioxide. Ventilation is the mechanical act of breathing accomplished by

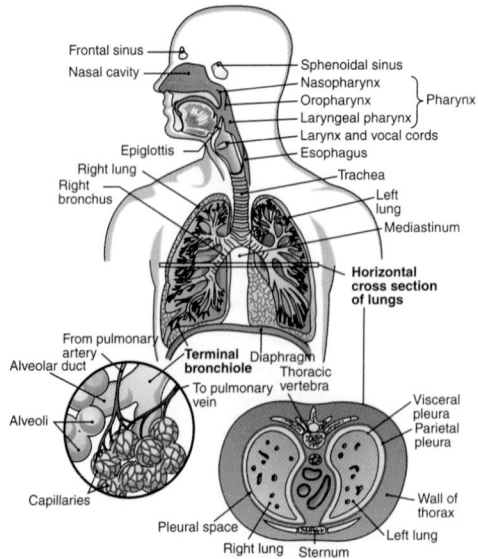

FIGURE 15-5   Major structures of the respiratory system.

expansion of the chest, both vertically and horizontally. Vertical expansion is accomplished through contraction of the diaphragm. Horizontal expansion occurs as the intercostal muscles lift the sternum and elevate the ribs, resulting in an increase in anteroposterior (AP) diameter. As the chest cavity enlarges, a slight negative pressure is created in the lungs, causing air to flow into the lungs called **inspiration. Expiration** is mostly passive occurring as the intercostal muscles and the diaphragm relax. As the diaphragm relaxes, it assumes a domed shape, decreasing the chest cavity size and creating a positive pressure, forcing air out of the lungs.

Nursing Assessment

COLLECTING SUBJECTIVE DATA

Interview Questions

Difficulty breathing? Timing? Associated factors? Precipitating factors? Relieving factors? Difficulty breathing when sleeping? Use of more than one pillow to sleep? Snoring? Coughing (productive, nonproductive)? Sputum (type, amount, color)? Allergies? Dyspnea or shortness of breath (at rest or on exertion)? If yes, have client use self-assessment tool at https://www.copdfoundation .org/downloads/COPD_PDF_Screener.pdf; this tool will help determine the client's risk level for chronic obstructive pulmonary disease (COPD) and need for a referral. Scores of 5 to 10 indicate a high risk of COPD, whereas scores of 0 to 4 indicate a low risk of COPD. Chest pain*? Location, timing? Associated factors? Precipitating factors? Relieving factors? History of asthma, bronchitis, emphysema, tuberculosis? Exposure to environmental inhalants (chemicals, fumes)? History of smoking (amount and length of time)? Efforts to quit? Travel to high-risk areas such as Mainland China; Hong Kong; Hanoi, Vietnam; Singapore; or Toronto, Canada? (Travel to these locations may have exposed the client to severe acute respiratory syndrome (SARS) or COVID-19.)

Risk Factors

Risk for respiratory disease related to smoking, immobilization or sedentary lifestyle, aging, environmental exposures, and morbid obesity; risk for lung cancer related to cigarette smoking and genetic predisposition, asbestos, or radon exposure.

---

*Immediately assess any reports of chest pain further to determine if the pain is due to cardiac ischemia, which is a medical emergency that requires immediate assessment and intervention. If not treated immediately, a lack of oxygen to the heart leads to damage and eventual death of heart muscle.

COLLECTING OBJECTIVE DATA

Equipment Needed

- Examination gown and drape
- Gloves and mask if indicated
- Stethoscope
- Tape measure with centimeters
- Marking pen
- Light source

Physical Assessment

Review Figures 15-1 to 15-5 for anatomy of the thorax and lungs. Expose anterior, posterior, and lateral chest with client in sitting position. Locate landmarks (see Fig. 15-3). Drape anterior chest and use finger pads or palms to palpate posterior chest. Have client fold arms across anterior chest and lean forward to increase area of lungs. First palpate, percuss, and auscultate the posterior lungs and thorax while the client is sitting. Then palpate, percuss, and auscultate lateral lungs and thorax while the client is in the supine position.

INSPECTION

ASSESSMENT PROCEDURE	NORMAL FINDINGS	ABNORMAL FINDINGS
Inspect anterior, posterior, and lateral thorax for the following: • Color • Intercostal spaces • Chest symmetry • Rib slope • Respiration patterns (rate, rhythm, depth)	• Pink • Even and relaxed • Equal • <90 degrees downward • Even, 14–20 per minute, unlabored ᗺᗺᗺᗺ	• Pallor, cyanosis • Bulging, retracting • Unequal • Horizontal or ≥90 degrees • Uneven, labored, <12 per minute or >20 per minute, shallow, deep. See Abnormal Findings 15-1 for altered respiration patterns.

ASSESSMENT PROCEDURE	NORMAL FINDINGS	ABNORMAL FINDINGS
• AP to lateral diameter	• 1:2 ratio (Fig. 15-6) 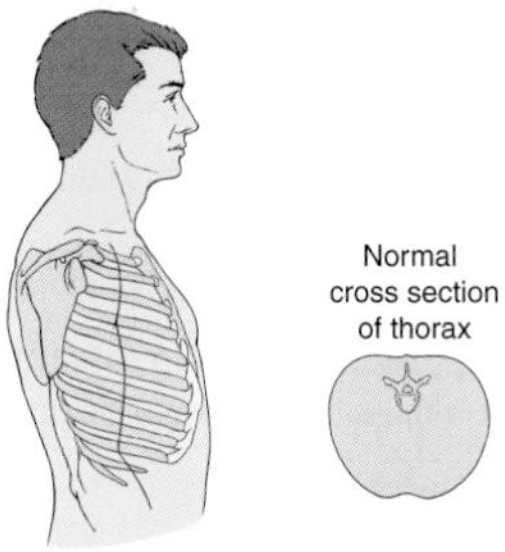 FIGURE 15-6 Cross section of thorax.	• >1:2 ratio (barrel chest seen in emphysema; Fig. 15-7) or <1:2 ratio 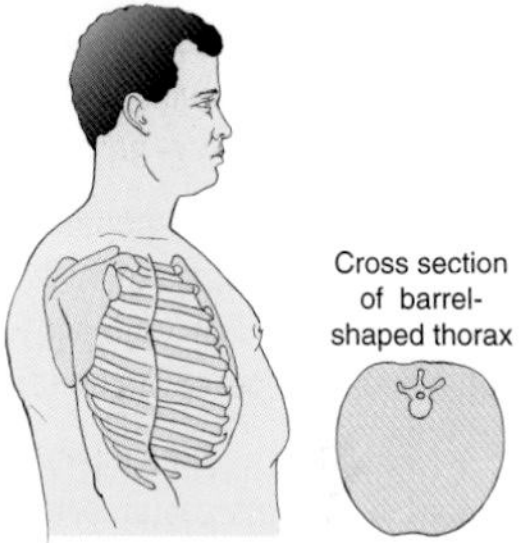 FIGURE 15-7 Cross section of barrel-shaped thorax.
• Shape and position of sternum • Position of trachea • Chest expansion	• Level with ribs • Midline • 7.6 cm (3 in.) with deep inspiration	• Depressed or projecting • Deviated to one side • <7.6 cm (3 in.) with deep inspiration. Decreased chest excursion is seen with COPD.

(Continued on following page)

PALPATION		
ASSESSMENT PROCEDURE	**NORMAL FINDINGS**	**ABNORMAL FINDINGS**
Palpate thorax at three levels for the following:		
• Sensation	• No pain or tenderness	• Pain, tenderness. Pain over thorax is seen with inflamed fibrous connective tissue; pain over intercostal area is seen with inflamed pleura.
• Vocal fremitus as client says "99"	• Vibration decreased over periphery of lungs and increased over major airways	• Vibration increased over lung with consolidation; vibration decreased over airway with obstruction, pleural effusion, or pneumothorax
Palpate thorax for thoracic expansion by the following methods:	5.08–7.62 cm (2–3 in.) symmetrical thoracic expansion	Less than 5.08–7.62 cm (2–3 in.) thoracic expansion; asymmetrical expansion seen with atelectasis or pneumonia.
• Place hands on posterior thorax at level of 10th vertebra. Gently press skin between thumbs and have client take deep breath. Observe thumb movement (Fig. 15-8A).	• Symmetrical expansion (thumbs move apart equal distance in both directions)	• Asymmetrical expansion (thumb movement apart is unequal)
• Anteriorly, press skin together at lower sternum and have client take deep breath. Observe thumb movement (Fig. 15-8B).	• Symmetrical expansion (thumbs move apart equal distance in both directions)	• Asymmetrical expansion (thumb movement apart is unequal)

ASSESSMENT PROCEDURE	NORMAL FINDINGS	ABNORMAL FINDINGS

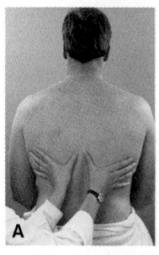 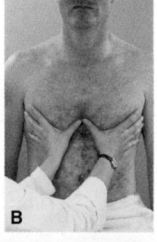

FIGURE 15-8 Palpation of thoracic expansion. (**A**) Posterior. (**B**) Anterior (Photo by B. Proud).

PERCUSSION

ASSESSMENT PROCEDURE	NORMAL FINDINGS	ABNORMAL FINDINGS
Use mediate percussion over shoulder apices and intercostal spaces. Compare both for symmetry of percussion notes, while moving from apex to base of lungs (see Fig. 15-9).		
Percuss over shoulder apices and at posterior, anterior, and lateral intercostal spaces as illustrated (see Fig. 15-9A, B). See Figure 15-4 to determine which lung areas are being percussed.	Resonance (Fig. 15-9C,D)	Hyperresonance is heard over emphysematous lungs; dullness heard over solid masses or fluid, (e.g., in lobar pneumonia, pleural effusion, or tumor).

(Continued on following page)

ASSESSMENT PROCEDURE	NORMAL FINDINGS	ABNORMAL FINDINGS

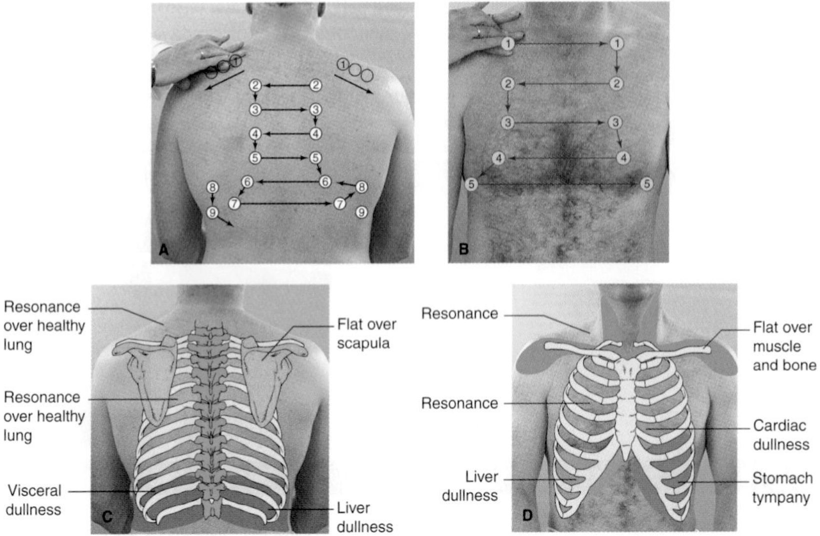

FIGURE 15-9 Intercostal landmarks for percussion and auscultation of thorax. (**A**) Posterior. (**B**) Anterior. (**C**) Normal percussive notes (posterior). (**D**) Normal percussive notes (anterior).

PERCUSSION (continued)		
ASSESSMENT PROCEDURE	**NORMAL FINDINGS**	**ABNORMAL FINDINGS**
Percuss for posterior, diaphragmatic excursions bilaterally (Fig. 15-10).	Diaphragm descends 3–6 cm from T10 (with full expiration held) to T12 (with full inspiration held).	Diaphragm descends <3 cm owing to atelectasis of lower lobes, emphysema, ascites, or tumors.

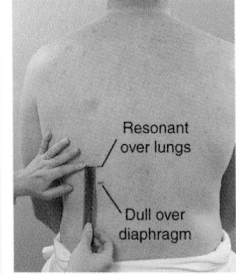

Resonant over lungs

Dull over diaphragm

FIGURE 15-10 Percussing bilaterally for diaphragmatic excursions.

AUSCULTATION

Using diaphragm of stethoscope, exert firm pressure over intercostal space. Instruct client to take slow, deep breaths through the mouth. Listen for two full breaths and compare symmetrical sides of thorax while moving stethoscope from apex to base of lungs.

(Continued on following page)

ASSESSMENT PROCEDURE	NORMAL FINDINGS	ABNORMAL FINDINGS
Auscultate breath sounds over the following: • Trachea 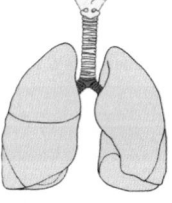	• Bronchial (loud, tubular) breath sounds heard over trachea; expiration longer than inspiration; short silence between inspiration and expiration. Bronchial breath sounds	• Bronchial sounds heard over lung periphery.
• Large-stem bronchi	• Bronchovesicular breath sounds heard over main-stem bronchi: Below clavicles and between scapulae (inspiratory phase equal to expiratory phase). 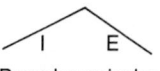Bronchovesicular breath sounds	• Bronchovesicular breath sounds heard over lung periphery.

ASSESSMENT PROCEDURE	NORMAL FINDINGS	ABNORMAL FINDINGS
• Lung periphery	• Vesicular (low, soft, breezy) breath sounds heard over lung periphery (inspiration longer than expiration).	• Decreased breath sounds with obstruction, pleural thickening, pleural effusion, or pneumothorax.
Auscultate breath sounds for adventitious sounds (crackles, wheezes). If an abnormal sound is heard, ask client to cough. Note if adventitious sound is still present or if it cleared with cough.	Lungs clear to auscultation on inspiration and expiration.	Crackles, wheezes, and pleural friction rubs are described in Abnormal Findings 15-2.
Auscultate for altered voice sounds over lung periphery where any previous lung abnormality is noted.		
• Bronchophony (client says "99" while examiner auscultates).	• Sounds muffled and indistinct	• Sounds loud and clear over consolidation from pneumonia, atelectasis, or tumor.
• Whispered pectoriloquy (client whispers "one, two, three" while examiner auscultates).	• Sounds muffled, faint, and indistinct	• Sounds loud and clear over areas of consolidation.
• Egophony (client says "ee" while examiner auscultates).	• Sounds like muffled long "e"	• Sounds like "ay" over areas of consolidation or compression.

ABNORMAL FINDINGS	15-1	**Altered Respiration Patterns**	
Type	Description	Pattern	Clinical Indication
Tachypnea	>24 per minute and shallow	⋀⋀⋀⋀⋀⋀	May be a normal response to fever, anxiety, or exercise.
			Can occur with respiratory insufficiency, alkalosis, pneumonia, or pleurisy.
Bradypnea	<10 per minute and regular	⋀_⋀_⋀	May be normal in well-conditioned athletes.
			Can occur with medication-induced depression of the respiratory center, diabetic coma, or neurologic damage.
Hyperventilation	Increased rate and increased depth	⋀⋀⋀⋀⋀⋀⋀	Usually occurs with extreme exercise, fear, or anxiety.
			Kussmaul respiration is a type of hyperventilation associated with diabetic ketoacidosis. Other causes of hyperventilation include disorders of the central nervous system, an overdose of the drug salicylate, or severe anxiety.

Hypoventilation	Decreased rate, decreased depth, irregular pattern		Usually associated with overdose of narcotics or anesthetics.
Cheyne–Stokes respiration	Regular pattern characterized by alternating periods of deep, rapid breathing followed by periods of apnea		May result from severe congestive heart failure, drug overdose, increased intracranial pressure, or renal failure. May be noted in older adults during sleep, not related to any disease process.
Biot respiration	Irregular pattern characterized by varying depth and rate of respirations followed by periods of apnea		May be seen with meningitis or severe brain damage.

ABNORMAL FINDINGS	15-2	Adventitious Breath Sounds		
Abnormal Sound		**Characteristics**	**Source**	**Associated Conditions**
Discontinuous Sounds				
Crackles (fine)		High-pitched, short, popping sounds heard during inspiration and not cleared with coughing; sounds are discontinuous and can be simulated by rolling a strand of hair between your fingers near your ear.	Inhaled air suddenly opens the small deflated air passages that are coated and sticky with exudate.	Crackles occurring late in inspiration are associated with restrictive diseases such as pneumonia and congestive heart failure. Crackles occurring early in inspiration are associated with obstructive disorders such as bronchitis, asthma, or emphysema.
Crackles (coarse)		Low-pitched, bubbling, moist sounds that may persist from early inspiration to early expiration; also described as softly separating Velcro.	Inhaled air comes into contact with secretions in the large bronchi and trachea.	May indicate pneumonia, pulmonary edema, and pulmonary fibrosis. "Velcro rales" of pulmonary fibrosis are heard louder and closer to stethoscope, usually do not change location, and are more common in clients with long-term COPD.

Continuous Sounds
Pleural friction rub

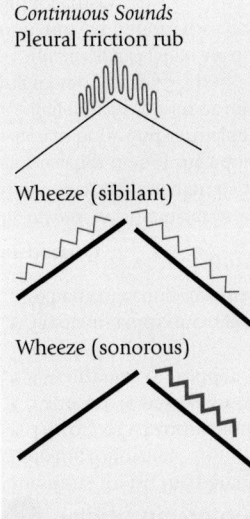

	Low-pitched, dry, grating sound; sound is much like crackles, only more superficial and occurring during both inspiration and expiration.	Sound is the result of rubbing of two inflamed pleural surfaces.	Pleuritis
Wheeze (sibilant)	High-pitched, musical sounds heard primarily during expiration but may also be heard on inspiration.	Air passes through constricted passages (caused by swelling, secretions, or tumor).	Sibilant wheezes are often heard in cases of acute asthma or chronic emphysema.
Wheeze (sonorous)	Low-pitched snoring or moaning sounds heard primarily during expiration but may be heard throughout the respiratory cycle. These wheezes may clear with coughing.	Same as sibilant wheeze. The pitch of the wheeze cannot be correlated with the size of the passageway that generates it.	Sonorous wheezes are often heard in cases of bronchitis or single obstructions and snoring before an episode of sleep apnea. *Stridor* is a harsh honking wheeze with severe broncholaryngospasm, such as occurs with croup.

PEDIATRIC VARIATIONS

Questions to ask the parents when collecting *subjective data* include the following.

- History of wheezing, asthma, or other breathing problems?
- Exposure to passive smoke?
- Occurrence of sudden infant death syndrome (SIDS) in family?
- Frequent colds or congestion?

When collecting *objective data*, note the following.

Inspection

In infants, AP diameter is equal to transverse diameter (1:1)—shape is nearly circular. By the age of 5 to 6 years, the AP diameter reaches that of the adult 1:2 or 5:7 ratio. Chest wall is thin, whereas bony and cartilaginous rib cage is soft and pliant.

Respirations should be unlabored and quiet; rate varies according to age (Table 15-1).

Infants and children are diaphragmatic breathers (with inspiration and expiration, the chest and abdominal walls will rise and fall together).

TABLE 15-1   Respiratory Rates in Children

Age	Normal Respiratory Rate (breaths/minute)
Infant	25–55
Toddler	20–30
Preschooler	20–25
School age	14–26
Adolescent	12–20

Adapted with permission from Kyle, T., & Carman, S. (2021). *Essentials of pediatric nursing* (4th ed., Table 10.3). Wolters Kluwer.

Infants have irregular respiratory patterns. As the infant gets older, the infant will develop a regular rhythm. Use of accessory muscles, nasal flaring, and grunting is not normal in the infant or child.

Percussion

In infants and young children, findings are normally hyperresonant throughout because of thinness of chest wall. Any decrease in resonance is equal to dullness in the adult.

Auscultation

Use the bell or small diaphragm to localize findings, especially in infants and young children. Breath sounds will be louder and harsher owing to close proximity to origin of sounds from thin chest wall. Adventitious lung sounds are not normal in the infant or child. Excessive secretions in the nose and pharynx may transmit noise to this area when auscultating the lungs. Attempt to clear this by having the child cough, clear the throat, or have the nurse suction the child to clear excessive secretions in the upper airway. Repeat auscultation of the lungs following this.

 GERIATRIC VARIATIONS

- Increase in normal respiratory rate (16–25 breaths/min)
- Loss of elasticity, fewer functional capillaries, and loss of lung resiliency
- Decreased ability to cough effectively due to weaker muscles and rigid thoracic wall
- Accentuated dorsal curve (kyphosis) of thoracic spine
- Sternum and ribs may be more prominent owing to loss of subcutaneous fat
- Decreased thoracic expansion due to calcification of costal cartilages and loss of the accessory musculature
- Increased diaphragmatic breathing due to anatomic changes
- Hyperresonance of thorax due to age-related emphysemic changes
- Decreased breath sounds and increased retention of mucus due to decreased pulmonary function
- Increased AP diameter (up to 5:7 AP-to-transverse diameter ratio) due to loss of resiliency and loss of skeletal muscle strength

 CULTURAL VARIATIONS

- Thoracic cavity size varies among cultural groups. Although there are definite differences in thorax size across ethnic groups, thorax size does not account for ethnic differences in lung function. Ethnic lung function differences are still being investigated (Saad et al., 2017).
- Cyanosis in dark-skinned people does not necessarily appear as bluish skin, but may appear as dullness or lifelessness of the perioral, conjunctival, and nail bed areas.
- Histoplasmosis, a systemic fungal disease, is common throughout the world, but in the United States, it is most common in the soils of the central and eastern states, especially around the Ohio and Mississippi River valleys (Centers for Disease Control and Prevention [CDC], 2018).

- Lung cancer is the second leading cause of cancer death in the United States for both males and females (American Cancer Society [ACS], 2020). Lung cancer consists of two types: small cell lung cancer (SCLC) and non–small cell lung cancer (NSCLC). SCLC accounts for 13% of cases, and NSCLC for 84% of cases. Black men and women are more likely to develop and die of lung cancer than White, Hispanic, or Asian men and women, although their exposure to cigarette smoke is lower (American Lung Association [ALA], 2020).

POSSIBLE COLLABORATIVE PROBLEMS—RISK OF

- Respiratory insufficiency/failure
- Pneumonia
- Pulmonary edema
- Airway obstruction/atelectasis
- Laryngeal edema
- Pleural effusion
- Atelectasis
- Asthma
- COPD
- Oxygen toxicity
- Carbon dioxide toxicity
- Pneumothorax
- Respiratory acidosis
- Respiratory alkalosis
- Tracheal necrosis
- Tracheobronchial
- Constriction

Teaching Tips for Selected Client Concerns

Client Concern: *Opportunity to improve respiratory health associated with client questions regarding improving respiratory health*

Encourage client to participate in a daily exercise program and to eat a healthy, low-cholesterol diet with adequate vitamin E and lutein. Provide client with information on the risks of secondhand smoke and how to decrease one's exposure. Encourage client not to start smoking and to limit exposure to air pollution and dangerous substances. The Indoor Air Quality Information Clearinghouse list of hotlines can be accessed at https://www.epa.gov/home/epa-hotlines.

 Client Concern: *Poor airway clearance and decreased oxygenation associated with shallow coughing, thickened mucus, and chronic lung damage*

Instruct client on effective deep breathing and coughing. Encourage liquid intake of 2 to 3 quarts/day. Caution client to use protective measures to prevent spread of infections.

Teach client diaphragmatic and pursed-lip breathing.

Provide literature on environmental control. Assess whether client has equipment to deal with emergencies (e.g., asthma inhaler, adrenaline kit). If allergy is produced by unknown food, assist client with keeping a diary of allergy attacks to determine cause.

Client Concern: *Poor gas exchange associated with smoking and/or frequent exposure to air pollution or dangerous substances*

Explain effects of smoking and how it is a primary risk factor for lung cancer. Assess client's desire to quit and refer to community agencies for self-help on smoking cessation programs. Discuss alternate methods of coping. Encourage wearing of mask if job requires exposure to dangerous inhalants.

 Client Concern: *Poor ventilation associated with bronchospasm and increased pulmonary secretions*

Postural drainage and percussion may be used with children of various ages. Teach parents safety measures when using vaporizers. Teach alternate ways of humidifying air. For example, have parent run hot water in shower and close bathroom door. Sit with child in this room for approximately 10 minutes to liquefy secretions by steam (child must not be left alone in room). For spastic, croupy cough, nighttime exposure to cold air outdoors is beneficial. *If child has asthma:* The number of asthma attacks should decrease over time as the child gets older. Assist parents with letting the child have more independence and avoiding overprotection. However, the child and parent must understand that an asthma attack can be an emergent situation if not controlled in a timely manner. Teach family how to decrease allergens (e.g., dust) in home by using smooth surfaces that are easy to clean.

 Client Concern: *Poor gas exchange of oxygen and/or carbon dioxide associated with poor muscle tone and decreased capacity to remove secretions secondary to direct pulmonary inefficiencies or decreased cardiac output to the lungs*

Teach client to inhale and relax stomach muscles, feeling their belly expand as their lungs fill with air. Encourage elderly to keep breathing in until they feel their chest expand with a deep breath. Hold the breath for a moment and exhale slowly, pulling belly in to feel the last bit of air leaving the lungs. Explain the importance of mobility and exercise to maintain adequate respiratory hygiene. Encourage client to discuss getting a yearly flu shot with their primary care provider.

References

American Cancer Society. (2020). *Key statistics for lung cancer.* https://www.cancer.org/cancer/lung-cancer/about/key-statistics.html

American Lung Association. (2020). *Lung cancer fact sheet.* https://www.lung.org/lung-health-diseases/lung-disease-lookup/lung-cancer/resource-library/lung-cancer-fact-sheet

Centers for Disease Control and Prevention. (2018). *Histoplasmosis.* https://www.cdc.gov/fungal/diseases/histoplasmosis/index.html

Saad, N., Patel, J., Minelli, C., & Burney, P. (2017). Explaining ethnic disparities in lung function among young adults: A pilot investigation. *PLoS ONE, 12*(6), e0178962. https://doi.org/10.1371/journal.pone.0178962

ASSESSING BREASTS AND LYMPHATIC SYSTEM

16

Structure and Function

The breasts are paired mammary glands that lie over the muscles of the anterior chest wall, anterior to the pectoralis major and serratus anterior muscles (Fig. 16-1). The male and female breasts are similar until puberty, when female breast tissue enlarges in response to hormones.

For assessment purposes, the breasts are divided into *four quadrants* by drawing horizontal and vertical imaginary lines that intersect at the nipple (Fig. 16-2).

The skin of the breasts is smooth and varies in color. The nipple contains the tiny openings of the *lactiferous ducts.* The areola surrounds the nipple and contains elevated sebaceous glands (*Montgomery glands*).

Female breasts consist of three types of tissue: glandular, fibrous, and fatty (adipose; Fig. 16-3). The amount of glandular, fibrous, and fatty tissue varies according to various factors, including the client's age, body build, nutritional status, hormonal cycle, and whether she is pregnant or lactating.

The major *axillary lymph nodes* consist of the *anterior* (pectoral), *posterior* (subscapular), *lateral* (brachial), *central* (midaxillary), *supraclavicular,* and *infraclavicular nodes* (Fig. 16-4).

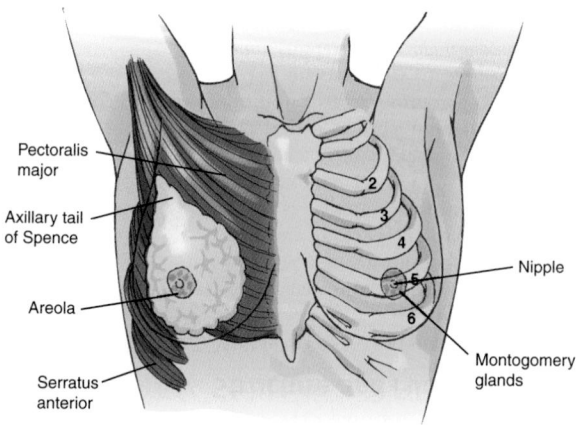

FIGURE 16-1 Anatomic breast landmarks and their position in the thorax.

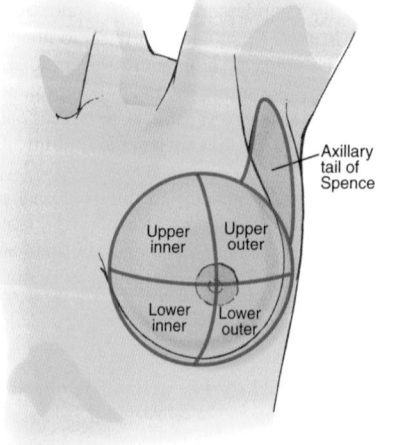

FIGURE 16-2 Breast quadrants. The upper outer quadrant is the area most targeted by breast cancer.

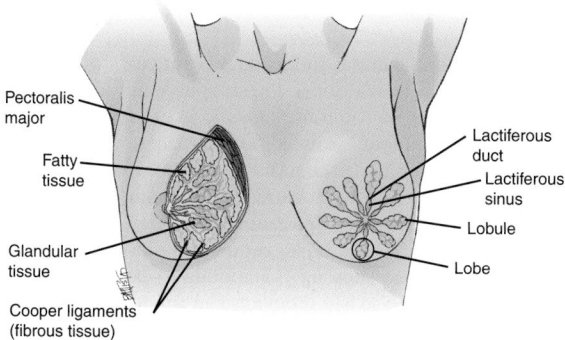

FIGURE 16-3 Internal anatomy of the breast.

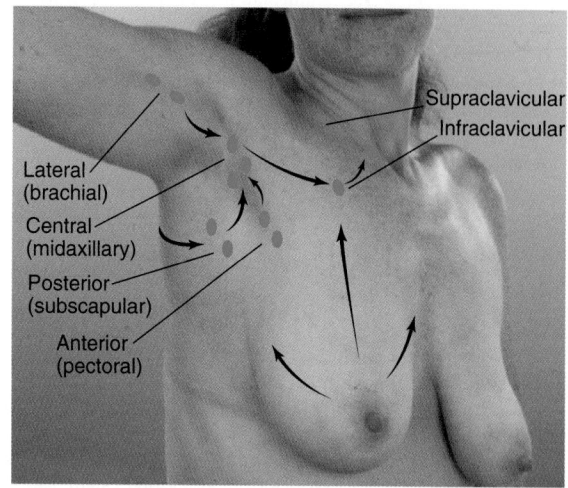

FIGURE 16-4 The lymph nodes drain impurities from the breasts (arrows show direction).

Nursing Assessment

COLLECTING SUBJECTIVE DATA

Interview Questions

Any lumps or lesions (location, size) or swelling in breasts? Change in size or firmness? Redness, warmth, or dimpling of breasts? Tenderness? Pain? Timing in menstrual cycle? Change in position of nipple or nipple discharge? Amount and character of discharge? Age of first menstruation? Age of client when they gave birth to children (if applicable)? Previous breast surgeries? History of breast cancer in family? Self-care: breast self-examination (BSE; frequency and time performed)? Taking any hormones, contraceptives, or antipsychotic agents, sedatives, opioid medications or medicines for high blood pressure, herbal supplements? Exposure to radiation, benzene, or asbestos? Amount of coffee, tea, or cola (or other forms of caffeine) consumed each day? Milk intake: amount, how often, and over how many years? Diet and daily exercise routine? Last breast examination? Last mammogram?

Risk Factors

Risk for breast cancer related to increasing age, personal history of breast cancer, family history of breast cancer, early menarche and late menopause, no natural children, first child after age 30 years, no history of breastfeeding, excessive weight (especially weight gain as an adult), higher education and socioeconomic status, regular alcohol intake (2–5 drinks daily), previous breast irradiation, hormone replacement with progesterone, no or poor BSE, poor screening, lack of adequate physical activity (45–60 minutes at least 5 days/week).

Use the risk tool available at http://www.cancer.gov/bcrisktool/ to calculate client's level of risk for developing breast cancer.

COLLECTING OBJECTIVE DATA

Equipment Needed

- Centimeter ruler
- Small pillow
- BSE guide to give to client (see Box 16-1)
- Gloves and slide for specimen if nipple discharge is present

Physical Assessment

Review Figures 16-1 to 16-4 for anatomy of the breasts and regional lymphatics.

Keep in mind that the breast examination may evoke fear, anxiety, or embarrassment that may influence the client's ability to discuss the condition of the breasts and BSE. Men with gynecomastia may be embarrassed to have what they consider a "female condition." Explain the steps and purpose of the examination. Warm

your hands. Remember it is important to carefully perform the breast examination on male as well as female clients.

BOX 16-1 BREAST SELF-EXAMINATION

BSE has become controversial because the benefits of survival rate may not outweigh the harm of performing unnecessary biopsies (ACS, 2020b). It may be useful if used in combination with regular physical examinations by a primary care provider, mammography, ultrasound, and magnetic resonance imaging (MRI) as needed. Each screening method has its benefits and disadvantages. BSE is an easy and inexpensive method that may help find breast cancer early, when it is most treatable. It is the choice of the individual whether or not to perform BSE. If the client values the benefits more the potential harm, they may want information on how to perform the BSE as follows.

It is important to explain to the client to not hesitate to call their primary care provider or gynecologist if they notice any breast changes or lumps. Most breast lumps are benign. Developing a routine can help the client to get to know the characteristics and texture of their breasts. Making notes can also help detect any changes.

Instructions for Client Who Chooses to Perform BSE

1. Inspect your breasts standing in front of mirror and raising your arms over your head. Observe size, shape, and color. Note any

swelling, discolorations, dimpling, or nipple drainage by gently squeezing each nipple (usually, there is no drainage).

Notify your primary care provider of any changes you see—any dimpling, bulging, nipple discharge or inversion of the skin, any redness, pain or discomfort, rash, or swelling.

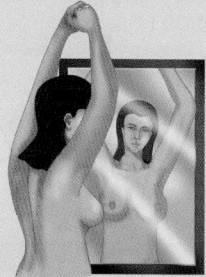

(Continued on following page)

BOX 16-1   BREAST SELF-EXAMINATION (continued)

2. Repeat step #1 standing in front of the mirror, except place your hands on your hips.

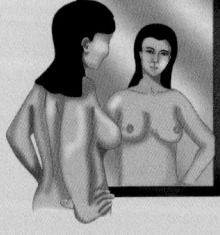

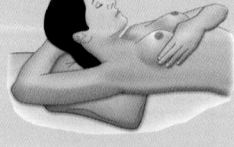

4. **Repeat feeling your entire breasts** as described in step #3 while standing. This may be easiest to do while showering. Hold your right arm up while feeling with your left fingers. Feel under your armpit with elbow slightly bent to make skin less taut. Repeat on the other side.

3. Lie down with a small pillow under your head and your right arm, with your right arm under your head, while you use your left hand to feel your right breast. Use your left hand's finger pads to feel your right breast, using mild, then moderate, then firm pressure down to your ribcage. Cover all of your breast in a vertical, circular, or wedge pattern, as seen in Figure 16-6. Then, change your position so that you can feel your left breast using your right hand in the same manner.

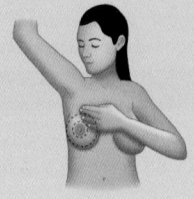

For information about what to do if you find a lump, go to https://www.breastcancer.org/symptoms/testing/types/self_exam.

ASSESSMENT PROCEDURE	NORMAL FINDINGS	ABNORMAL FINDINGS

INSPECTION

Inspect the breasts with the client in a sitting position with arms at sides, arms overhead, hands pressed on hips, palms pressed together, and arms extended straight ahead as client leans forward (Fig. 16-5). Also inspect the areolae and nipples.

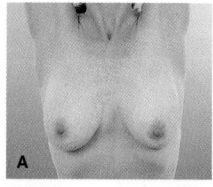
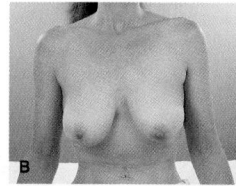
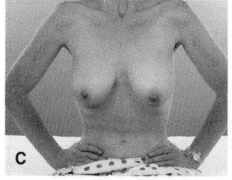
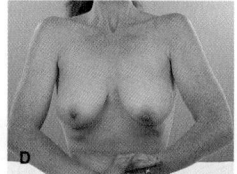
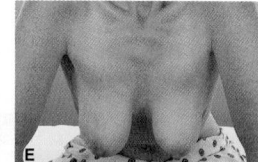

FIGURE 16-5 (A) Arms over head. **(B)** Arms at side. **(C)** Arms pressed on hips. **(D)** Hands pressed together. **(E)** Leaning forward, arms extended.

(Continued on following page)

ASSESSMENT PROCEDURE	NORMAL FINDINGS	ABNORMAL FINDINGS
INSPECTION (*continued*)		
Observe **breasts** for the following:		
• Size and symmetry	• Relatively equal with slight variation	• Recent change to unequal size. Recent increase in size of one breast may indicate inflammation or abnormal growth.
• Shape	• Round and pendulous	• Retraction or dimpling (Abnormal Findings 16-1) may be due to fibrosis and may indicate a malignant tumor.
• Color	• Pink; striae with age and pregnancy	• Redness, inflammation, blue hue, increased venous engorgement.
• Skin surface	• Smooth	• Retraction, dimpling, enlarged pores, *peau d'orange* (seen in metastatic breast disease due to edema from blocked lymphatic drainage; see Abnormal Findings 16-1), edema, lumps, lesions, rashes, ulcers.
Observe **areolae and nipples** for the following:		
• Size	• Relatively the same, slight variation	• Large variation

ASSESSMENT PROCEDURE	NORMAL FINDINGS	ABNORMAL FINDINGS
• Color	• Pink to dark brown (varies with skin and hair color)	• Inflamed
• Shape	• Round, oval, everted	• Inversion, if it occurs after maturation or changes with movement. Recent retraction of previously everted nipple suggests malignancy.
• Discharge	• None; clear yellow 2 days after childbirth	• Foul, purulent, sanguineous drainage. Any spontaneous discharge needs to be referred for further evaluation.
• Texture	• Small Montgomery tubercles present	• Lesions, rashes, ulcers. Peau d'orange skin is seen with carcinoma. Red, scaly, crusty areas are indicative of *Paget disease* (see Abnormal Findings 16-1).

PALPATION

Use the flat pads of three fingers to compress tissue against breast wall gently. Palpate with client sitting. Then have client lie down and place arm of side being examined overhead with small pillow under upper back. Palpate in circular motion starting at the 12-o'clock position and moving in concentric rings inward to areola and nipple (Fig. 16-6A). Bimanual palpation may be used in large-breasted clients. A wedge (Fig. 16-6B) or vertical (Fig. 16-6C) pattern may be used if preferred.

(Continued on following page)

ASSESSMENT PROCEDURE	NORMAL FINDINGS	ABNORMAL FINDINGS

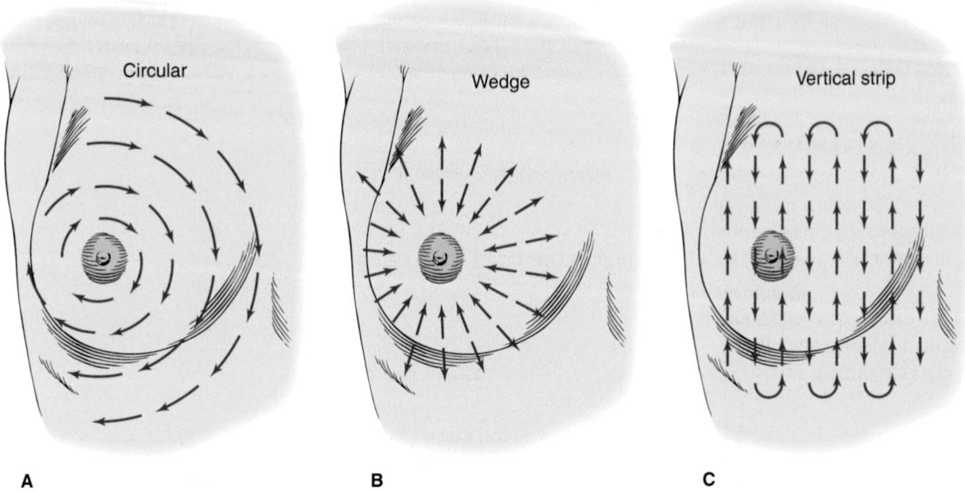

A

B

C

FIGURE 16-6 Patterns for breast palpation. Arrows indicate direction and areas for palpation. **(A)** Circular or clockwise. **(B)** Wedge. **(C)** Vertical strip.

ASSESSMENT PROCEDURE	NORMAL FINDINGS	ABNORMAL FINDINGS
Palpate **breasts** for the following.		
• Temperature	• Warm	• Erythema; heat indicates inflammation if client is not lactating or has not just given birth.
• Elasticity	• Elastic	• Lumpy
• Tenderness	• Nontender; slightly tender (tenderness and fullness may occur before menses)	• Painful
• Masses (note size, shape, mobility, consistency, and location according to quadrant; see Fig. 16-2).	• Bilateral firm inframammary transverse ridge at base of breasts	• Masses or nodules. Malignant tumors are most often found in upper outer quadrant of breast and are usually unilateral with irregular, poorly delineated borders; hard; immobile, and fixed to surrounding tissues. *Fibroadenomas* (benign) are usually 1–5 cm, round or oval, mobile, firm, solid, elastic, nontender, and single or multiple in one or both breasts. *Fibrocystic disease* (benign) consists of bilateral, multiple, firm, regular, rubbery, mobile nodules with well-demarcated borders (see Abnormal Findings 16-2).

(Continued on following page)

ASSESSMENT PROCEDURE	NORMAL FINDINGS	ABNORMAL FINDINGS
Palpate **nipple** gently for discharge (Fig. 16-7). 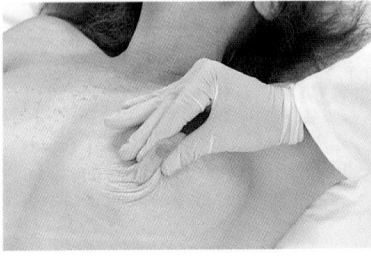 **FIGURE 16-7** Palpating nipples for masses and discharge.	• None; clear yellow 2 days after childbirth.	• Unilateral serous, serosanguineous, clear, yellow, dark red. Discharge may be seen in endocrine disorders and with some medications, such as antihypertensives, antidepressants, and estrogen. Discharge from one breast may indicate benign intraductal papilloma, fibrocystic disease, or breast cancer.
• Palpate **lymph nodes** in the following areas: supraclavicular, subclavian, intermediate, brachial, scapular, mammary, internal mammary (see Fig. 16-4).	• None palpable ($<$1 cm)	• Palpable lymph nodes ($>$1 cm)

MALE VARIATIONS

Although rare, men can have breast cancer, which may not be caught until the late stages, because many in society are unaware of its occurrence in men (American Cancer Society [ACS], 2020a).

Inspect and palpate breast with client seated, arms at sides. Palpate lymph nodes. No swelling, ulcerations, or nodules should be noted. Flat disc of undeveloped breast tissue under nipple is normally palpated. Soft fatty tissue enlargement seen in obesity. Gynecomastia (Fig. 16-8) and a smooth, firm movable disc of glandular tissue may be seen in one breast during puberty for a short time and may be seen in hormonal imbalances (disease or medication induced) and drug abuse. Irregular, hard nodules are seen in malignancy.

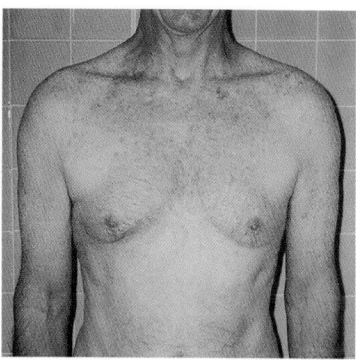

FIGURE 16-8 Gynecomastia.

ABNORMAL FINDINGS 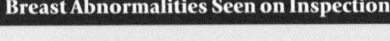 **16-1** **Breast Abnormalities Seen on Inspection**

PEAU D'ORANGE
Resulting from edema, an orange-peel appearance of the breast is associated with cancer.

PAGET DISEASE
Redness and flaking of the nipple may be seen early in Paget disease and then disappear. However, further assessment is needed as this does not mean the disease is gone. Tingling, itching, increased sensitivity, burning, discharge, and pain in the nipple are late signs of Paget disease. It may occur in both breasts, but is rare.

NIPPLE INVERSION FROM BREAST CANCER
Nipple inversion may suggest malignancy.

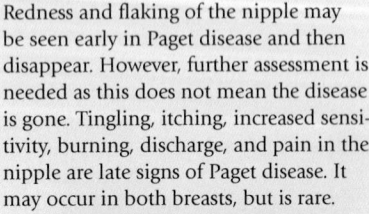

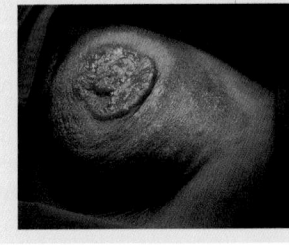

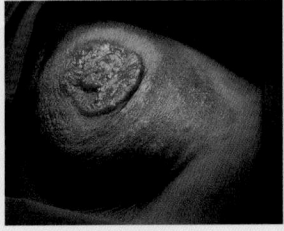

RETRACTED BREAST TISSUE

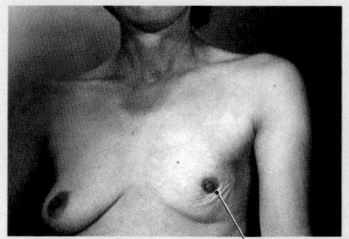

Skin, areola, and
nipple retraction

MASTITIS

Reddened, painful area on breast warm
to palpation.

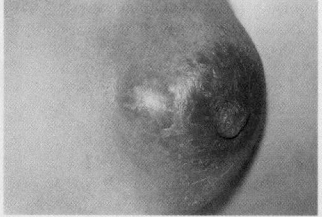

MASTECTOMY

(A) Radical mastectomy. (B) Modified
radical mastectomy.

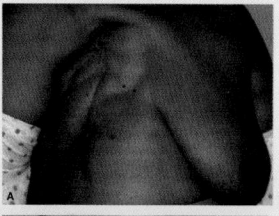

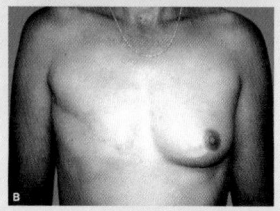

(*Continued on following page*)

ABNORMAL FINDINGS

| ABNORMAL FINDINGS | **16-1** | **Breast Abnormalities Seen on Inspection (*continued*)** |

CARCINOMA OF THE BREAST (NOTE BULGING AND SKIN CHANGES)

GYNECOMASTIA

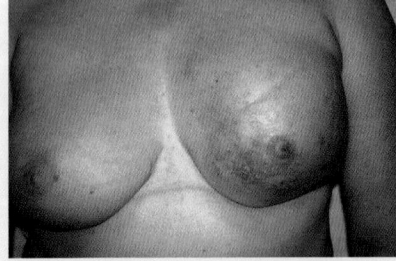

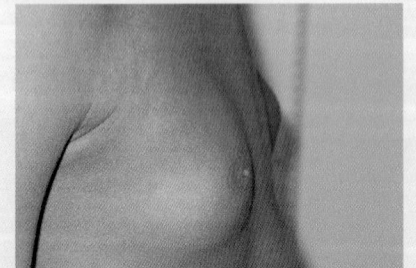

Photo credits: Retracted breast tissue, carcinoma of the breast, and gynecomastia, reprinted with permission from Jensen, S. (2019). *Nursing health assessment: A best practice approach* (3rd ed., Table 19-4 (part)). Wolters Kluwer; nipple inversion from breast cancer, reprinted with permission from Harris, J. R., Lippman, M. E., Morrow, M., & Osborne, C. K. (2014). *Diseases of the breast* (5th ed.). Lippincott Williams & Wilkins; mastitis, reprinted with permission from Hatfield, N. T., & Kincheloe, C. (2017). *Introductory maternity and pediatric nursing* (4th ed.). Wolters Kluwer; mastectomy, reprinted with permission from Berek, J. S., Hacker, N. F. (2014). *Berek and Hacker's gynecologic oncology* (6th ed.). Lippincott, Williams & Wilkins.

ABNORMAL FINDINGS | **16-2** | **Abnormalities Noted on Palpation of the Breasts**

Whereas some abnormalities of the breast are readily apparent, such as peau d'orange and Paget disease, some breast internal changes are detected only by palpation and mammography. The following illustrations represent breast abnormalities characteristic of tumors, fibroadenomas, and benign disease (fibrocystic breasts).

CANCEROUS TUMORS

These are irregular, firm, hard, undefined masses that may be fixed or mobile. They are not usually tender and usually occur after age 50.

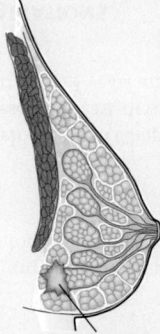

Tumor

FIBROADENOMAS

These lesions are lobular, ovoid, or round. They are firm, well defined, seldom tender, and usually singular and mobile. They occur more commonly between puberty and menopause.

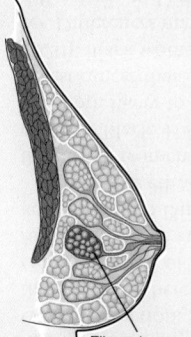

Fibroadenoma

BENIGN BREAST DISEASE

Also called *fibrocystic breast disease*, benign breast disease is marked by round, elastic, defined, tender, and mobile cysts. The condition is most common from age 30 to menopause, after which it decreases.

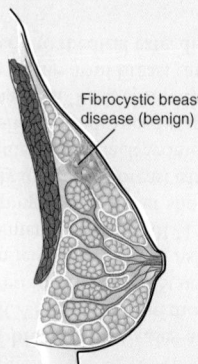

Fibrocystic breast disease (benign)

🐴 PEDIATRIC VARIATIONS

Subjective Data

Age of menarche? Asymmetrical breast growth? Girls prior to puberty: pain or discomfort? Boys during adolescence: abnormal increase in size?

Objective Data

See normal breast development in Chapter 23, Table 23-1, which varies with age. Adolescent breast development is usually seen between the ages of 10 and 13 years and takes about 3 years for full development.

🪑 GERIATRIC VARIATIONS

- Breasts pendulous, atrophied, and less firm owing to a decrease in estrogen levels.
- May have smaller, flatter nipples that are less erectile on stimulation. Nipples may retract, but will evert with gentle pressure.
- Breasts may feel more granular, with more fibrotic tissue.

🌍 CULTURAL VARIATIONS

Genetic variation: About 5% to 10% of breast cancer cases are thought to be hereditary. *BRCA1* and *BRCA2* genes are the most common cause of hereditary breast cancer. In the United States, *BRCA* mutations are found most often in Jewish women of Ashkenazi (Eastern Europe) origin (Basser Center for BRCA, 2017).

Studies of ethnic variation in developing breast cancer show that White women are slightly more likely to develop breast cancer than Black, Hispanic, and Asian women, but Black women are more likely to develop more aggressive and advanced-stage breast cancer that is diagnosed at a young age ("Race/ethnicity," 2020). Black women are also more likely to die from breast cancer. Differences may be due to varying access to medical care, diet differences, and other lifestyle issues.

POSSIBLE COLLABORATIVE PROBLEMS—RISK OF

- Infection (abscess)
- Hematoma
- Fibrocystic disease
- Breast cancer

Teaching Tips for Selected Client Concerns

***Client Concern:** Opportunity to enhance breast health and early detection of lumps or lesions associated with request to learn BSE*

- The U.S. Preventive Services Task Force (USPSTF) recommends against teaching BSE because current evidence is insufficient to assess the additional benefits and harms of clinical breast examination (CBE) beyond screening mammography in women aged 75 years or older. The American College of Obstetricians and Gynecologists (ACOG, 2017) recommended against BSE for women at average risk for breast cancer. However, BSE used for breast awareness, when no particular systematic approach to regular examination is taken, was recommended. Many organizations now advise an alternative called "breast self-awareness" (becoming familiar with the appearance, feel, and shape of one's breasts and nipples). For higher risk individuals, BSE is an option for women starting in their 20s (Box 16-1). Women should report any breast changes to their health professional right away.

- Teach Clients
  - Women and men can have breast cancer; both should note any changes in breast size, shape, or tissue consistency and report to health care provider.
  - Inform clients of different screening recommendations and advise them to talk with their health care provider to determine the best screening protocol for them (see screening recommendations under Screening).
- Teach Risk Factors for Breast Cancer
  - Get intentional physical exercise for least 45–60 minutes per day for 5 days per week or more.
  - Avoid alcohol intake of more than one alcoholic beverage per day (e.g., 6-oz glass of wine).
  - Avoid excessive weight gain, especially as an adult and especially after menopause.
  - Be aware of increased risk if client has no children or had first child after 30 years of age.
  - Note breast consistency and be aware that denser breasts increase risk; women with denser breast tissue should work with their health care provider to establish a recommendation for screening patterns.

- Consider family history of breast cancer and note risk if genetic kin, including father and brothers, have had breast cancer.
- Night shift work and exposure to secondhand smoke may be linked to increased risk for breast cancer.
- Avoid even dim light source while sleeping at night.
- Avoid drinking milk daily or in large quantities.
- Advise client to talk with health care provider after completing a formal breast cancer risk assessment such as the Gail model.

  Breast cancer risks for women at a younger age (Centers for Disease Control and Prevention [CDC], 2019):
- Relatives with breast cancer diagnosed before age 45
- Changes in *BRCA1* or *BRCA2* breast cancer genes or close relatives with those changes
- Ashkenazi Jewish heritage
- Prior radiation therapy to breast or chest
- A history of breast cancer or certain other breast health problems, such as lobular carcinoma in situ (LCIS), ductal carcinoma in situ (DCIS), atypical ductal hyperplasia, or atypical lobular hyperplasia
- Mammography shows dense breasts

- **Teach Recommendations for Breast examinations**
  - Mammogram is the screening of choice for breast cancer, and the 3D mammogram is recommended when available (MD Anderson, 2020). The 3D mammogram takes multiple images to provide a 3D picture of the breast.
  - Screening recommendations for breast cancer have become more uniform. Recommended screening guidelines from ACS and USPSTF:
- **ACS (2018)**
  - Mammography is a choice between 40 and 44 years.
  - Mammography yearly for women between 45 and 54 years of age
  - Mammography every 2 years for women aged 55 years and older
- **USPSTF (2016)**
  - Mammography yearly for women between 50 and 74 years of age
  - Mammography between 40 and 49 is an individual choice.
  - Mammography after 75 has no evidence of benefit.

- **The Canadian Task Force on Preventive Health Care** (2019) recommended personal choice for women between 40 and 49 years of age; for those 50–69 years, a mammogram every 2–3 years; for those between 70 and 74 years, a mammogram every 2 years. There was no recommendation for women beyond 74 years.

References

American Cancer Society. (2018). *American Cancer Society guidelines for the early detection of cancer: Breast cancer.* https://www.cancer.org/healthy/find-cancer-early/cancer-screening-guidelines/american-cancer-society-guidelines-for-the-early-detection-of-cancer.html

American Cancer Society. (2020a). *About breast cancer in men.* https://www.cancer.org/cancer/breast-cancer-in-men/about.html

American Cancer Society. (2020b). *American Cancer Society recommendations for early detection of breast cancer.* https://www.cancer.org/cancer/breast-cancer/screening-tests-and-early-detection/american-cancer-society-recommendations-for-the-early-detection-of-breast-cancer.html

American College of Obstetricians & Gynecologists. (2017). *Breast cancer risk assessment and screening in average-risk women.* https://www.acog.org/clinical/clinical-guidance/practice-bulletin/articles/2017/07/breast-cancer-risk-assessment-and-screening-in-average-risk-women

Basser Center for BRCA. (2017). *BRCA1 and BRCA2 in the Ashkenazi Jewish community.* https://www.basser.org/sites/default/files/2018-05/Basser%20Ashkenazi%20Jewish%20Fact%20Sheet%202017.pdf

Canadian Task Force on Preventive Health Care (2019). *Breast cancer update (2018).* https://canadiantaskforce.ca/guidelines/published-guidelines/breast-cancer-update/

Centers for Disease Control and Prevention. (2019). *Risk factors for breast cancer at a young age.* https://www.cdc.gov/cancer/breast/young_women/bringyourbrave/breast_cancer_young_women/risk_factors.htm?s_cid=byb_sem_013

MD Anderson Cancer Center. (2020). *3D mammogram: What you should know.* https://www.mdanderson.org/publications/focused-on-health/FOH-3D-mammography.h19-1589835.html

Race/ethnicity. (2020). https://www.breastcancer.org/risk/factors/race_ethnicity

U.S. Preventive Services Task Force. (2016). *Breast cancer: Screening.* https://www.uspreventiveservicestaskforce.org/uspstf/recommendation/breast-cancer-screening

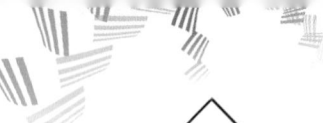

17 ASSESSING HEART AND NECK VESSELS

Structure and Function Overview

HEART AND GREAT VESSELS

The heart is a hollow, muscular, four-chambered organ located in the middle of the thoracic cavity between the lungs in the space called the *mediastinum*. It is about the size of a clenched fist and weighs approximately 255 g (9 oz) in women and 309 g (10.9 oz) in men. The heart extends vertically from the second to the fifth intercostal space (ICS) and horizontally from the right edge of the sternum to the left midclavicular line (MCL). The heart can be described as an inverted cone. The upper portion, near the second ICS, is the base, and the lower portion, near the fifth ICS and the left MCL, is the apex. The anterior chest area that overlies the heart and great vessels is called the *precordium* (Fig. 17-1).

The large veins and arteries leading directly to and away from the heart are referred to as the *great vessels*. The *superior and inferior venae cavae* return blood to the right atrium from the upper and lower torso, respectively. The *pulmonary artery* exits the right ventricle, bifurcates, and carries blood to the lungs. The *pulmonary veins* (two from each lung) return oxygenated blood to the left atrium. The *aorta* transports oxygenated blood from the left ventricle to the body (Fig. 17-2).

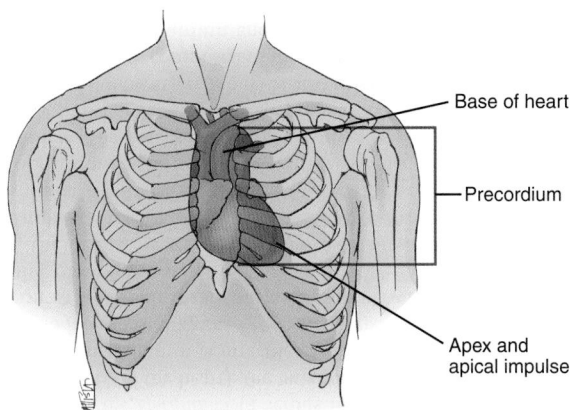

FIGURE 17-1 The heart and major blood vessels lie centrally in the chest behind the protective sternum.

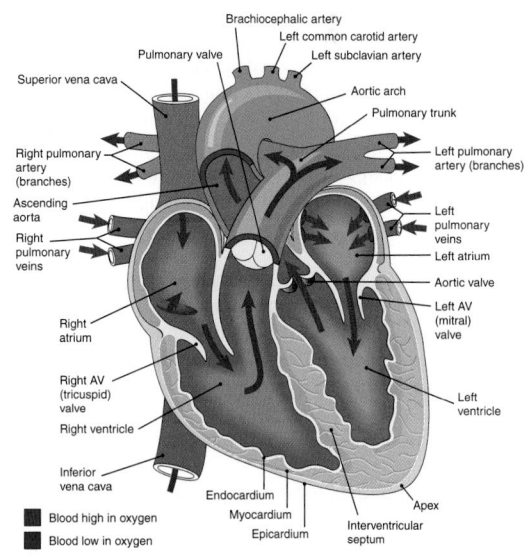

FIGURE 17-2 Heart chambers, valves, and direction of circulatory flow. AV, atrioventricular.

The heart coverings and walls consist of a *pericardium* (a tough, inextensible, loose-fitting, fibroserous sac that attaches to the great vessels and surrounds the heart); the *parietal pericardium* (a serous membrane that secretes a small amount of pericardial fluid that allows for smooth, friction-free movement of the heart); the *epicardium* (a serous membrane that covers the outer surface of the heart); the *myocardium* (the thickest layer of the heart made up of contractile cardiac muscle cells); and the *endocardium* (a thin layer of endothelial tissue that forms the innermost layer of the heart and is continuous with the endothelial lining of blood vessels).

The heart consists of four chambers or cavities: two upper chambers, the *right and left atria*, and two lower chambers, the *right and left ventricles*. One-way valves that direct the flow of blood through the heart protect the entrance and exit of each ventricle. The *atrioventricular* (AV) valves are located at the entrance into the ventricles. There are two AV valves: the tricuspid valve and the bicuspid, which is also called the *mitral valve*. The tricuspid valve is composed of three cusps or flaps and is located between the right atrium and the right ventricle; the bicuspid (mitral) valve is composed of two cusps or flaps and is located between the left atrium and the left ventricle.

Open AV valves allow blood to flow from the atria into the ventricles. However, as the ventricles begin to contract, the AV valves snap shut, preventing the regurgitation of blood into the atria.

The *semilunar valves* are located at the exit of each ventricle at the beginning of the great vessels. Each valve has three cusps or flaps that look like half-moons, hence the name "semilunar." There are two semilunar valves: the pulmonic valve is located at the entrance of the pulmonary artery as it exits the right ventricle, and the aortic valve is located at the beginning of the ascending aorta as it exits the left ventricle (see Fig. 17-2).

ELECTRICAL CONDUCTION SYSTEM OF THE HEART

Cardiac muscle cells have a unique inherent ability to spontaneously generate electrical impulses and conduct them through the heart. The generation and conduction of electrical impulses by specialized sections of the myocardium regulate the events associated with the filling and emptying of the cardiac chambers. The process is called the *cardiac cycle*. The *sinoatrial (SA) node*, located on the posterior wall of the right atrium, generates impulses (at a rate of 60–100 per minute) that cause the atria to contract simultaneously, sending blood into the ventricles. The current, initiated by the SA node, is conducted across the atria to the *AV node* located in the lower interatrial septum. The AV node slightly delays incoming electrical impulses from the atria and then relays the impulse to the AV bundle (bundle of His) in the upper interventricular septum. The electrical impulse then travels down the right and left bundle branches and the *Purkinje fibers* in the myocardium of both ventricles, causing them to contract almost simultaneously. Although the SA node functions as the "pacemaker of the heart," this activity shifts to other areas of the conduction system, such as the *bundle of His* (with an inherent discharge of 40–60 per minute), if the SA node cannot function.

PRODUCTION OF HEART SOUNDS

Heart sounds are produced by valve closure. The opening of valves is silent. Normal heart sounds, characterized as "lub dub" (S_1 and S_2), and, occasionally, extra heart sounds and murmurs can be auscultated with a stethoscope over the precordium, the area of the anterior chest overlying the heart and great vessels.

The first heart sound (S_1) is the result of closure of the AV valves—the mitral and tricuspid valves. S_1 correlates with the beginning of systole (Fig. 17-3). If heard as two sounds, the first component represents mitral valve closure (M_1) and the second component represents tricuspid closure (T_1).

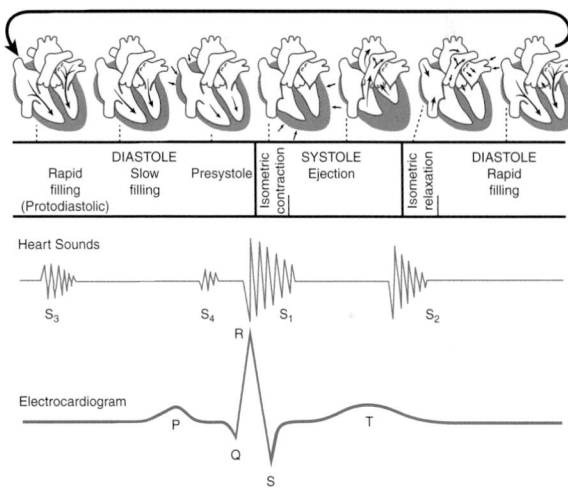

FIGURE 17-3 The cardiac cycle consists of filling and ejection. Heart sounds S_2, S_3, and S_4 are associated with diastole, whereas S_1 is associated with systole. The electrical activity of the heart is measured throughout diastole and systole by electrocardiography.

The second heart sound (S_2) results from closure of the semilunar valves (aortic and pulmonic) and correlates with the beginning of diastole. S_2 ("dub") is also usually heard as one sound, but may be heard as two sounds. If S_2 is heard as two sounds, the first component represents aortic valve closure (A_2) and the second component represents pulmonic valve closure (P_2).

NECK VESSELS

The internal jugular veins lie deep and medial to the sternocleidomastoid muscle. The external jugular veins lie lateral to the sternocleidomastoid muscle and above the clavicle. The jugular veins return blood to the heart from the head and neck by way of the superior vena cava.

The level of the jugular venous pressure reflects right atrial (central venous) pressure and right ventricular diastolic filling pressure. Right-sided heart failure raises pressure and volume, thus raising jugular venous pressure. *Decreased jugular venous pressure* occurs with reduced left ventricular output or blood volume. The right internal jugular vein is most directly connected to the right atrium and provides the best assessment of pressure changes. Components of the jugular venous pulse are as follows:

- a wave—reflects rise in atrial pressure that occurs with atrial contraction.
- x descent—reflects right atrial relaxation and descent of the

- v wave—reflects right atrial filling, increased volume, and increased atrial pressure.
- y descent—reflects right atrial emptying into the right ventricle and decreased atrial pressure.

Nursing Assessment

COLLECTING SUBJECTIVE DATA

Interview Questions

Chest pain—onset? Location? Radiation? Quality? Rating on scale of 1 to 10 (10 being the worst)? Duration? How often? See Table 17-1 for a description of various types of cardiovascular pain.

What brings it on? What relieves it? Does activity make it worse? Does it have a pattern or radiate? (See Figs. 17-4 and 17-5.) Are there any other associated symptoms, such as nausea, vomiting, sweating? Irregular heartbeat, palpitations? Does your heart pound or beat too fast? Does your heart skip or jump? Difficulty breathing or shortness of breath? Dizziness? Light-headedness? Swelling in feet, ankles or legs? Heart burn—Onset? How often? Relief? History of heart defect? Murmur? Rheumatic fever? Heart surgery? Cardiac balloon interventions? Last electrocardiogram and results? Cholesterol levels? Medica-

TABLE 17-1 **Description of Various Types of Cardiovascular Pain**

Problem/Condition	Description using COLDSPA
Angina (myocardial ischemia)	C: tight pressing, heavy O: Discomfort occurring often with exertion L: Across the chest and may radiate to shoulders, jaws, neck, or upper abdomen D: Lasts up to 20 minutes S: Mild to moderate pain P: May be relieved with nitroglycerine A: May occur with difficulty breathing, nausea, or sweating
Myocardial infarction (irreversible heart damage because of myocardial ischemia)	C: Heavy, tight pressing O: Discomfort occurring with or without exertion L: Across the chest and may radiate to shoulders, jaws, neck, or upper abdomen D: Lasts 20 minutes up to hours S: Often moderate to severe pain P: Rest does not relieve A: May occur with nausea, vomiting, weakness, and sweating

(Continued on following page)

TABLE 17-1 **Description of Various Types of Cardiovascular Pain** (*continued*)

Problem/Condition	Description using COLDSPA
Aortic dissecting aneurysm (tear in the wall lining the aorta)	C: Tearing, ripping sensation O: Abrupt L: In chest radiating to neck, back, or abdomen D: Lasting for hours S: Severe P: Aggravated by hypertension. Relieved only with treatment A: Also seen with difficulty swallowing, hoarseness, leg pain, and syncope
Pericarditis (inflammation of the parietal pleura next to the pericardium)	C: Sharp, stabbing, pounding feeling when heart beats O: Ongoing L: Pericardial pain radiating to shoulders or neck D: Ongoing S: Severe P: Aggravated by breathing position changes, coughing, and may be relieved with sitting forward A: May also be seen with fever, weakness, tiredness, coughing, trouble breathing, and/or pain when swallowing

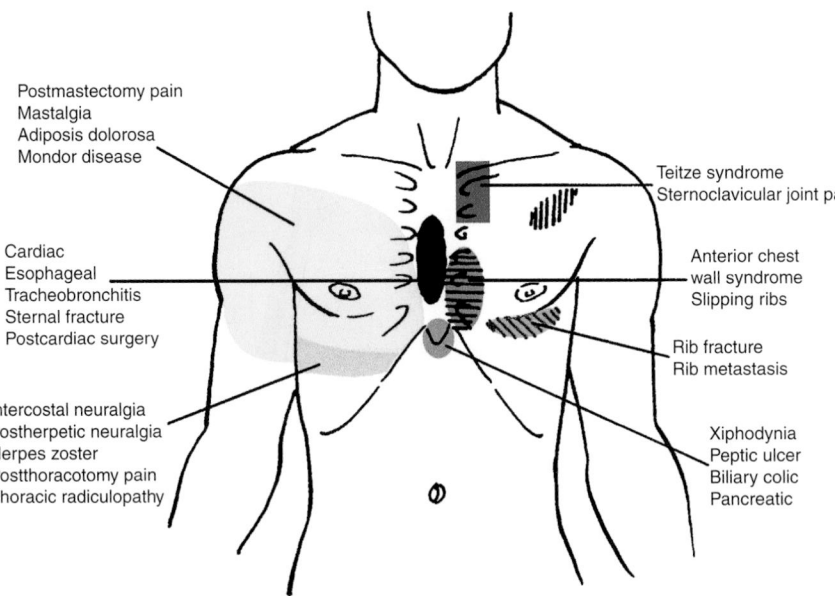

Postmastectomy pain
Mastalgia
Adiposis dolorosa
Mondor disease

Teitze syndrome
Sternoclavicular joint pain

Cardiac
Esophageal
Tracheobronchitis
Sternal fracture
Postcardiac surgery

Anterior chest
wall syndrome
Slipping ribs

Intercostal neuralgia
Postherpetic neuralgia
Herpes zoster
Postthoracotomy pain
Thoracic radiculopathy

Rib fracture
Rib metastasis

Xiphodynia
Peptic ulcer
Biliary colic
Pancreatic

FIGURE 17-4 Common sites of anterior chest wall pain because of chest wall structures or referred pain. (Reprinted with permission from Ballantyne, J. C., Fishman, S. M., Rathmell, J. P. [2019]. *Bonica's management of pain* [5th ed.]. Wolters Kluwer.)

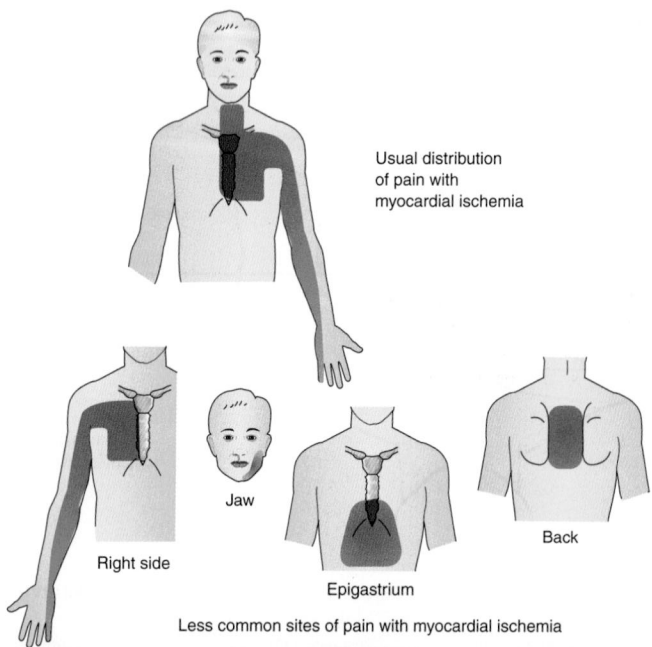

Usual distribution of pain with myocardial ischemia

Jaw

Right side

Epigastrium

Back

Less common sites of pain with myocardial ischemia

FIGURE 17-5 Pain patterns with myocardial ischemia. The usual distribution of pain is referral to all or part of the sternal region, the left side of the chest, the neck, and down the ulnar side of the left forearm and hand. With severe ischemic pain, the right side of the chest and right arm are often involved as well, although isolated involvement of these areas is rare. Other sites sometimes involved, either alone or together with pain in other sites, are the jaw, epigastrium, and back. (Reprinted with permission from Rosdahl, C. B., & Kowalski, M. T. [2017]. *Textbook of basic nursing* [11th ed.]. Wolters Kluwer Health, Lippincott Williams & Wilkins.)

hypertension, myocardial infarction, coronary heart disease, elevated cholesterol levels, or diabetes mellitus? Smoking? Packs per day? Over how many years? Attempts and/or desire to quit? Twenty-four-hour dietary recall? Alcohol consumption each day? Form of exercise? How often? Any change in activities of daily living over the last 5 years? Over the last 10 years? Ability to care for self? Any activities limited because of chest pain, shortness of breath, or fatigue? Effects of heart disease on sexual activities? Number of pillows used to sleep on at night? Daily stressors? Forms of relaxation? Fears regarding heart disease?

◎ CLINICAL TIP
It should be assumed that chest pain is due to cardiac ischemia until determined otherwise through a thorough assessment. This may be life threatening because of lack of oxygen, causing damage to cells in the heart muscle. This is a medical emergency.

Risk Factors

Risk for coronary heart disease related to hypertension, increased low-density lipoprotein (LDL) cholesterol and decreased high-density lipoprotein cholesterol, diabetes mellitus, minimal exercise, cigarette smoking, diet high in saturated fat and trans fatty acids, postmenopausal without estrogen replacement (in females), family history, and upper body obesity.

COLLECTING OBJECTIVE DATA

Equipment Needed

- Stethoscope with bell and diaphragm
- Alcohol swab to clean ear and end pieces of stethoscope
- Watch with a second hand
- Small pillow
- Penlight or movable examination light
- Centimeter rulers (two)

Physical Assessment

See Figure 17-2 for a diagram of the heart chambers, valves, and circulation. Additional data gathered during assessment of the blood pressure, skin, nails, head, thorax and lungs, and peripheral pulses all play a part in the complete cardiovascular assessment. Provide the client with as much modesty as possible. Explain that the client will need to move to different positions to facilitate auscultation of heart sounds. Tell the client you will be listening to the heart in several areas and that this does not necessarily mean that anything is wrong. *Note: If a client has large breasts, ask them to pull the breast upward and to the side when you are auscultating for heart sounds.*

NECK VESSELS

ASSESSMENT PROCEDURE	NORMAL FINDINGS	ABNORMAL FINDINGS
Inspection		
Observe the **jugular venous pulse.** Inspect the jugular venous pulse by standing on the right side of the client. The client should be in a supine position with the torso elevated 30–45 degrees. Make sure the head and torso are on the same plane. Ask the client to turn the head slightly to the left. Shine a tangential light source onto the neck to increase visualization of pulsations as well as shadows. Next, inspect the suprasternal notch or the area around the clavicles for pulsations of the internal jugular veins. ***Note:*** *Be careful not to confuse pulsations of the carotid arteries with pulsations of the internal jugular veins.*	The jugular venous pulse is not normally visible with the client sitting upright. This position fully distends the vein, and pulsations may or may not be discernible.	Fully distended jugular veins with the client's torso elevated more than 45 degrees indicate increased central venous pressure that may be the result of right ventricular failure, pulmonary hypertension, pulmonary emboli, or cardiac tamponade. Distention of jugular vein on one side may be caused by a kink or aneurysm.

ASSESSMENT PROCEDURE	NORMAL FINDINGS	ABNORMAL FINDINGS
Evaluate **jugular venous pressure** (Fig. 17-6). Evaluate jugular venous pressure by watching for distention of the jugular vein. It is normal for the jugular veins to be visible when the client is supine. To evaluate jugular vein distention, position the client in a supine position with the head of the bed elevated 30, 45, 60, and 90 degrees. At each increase of the elevation, have the client's head turned slightly away from the side being evaluated. Using tangential lighting, observe for distention, protrusion, or bulging. *Note: In acute care settings, a more accurate way to measure jugular pressure is by use of invasive cardiac monitors (pulmonary artery catheters) to precisely measure pressures* (Kelly & Rabbani, 2013).	The jugular vein should not be distended, bulging, or protruding at 45 degrees or greater. 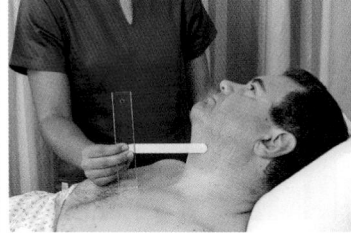 **FIGURE 17-6** Assessing jugular venous pressure.	Distention, bulging, or protrusion at 45, 60, or 90 degrees may indicate right-sided heart failure. Document at which positions (45, 60, and/or 90 degrees) you observe distention. Clients with obstructive pulmonary disease may have elevated venous pressure only during expiration. An inspiratory increase in venous pressure, called Kussmaul sign, may occur in clients with severe constrictive pericarditis.

(Continued on following page)

NECK VESSELS (*continued*)

ASSESSMENT PROCEDURE	NORMAL FINDINGS	ABNORMAL FINDINGS
Auscultation		
Auscultate the **carotid arteries**. Auscultate the carotid arteries if the client is middle-aged or older or if you suspect cardiovascular disease. Place the bell of the stethoscope over the carotid artery and ask the client to hold their breath for a moment so breath sounds do not conceal any vascular sounds (Fig. 17-7). *Note: Always auscultate the carotid arteries before palpating because palpation may increase or slow the heart rate, changing the strength of the carotid impulse heard.*	No blowing, swishing, or other sounds are heard. 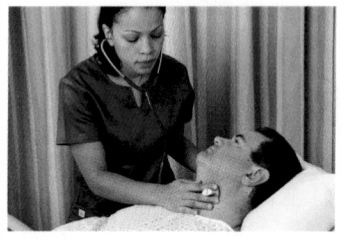 **FIGURE 17-7** Auscultating the carotid arteries.	A *bruit*, a blowing or swishing sound caused by turbulent blood flow through a narrowed vessel, is indicative of occlusive arterial disease. However, if the artery is more than two-thirds occluded, a bruit may not be heard. Pulse inequality may indicate arterial constriction or occlusion in one carotid. Weak pulses may indicate *hypovolemia*, shock, or decreased cardiac output. A bounding, firm pulse may indicate *hypervolemia* or increased cardiac output. Variations in strength from beat to beat or with respiration are abnormal and may indicate a variety of problems. A delayed upstroke may indicate *aortic stenosis.*

ASSESSMENT PROCEDURE	NORMAL FINDINGS	ABNORMAL FINDINGS
	Pulses are equally strong: a 2+ or normal with no variation in strength from beat to beat. Contour is normally smooth and rapid on the upstroke and slower and less abrupt on the downstroke. The strength of the pulse is evaluated on a scale from 0 to 4 as follows: **Pulse Amplitude Scale** 0 = absent 1+ = weak 2+ = normal 3+ = increased 4+ = bounding	
Palpation		
Palpate the **carotid arteries.** Palpate each carotid artery alternately by placing the pads of the index and middle fingers medial to the sternocleidomastoid muscle on the neck (Fig. 17-8). Note amplitude and contour of the pulse, elasticity of the artery, and any thrills.	Arteries are elastic and no thrills are noted. Pulses are equally strong: a 2+ or normal with no variation in strength from beat to beat. Contour is normally smooth and rapid on the upstroke and slower and less abrupt on the downstroke.	Loss of elasticity may indicate *arteriosclerosis.* Thrills may indicate a narrowing of the artery. Pulse inequality may indicate arterial constriction or occlusion in one carotid. Weak pulses may indicate hypovolemia, shock, or decreased cardiac output.

(Continued on following page)

NECK VESSELS (continued)		
ASSESSMENT PROCEDURE	**NORMAL FINDINGS**	**ABNORMAL FINDINGS**
Palpation		
Note: Palpate the carotid arteries individually because bilateral palpation could result in reduced cerebral blood flow. *Be cautious with older clients because atherosclerosis may have caused obstruction and compression may easily block circulation.* 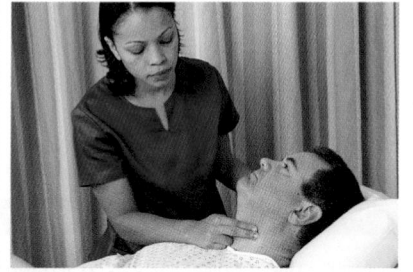 **FIGURE 17-8** Palpating the carotid arteries.	The strength of the pulse is evaluated on a scale from 0 to 4 as follows: **Pulse Amplitude Scale** 0 = absent 1+ = weak 2+ = normal 3+ = increased 4+ = bounding	A bounding, firm pulse may indicate hypervolemia or increased cardiac output. Variations in strength from beat to beat or with respiration are abnormal and may indicate a variety of problems. A delayed upstroke may indicate aortic stenosis.

HEART AND GREAT VESSELS

Inspection

Inspect chest to identify landmarks that aid in assessment of the heart (Fig. 17-9). Check for visibility of point of maximum impulse (PMI) and any abnormal pulsations.

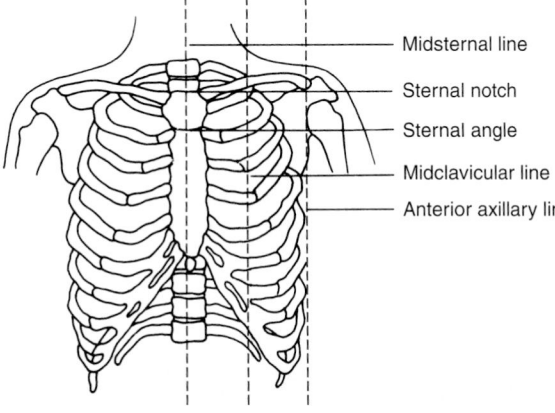

- Midsternal line
- Sternal notch
- Sternal angle
- Midclavicular line
- Anterior axillary line

FIGURE 17-9 Landmarks of the chest.

(*Continued on following page*)

HEART AND GREAT VESSELS (*continued*)

ASSESSMENT PROCEDURE	NORMAL FINDINGS	ABNORMAL FINDINGS
Inspect for any pulsations on anterior chest over heart. With the client in supine position with the head of the bed elevated between 30 and 45 degrees, stand on the client's right side and look for the apical impulse and any abnormal pulsations. *Note: The apical impulse was originally called the PMI. However, this term is no longer used because a maximal impulse may occur in other areas of the precordium as a result of abnormal conditions.*	The apical impulse may or may not be visible. If apparent, it would be in the mitral area (left midclavicular line, fourth or fifth intercostal space). The apical impulse is a result of the left ventricle moving outward during systole.	• Pulsations, which may also be called heaves or lifts, other than the apical pulsation are considered abnormal and should be evaluated. A heave or lift may occur as the result of an enlarged ventricle from an overload of work.

Palpation

The client should be lying down. Palpate using the fingertips and palmar surfaces of fingers in an organized fashion, beginning in the aortic area and moving down the chest toward the tricuspid area (Fig. 17-10).

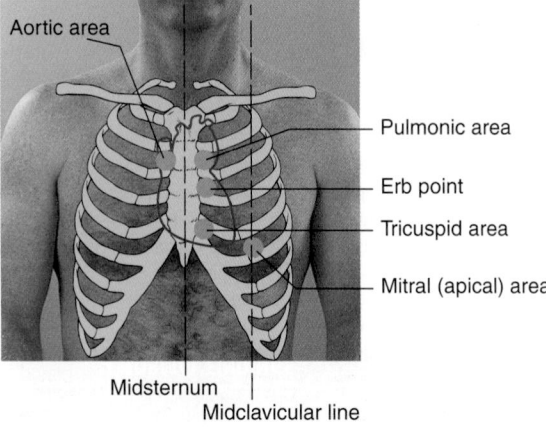

FIGURE 17-10 Areas to palpate and auscultate on the chest.

(*Continued on following page*)

HEART AND GREAT VESSELS (*continued*)

ASSESSMENT PROCEDURE	NORMAL FINDINGS	ABNORMAL FINDINGS
Palpate the **apical impulse**. Remain on the client's right side and ask the client to remain supine. Use one or two finger pads to palpate the apical impulse in the mitral area (fourth or fifth intercostal space at the midclavicular line). You may ask the client to roll to the left side to better feel the impulse using your finger pads (Fig. 17-11). *Note: If this apical pulsation cannot be palpated, have the client assume a left lateral position. This displaces the heart toward the left chest wall and relocates the apical impulse farther to the left.*	The apical impulse is palpated in the mitral area and may be the size of a nickel (1–2 cm). Amplitude is usually small—like a gentle tap. The duration is brief, lasting through the first two-thirds of systole and often less. In obese clients or clients with large breasts, the apical impulse may not be palpable.	The apical impulse may be impossible to palpate in clients with pulmonary emphysema. If the apical impulse is larger than 1–2 cm, displaced, more forceful, or of longer duration, suspect cardiac enlargement.

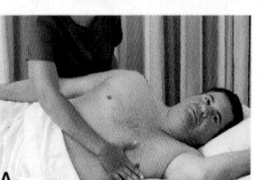

FIGURE 17-11 Locate the apical impulse with the palmar surface (**A**) and then palpate the apical pulse with the finger pad (**B**).

Palpate for **abnormal pulsations**. Use your palmar surfaces to palpate the apex, left sternal border, and base.	No pulsations or vibrations are palpated in the areas of the apex, left sternal border, or base.	A thrill or a pulsation is usually associated with a grade IV or higher murmur.

ASSESSMENT PROCEDURE	NORMAL FINDINGS	ABNORMAL FINDINGS
Percussion		
Percussion may be done to define cardiac borders by identifying areas of dullness, but it is generally unreliable. Size of heart can be more accurately determined by chest x-ray.		
Auscultation		
Auscultate in an orderly, systematic fashion beginning with the aortic area. Move across and then down the chest. Focus on one sound at a time. Auscultate each area with the stethoscope diaphragm applied firmly to the chest. Repeat the sequence using the stethoscope bell applied lightly to the chest. Auscultate with the client in the supine position. Then listen specifically over the apex with the bell while client is in the left lateral position. Assist client to a sitting position and auscultate the pericardium with the diaphragm. Then have the client lean forward and exhale while you listen over the aortic area with the diaphragm.		
Auscultate **heart rate and rhythm.** Place the diaphragm of the stethoscope at the apex and listen closely to the rate and rhythm of the apical impulse.	Rate should be 60–100 beats/min, with regular rhythm. A regularly irregular rhythm, such as sinus arrhythmia when the heart rate increases with inspiration and decreases with expiration, may be normal in young adults. Resting pulse rate (RPR) varies by age, fitness level, gender, ethnicity/racial background, and other factors (El-Wazir, 2019).	Bradycardia (<60 beats/min) or tachycardia (>100 beats/min) may result in decreased cardiac output. Refer clients with irregular rhythms (e.g., premature atrial contraction or premature ventricular contractions, atrial fibrillation, atrial flutter with varying blocks) for further evaluation. These types of irregular patterns may predispose the client to decreased cardiac output, heart failure, or emboli.

(Continued on following page)

HEART AND GREAT VESSELS (*continued*)

ASSESSMENT PROCEDURE	NORMAL FINDINGS	ABNORMAL FINDINGS
If you detect an irregular rhythm, auscultate for a pulse rate deficit. This is done by palpating the radial pulse while you auscultate the apical pulse. Count for a full minute.	The radial and apical pulse rates should be identical.	A pulse deficit (difference between the apical and peripheral/radial pulses) may indicate atrial fibrillation, atrial flutter, premature ventricular contractions, and varying degrees of heart block.

Auscultate to identify S_1 and S_2 (Fig. 17-12). Auscultate the first heart sound (S_1 or "lub") and the second heart sound (S_2 or "dub"). Remember these two sounds make up the cardiac cycle of systole and diastole. S_1 starts systole, and S_2 starts diastole. The space, or systolic pause, between S_1 and S_2 is of short duration (thus S_1 and S_2 occur very close together); the space, or diastolic pause, between S_2 and the start of another S_1 is of longer duration.

Note: If you are experiencing difficulty differentiating S_1 from S_2, palpate the carotid pulse: the harsh sound that you hear from the carotid pulse is S_1

S_1 corresponds with each carotid pulsation and is loudest at the apex of the heart. S_2 immediately follows after S_1 and is loudest at the base of the heart.

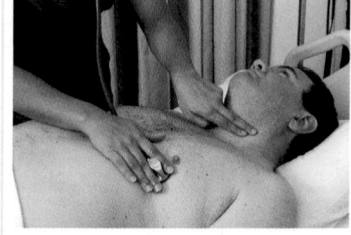

FIGURE 17-12 Palpating the carotid pulse while auscultating S_1.

ASSESSMENT PROCEDURE	NORMAL FINDINGS	ABNORMAL FINDINGS
Listen to S_1. Use the diaphragm of the stethoscope to best hear S_1 (Fig. 17-13). 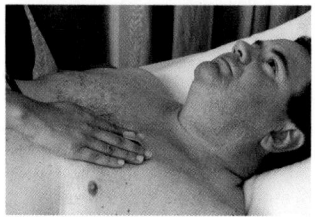 **FIGURE 17-13** Auscultating S_2.	A distinct sound is heard in each area but is loudest at the apex. May become softer with inspiration. A split S_1 may be heard normally in young adults at the left lateral sternal border.	Accentuated, diminished, varying, or split S_1 are all abnormal findings.
Listen to S_2. Use the diaphragm of the stethoscope (see Figs. 17-12 and 17-13). Ask the client to breathe regularly. *Note: Do not ask the client to hold their breath. Breath holding will cause any normal or abnormal split to subside.*	Distinct sound is heard in each area but is loudest at the base. A split S_2 (into two distinct sounds of its components—A_2 and P_2) is normal and termed *physiologic splitting*. It is usually heard late in inspiration at the second or third left interspaces.	Any split S_2 heard in expiration is abnormal.

(Continued on following page)

HEART AND GREAT VESSELS (*continued*)

ASSESSMENT PROCEDURE	NORMAL FINDINGS	ABNORMAL FINDINGS
Auscultate for **extra heart sounds.** Use the diaphragm first, then the bell to auscultate over the entire heart area. Note the characteristics (e.g., location, timing) of any extra sound heard. Auscultate during the systolic pause (space heard between S_1 and S_2). Auscultate during the diastolic pause (space heard between end of S_2 and the next S_1). *Note: While auscultating, keep in mind that development of a pathologic S_3 may be the earliest sign of heart failure.*	Normally no sounds are heard. A physiologic S_3 (Fig. 17-14) heart sound is a benign finding commonly heard at the beginning of the diastolic pause in children, adolescents, and young adults. It is rare after age 40. The physiologic S_3 usually subsides upon standing or sitting up. A physiologic S_4 heart sound (Fig. 17-15) may be heard near the end of diastole in well-conditioned athletes and in adults older than age 40 or 50 with no evidence of heart disease, especially after exercise.	Ejection sounds or clicks (e.g., a midsystolic click associated with mitral valve prolapse). A friction rub may also be heard during the systolic pause. A pathologic S_3 (ventricular gallop) may be heard with ischemic heart disease, hyperkinetic states (e.g., anemia), or restrictive myocardial disease. A pathologic S_4 (atrial gallop) toward the left side of the precordium may be heard with coronary artery disease, hypertensive heart disease, cardiomyopathy, and aortic stenosis. A pathologic S_4 toward the right side of the precordium may be heard with pulmonary hypertension and pulmonic stenosis. S_3 and S_4 pathologic sounds together create a quadruple rhythm, which is called a *summation gallop.* Opening snaps occur early in diastole and indicate mitral valve stenosis. A friction rub may also be heard during the diastolic pause.

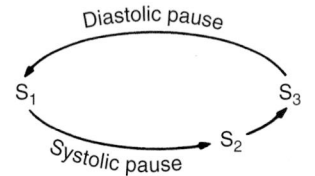

FIGURE 17-14 S_3 heart sound.

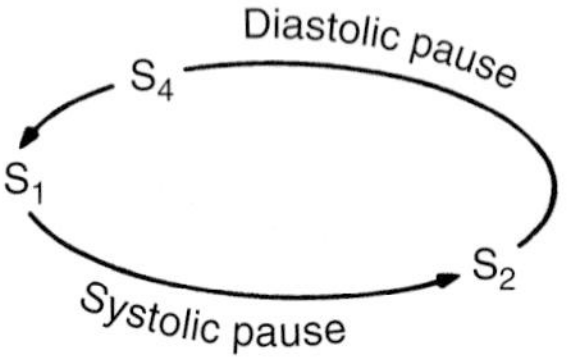

FIGURE 17-15 S_4 heart sound.

ASSESSMENT PROCEDURE	NORMAL FINDINGS	ABNORMAL FINDINGS
Auscultate for **murmurs.** A murmur is a swishing sound caused by turbulent blood flow through the heart valves or great vessels. Auscultate for murmurs across the entire heart area. Use the diaphragm and the bell of the stethoscope in all areas of auscultation because murmurs have a variety of pitches. Also auscultate with the client in different positions as described in the next section because some murmurs occur or subside according to the client's position.	Normally no murmurs are heard. However, innocent and physiologic midsystolic murmurs may be present in a healthy heart. See Table 17-2 for classification of murmurs.	Pathologic midsystolic, pansystolic, and diastolic murmurs. See Table 17-2 for classification of murmurs.

TABLE 17-2   **Gradations of Systolic Murmurs**

Grade	Description
Grade 1/6	Softer in volume than S_1 and S_2, very faint
Grade 2/6	Equal in volume to S_1 and S_2, quiet, but heard immediately
Grade 3/6	Louder in volume than S_1 and S_2, moderately loud
Grade 4/6	Louder in volume than S_1 and S_2, *with palpable thrill*
Grade 5/6	Louder in volume than S_1 and S_2, with *thrill*; may be heard when the stethoscope is partly off the chest
Grade 6/6	Louder in volume than S_1 and S_2, with *thrill*; may be heard with stethoscope entirely off the chest

Reprinted with permission from Bickley, L. S., Szilagyi, P. G., Hoffman, R. M., & Soriano, R. P. (2021). *Bates' guide to physical examination and history taking* (13th ed., Box 16-14). Wolters Kluwer.

(Continued on following page)

HEART AND GREAT VESSELS (*continued*)		
ASSESSMENT PROCEDURE	**NORMAL FINDINGS**	**ABNORMAL FINDINGS**
Auscultate **with the client assuming other positions.** Ask the client to assume a left lateral position. Use the bell of the stethoscope and listen at the apex of the heart.	S_1 and S_2 heart sounds are normally present.	An S_3 or S_4 heart sound or a murmur of mitral stenosis that was not detected with the client in the supine position may be revealed when the client assumes the left lateral position.
Ask the client to sit up, lean forward, and exhale. Use the diaphragm of the stethoscope and listen over the apex and along the left sternal border.	S_1 and S_2 heart sounds are normally present.	Murmur of aortic regurgitation may be detected when the client assumes this position.

PHYSICAL ASSESSMENT	
ASSESSMENT PROCEDURE	**NORMAL FINDINGS AND VARIATIONS**
Inspect **chest wall** in semi-Fowler position from an angle for PMI.	PMI is easily visible because heart is larger in proportion to chest size (Fig. 17-16). Heart lies more horizontally up to age 5–6 years. Thus, the PMI may be lateral to the MCL.

ASSESSMENT PROCEDURE	NORMAL FINDINGS AND VARIATIONS

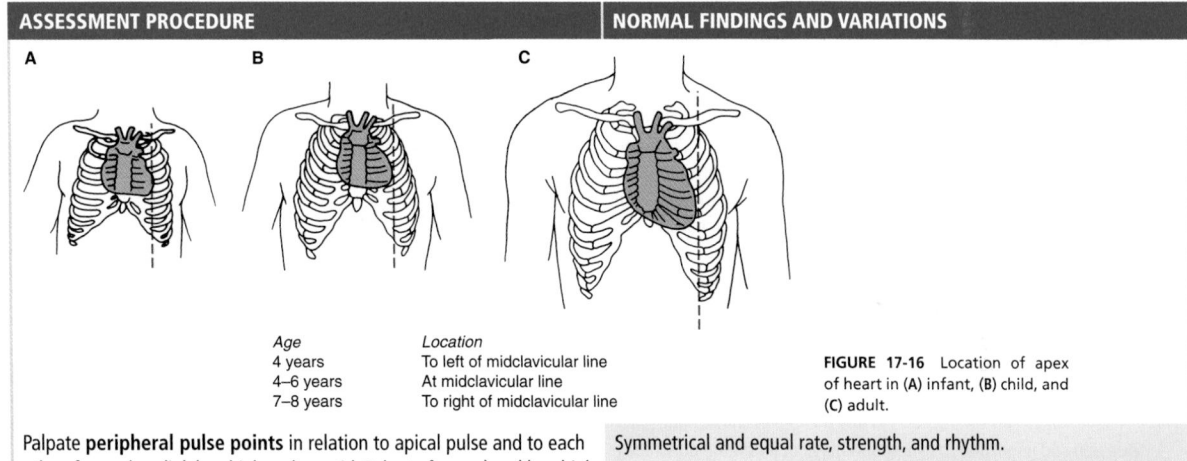

Age	Location
4 years	To left of midclavicular line
4–6 years	At midclavicular line
7–8 years	To right of midclavicular line

FIGURE 17-16 Location of apex of heart in (A) infant, (B) child, and (C) adult.

Palpate **peripheral pulse points** in relation to apical pulse and to each other: femoral, radial, brachial, and carotid. Palpate femoral and brachial pulses at the same time.	Symmetrical and equal rate, strength, and rhythm.

(Continued on following page)

PHYSICAL ASSESSMENT

ASSESSMENT PROCEDURE	NORMAL FINDINGS AND VARIATIONS
Percuss **heart size.** *Note: This is rarely done owing to inaccuracy of the method.* Auscultate **S_1 and S_2** at:	Percussion area is slightly larger because of horizontal position and overlying thymus gland.
Pulmonic area (Erb point).	S_1 is louder than S_2, or S_2 is louder than S_1. Splitting of S_2 is heard best at Erb point (25% to 33% of all children). This is a frequent site of *innocent murmurs* (grade 3 or lower), which are common throughout childhood. They are of short duration with no transmission to other areas; are low pitched, musical, or of groaning quality that is variable in intensity in relation to position, respiration, activity, fever, and anemia with no other associated signs of heart disease. Other murmurs may indicate pathology.
Tricuspid area	S_1 louder, preceding S_2
Mitral area	S_1 loudest
Auscultate for sinus arrhythmia	Varies with respiration; very common and disappears with age. Heart rate may increase with inhaling and decrease with exhaling. If a child holds their breath, rhythm will become regular.
Auscultate for pulse rate	See Table 17-3 for normal pediatric pulse rates.

TABLE 17-3   **Average Heart Rate of Infants and Children at Rest**

Age	Average Rate (beats/min)	Range (1st to 99th Percentile)
Birth	140	90–165
First 6 months	130	80–175
6–12 months	115	90–170
1–2 years	110–120	88–155
2–6 years	100–110	65–140
6–10 years	75–90	52–130

Reprinted with permission from Bickley, L. S., Szilagyi, P. G., Hoffman, R. M., & Soriano, R. P. (2021). *Bates' guide to physical examination and history taking* (13th ed., Box 25-34). Wolters Kluwer.

 PEDIATRIC VARIATIONS

Interview Questions

In addition to the focus questions for adults, inquire about the following: Mother's use of therapeutic drugs or drug abuse during pregnancy? Poor weight gain? Signs of delayed development (e.g., slowed social development, language development, or motor skills)? Difficulty in feeding (breast, bottle, acceptance of new foods)? Inability to tolerate physical activity or play with peers? Squatting behavior? Excessive irritability or crying? Circumoral cyanosis or central cyanosis?

See Table 17-3 for average heart rates of infants and children.

 GERIATRIC VARIATIONS

- Be cautious with palpating carotid arteries in older clients because atherosclerosis may have caused obstruction and compression may easily block circulation.
- Thickening of heart walls
- Decreased elasticity of heart and arteries; reduced pumping ability of heart
- Decreased cardiac output and cardiac reserve
- Apical impulse may be difficult to palpate because of increased anteroposterior chest diameter.
- Location of heart sounds and PMI may be varied owing to kyphosis or scoliosis.
- Early and soft systolic murmurs are common.
- Atrial fibrillations often occur.
- Reduced maximum heart rate

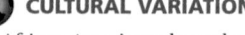

CULTURAL VARIATIONS

- African Americans have the world's highest rates of hypertension, with 40% of non-Hispanic African American men and women having hypertension (AHA, 2016). Their hypertension develops earlier in life and is more severe than other ethnic groups. As for cholesterol, Hispanic males have the highest LDL cholesterol worldwide, followed by White women, and Asians have the lowest levels (AHA, 2019a).

- Hispanics and Blacks have increasing stiffness of carotid arteries with age in comparison to Whites. As they age, Hispanics have an increased carotid diameter, which is not seen in Whites and Blacks (Markert et al., 2011). The widening of the carotid diameter in Hispanics may account for their significantly reduced rate of mortality from ischemic stroke than the rate for non-Hispanic Whites.

- In the United States, heart disease causes more deaths than other conditions among all ethnic groups. However, all cardiovascular diseases are higher in the southern states; therefore, that region is sometimes referred to as the "Stroke Belt" (Moawad, 2020).

- Surprisingly, in what has been called the "Hispanic paradox," those of Hispanic ethnicity have a higher prevalence of diabetes and obesity—and higher death rates related to diabetes, chronic liver disease/cirrhosis, and environmental conditions conducive to disease—compared with Whites but have a lower overall cardiovascular disease and mortality rate by 2 years than Whites (CDC, 2015).

POSSIBLE COLLABORATIVE PROBLEMS—RISK OF

Decreased cardiac output	Congenital heart disease
Congestive heart failure	Endocarditis
Myocardial ischemia	Angina
Cardiogenic shock	Dysrhythmia

Teaching Tips for Selected Client Concerns

Client Concern: *Fear of developing heart disease associated with family history of heart disease*

Explain what you are doing when auscultating so the client won't become alarmed by the amount of time you are taking. Explain that vigorous exercise (20–30 minutes three times a week) may decrease serum triglycerides and cholesterol, and therefore may prevent heart disease by increasing the working capabilities of the body and heart capillaries. Advise client to have a complete physical examination before starting a new fitness program.

Client Concern: *Impaired sexual activities associated with fear of injury related to postmyocardial infarction*

Instruct client to discuss limitations on sexual activities as recommended by the physician. (Usually, a client can safely engage in sexual intercourse by the time they are permitted to walk up a flight of stairs.)

***Client Concern:** Lack of information and knowledge for preventing coronary heart disease*

Teach client the following dietary and lifestyle guidelines (American Heart Association, 2017):

- Choose a diet that emphasizes intake of vegetables, fruits, and whole grains; includes low-fat dairy products, poultry, fish, legumes, nontropical vegetable oils, and nuts; and limits intake of sweets, sugar-sweetened beverages, and red meats (AHA, 2017).
- A diet high in fat and cholesterol and low in fruits and vegetables increases the chance of fatty plaque formation in the coronary vessels, which increases the chance of cardiovascular disease.
- Excessive intake of alcohol has been linked to hypertension. Three drinks at one sitting raises blood pressure. More than two drinks per day for men under 65, or one drink per day for women and men over 65, is associated with high blood pressure and other diseases (Mayo Clinic, 2019).

- Reduce elevated cholesterol (through diet, activity, or per medication, if prescribed).
- Lower blood pressure (through weight loss and increased activity).
- Increase physical activity; participate in at least moderate physical activity daily.
- Work to achieve or maintain a healthy weight for height.
- Manage diabetes if diagnosed.
- Limit alcohol intake to an average of one to two drinks per day for men and one drink per day for women. AHA (2019c) defined a drink as one 12 oz. beer, 4 oz. of wine, 1.5 oz. of 80-proof spirits, or 1 oz. of 100-proof spirits.
- Practice stress-reducing techniques such as exercise, relaxation, meditation, yoga, recreational and diversional activities from everyday work, hobbies, and so forth.
- Do not smoke tobacco, and avoid secondhand smoke.
- Refer to Agency for Healthcare Research and Quality (AHRQ). (2012). 5 Major steps to intervention (the "5 A's"). Available at https://www.ahrq.gov/prevention/guidelines/tobacco/5steps .html#:~:text=The%20five%20major%20steps%20to,every% 20patient%20at%20every%20visit.&text=Advise%20%2D%20 In%20a%20clear%2C%20strong,every%20tobacco%20user% 20to%20quit.

Client Concern: Decreased oxygenation of cardiac tissues associated with excessive activity and congestive heart failure

Teach the client to follow physician's activity recommendations. Teach the client to cluster low-energy tasks (walk to bathroom, brush teeth, gather clothes, return to chair before putting on clothes). Teach the client to space higher energy tasks with adequate rest periods. Teach the client to take radial pulse and follow the physician's recommendations for maximum pulse rate with activity.

Client Concern: Opportunity to enhance effects of prescribed cardiovascular medications

Teach client correct method for taking pulse. Instruct on heart rate necessary for taking prescribed medication.

Teach self-monitoring of heart rate or blood pressure, which is recommended if the client is taking cardiotonic or antihypertensive medications. A demonstration is necessary to ensure appropriate technique.

The AHA (2019b) recommends blood pressure screening starting at age 20 (at each healthcare visit and at least once a year if blood pressure is less than 120/80 mmHg) and fasting lipoprotein profile (cholesterol and triglycerides; baseline and every 4–6 years).

Client Concern: Opportunity to enhance exercise habits associated with requests and questions regarding primary care provider's recommended exercise plan

A sedentary lifestyle is a known modifiable risk factor contributing to heart disease. Aerobic exercise three times per week for 30 minutes is more beneficial than anaerobic exercise or sporadic exercise in preventing heart disease.

Teach the client to seek physician's recommendation regarding an exercise plan and describe the following guidelines for healthy individuals (American Heart Association, 2018). Healthy adults ages 18 to 65 years need moderate physical activity for a minimum of 30 minutes on 5 days per week or vigorous-intensity aerobic activity for a minimum of 20 minutes on 3 days per week. Combinations of moderate- and vigorous-intensity activity can be performed to meet this recommendation. In addition, every adult should perform activities that maintain or increase muscular strength and endurance a minimum of 2 days each week.

Client Concern: Fear associated with unknown outcomes of newly diagnosed cardiac defect in child

Explain to the parents and the child in simple, comprehensive terms information regarding the new diagnosis. Explain all procedures to family and child prior to the event. Encourage family to spend time alone with child to provide comfort and support to the child. Bring items from home for the child while hospitalized for the comfort of the child (special toy, blanket, etc.). Use play therapy to encourage the child to ask questions and to assist the child in understanding what is happening at the time.

References

American Heart Association. (2016). *High blood pressure and African Americans.* https://www.heart.org/en/health-topics/high-blood-pressure/why-high-blood-pressure-is-a-silent-killer/high-blood-pressure-and-african-americans

American Heart Association. (2017). *The American Heart Association's diet and lifestyle recommendations.* https://www.heart.org/HEARTORG/HealthyLiving/HealthyEating/Nutrition/The-American-Heart-Associations-Diet-and-Lifestyle-Recommendations_UCM_305855_Article.jsp

American Heart Association. (2019a). *Ethnicity a 'risk-enhancing' factor under new cholesterol guidelines.* https://www.heart.org/en/news/2019/01/11/ethnicity-a-risk-enhancing-factor-under-new-cholesterol-guidelines

American Heart Association. (2019b). *Heart-health screenings.* https://www.heart.org/en/health-topics/consumer-healthcare/what-is-cardiovascular-disease/heart-health-screenings

American Heart Association. (2019c). *Is drinking alcohol a part of a healthy lifestyle?* https://www.heart.org/en/healthy-living/healthy-eating/eat-smart/nutrition-basics/alcohol-and-heart-health

Centers for Disease Control and Prevention. (2015). Vital signs: Leading causes of death, prevalence of diseases and risk factors, and use of health services among Hispanics in the United States—2009-2013. *Morbidity and Mortality Weekly Reports (MMWR), 64*(17), 469–478.

El-Wazir. (2019). Cardiac autonomic function in different ethnic groups. *Physiology News Magazine, Summer* (115). Available at https://www.physoc.org/magazine-articles/cardiac-autonomic-function-in-different-ethnic-groups-is-heart-rate-variability-the-same-in-different-populations/ DOI: https://doi.org/10.36866/pn.115.44

Kelly, C. & Rabbani, L. (2013). Pulmonary-artery catheterization. *New England Journal of Medicine*, 369, e35. Available at https://www.nejm.org/doi/full/10.1056/NEJMvcm1212416

DOI: 10.1056/NEJMvcm1212416

Markert, M., Della-Monte, D., Cabral, D., Roberts, E., Gardener, H., Dong, C., Wright C. B., Elkind, M. S. V., Sacco, R. L. & Rundek, T. (2011). Ethnic differences in carotid artery diameter and stiffness: The Northern Manhattan study. *Atherosis, 219*(2), 827–832. https://www.ncbi.nlm.nih.gov/pmc/articles/PMC3226921/#__ffn_sectitle

Mayo Clinic. (2019). *Alcohol: Does it affect blood pressure?* https://www.mayoclinic.org/diseases-conditions/high-blood-pressure/expert-answers/blood-pressure/faq-20058254

Moawad, H. (2020). *The United States stroke belt: Why more strokes happen in the southern states.* https://www.verywellhealth.com/united-states-stroke-belt-4068563

ASSESSING PERIPHERAL VASCULAR SYSTEM

Structure and Function Overview

The peripheral vascular system, composed of arteries, capillaries, and veins, carries blood to and from the heart and contributes to regulating blood pressure and to exchanging oxygen, nutrients, and waste materials between the blood and tissue in the capillary network. The lymphatic system filters and returns tissue fluid back to the venous circulation.

Arteries carry blood from the heart to the capillaries. Artery walls are thicker and stronger than veins and contain elastic fibers to accommodate stretching as blood surges through the vessels. Each heartbeat forces a surge of blood through the arterial vessels under high pressure, which is the arterial pulse. These pulses that can be palpated include the brachial pulse, radial pulse, ulnar pulse, femoral pulse, popliteal pulse, posterior tibial pulse, and dorsalis pedal pulse (Fig. 18-1). Assessment of the carotid pulse is discussed in Chapter 17: Assessing Heart and Neck Vessels.

CAPILLARY BED AND FLUID EXCHANGE

Capillaries, very small blood vessels, form the connecting network between the arterial and venous circulation, known as *arterioles* and *venules*. This network allows balance between the vascular and interstitial

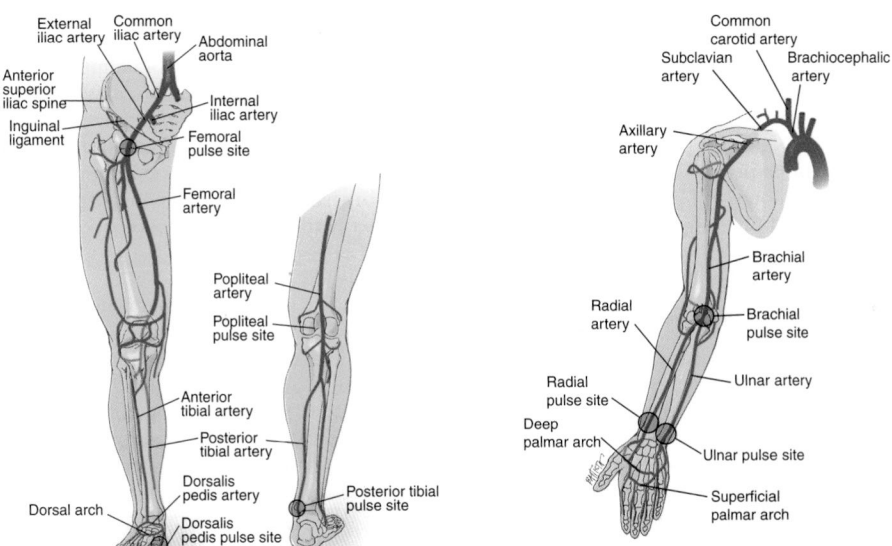

FIGURE 18-1 Major arteries of the arms and legs.

spaces. The arterial vessels transport oxygen, water, and nutrients to microscopic capillaries (Fig. 18-2). Hydrostatic pressure is the mechanism by which interstitial fluid diffuses out of the capillaries into the tissue space to release oxygen, water, and nutrients and pick up waste products. Fluid reenters the capillaries by osmotic pressure and is transported away from the tissues and interstitial spaces by venous circulation. *Lymphatic capillaries* function to remove excess fluid left behind in the interstitial spaces to maintain the balance of interstitial fluid and prevent edema.

VEINS

Veins, blood vessels that carry deoxygenated, nutrient-depleted, waste-laden blood from the tissues back to the heart, contain 70% of the body's blood volume. The veins of the arms, upper trunk, head, and neck carry blood to the superior vena cava, where it passes into the right atrium. Blood from the lower trunk and legs drains upward into the inferior vena cava. This is a low-pressure system with no force to propel blood forward. The upward flow of blood back to the heart is a result of one-way valves in the veins, skeletal muscle contraction, and the pressure gradient in the chest and abdomen that occurs with breathing. Problems with any of these mechanisms can impede venous return, resulting in venous stasis and edema in the lower extremities. Venous walls are thinner with a larger diameter than arteries. There are two *deep veins* in the leg: the *femoral vein* and *popliteal vein*. The *superficial veins* are the *great and small saphenous veins*. *Perforator veins* connect the superficial veins with the deep veins (Fig. 18-3). Assessment of the jugular vein is discussed in Chapter 17: Assessing Heart and Neck Vessels.

LYMPHATIC SYSTEM

The *lymphatic system*, a complex vascular system composed of *lymphatic capillaries*, *lymphatic vessels*, and *lymph nodes*, drains excess fluid and plasma proteins from tissues, returning them back to the venous system to prevent edema. Fluids and proteins are absorbed into the *lymphatic vessels* by *lymphatic capillaries*, which form larger vessels that pass through *lymph nodes*, where microorganisms, foreign materials, dead cells, and abnormal cells are trapped and destroyed. After the lymph is filtered, it travels to either the *right lymphatic duct*, which drains the upper right side of the body, or the *thoracic duct*, which drains the rest of the body back into the venous system through *subclavian veins* (Fig. 18-4).

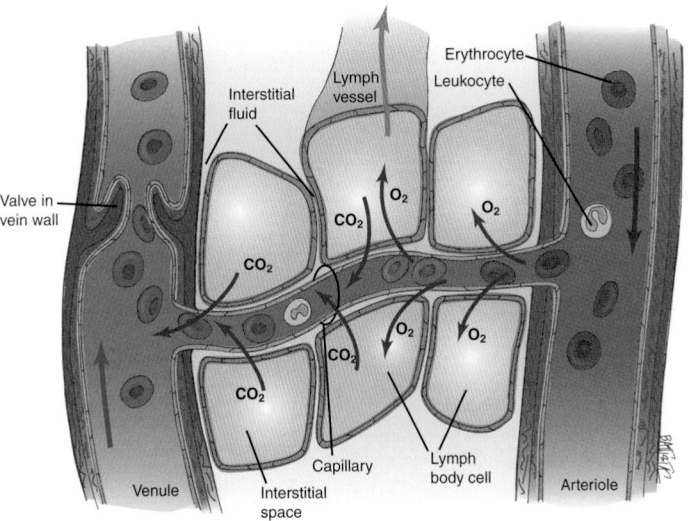

FIGURE 18-2 Normal capillary circulation ensures removal of excess fluid (edema) from the interstitial spaces as well as delivery of oxygen and nutrients and removal of carbon dioxide.

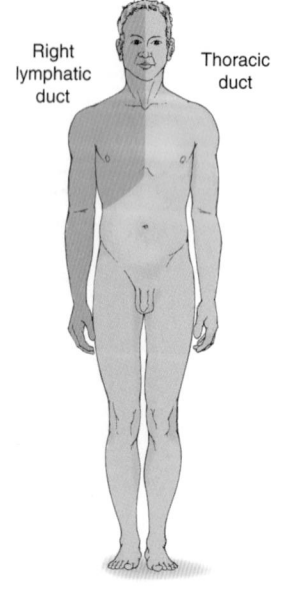

FIGURE 18-3 Major veins of the legs.

FIGURE 18-4 Lymphatic drainage.

This filtering defends the body against microorganisms and absorbs fats (lipids) from the small intestine into the bloodstream. The *superficial lymph nodes* assessed in this chapter include the *epitrochlear nodes* and the *superficial inguinal nodes*. The *epitrochlear nodes* drain the lower arm and hand. Lymph from the remainder of the arm and hand drains to the axillary lymph nodes. The *superficial inguinal nodes* drain the legs, external genitalia, and lower abdomen and buttocks (Fig. 18-5).

Nursing Assessment

COLLECTING SUBJECTIVE DATA

Interview Questions

Any changes in skin color, texture, or temperature? Pain in calves, feet, buttocks, or legs? What aggravates the pain? Walking? Sitting for long periods? Standing for long periods? Does it awaken you? What relieves the pain? Elevating legs? Rest? Lying down? Is there associated coldness, cyanosis, edema, varicosities, paresthesia, or tingling in legs or feet? Any leg veins that are rope-like, bulging, or contorted? Any sores on legs? Location? Size? Appearance? Onset? Duration? Delayed healing of sores? If client is male: Any changes in sexual activity? History of heart or

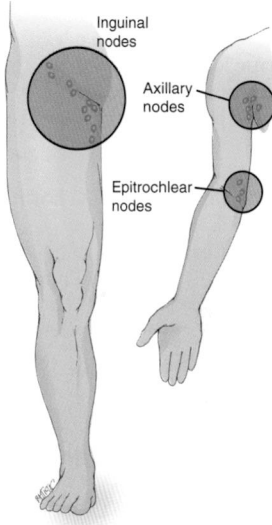

FIGURE 18-5 Superficial lymph nodes of the arms and legs.

blood vessel surgery? Family history of diabetes, hypertension, coronary artery disease, or elevated cholesterol or triglyceride levels? Is client taking any drugs that may mimic arterial insufficiency? Self-care activities: Does client have well-fitting shoes? Does client wear constricting garments or hosiery? In what type of chair does client usually sit? Does client cross legs frequently? What amount and type of exercise does the client do? Does client smoke? Amount and for how long?

Risk Factors

Risks for arterial peripheral vascular disease (PVD) related to tobacco smoking, age greater than 50 years (if client has a history of diabetes or other risk factors then age *less than* 50 years is a risk factor), family history of hypertension, coronary or PVD.

Risks for venous PVD include pregnancy, prolonged standing, limited physical activity/poor physical fitness, congenital or acquired vein wall weakness, female gender, increasing age, genetics (e.g., African American), obesity, lack of dietary fiber, use of constricting corsets/clothes.

COLLECTING OBJECTIVE DATA

Equipment Needed

- Stethoscope
- Sphygmomanometer
- Doppler
- Tape measure (paper)
- Cotton (to detect light touch)
- Paper clip (tip used to detect sharp sensation—safer than pin tip)
- Tuning fork (to detect vibratory sensation)

Physical Assessment

After explaining what assessments you will be making, provide privacy while the client changes into an examination gown. See Figures 18-1 and 18-3 for diagrams of major arteries and veins.

INSPECTION AND PALPATION OF CIRCULATION TO HANDS AND ARMS

ASSESSMENT PROCEDURE	NORMAL FINDINGS	ABNORMAL FINDINGS
Arms		
Inspection		
Observe **arm size and venous pattern**; also look for **edema**. If there is an observable difference, measure bilaterally the circumference of the arms at the same locations with each remeasurement and record findings in centimeters. ◎ **CLINICAL TIP** Mark locations on arms with a permanent marker to ensure the exact same locations are used with each reassessment.	Arms are bilaterally symmetric with minimal variation in size and shape. No edema or prominent venous patterning.	Lymphedema (Abnormal Findings 18-1) results from blocked lymphatic circulation, which may be caused by breast surgery. It usually affects one extremity, causing induration and nonpitting edema. Prominent venous patterning with edema may indicate venous obstruction (Table 18-1).
Observe **coloration of the hands and arms**.	Color varies depending on the client's skin tone, although color should be the same bilaterally (see Chapter 14 for more information).	Raynaud, a vascular disorder (Abnormal Findings 18-1) caused by vasoconstriction or vasospasm of the fingers or toes, is characterized by rapid changes of color (pallor, cyanosis, and redness), swelling, pain, numbness, tingling, burning, throbbing, and coldness. Commonly occurs bilaterally; symptoms last minutes to hours.

(Continued on following page)

INSPECTION AND PALPATION OF CIRCULATION TO HANDS AND ARMS (*continued*)

ASSESSMENT PROCEDURE	NORMAL FINDINGS	ABNORMAL FINDINGS
Palpation		
Palpate the client's **fingers, hands, and arms** and note the **temperature**.	Skin is warm to the touch bilaterally from fingertips to upper arms.	A cool extremity may be a sign of arterial insufficiency. Cold fingers and hands, for example, are common findings with Raynaud.
Palpate to assess **capillary refill time**. Compress the nailbed until it blanches. Release the pressure and calculate the time it takes for color to return. This test indicates peripheral perfusion and reflects cardiac output. *Note: Inaccurate findings may result if the room is cool, if the client has edema, has anemia, or if the client recently smoked a cigarette.*	Capillary beds refill (and, therefore, color returns) in 2 seconds or less.	Capillary refill time exceeding 2 seconds may indicate vasoconstriction, decreased cardiac output, shock, arterial occlusion, or hypothermia.
Palpate the **radial pulse.** Gently press the radial artery against the radius (Fig. 18-6). Note elasticity and strength. Assess pulse amplitude (Box 18-1). *Note: For difficult-to-palpate pulses, use a Doppler ultrasound device.*	Radial pulses are bilaterally strong (2+). Artery walls have a resilient quality (bounce).	Increased radial pulse volume indicates a hyperkinetic state (4+ or bounding pulse). Diminished (1+) or absent (0) pulse suggests partial or complete arterial occlusion (which is more common in the legs than the arms). The pulse could also be decreased from Buerger disease or scleroderma.

ASSESSMENT PROCEDURE	**NORMAL FINDINGS**	**ABNORMAL FINDINGS**
Palpate the **ulnar pulses.** Apply pressure with your first three fingertips to the medial aspects of the inner wrists. The ulnar pulses are not routinely assessed because they are located deeper than the radial pulses and are difficult to detect. Palpate the ulnar arteries if you suspect arterial insufficiency (Fig. 18-7).	The ulnar pulses may not be detectable.	Obliteration of the pulse may result from compression by external sources, as in compartment syndrome. Lack of resilience or inelasticity of the artery wall may indicate arteriosclerosis.

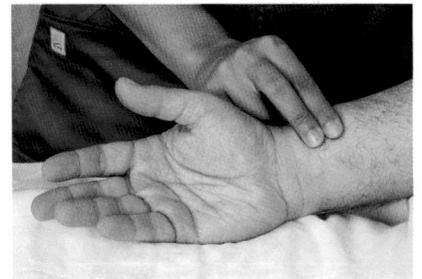

FIGURE 18-6   Palpating the radial pulse.

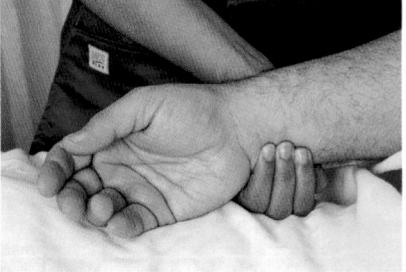

FIGURE 18-7   Palpating the ulnar pulse.

(Continued on following page)

INSPECTION AND PALPATION OF CIRCULATION TO HANDS AND ARMS (*continued*)

ASSESSMENT PROCEDURE	NORMAL FINDINGS	ABNORMAL FINDINGS
Palpate the **brachial pulses** if you suspect **arterial insufficiency.** Place the first three fingertips of each hand at the client's right and left medial antecubital creases. Alternatively, palpate the brachial pulse in the groove between the biceps and triceps. Assess pulse amplitude (see Box 18-1).	Brachial pulses have equal strength bilaterally.	Brachial pulses are increased, diminished, or absent.
Palpate the **epitrochlear lymph nodes.** Take the client's left hand in your right hand as if you were shaking hands. Flex the client's elbow about 90 degrees. Use your left hand to palpate behind the elbow in the groove between the biceps and triceps muscles (Fig. 18-8). If nodes are detected, evaluate for size, tenderness, and consistency. Repeat palpation on the opposite arm.	Normally, epitrochlear lymph nodes are not palpable.	Enlarged epitrochlear lymph nodes may indicate an infection in the hand or forearm, or they may occur with generalized lymphadenopathy. Enlarged lymph nodes may also occur because of a lesion in the area.

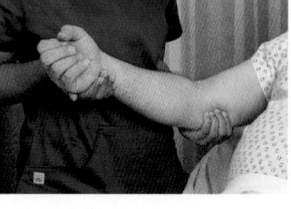

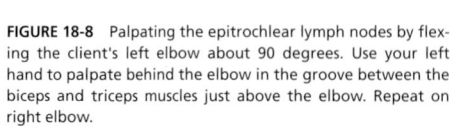

FIGURE 18-8 Palpating the epitrochlear lymph nodes by flexing the client's left elbow about 90 degrees. Use your left hand to palpate behind the elbow in the groove between the biceps and triceps muscles just above the elbow. Repeat on right elbow.

ASSESSMENT PROCEDURE	NORMAL FINDINGS	ABNORMAL FINDINGS
Perform the **Allen test** to evaluate patency of the radial or ulnar arteries when patency is questionable or before such procedures as a radial artery puncture. First assess ulnar patency. Have the client rest the hand palm side up on the examination table and make a fist. Then use your thumbs to occlude the radial and ulnar arteries (Fig. 18-9A).	Pink coloration returns to the palms within 3 to 5 seconds if the ulnar artery is patent.	With arterial insufficiency or occlusion of the ulnar artery, pallor persists.
Continue pressure to keep both arteries occluded and have the client release the fist (Fig. 18-9B).		
Note that the palm remains pale. Release the pressure on the ulnar artery and watch for color to return to the hand. To assess radial patency, repeat the procedure as before, but at the last step, release pressure on the radial artery (Fig. 18-9C).	Pink coloration returns within 3 to 5 seconds if the radial artery is patent.	With arterial insufficiency or occlusion of the radial artery, pallor persists.

(Continued on following page)

INSPECTION AND PALPATION OF CIRCULATION TO HANDS AND ARMS (*continued*)		
ASSESSMENT PROCEDURE	**NORMAL FINDINGS**	**ABNORMAL FINDINGS**
Note: Opening the hand into exaggerated extension may cause persistent pallor (false-positive Allen test).		

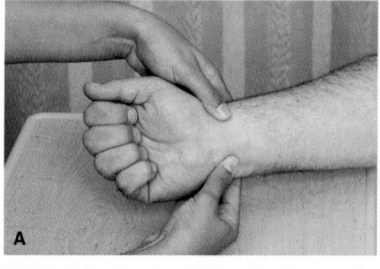 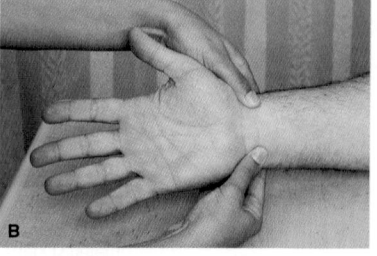 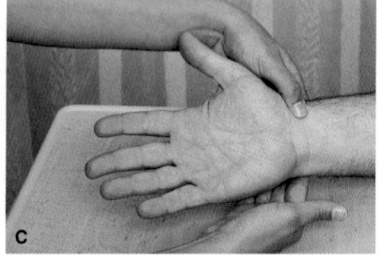

FIGURE 18-9 Allen test. **(A)** Have the client rest the hand palm side up on the examination table and then make a fist. Use your thumbs to occlude the radial and ulnar arteries. **(B)** Continue pressure to keep both arteries occluded and have the client release the fist. Note that the palm remains pale. **(C)** Release the pressure on the ulnar artery and watch for color to return to the hand. To assess radial patency, repeat the procedure as before, but as the last step, release pressure on the radial artery.

INSPECTION AND PALPATION OF CIRCULATION TO FEET AND LEGS

ASSESSMENT PROCEDURE	NORMAL FINDINGS	ABNORMAL FINDINGS

Ask the client to lie supine. Drape the groin area and place a pillow under client's head.

Observe **skin color** while inspecting **both legs from the toes to the groin.**

Pink color for lighter-skinned clients and pink or red tones visible under darker-pigmented skin. There should be no changes in pigmentation.

Pallor, especially when elevated, and rubor, when dependent, suggest arterial insufficiency. Dark-colored toes and blisters are seen with arterial insufficiency and gangrene (which causes dry, shriveled skin changing from blue to black before sloughing off) (Abnormal Findings 18-1). Cyanosis when dependent suggests venous insufficiency. A rusty, ruddy, or brownish pigmentation (rubor) around the ankles indicates venous insufficiency. (Refer to Tables 18-2 and 18-3 to differentiate between venous insufficiency and arterial insufficiency.) See Figure 18-10A and B.

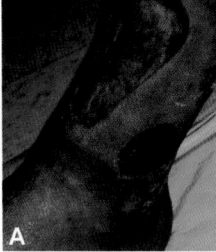 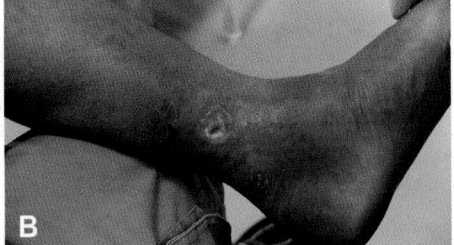

FIGURE 18-10 **(A)** Characteristic ulcer of arterial insufficiency. **(B)** Characteristic ulcer of venous insufficiency. (Part A reprinted with permission from Berg, D., & Worzala, K. [2006]. *Atlas of adult physical diagnosis*. Lippincott Williams & Wilkins.)

(Continued on following page)

INSPECTION AND PALPATION OF CIRCULATION TO FEET AND LEGS (*continued*)

ASSESSMENT PROCEDURE	NORMAL FINDINGS	ABNORMAL FINDINGS
Inspect top and bottom of feet for lesions or ulcers. Palpate for sensation.	Feet are free of lesions or ulcerations. Client has bilateral equal sensation to both feet.	Ulcers of the feet may be seen with diabetic neuropathy, neurologic disorders, or Hansen disease (Abnormal Findings 18-2).
Inspect for edema. Inspect the legs for unilateral or bilateral edema. Note veins, tendons, and bony prominences. If the legs appear asymmetric, use a centimeter tape to measure in four different areas: circumference at mid-thigh, largest circumference at the calf, smallest circumference above the ankle, and across the forefoot. Compare both extremities at the same locations. *Note: Taking a measurement in centimeters from the patella to the location to be measured can aid in getting the exact location on both legs. If additional readings are necessary, use a felt-tipped pen to ensure exact placement of the measuring tape.*	Identical size and shape bilaterally; no swelling or atrophy.	Bilateral edema may be detected by the absence of visible veins, tendons, or bony prominences. Bilateral edema usually indicates a systemic problem (such as heart failure or chronic venous insufficiency) or a local problem (such as lymph edema, which tends to be unilateral) (Dean et al., 2019). Bilateral edema may also be caused by prolonged standing or sitting (orthostatic edema). Unilateral edema is characterized by a 1-cm difference in measurement at the ankles or a 2-cm difference at the calf, and a swollen extremity. It is usually caused by venous stasis due to insufficiency or an obstruction (Abnormal Findings 18-3). It may also be caused by lymphedema. A difference in measurement between legs may also be due to muscular atrophy. Muscular atrophy usually results from disuse due to stroke or from being in a cast for a prolonged time.

ASSESSMENT PROCEDURE	NORMAL FINDINGS	ABNORMAL FINDINGS
Inspect distribution of hair on legs.	Hair covers the skin on the legs and appears on the dorsal surface of the toes.	Loss of hair on the legs suggests arterial insufficiency. Often, thin, shiny skin is noted as well.
Inspect for lesions or ulcers.	Legs are free of lesions or ulcerations.	Ulcers with smooth, even margins that occur at pressure areas, such as the toes and lateral ankle, result from arterial insufficiency. Ulcers with irregular edges, bleeding, and possible bacterial infection that occur on the medial ankle result from venous insufficiency (see Fig. 10A and B and Abnormal Findings 18-3).
Palpate **edema.** If edema is noted during inspection, palpate the area to determine if it is pitting or nonpitting. Press the edematous area with the tips of your fingers, hold for a few seconds, then release.	No edema (pitting or nonpitting) present in the legs.	If the depression does not rapidly refill and the skin remains indented on release, pitting edema is present. It is associated with systemic problems, such as heart failure or hepatic cirrhosis; local causes such as venous stasis due to insufficiency or obstruction; or prolonged standing or sitting (orthostatic edema). A 1+ to 4+ scale is used to grade the severity of pitting edema, with 4+ being most severe (Fig. 18-11).

(*Continued on following page*)

INSPECTION AND PALPATION OF CIRCULATION TO FEET AND LEGS (*continued*)

ASSESSMENT PROCEDURE	NORMAL FINDINGS	ABNORMAL FINDINGS

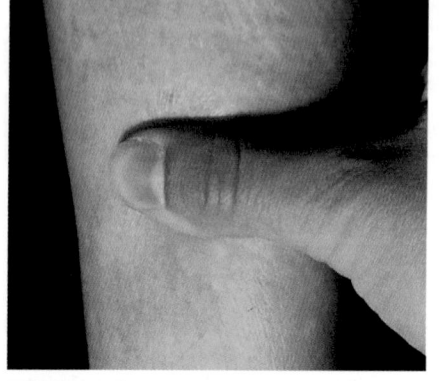 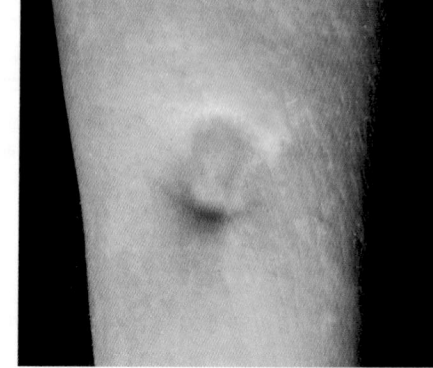

FIGURE 18-11 Pitting edema.

ASSESSMENT PROCEDURE	NORMAL FINDINGS	ABNORMAL FINDINGS
Palpate bilaterally for temperature of the feet and legs. Use the backs of your fingers. Compare your findings in the same areas bilaterally. Note location of any changes in temperature.	Toes, feet, and legs are equally warm bilaterally.	Generalized coolness in one leg or change in temperature from warm to cool as you move down the leg suggests arterial insufficiency. Increased warmth in the leg may be caused by superficial thrombophlebitis resulting from a secondary inflammation in the tissue around the vein. *Note: Bilateral coolness of the feet and legs may suggest room is too cool, client recently smoked a cigarette, or client is anemic or anxious. These factors cause vasoconstriction.*
Palpate the **superficial inguinal lymph nodes.** First, expose the client's inguinal area, keeping the genitals draped. Feel over the upper medial thigh for the vertical and horizontal groups of superficial inguinal lymph nodes. If detected, determine size, mobility, and tenderness. Repeat palpation on the opposite thigh.	Nontender, movable lymph nodes up to 1 or even 2 cm are commonly palpated.	Lymph nodes larger than 2 cm with or without tenderness (lymphadenopathy) may be from a local infection or generalized lymphadenopathy. Fixed nodes may indicate malignancy.

(Continued on following page)

INSPECTION AND PALPATION OF CIRCULATION TO FEET AND LEGS (*continued*)

ASSESSMENT PROCEDURE	NORMAL FINDINGS	ABNORMAL FINDINGS
Palpate the **femoral pulses.** Ask the client to bend the knee and move it out to the side. Press deeply and slowly below and medial to the inguinal ligament. Use two hands if necessary. Release pressure until you feel the pulse. Repeat palpation on the opposite leg. Compare pulse amplitude (Box 18-1) bilaterally (Fig. 18-12).	Femoral pulses strong and equal bilaterally.	Weak or absent femoral pulses indicate partial or complete arterial occlusion.
Auscultate the **femoral pulses.** If arterial occlusion is suspected in the femoral pulse, position the stethoscope over the femoral artery and listen for bruits. Repeat for other artery (Fig. 18-13).	No sounds auscultated over the femoral arteries.	Bruits over one or both femoral arteries suggest partial obstruction of the vessel and diminished blood flow to the lower extremities.

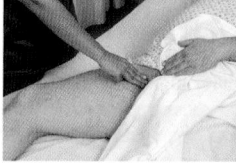 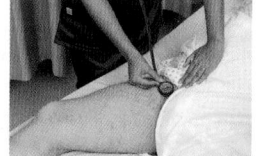

FIGURE 18-12 Palpating the femoral pulse.

FIGURE 18-13 Auscultating the femoral pulse to detect bruits.

ASSESSMENT PROCEDURE	NORMAL FINDINGS	ABNORMAL FINDINGS
Palpate the **popliteal pulses.** Ask the client to raise (flex) the knee partially. Place your thumbs on the knee while positioning your fingers deep in the bend of the knee. Apply pressure to locate the pulse. It is usually detected lateral to the medial tendon (Fig. 18-14). Assess pulse amplitude (see Box 18-1). *Note: If you cannot detect a pulse, try palpating with the client in a prone position. Partially raise the leg, and place your fingers deep in the bend of the knee. Repeat palpation in opposite leg and note amplitude bilaterally. With continued difficulty, use a Doppler device to assess pulses.*	It is not unusual for the popliteal pulse to be difficult or impossible to detect, and yet for circulation to be normal.	Although normal popliteal arteries may be nonpalpable, an absent pulse may also be the result of an occluded artery. Further circulatory assessment such as temperature changes, skin color differences, edema, hair distribution variations, and dependent rubor (dusky redness) distal to the popliteal artery assists in determining the significance of an absent pulse. Cyanosis may be present yet more subtle in darker-skinned clients (Mann, 2013).

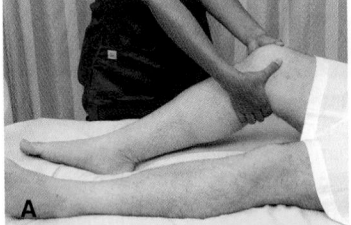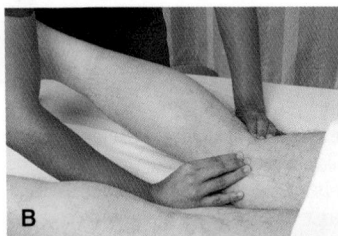

FIGURE 18-14 Palpating the popliteal pulse with the client (**A**) supine and (**B**) prone. If you cannot detect a pulse, try palpating with the client in a prone position. Partially raise the leg and place your fingers deep in the bend of the knee. Repeat palpation in opposite leg and note amplitude bilaterally.

(Continued on following page)

INSPECTION AND PALPATION OF CIRCULATION TO FEET AND LEGS (*continued*)

ASSESSMENT PROCEDURE	NORMAL FINDINGS	ABNORMAL FINDINGS
Palpate the **dorsalis pedis pulses.** Dorsiflex the client's foot and apply light pressure lateral to and along the side of the extensor tendon of the big toe. The pulses of both feet may be assessed at the same time to aid in making comparisons. Assess pulse amplitude (see Box 18-1) bilaterally (Fig. 18-15). *Note: It may be difficult or impossible to palpate a pulse in an edematous foot. A Doppler ultrasound device may be useful in this situation.*	Dorsalis pedis pulses are bilaterally strong. This pulse is congenitally absent in 5% to 10% of the population.	A weak or absent pulse may indicate impaired arterial circulation. Further circulatory assessments (temperature and color) are warranted to determine the significance of an absent pulse.

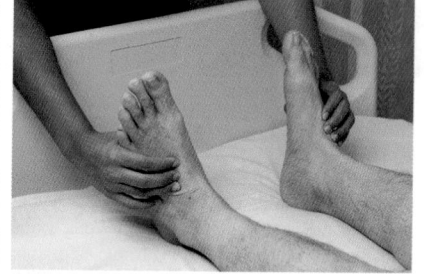

FIGURE 18-15 Palpating the dorsalis pedis pulse.

ASSESSMENT PROCEDURE	NORMAL FINDINGS	ABNORMAL FINDINGS
Palpate the **posterior tibial pulses.** Palpate behind and just below the medial malleolus (in the groove between the ankle and the Achilles tendon) (Fig. 18-16). Palpating both posterior tibial pulses at the same time aids in making comparisons. Assess pulse amplitude (see Box 18-1) bilaterally. *Note: Edema in ankles may make it difficult to palpate a posterior tibial pulse. A Doppler may be useful to assess the pulse.*	The posterior tibial pulses should be strong bilaterally. However, in about 15% of healthy clients, the posterior tibial pulses are absent. 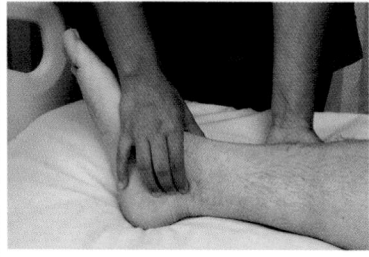 **FIGURE 18-16** Palpating the posterior tibial pulse.	A weak or absent pulse indicates partial or complete arterial occlusion.

(Continued on following page)

INSPECTION AND PALPATION OF CIRCULATION TO FEET AND LEGS (*continued*)

ASSESSMENT PROCEDURE	NORMAL FINDINGS	ABNORMAL FINDINGS
Inspect for **varicosities and thrombophlebitis.** Ask the client to stand because varicose veins may not be visible when the client is supine and not as pronounced when the client is sitting. As the client is standing, inspect for superficial vein thrombophlebitis. To fully assess for a suspected phlebitis, lightly palpate for tenderness. If superficial vein thrombophlebitis is present, note redness or discoloration on the skin surface over the vein.	Veins are flat and barely seen under the surface of the skin.	Varicose veins may appear as distended, nodular, bulging, and tortuous, depending on severity. Varicosities are common in the anterior lateral thigh, lower leg, the posterior lateral calf, and anus (known as hemorrhoids). Varicose veins (Abnormal Findings 18-3) result from incompetent valves in the veins, weak vein walls, or an obstruction above the varicosity. Despite venous dilation, blood flow is decreased and venous pressure is increased. Superficial vein thrombophlebitis is marked by redness, thickening, and tenderness along the vein. Aching or cramping may occur with walking. Swelling and inflammation are often noted.

Diagnostic testing, such as venous Doppler ultrasound of the legs, and referral are indicated for a definitive diagnosis. |

ASSESSMENT PROCEDURE	NORMAL FINDINGS	ABNORMAL FINDINGS
Special Tests for Arterial or Venous Insufficiency		
Perform **position change test for arterial insufficiency.** If pulses in the legs are weak, further assessment for arterial insufficiency is warranted. The client should be in a supine position. Place one forearm under both of the client's ankles and the other forearm underneath the knees. Raise the legs about 12 inches above the level of the heart. As you support the client's legs, ask the client to pump the feet up and down for about a minute to drain the legs of venous blood, leaving only arterial blood to color the legs. At this point, ask the client to sit up and dangle legs off the side of the examination table. Note the color of both feet and the time it takes for color to return (Fig. 18-17). *Note: This assessment maneuver will not be accurate if the client has PVD of the veins with incompetent valves.*	Feet pink to slightly pale in color in the light-skinned client with elevation. Inspect the soles in the dark-skinned client, although it is more difficult to see subtle color changes in darker skin. When the client sits up and dangles the legs, a pinkish color returns to the tips of the toes in 10 seconds or less. The superficial veins on top of the feet fill in 15 seconds or less. Normal responses with absent pulses suggest that an adequate collateral circulation has developed around an arterial occlusion.	Marked pallor with legs elevated is an indication of arterial insufficiency. Return of pink color that takes longer than 10 seconds and superficial veins that take longer than 15 seconds to fill suggest arterial insufficiency. Persistent rubor (dusky redness) of toes and feet with legs dependent also suggests arterial insufficiency (see Abnormal Findings 18-1).

(Continued on following page)

INSPECTION AND PALPATION OF CIRCULATION TO FEET AND LEGS (*continued*)

ASSESSMENT PROCEDURE	NORMAL FINDINGS	ABNORMAL FINDINGS

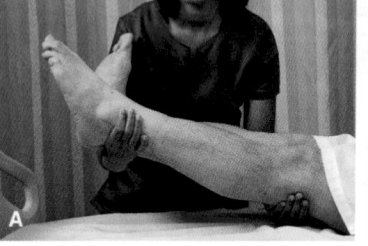 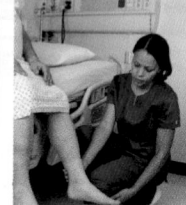

FIGURE 18-17 Testing for arterial insufficiency by (**A**) elevating the legs and then (**B**) having the client dangle the legs.

Manual compression test

If the client has varicose veins, perform manual compression to assess the competence of the vein's valves. Ask the client to stand. Firmly compress the lower portion of the varicose vein with one hand. Place your other hand 6–8 in. above your first hand. Feel for a pulsation to your fingers in the upper hand (Fig. 18-18). Repeat this test in the other leg if varicosities are present.	No pulsation is palpated if the client has competent valves.	You will feel a pulsation with your upper fingers if the valves in the veins are incompetent.

ASSESSMENT PROCEDURE	NORMAL FINDINGS	ABNORMAL FINDINGS
Trendelenburg test If the client has varicose veins (Abnormal Findings 18-3), perform the Trendelenburg test to determine the competence of the saphenous vein valves and the retrograde (backward) filling of the superficial veins. The client should lie supine. Elevate the client's leg 90 degrees for about 15 seconds or until the veins empty. With the leg elevated, apply a tourniquet to the upper thigh. *Note: Arterial blood flow is not occluded if there are arterial pulses distal to the tourniquet.* Assist the client to a standing position and observe for venous filling. Remove the tourniquet after 30 seconds and watch for sudden filling of the varicose veins from above.	Saphenous vein fills from below in 30 seconds. If valves are competent, there will be no rapid filling of the varicose veins from above (retrograde filling) after removal of tourniquet. 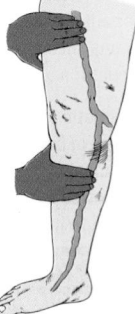 **FIGURE 18-18** Performing manual compression to assess competence of venous valves in clients with varicose veins.	Filling from above with the tourniquet in place and the client standing suggests incompetent valves in the saphenous vein. Rapid filling of the superficial varicose veins from above after the tourniquet has been removed also indicates retrograde filling past incompetent valves in the veins.

(Continued on following page)

INSPECTION AND PALPATION OF CIRCULATION TO FEET AND LEGS (*continued*)

ASSESSMENT PROCEDURE	NORMAL FINDINGS	ABNORMAL FINDINGS
Determine ankle–brachial index (ABI), also known as ankle–brachial pressure index (ABPI). Although this **advanced skill** is usually performed in a cardiovascular center, it is important to know how the test is performed and the implications. If the client has symptoms of arterial occlusion, the ABPI should be used to compare upper- and lower-limb systolic blood pressure. The ABI is the ratio of the ankle systolic blood pressure to the arm (brachial) systolic blood pressure: $$\frac{\text{Systolic ankle pressure}}{\text{Systolic brachial pressure}} = \text{ABI Index}$$ The ABI is considered an accurate objective assessment for determining the degree of peripheral arterial disease (PAD). It detects decreased systolic pressure distal to the area of stenosis or arterial narrowing and allows the nurse to quantify this measurement.	Generally, the ankle pressure in a healthy person is the same or slightly higher than the brachial pressure, resulting in an ABI of approximately 1, or no arterial insufficiency. A normal resting ABI is 1.0 to 1.4. This means that client's ankle blood pressure is the same or greater than the brachial arm pressure and that there is no significant narrowing or blockage of blood flow (Aboyans et al., 2012).	Early recognition of cardiovascular disease, even in asymptomatic people, can be determined using ABI measurements. People who smoke, are physically inactive, have a body mass index >30, or are hypertensive are more likely to have an abnormal ABI, suggesting PAD (Patel et al., 2018). If the ABI is 0.91 to 1.00, it is considered borderline abnormal. Abnormal values for the resting ABI are 0.9 or lower and 1.40 or higher; both of these indicate an increased chance of narrowed arteries in various areas of the body and increase one's risk of having a heart attack or stroke (Aboyans et al., 2012; My Cleveland Clinic, 2019). Abnormal values for the resting ABI are often associated with diabetes mellitus, chronic renal failure, and hyperparathyroidism. Medial calcific sclerosis produces falsely elevated ankle pressure by making the vessels noncompressible.

TABLE 18-1 **Stages of Lymphedema**

Grade	Description
Stage 0 Subclinical stage	No obvious signs or symptoms. Impaired lymph drainage is subclinical. Lymphedema (LE) may be present for months to years before progressing to later stages. Edema is not evident.
Stage I Mild stage	Swelling is present. Affected area pits with pressure. Elevation relieves swelling. Skin texture is smooth.
Stage II Moderate stage	Accumulation of fluid. Skin may look tight, shiny, and tissue may have a spongy feel. Pitting may or may not be present as tissue fibrosis (hardening) begins to develop. Elevation does not alleviate the swelling. Hair loss or nail changes may be experienced in affected extremity. This is an irreversible stage, but dermal fibrosis may improve with prolonged treatment.
Stage III Severe stage	LE has progressed to the lymphostatic elephantiasis stage, at which the limb is very large. Affected area is nonpitting, often with permanent edema. Skin folds develop. At increased risk for recurrent cellulitis, infections (lymphangitis), or ulcerations. Affected limb may ooze fluid. Elevation will not alleviate symptoms.

Adapted from LymphCare (2020). Stages of lymphedema. Available at https://www.lymphcareusa.com/professional/lymph-a-what/what-is-lymphedema/stages-0-3.html

BOX 18-1   ASSESSING PULSE STRENGTH

Palpation of the pulses in the peripheral vascular examination is typically to assess amplitude or strength. Pulse amplitude is graded on a 0 to 4+ scale, with 4+ being the strongest. Elasticity of the artery wall may also be noted during the peripheral vascular examination, by palpating for a resilient (bouncy) quality rather than a more rigid arterial tone, whereas pulse rate and rhythm are best assessed during examination of the heart and neck vessels.

PULSE AMPLITUDE

Pulse amplitude is typically graded as 0 to 4+:

Rating	Description
0	Absent
1+	Weak, diminished (easy to obliterate)
2+	Normal (obliterate with moderate pressure)
3+	Strong (obliterate with firm pressure)
4+	Bounding (unable to obliterate)

TABLE 18-2   Comparison of Arterial and Venous Insufficiency

	Arterial Insufficiency	Venous Insufficiency
Pulse	Decreased or absent	Present
Color	Pale on elevation, dusky rubor on dependency	Pink to cyanotic, brown pigment at ankles
Temperature	Cool, cold	Warm
Edema	None	Present
Skin	Shiny skin, thick nails, absence of hair, ulcers on toes, gangrene may develop	Ulcers on ankles; discolored, scaly
Sensation	Leg pain aggravated by exercise and relieved with rest; pressure or cramps in buttocks or calves during walking, paresthesias	Leg pain aggravated by prolonged standing or sitting, relieved by elevation of legs, lying down, or walking; also relieved with use of support hose

TABLE 18-3 **Characteristics of Arterial and Venous Insufficiency and Resulting Ulcers**

Characteristic	Arterial	Venous
General Characteristics		
Pain	Intermittent claudication to sharp, unrelenting, constant	Aching, cramping
Pulses	Diminished or absent	Present, but may be difficult to palpate through edema
Skin characteristics	Dependent rubor—elevation pallor of foot, dry, shiny skin, cool-to-cold temperature, loss of hair over toes and dorsum of foot, nails thickened and ridged	Pigmentation in gaiter area (area of medial and lateral malleolus), skin thickened and tough, may be reddish blue, frequently associated dermatitis
Ulcer Characteristics		
Location	Tip of toes, toe webs, heel or other pressure areas if confined to bed	Medial malleolus; infrequently lateral malleolus or anterior tibial area
Pain	Very painful	Minimal pain if superficial or may be very painful
Depth of ulcer	Deep, often involving joint space	Superficial
Shape	Circular	Irregular border
Ulcer base	Pale to black and dry gangrene	Granulation tissue—beefy red to yellow fibrinous in chronic long-term ulcer
Leg edema	Minimal unless extremity kept in dependent position constantly to relieve pain	Moderate to severe

Adapted with permission from Hinkle, J., & Cheever, K. (2017). *Brunner & Suddarth's textbook of medical-surgical nursing* (14th ed., Table 30-1). Wolters Kluwer.

ABNORMAL FINDINGS | **18-1** | **Abnormal Arterial Findings**

NECROTIC GREAT TOE WITH BLISTERS ON TOES AND FOOT

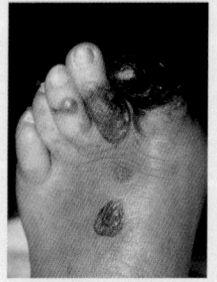

Arterial ulcer. Great toe is necrotic with blisters on the toes and foot seen in arterial insufficiency.

RAYNAUD DISEASE

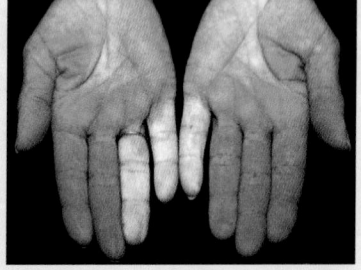

Dramatic blanching of fingers on both hands in Raynaud phenomenon.

Photo credits: Necrotic big toe, reprinted with permission from Baranoski, S., & Ayello, E. (2015). *Wound care essentials.* Wolters Kluwer; Raynaud disease, reprinted with permission from Craft, N., Fox, L. P., Goldsmith, L. A., Papier, A., Birnbaum, R., Mercurio, M. G., Miller, D., Rajendran, P., Rosenblum, M., Taylor, E., Tumeh, P. C. (2015). *VisualDx: Essential adult dermatology.* Wolters Kluwer.

NEUROPATHIC ULCER

Photo credit: Reprinted with permission from Pellico, L. H. (2013). *Focus on adult health*. Wolters Kluwer.

ABNORMAL FINDINGS 18-3 Abnormal Venous Findings

SUPERFICIAL THROMBOPHLEBITIS

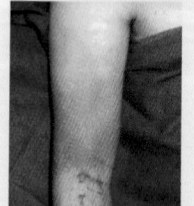

Superficial thrombophlebitis resulting from thrombus formation in the superficial veins. Often seen with unilateral localized pain, achiness, edema, redness, and warmth to touch.

LYMPHEDEMA

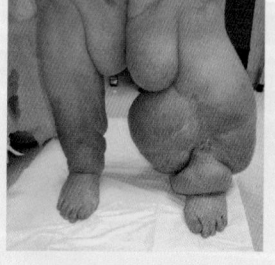

A 44-year-old female with massive localized lymphedema.

VARICOSE VEINS ON A FEMALE'S LEGS

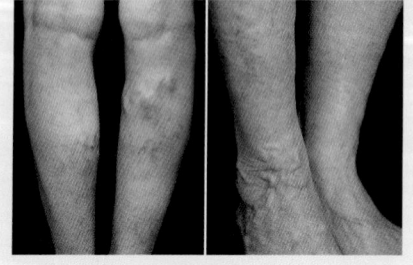

Photo credits: Superficial thrombophlebitis, Reprinted with permission from Jensen, S. (2015). *Nursing health assessment: A best practice approach.* Wolters Kluwer; lymphedema, reprinted with permission from Baranoski, S., & Ayello, E. (2015). *Wound care essentials. Wolters Kluwer.*)

GERIATRIC VARIATIONS

- Hair loss of lower extremities occurs with aging and may not be an absolute sign of arterial insufficiency.
- Inspect for rigid, tortuous veins and arteries (decreased venous return and competency) because varicosities are common in older adults.
- Prominent, bulging veins are common. Varicosities are common in the older adult and are considered a problem only if ulcerations, signs of thrombophlebitis, or cords are present. Cords are nontender, palpable veins having a rubber tubing consistency (see Abnormal Findings 18-3).
- Blood pressure increases as elasticity decreases in arteries with proportionately greater increase in systolic pressure, resulting in a widening of pulse pressure.
- Older clients with arterial disease may not have the classic symptoms of intermittent claudication but may experience coldness, color change, numbness, and abnormal sensations.

 CULTURAL VARIATIONS

- African Americans in the United States have higher rates of PAD than Whites and Hispanics (NHLBI, 2019).

- VenousNews (2019) reported the highest rate of venous insufficiency is in White women but noted significant differences in incidence and prevalence when comparing racial groups and increasing age.
- African Americans have a higher number of lower leg veins than do Whites. This may account for the lower prevalence rates of varicose veins in people of African descent (1%–2%) when compared to those of Whites (10%–18%) (Caggiati, 2013).
- However, PAD was more prevalent in African Americans and lower in Asian Americans as compared to Whites (Vitalis et al., 2017).

POSSIBLE COLLABORATIVE PROBLEMS—RISK OF

- Hypertension
- Thrombophlebitis
- Arterial insufficiency
- Peripheral neuropathy
- Thrombosis/emboli
- Venous insufficiency
- Edema
- Gangrene
- Vasospasms
- Claudication
- Stasis ulcers

Teaching Tips for Selected Client Concerns and Collaborative Problems

Client Concern: *Poor skin integrity (leg ulcers) associated with arterial venous insufficiency*

Teach Client

- Importance of exercise and diet (eat foods high in protein, vitamins A and C, and zinc to promote healing, unless contraindicated by other therapies) to aid healing of leg ulcers. Explain importance of keeping area clean and dry.
- Importance of rest, avoidance of restrictive clothing, elevation of extremities to reduce edema, and proper diet to aid healing of leg ulcers.

Client Concern: *Risk for decreased tissue perfusion associated with PVD*

Teach Client

- How to assess condition of extremities (color, temperature, sensation, movement, swelling).
- Quit smoking if you're a smoker; seek a smoking cessation program.

- If you have diabetes, keep your blood sugar in good control.
- Exercise regularly. Aim for 30 minutes at least three times a week with approval of health care provider.
- Maintain normal cholesterol and blood pressure levels.
- Eat a well-rounded diet and foods that are low in saturated and trans fats.
- Maintain a healthy weight.
- Ask your health care provider about screening with an ABI measurement once you reach 50 years of age or if you have risk factors for PAD.
- If you have Raynaud, it may often be controlled with minor lifestyle changes, such as keeping hands and feet warm and dry, preventing dryness and cracking of skin, quitting smoking, learning to manage stress, and exercising (if outside only with medical advice in cold weather).
- Follow health care providers' orders for any prescribed medications.

Risk for Peripheral Vascular Disease

Teach client risk factors associated with PVD as follows (Matsushita et al., 2019; VascularNews, 2019):

- Smoking, diabetes, and/or a history of coronary heart disease or stroke increases lifetime risk up to five times.

- Diabetes
- Obesity (a body mass index over 30)
- High blood pressure
- High cholesterol
- Increasing age, especially after reaching 50 years of age
- A family history of PAD, heart disease, or stroke
- High levels of homocysteine, a protein component that helps build and maintain tissue

Teach client to discuss screening with primary care provider if at high risk. Screening methods for PAD involve physical examination of pulses in feet and legs, ABI (comparison of blood pressure at ankle with blood pressure at arm), ultrasound (including Doppler to detect blood flow through blood vessels), angiography, and blood tests for cholesterol and triglycerides (Mayo Clinic, 2018). The most common screening method is the ABI.

Possible Collaborative Problem: Risk for Hypertension

Explain the effects of diet (low fat and low cholesterol), reduction of stress, vigorous exercise, not smoking, and decreased use of alcohol on promotion of adequate circulation. Blood pressure

checks should be done on a regular basis. Blood pressures of 120 to 139/80 to 89 mmHg are considered prehypertensive and require lifestyle modification (Seventh Report of the Joint National Committee on Prevention, Detection, and Treatment of High Blood Pressure, 2003). Refer any client with a reading greater than or equal to 140/90 mmHg for treatment.

References

Aboyans, V., Criqui, M., Abraham, P., Allison, M., Creager, M., Diehm, C., Fowkes, F. G. R., Hiatt, W. R., Jönsson, B., Lacroix, P., Marin, B., McDermott, M. M., Norgren, L. Pande R. L., Preux, P.-M., Stoffers, H. E. J., Treat-Jacobson, D., American Heart Association Council on Peripheral Vascular Disease., Council on Epidemiology and Prevention., Council on Clinical Cardiology., Council on Cardiovascular Nursing., Council on Cardiovascular Radiology and Intervention., & Council on Cardiovascular Surgery and Anesthesia. (2012). Measurement and interpretation of the ankle-brachial index: A scientific statement from the American Heart Association. *Circulation, 126*(24), 2890–2909.

Caggiati, A. (2013). The venous valves of the lower limbs. *Phlebolymphology, 20*(2), 87–95. https://www.phlebolymphology.org/wp-content/uploads/2014/09/Phlebolymphology78.pdf

Dean, S., Valenti, E., Hock, K., Leffler, J., Compston, A., & Abraham, W. (2019). The clinical characteristics of lower extremity lymphedema in

440 patients. *Journal of Vascular Surgery, Venous and Lymphatic Disorders,* 8(5), 851-859. https://doi.org/10.1016/j.jvsv.2019.11.014

Mann, A. R. (2013). *Handbook for focus on adult health medical-surgical nursing,* Wolters Kluwer Health/Lippincott Williams & Wilkins.

Matsushita, K., Sang, Y., Ning, H., Ballew, S., Chow, E., Grams, M., Selvin, E., Allison, M., Criqui, M., Coresh, J., Lloyd-Jones, D. M., & Wilkins, J. (2019). Lifetime risk of lower-extremity peripheral artery disease defined by ankle-brachial index in the United States. *Journal of the America Heart Association, 8,* e012177. https://doi.org/10.1161/JAHA.119.012177

Mayo Clinic. (2018). *Peripheral artery disease (PAD).* https://www.mayoclinic.org/diseases-conditions/peripheral-artery-disease/symptoms-causes/syc-20350557

My Cleveland Clinic. (2019). *Ankle-brachial index.* https://my.clevelandclinic.org/health/diagnostics/17840-ankle-brachial-index-abi#:~:text=The%20ABI%20itself%20is%20the,1.0%20and%201.4%20is%20normal

National Heart, Lung, and Blood Institute. (2019). *Risk of peripheral artery disease significantly higher in African-Americans.* https://www.nhlbi.nih.gov/news/2019/risk-peripheral-artery-disease-significantly-higher-african-americans

Patel, K., Jones, P., Ellerbeck, E., Buchanan, D., Chan, P., Pacheco, C., Moneta, G., Spertus, J. A., & Smolderen, K. (2018). Underutilization of evidence-based smoking cessation support strategies despite high smoking addiction burden in peripheral artery disease specialty care: Insights from the international PORTRAIT registry. *Journal of the American Heart Association, 7*(20), e010076. https://www.ahajournals.org/doi/10.1161/JAHA.118.010076

Seventh Report of the Joint National Committee on Prevention, Detection, and Treatment of High Blood Pressure. (2003). *Hypertension, 42,* 1206-1252. DOI: https://doi.org/10.1161/01.HYP.0000107251.49515.c2 Available at https://www.ahajournals.org/doi/10.1161/01.HYP.0000107251.49515.c2

VascularNews. (2019). *Peripheral artery disease risk hinges on health factors and demographics, including race.* https://vascularnews.com/peripheral-arterial-disease-risk-hinges-on-health-factors-and-demographics-including-race/

Vitalis, A., Lip, G., Kay, M., Vohra, R., & Shantsila, A. (2017). Ethnic differences in the prevalence of peripheral arterial disease: A systematic review and meta-analysis. *Expert Review of Cardiovascular Therapy, 15*(4), 327–338. https://doi.org/10.1080/14779072.2017.1305890

VenousNews. (2019). *US study finds racial disparities in outcomes of superficial vein treatments.* https://venousnews.com/racial-disparities-superficial-vein-treatments/

19 > ASSESSING ABDOMEN

Structure and Function Overview

The abdomen is bordered superiorly by the costal margins, inferiorly by the symphysis pubis and inguinal canals, and laterally by the flanks. It is important to understand the anatomic divisions known as the abdominal quadrants, the abdominal wall muscles, the internal anatomy of the abdominal cavity, and the abdominal vasculature in order to perform an adequate assessment of the abdomen.

ABDOMINAL QUADRANTS

The abdomen is divided into four quadrants for purposes of physical examination. These are termed the right upper quadrant (RUQ), right lower quadrant (RLQ), left lower quadrant (LLQ), and left upper quadrant (LUQ) (Fig. 19-1). Note which organs are located within each quadrant (Box 19-1).

ABDOMINAL WALL MUSCLES

The abdominal contents are enclosed externally by the abdominal wall musculature, which includes three layers of muscle extending from the back, around the flanks, and to the front. The outermost layer is the external abdominal oblique, the middle layer is the internal abdominal oblique, and the innermost layer is the transverse abdominis (Fig. 19-2).

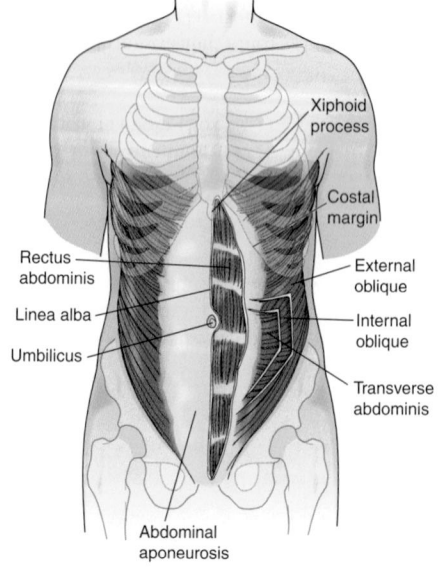

FIGURE 19-1 Abdominal quadrants.

FIGURE 19-2 Abdominal wall muscles.

BOX 19-1 LOCATING ABDOMINAL STRUCTURES BY QUADRANTS

RUQ

Ascending and transverse colon
Duodenum
Gallbladder
Hepatic flexure of colon
Liver
Pancreas (head)
Pylorus (the small bowel—or ileum—traverses all quadrants)
Right adrenal gland
Right kidney (upper pole)
Right ureter

RLQ

Appendix
Ascending colon
Cecum
Right kidney (lower pole)
Right ovary and tube
Right ureter
Right spermatic cord

LUQ

Left adrenal gland
Left kidney (upper pole)
Left ureter
Pancreas (body and tail)
Spleen
Splenic flexure of colon
Stomach
Transverse ascending colon

LLQ

Left kidney (lower pole)
Left ovary and tube
Left ureter
Left spermatic cord
Sigmoid colon

MIDLINE

Bladder
Uterus
Prostate gland

INTERNAL ABDOMINAL STRUCTURES

A thin, shiny, serous membrane lines the abdominal cavity and provides a protective covering (parietal peritoneum) for most of the internal abdominal organs (visceral peritoneum). Within the abdominal cavity are structures of several different body systems—gastrointestinal (GI), reproductive (female), lymphatic, and urinary. These structures are typically referred to as the abdominal viscera and can be divided into two types—solid viscera and hollow viscera. Solid viscera are those organs that maintain their shape consistently—the liver, pancreas, spleen, adrenal glands, kidneys, ovaries, and uterus. The hollow viscera consist of structures that change shape depending on their contents. These include the stomach, gallbladder, small intestine, colon, and bladder.

Solid Viscera

The liver is the largest solid organ in the body. It is located below the diaphragm in the RUQ of the abdomen (Fig. 19-3). The pancreas, located mostly behind the stomach, deep in the upper abdomen, is normally not palpable (see Figs. 19-3 and 19-4). The spleen is approximately 7 cm wide and is located above the left kidney, just below the diaphragm at the level of the 9th, 10th, and 11th ribs (see Fig. 19-3). This soft, flat structure is normally

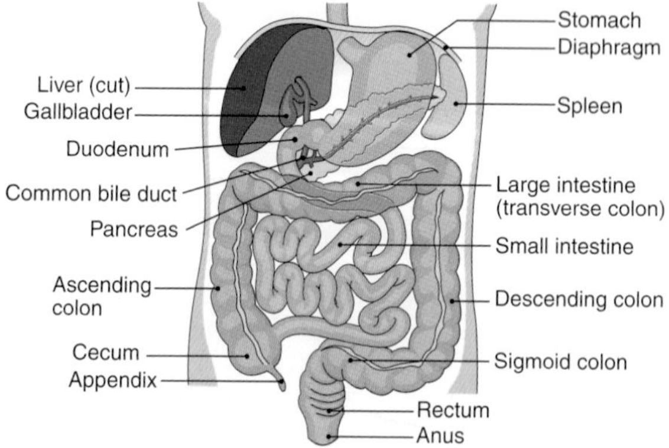

FIGURE 19-3 Abdominal viscera.

not palpable. The kidneys are located high and deep under the diaphragm (see Fig. 19-4).

The pregnant uterus may be palpated above the level of the symphysis pubis in the midline (see Fig. 19-4). The ovaries are located in the RLQ and LLQ and are normally palpated during a bimanual examination of the internal genitalia.

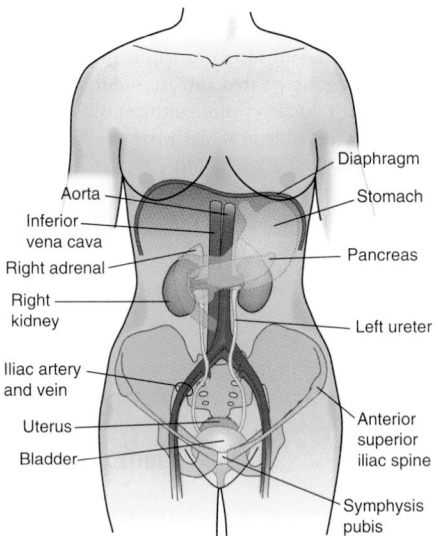

FIGURE 19-4 Abdominal and vascular structures (aorta and iliac artery and vein).

Hollow Viscera

The stomach is a distensible, flask-like organ located in the LUQ, just below the diaphragm and in between the liver and the spleen. The stomach is not usually palpable (see Fig. 19-3).

The gallbladder, a muscular sac approximately 10 cm long, is not normally palpated because it is difficult to distinguish between the gallbladder and the liver (see Fig. 19-3).

The small intestine is actually the longest portion of the digestive tract (approximately 7 m long). The small intestine, which lies coiled in all four quadrants of the abdomen, is not normally palpated (see Fig. 19-3).

The colon, or large intestine, has a wider diameter than the small intestine (approximately 6 cm) and is approximately 1.4 m long. The colon is composed of three major sections: ascending, transverse, and descending.

The sigmoid colon is often felt as a firm structure on palpation, whereas the cecum and ascending colon may feel softer. The transverse and descending colon may also be felt on palpation (see Fig. 19-3).

The urinary bladder is a distensible muscular sac located behind the pubic bone in the midline of the abdomen. A bladder filled with urine may be palpated in the abdomen above the symphysis pubis (see Fig. 19-4).

VASCULAR STRUCTURES

The abdominal organs are supplied with arterial blood by the abdominal aorta and its major branches. Pulsations of the aorta are frequently visible and palpable midline in the upper abdomen (see Fig. 19-4).

COLLECTING SUBJECTIVE DATA

Interview Questions

Abdominal pain? Character? Onset? Location? Duration? Severity? Relieving and aggravating factors? Associated factors? (See Abnormal Findings 19-1.) Indigestion? Nausea? Vomiting? Precipitating/relieving factors? Change in appetite? Associated weight loss? Change in bowel elimination? Describe. Constipation? Diarrhea? Associated symptoms? Any past GI disorders (ulcers, gastroesophageal reflux, inflammatory or obstructive bowel, pancreatitis, gallbladder or liver disease, diverticulosis, appendicitis, history of viral hepatitis)? Family history of colon, stomach, pancreatic, liver, kidney, or bladder cancer? Use of medications—aspirin, ibuprofen, anti-inflammatory drugs, steroids? Chronic use of antacids or histamine-2 blockers? GI diagnostic tests? Surgeries? Health practices: usual diet? Exercise? Use of alcohol? Use of caffeine, typical dietary and fluid intake (24-hour recall)? Effects of GI problems on activities of lifestyle? Current life stressors?

Risk Factors

- Risk for hepatitis B virus (HBV) exposure related to contact in population of high HBV endemicity, sexual contact with carriers, intravenous drug abusers, heterosexuals who have had more than one sex partner in the past 6 months, males who have sex with other males, people with hemophilia, people undergoing hemodialysis, international travelers in high-risk HBV areas, healthcare workers, long-term prison inmates.
- Risk for gallbladder cancer related to female gender after menopause, increased parity, obesity, chronic inflammation or other diseases of the gallbladder or biliary system, and chronic infections of *Helicobacter pylori* or *Salmonella*.
- Risk for colon cancer related to age greater than 50 years; family or personal history of colorectal cancer; history of endometrial, breast, or ovarian cancer; history of inflammatory bowel disease or polyps; diet low in fiber and high in fat; African American ethnicity; sedentary lifestyle; heavy alcohol intake; or past radiation treatments for other cancers.

COLLECTING OBJECTIVE DATA

Equipment Needed

- Stethoscope (warm the diaphragm and bell)
- Centimeter ruler
- Marking pen
- Small pillow

Physical Assessment

Review Figures 19-1 to 19-4 for a diagram of landmarks of the abdomen.

Assessment of the abdomen differs from other assessments in that inspection and auscultation precede percussion and palpation. This sequence allows accurate assessment of bowel sounds and delays more uncomfortable maneuvers until last. The client is placed in the supine position, with small pillows under the head and knees. The abdomen is exposed from the breasts to the symphysis pubis.

Examiner should warm hands and have short fingernails. Stand at the client's right side and carry out assessment systematically, beginning with the LUQ and progressing clockwise through the four abdominal quadrants (see Fig. 19-1). The client's bladder should be empty.

INSPECTION		
ASSESSMENT PROCEDURE	**NORMAL FINDINGS**	**ABNORMAL FINDINGS**
Inspect the **skin** for the following:		
• Color	• Normally paler, with white striae	• Purple flank color (Grey Turner sign) seen with bleeding within the abdominal wall • Dark bluish-pink striae are associated with Cushing syndrome.

(Continued on following page)

INSPECTION (*continued*)

ASSESSMENT PROCEDURE	NORMAL FINDINGS	ABNORMAL FINDINGS
• Integrity	• No rashes or lesions.	• Striae may also be caused by ascites that stretches the skin. • Pale and taut with ascites, which may result from liver failure or liver disease • Rashes, lesions • Changes in moles including size, color, and border symmetry. Bleeding moles or petechiae (reddish or purple lesions) may also be abnormal.
• Venous pattern	• Scattered fine veins may be visible. Blood in the veins located above the umbilicus flows toward the head; blood in the veins located below the umbilicus flows toward the lower body.	• Engorged, prominent veins seen with cirrhosis of the liver, inferior vena cava obstruction, portal hypertension, or ascites.
Perform the following special maneuver for **prominent abdominal veins:**		
• Compress a section of vein with two fingers next to each other, remove one finger, and observe for filling; repeat procedure, removing the other finger.	• Blood fills from upper to lower abdomen.	• Blood fills from lower to upper abdomen (obstructed inferior vena cava).

ASSESSMENT PROCEDURE	NORMAL FINDINGS	ABNORMAL FINDINGS
Inspect the **umbilicus** for the following:		
• Position	• Midline at lateral line • Sunken, centrally located	• Deviated from midline with pressure from a mass, hernia, enlarged organs, or fluid; everted with abdominal distention, umbilical hernia, or scar tissue.
• Color	• Pinkish	• Inflamed, crusted; bluish color (Cullen sign) seen in intra-abdominal hemorrhage
• Contour	• Recessed (inverted) or protruding no more than 0.5 cm and is round or conical	• An everted umbilicus is seen with abdominal distention. An enlarged, everted umbilicus suggests umbilical hernia.
Inspect **abdominal contour**. Sitting at the client's side, look across the abdomen at a level slightly higher than the client's abdomen (Fig. 19-5). Inspect the area between the lower ribs and pubic bone. Measure abdominal girth.	Abdomen is flat, rounded, or scaphoid (usually seen in thin adults); the abdomen should be evenly rounded.	A generalized protuberant or distended abdomen may be due to obesity, air (gas), or fluid accumulation. Distention below the umbilicus may be due to a full bladder, uterine enlargement, or an ovarian tumor or cyst. Distention of the upper abdomen may be seen with masses of the pancreas or gastric dilation. The major causes of abdominal distention are sometimes referred to as the "6 Fs": fat, feces, fetus, fibroids, flatulence, and fluid.

(Continued on following page)

INSPECTION (*continued*)

ASSESSMENT PROCEDURE	NORMAL FINDINGS	ABNORMAL FINDINGS
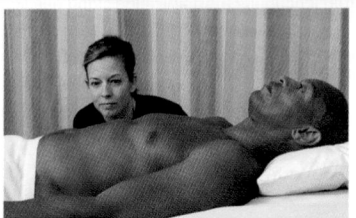 **FIGURE 19-5** View abdominal contour from the client's side.		A scaphoid (sunken) abdomen may be seen with severe weight loss or cachexia related to starvation or terminal illness.
Assess **abdominal symmetry**. Look at the abdomen as the client lies in a relaxed supine position.	Abdomen is symmetric.	Asymmetry may be seen with organ enlargement, large masses, hernia, diastasis recti, or bowel obstruction.
Observe **aortic pulsations**. Ultrasound has high sensitivity and specificity and is the preferred screening modality. Abdominal palpation has poor accuracy and is not recommended for screening (Agency for Healthcare Research and Quality, 2018).	A slight pulsation of the abdominal aorta, which is visible in the epigastrium, extends full length in thin people.	Vigorous, wide, exaggerated pulsations may be seen with abdominal aortic aneurysm (AAA). See Abnormal Findings 19-2 to 19-4.

ASSESSMENT PROCEDURE	NORMAL FINDINGS	ABNORMAL FINDINGS
Observe for **peristaltic waves.**	Normally, peristaltic waves are not seen, although they may be visible in very thin people as slight ripples on the abdominal wall.	Peristaltic waves are increased and progress in a ripple-like fashion from the LUQ to the RLQ with intestinal obstruction (especially small intestine). In addition, abdominal distention typically is present with intestinal wall obstruction.

AUSCULTATION

Note: *Using the diaphragm of a warm stethoscope, apply light pressure to auscultate for bowel sounds for up to 5 minutes in each quadrant. Use the bell to auscultate for vascular sounds.*

Auscultate for **bowel sounds.**	A series of intermittent, soft clicks and gurgles are heard at a rate of 5 to 30 per minute. Postoperatively, bowel sounds may resume gradually with the small intestine functioning normally in the first few hours post-op; stomach emptying takes 24 to 48 hours to recover, and the colon requires 3 to 5 days to recover propulsive activity.	"Hyperactive" bowel sounds that are rushing, tinkling, and high pitched (borborygmus) may be abnormal indicating very rapid motility heard in early bowel obstruction, gastroenteritis, diarrhea, or use of laxatives. "Hypoactive" and/or absent bowel sounds indicate diminished bowel motility. Common causes include paralytic ileus following abdominal surgery, inflammation of the peritoneum, or late bowel obstruction. May also occur in pneumonia.

(Continued on following page)

AUSCULTATION (*continued*)

ASSESSMENT PROCEDURE	NORMAL FINDINGS	ABNORMAL FINDINGS
Auscultate for **vascular sounds** (Fig. 19-6). Use the bell of the stethoscope to listen for bruits (low-pitched, murmur-like sounds) over the abdominal aorta and renal, iliac, and femoral arteries.	Bruits are not normally heard over abdominal aorta or renal, iliac, or femoral arteries. However, bruits confined to systole may be normal in some clients depending on other differentiating factors.	A bruit with both systolic and diastolic components occurs when blood flow in an artery is turbulent or obstructed. This may indicate an aneurysm or renal arterial stenosis (RAS). When blood flows through a narrow vessel, it makes a whooshing sound, called a bruit. However, the absence of this sound does not exclude the possibility of RAS. For a more accurate diagnosis, an ultrasound or an angiogram is needed.

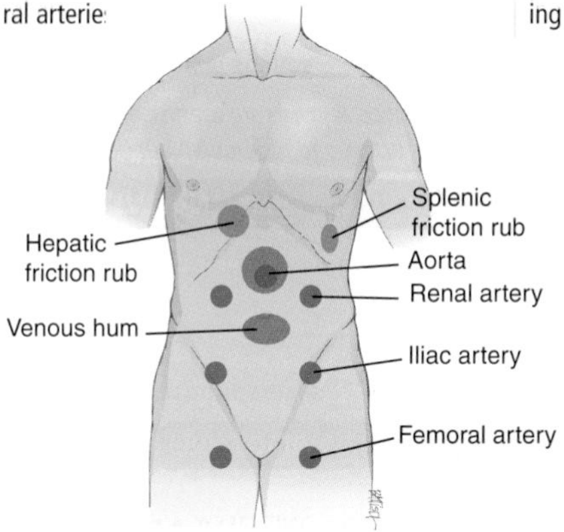

FIGURE 19-6 Vascular sounds and friction rubs can best be heard over these areas.

ASSESSMENT PROCEDURE	NORMAL FINDINGS	ABNORMAL FINDINGS
Note: Auscultating for vascular sounds is especially important if the client has hypertension or if you suspect arterial insufficiency to the legs.	*Note: If bruits are heard,* **do not palpate abdomen** *as it may indicate a narrowed vessel or aneurysm.*	
Listen for **venous hum**. Using the bell of the stethoscope, listen for a venous hum in the epigastric and umbilical areas.	Venous hum is not normally heard over the epigastric and umbilical areas.	Venous hums are rare. However, an accentuated venous hum heard in the epigastric or umbilical areas suggests increased collateral circulation between the portal and systemic venous systems, as in cirrhosis of the liver.
Auscultate for a **friction rub** over the liver and spleen. Listen over the right and left lower rib cage with the diaphragm of the stethoscope.	No friction rub over the liver or spleen is present.	Friction rubs are rare. If heard, they have a high-pitched, rough, grating sound produced when the large surface area of the liver or spleen rubs the peritoneum. They are heard in association with respiration.
		A friction rub heard over the lower right costal area is associated with hepatic abscess or metastases.
		A rub heard at the anterior axillary line in the lower left costal area is associated with splenic infarction, abscess, infection, or tumor.

(Continued on following page)

PERCUSSION

ASSESSMENT PROCEDURE	NORMAL FINDINGS	ABNORMAL FINDINGS

Note: Percussion notes will vary from dull to tympanic, with tympany dominating over the hollow organs. The hollow organs include the stomach, intestines, bladder, aorta, and gallbladder. Dull percussion notes will be heard over the liver, spleen, pancreas, kidneys, and uterus. Percuss from areas of tympany to dullness to locate borders of these solid organs.

Percuss abdomen in **all four quadrants** for percussion tones (notes); see Figure 19-7.	Generalized tympany predominates over the abdomen because of air in the stomach and intestines.	Increased dullness over enlarged organs; hyper-resonance over gaseous, distended abdomen.

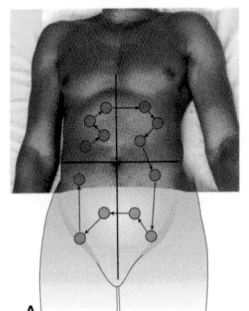

FIGURE 19-7 Abdominal percussion sequences may proceed clockwise or up and down over the abdomen. **(A)** Abdominal percussion pattern. **(B)** Abdominal percussion technique.

ASSESSMENT PROCEDURE	NORMAL FINDINGS	ABNORMAL FINDINGS
Percuss the **liver** for span as follows: • Percuss starting below umbilicus at client's right midclavicular line (MCL), and percuss upward until you hear dullness; mark this point. Percuss downward from lung resonance in the right MCL to dullness and mark this point.	Liver span is 6 to 12 cm (2.5–5 in.) in the right MCL (Fig. 19-8). The lower border of liver dullness is located at the costal margin to 1 to 2 cm below. On deep inspiration, the lower border of liver dullness may descend from 1 to 4 cm below the costal margin. **Note:** *Liver span is greater in men.*	• Liver span is greater than 12 cm in the right MCL with enlarged liver as seen in tumors, cirrhosis, abscess, and vascular engorgement. A liver in a lower position may be caused by emphysema, and a liver in a higher position may be caused by a mass, ascites, or paralyzed diaphragm.

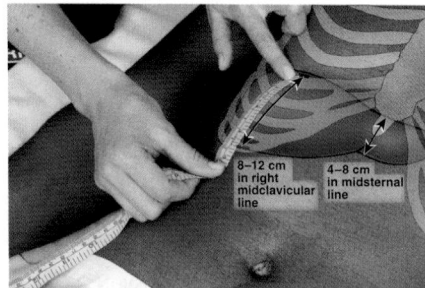

8–12 cm in right midclavicular line 4–8 cm in midsternal line

FIGURE 19-8 Normal liver span.

(Continued on following page)

PERCUSSION (*continued*)

ASSESSMENT PROCEDURE	NORMAL FINDINGS	ABNORMAL FINDINGS
• Repeat in midsternal line.	• Liver span is 4 to 8 cm in midsternal line.	• Liver span is greater than 8 cm in right midsternal line.

The Scratch test is a technique that can be used to ascertain the location and size of the liver and spleen. This test can be particularly useful if the abdomen is tense (rigid or guarded), distended, obese, or tender.

Mark a point on the right costal margin at the MCL. Place the diaphragm of the stethoscope on the xiphisternum. Use one finger to very lightly stroke the skin in transverse strokes parallel to where the liver edge is suspected. Advance strokes from the RLQ along the MCL line to the costal margin (Fig. 19-9). The sound will suddenly be transmitted through the stethoscope and increase in intensity. Mark the point of loudest intensity to estimate the liver's edge.

The normal liver span at the midsternal line (MSL) is 4 to 8 cm.

An enlarged liver may be roughly estimated (not accurately) when more intense sounds outline a liver span or borders outside the normal range. See Abnormal Findings 19-4.

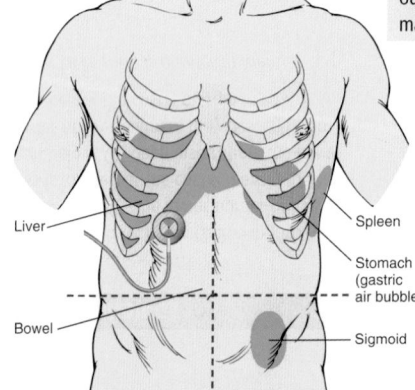

Liver — Spleen — Stomach (gastric air bubble) — Bowel — Sigmoid

FIGURE 19-9 The Scratch test. Use one finger to very lightly stroke the skin horizontally, starting at the umbilicus. Continue to stroke the skin moving toward the lower costal margin. The sound will suddenly be transmitted through the stethoscope and increase in intensity. This indicates the lower border of the liver.

ASSESSMENT PROCEDURE	NORMAL FINDINGS	ABNORMAL FINDINGS
Splenic percussion sign: Ask client to inhale deeply and hold breath; percuss lowest interspaces at the left anterior axillary line.	Percussion note remains tympanic on inhalation.	Percussion note becomes dull on inhalation.
Perform blunt percussion on the kidneys at the costovertebral angles (CVA) over the 12th rib (Fig. 19-10).	Normally, no tenderness or pain is elicited or reported by the client. The examiner senses only a dull thud.	Tenderness or sharp pain elicited over the CVA suggests kidney infection (pyelonephritis), renal calculi, or hydronephrosis.

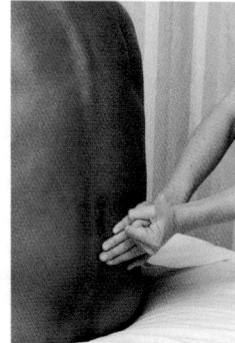

FIGURE 19-10 Performing blunt percussion over the kidney.

(Continued on following page)

PALPATION

Note: Light palpation precedes deep palpation to detect tenderness and superficial masses. Deep palpation is used to detect masses and size of organs.

Watch the client's facial expressions and body posture carefully to help assess pain. Examine tender areas last. Never use deep palpation over tender organs in clients with polycystic kidneys, after renal transplant, or after hearing an abnormal bruit. Use deep palpation with caution.

ASSESSMENT PROCEDURE	NORMAL FINDINGS	ABNORMAL FINDINGS
Lightly palpate all **four quadrants** for the following:		
• Tenderness	• Nontender	• Tender, painful with infection, inflammation, pressure from gaseous distention, tumors, or enlarged organs
• Consistency	• Soft, nontender	• Rigid, board-like
• Masses	• No masses	• Superficial masses (A superficial mass becomes more prominent against examiner's hand when client lifts head from examination table, whereas a deep abdominal mass does not.)

ASSESSMENT PROCEDURE	NORMAL FINDINGS	ABNORMAL FINDINGS
Do not palpate a pulsating midline mass as it may be a dissecting aneurysm that can rupture from the pressure of palpation. Also avoid deep palpation over tender organs as in the case of polycystic kidneys, Wilms tumor, transplantation, or suspected splenic trauma.		
Deeply palpate **all four quadrants** for the following:		
• Tenderness	• Mild tenderness over midline at xiphoid, cecum, and sigmoid colon	• Tenderness, severe pain seen with tumor, cyst, abscess, enlarged organ, aneurysm, or adhesions
• Guarding	• Voluntary guarding	• Involuntary guarding is seen with peritoneal irritation; right-sided guarding is seen with acute cholecystitis.
• Masses	• No masses, aorta, and feces in colon	• Masses

(Continued on following page)

PALPATION (*continued*)		
ASSESSMENT PROCEDURE	**NORMAL FINDINGS**	**ABNORMAL FINDINGS**
Palpate deeply for **liver border** at right costal margin (Assessment Guide 19-1) for the following:		
• Tenderness	• Nontender	• Tenderness seen in trauma or diseased liver
• Consistency	• Smooth, firm sharp edge and no masses	• Hard, firm liver may indicate cancer; nodularity may occur with tumors, metastatic cancer, late cirrhosis, or syphilis.
Palpate deeply for **splenic border,** using bimanual technique (see Assessment Guide 19-1). Check for the following:		
• Size	• Not normally palpable	• Enlarged and palpable with trauma, mononucleosis, blood disorders, and malignancies
		Caution: *To avoid traumatizing and possibly rupturing the organ, be gentle when palpating an enlarged spleen.*
• Tenderness	• Nontender	• Tender
Palpate deeply for the **kidneys** by using bimanual technique (Assessment Guide 19-2). Assess for the following:		
• Size	• Not normally palpable	• Enlarged and palpable owing to cyst, tumor, or hydronephrosis

ASSESSMENT PROCEDURE	NORMAL FINDINGS	ABNORMAL FINDINGS
• Tenderness	• Nontender	• Tender
• Masses	• No masses	• Masses
Special maneuvers for **ascites**:		
• Measure abdominal girth at the same point every day.	• No increase in abdominal girth.	• Increase in abdominal girth.
• Fluid wave test: The client should remain supine. Have assistant put lateral side of lower arm firmly on center of abdomen (Fig. 19-11). Firmly place palmar surfaces of fingers and hand on one side of abdomen. Tap with other hand on opposite side of abdominal wall.	• No fluid wave transmitted. 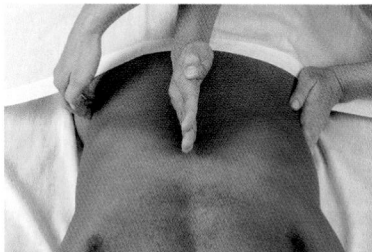 **FIGURE 19-11** Performing fluid wave test.	• Fluid wave palpated with ascites. Movement of a fluid wave against the resting hand suggests large amounts of fluid are present (ascites). • Because this test is not completely reliable, definitive testing by ultrasound is needed. • Ascites often is a sign of severe liver disease due to portal hypertension (high pressure in the blood vessels of the liver and low albumin levels).

(Continued on following page)

PALPATION (*continued*)		
ASSESSMENT PROCEDURE	**NORMAL FINDINGS**	**ABNORMAL FINDINGS**
• Shifting dullness: Place client in supine position and percuss from midline to flank, noting level of dullness. Then assist client to side position and percuss again for level of dullness (Fig. 19-12). *Note: This test is not always reliable, thus definitive testing by ultrasound is necessary.*	• Level of dullness does not change.	• Level of dullness is higher when client turns on side. (When ascites is present and the client is supine, the fluid assumes a dependent position and produces a dull percussion tone around the flanks. Air rises to the top, and tympany is percussed around the umbilicus. When the client turns onto one side and ascites is present, the fluid assumes a dependent position and air rises to the top.)

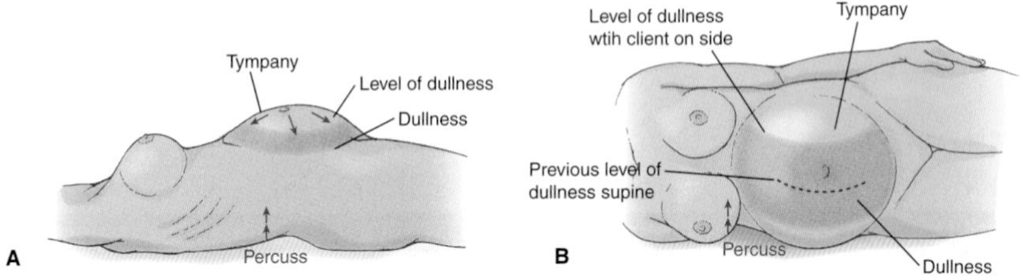

FIGURE 19-12 Percussing for level of dullness with (A) client supine and (B) client lying on side.

ASSESSMENT PROCEDURE	NORMAL FINDINGS	ABNORMAL FINDINGS
Special tests for **appendicitis/peritoneal irritation:** See Box 19-2 for summary of tests.		
• Assess for rebound tenderness. If the client has abdominal pain or tenderness, test for rebound tenderness by palpating deeply at 90 degrees into the abdomen halfway between the umbilicus and the anterior iliac crest (**McBurney Point**).	• No rebound tenderness is present.	• Client perceives sharp, stabbing pain as the examiner releases pressure from the abdomen (**Blumberg Sign**). It suggests peritoneal irritation (as from appendicitis). If the client feels pain at an area other than where you were assessing for rebound tenderness, consider that area as the source of the pain (see "Test for **referred rebound tenderness**").
• Then suddenly release pressure. Listen and watch for the client's expression of pain. Ask the client to describe which hurt more—the pressing in or the releasing—and where on the abdomen the pain occurred.		
Note: Test for rebound tenderness at the end of the examination because a positive response produces pain and muscle spasm that can interfere with the remaining examination.		
• Test for **referred rebound tenderness.** Palpate deeply in the LLQ and quickly release pressure (Fig. 19-13).	• No rebound pain is elicited.	• Pain in the RLQ during pressure in the LLQ is a positive **Rovsing Sign.** It suggests acute appendicitis.

(Continued on following page)

PALPATION (continued)

ASSESSMENT PROCEDURE	NORMAL FINDINGS	ABNORMAL FINDINGS
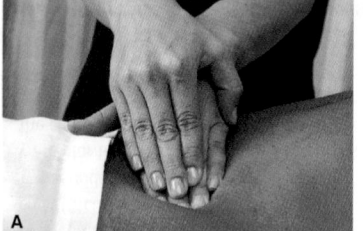 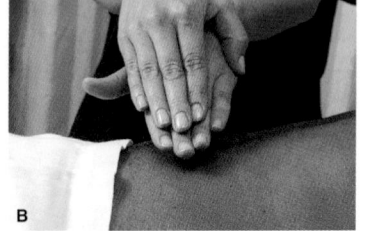 **FIGURE 19-13** Assessing for Rovsing Sign: (A) Palpating deeply. (B) Releasing pressure rapidly. *Note: Avoid continued palpation when test findings are positive for appendicitis because of the danger of rupturing the appendix.* • Assess for **Psoas Sign**. Ask the client to lie on the left side. Hyperextend the right leg of the client (Fig. 19-14).	• No abdominal pain is present.	• Pain in the RLQ (**Psoas Sign**) is associated with irritation of the iliopsoas muscle due to appendicitis (an inflamed appendix).

ASSESSMENT PROCEDURE	NORMAL FINDINGS	ABNORMAL FINDINGS
• Assess for **Obturator Sign.** Support the client's right knee and ankle. Flex the hip and knee, and rotate the leg internally and externally (Fig. 19-15).	• No abdominal pain is present.	• Pain in the RLQ indicates **irritation of the obturator muscle** due to appendicitis or a perforated appendix.
• Perform **Hypersensitivity Test.** Stroke the abdomen with a sharp object (e.g., broken cotton-tipped applicator or tongue blade) or grasp a fold of skin with your thumb and index finger and quickly let go. Do this several times along the abdominal wall.	• The client feels no pain and no exaggerated sensation.	• Pain or an exaggerated sensation felt in the RLQ is a positive skin **Hypersensitivity Test** and may indicate appendicitis.

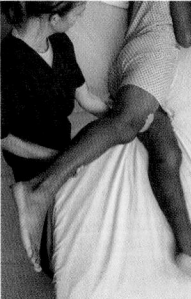

FIGURE 19-14 Test for Psoas Sign.

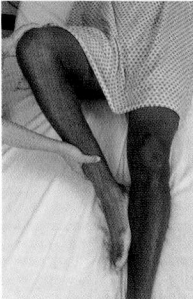

FIGURE 19-15 Test for Obturator Sign.

(Continued on following page)

PALPATION (*continued*)		
ASSESSMENT PROCEDURE	**NORMAL FINDINGS**	**ABNORMAL FINDINGS**
Test for **Cholecystitis**: • Assess RUQ pain or tenderness, which may signal cholecystitis (inflammation of the gallbladder). Press your fingertips under the liver border at the right costal margin and ask the client to inhale deeply.	• No increase in pain is present.	• Accentuated sharp pain that causes the client to hold their breath (inspiratory arrest) is a positive **Murphy Sign** and is associated with acute cholecystitis.

BOX 19-2	ABDOMINAL SIGNS	
Name	**Description**	**Cause**
Psoas Sign	Pain in RLQ when leg is hyperextended	Irritation of the iliopsoas muscle due to appendicitis (an inflamed appendix)
Obturator Sign	Pain in the RLQ when hip and knee are flexed and leg is rotated internally and externally	Irritation of the obturator muscle due to appendicitis or a perforated appendix
Murphy Sign	Pain elicited when pressure is applied under the liver border at the right costal margin and client inhales deeply	Inflammation of the gallbladder
Rovsing Sign	Pain in the RLQ during pressure in the LLQ	Acute appendicitis
Blumberg Sign	Abdominal pain or tenderness experienced when examiner tests for rebound tenderness by palpating deeply at 90 degrees into the abdomen one-halfway between the umbilicus and the anterior iliac crest (**McBurney Point**)	Peritoneal irritation

ABNORMAL FINDINGS   **19-1**   **Mechanisms and Sources of Abdominal Pain**

TYPES OF PAIN

Abdominal pain may be formally described as visceral, parietal, or referred.

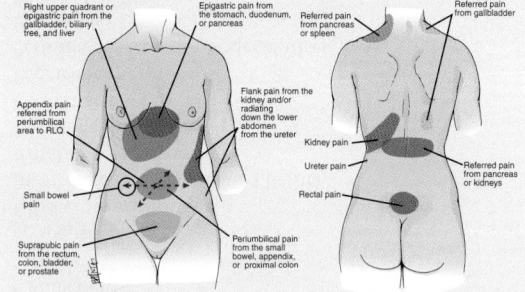

- *Visceral pain* occurs when hollow abdominal organs, such as the intestines, become distended or contract forcefully or when the capsules of solid organs such as the liver and

spleen are stretched. Poorly defined or localized and intermittently timed, this type of pain is often characterized as dull, aching, burning, cramping, or colicky.

- *Parietal pain* occurs when the parietal peritoneum becomes inflamed, as in appendicitis or peritonitis. This type of pain tends to localize more to the source and is characterized as a more severe and steady pain.

- *Referred pain* occurs at distant sites that are innervated at approximately the same levels as the disrupted abdominal organ. This type of pain travels, or refers, from the primary site and becomes highly localized at the distant site. The accompanying illustrations show common clinical patterns and referents of pain.

CHARACTER OF ABDOMINAL PAIN AND IMPLICATIONS

Dull, aching
 Appendicitis
 Acute hepatitis
 Biliary colic

(Continued on following page)

ABNORMAL FINDINGS	19-1	Mechanisms and Sources of Abdominal Pain (*continued*)

CHARACTER OF ABDOMINAL PAIN AND IMPLICATIONS (*continued*)

   Cholecystitis
   Cystitis
   Dyspepsia
   Glomerulonephritis
   Incarcerated or strangulated hernia
   Irritable bowel syndrome
   Hepatocellular cancer
   Pancreatitis
   Pancreatic cancer
   Perforated gastric or duodenal ulcer
   Peritonitis
   Peptic ulcer disease
   Prostatitis
Burning, gnawing
   Dyspepsia
   Peptic ulcer disease
Cramping ("crampy")
   Acute mechanical obstruction

   Appendicitis
   Colitis
   Diverticulitis
   Gastroesophageal reflux disease (GERD)
Pressure
   Benign prostatic hypertrophy
   Prostate cancer
   Prostatitis
   Urinary retention
Colicky
   Colon cancer
Sharp, knife-like
   Splenic abscess
   Splenic rupture
   Renal colic
   Renal tumor
   Ureteral colic
   Vascular liver tumor
Variable
   Stomach cancer

ABNORMAL FINDINGS   **19-2**   **Abdominal Distention**

With the exception of pregnancy, abdominal distention is usually considered an abnormal finding. Percussion may help determine the cause.

PREGNANCY (NORMAL FINDING)
Pregnancy is included here so that the examiner may differentiate it from abnormal findings.

It causes a generalized protuberant abdomen, protuberant umbilicus, a fetal heartbeat that can be heard on auscultation, percussible tympany over the intestines, and dullness over the uterus.

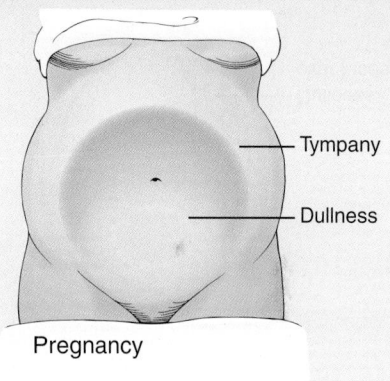

Pregnancy

(*Continued on following page*)

ABNORMAL FINDINGS · 19-2 · Abdominal Distention (*continued*)

FAT

Obesity accounts for most uniformly protuberant abdomens. The abdominal wall is thick, and tympany is the percussion tone elicited. The umbilicus usually appears sunken.

FECES

Hard stools in the colon appear as a localized distention. Percussion over the area discloses dullness.

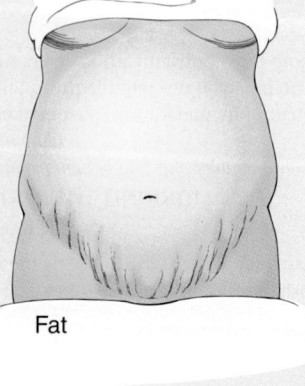

Fat

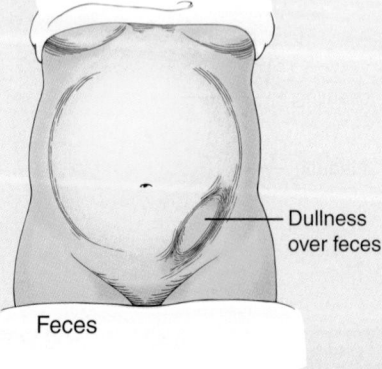

Dullness over feces

Feces

FIBROIDS AND OTHER MASSES
A large ovarian cyst or fibroid tumor appears as generalized distinction in the lower abdomen. The mass displaces bowel; thus, the percussion tone over the distended area is dullness, with tympany at the periphery. The umbilicus may be everted.

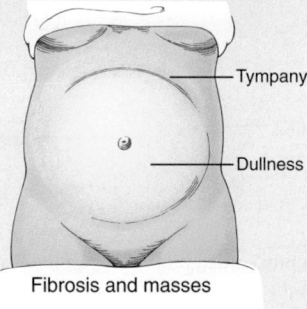

Fibrosis and masses

FLATUS
The abdomen distended with gas may appear as a generalized protuberance (as shown), or it may appear more localized. Tympany is the percussion tone over the area.

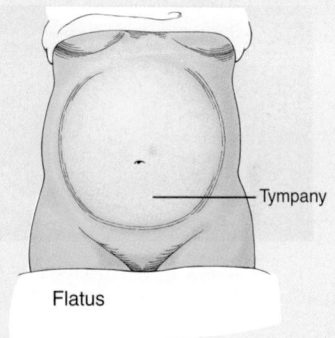

Flatus

(Continued on following page)

ABNORMAL FINDINGS

ABNORMAL FINDINGS | **19-2** | **Abdominal Distention** (*continued*)

ASCITIC FLUID

Fluid in the abdomen causes generalized protuberance, bulging flanks, and an everted umbilicus. Percussion reveals dullness over fluid (bottom of abdomen and flanks) and tympany over intestines (top of abdomen).

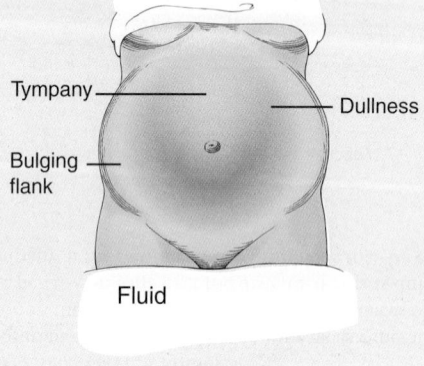

Tympany — Dullness

Bulging flank

Fluid

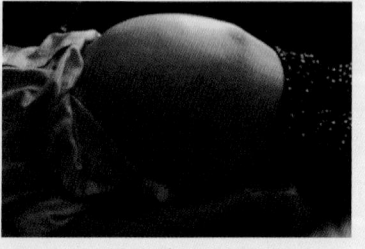

ABNORMAL FINDINGS 19-3 **Abdominal Bulges**

UMBILICAL HERNIA

An umbilical hernia results from the bowel protruding through a weakness in the umbilical ring. This condition occurs more frequently in infants but also occurs in adults.

EPIGASTRIC HERNIA

An epigastric hernia occurs when the bowel protrudes through a weakness in the linea alba. The small bulge appears midline between the xiphoid process and the umbilicus. It may be discovered only on palpation.

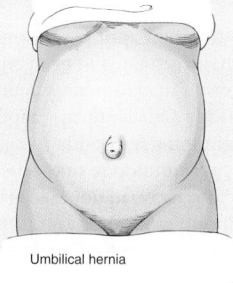

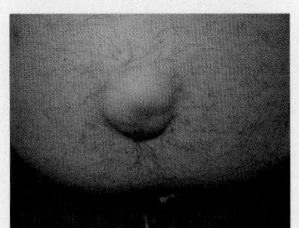

Umbilical hernia

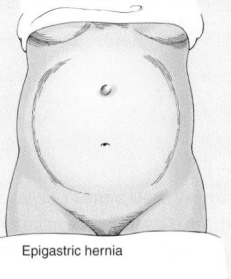

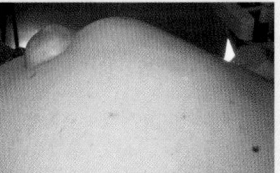

Epigastric hernia

(*Continued on following page*)

ABNORMAL FINDINGS

ABNORMAL FINDINGS 19-3 Abdominal Bulges (*continued*)

DIASTASIS RECTI
Diastasis recti occurs when the bowel protrudes through a separation between the two rectus abdominis muscles. It appears as a midline ridge. The bulge may appear only when the client raises the head or coughs. The condition is of little significance.

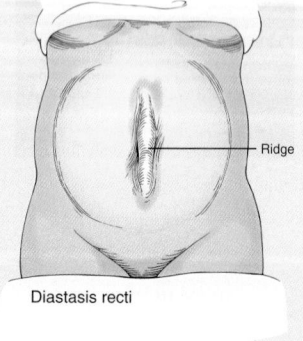

Ridge

Diastasis recti

INCISIONAL HERNIA
An incisional hernia occurs when the bowel protrudes through a defect or weakness resulting from a surgical incision. It appears as a bulge near a surgical scar on the abdomen.

Incisional hernia

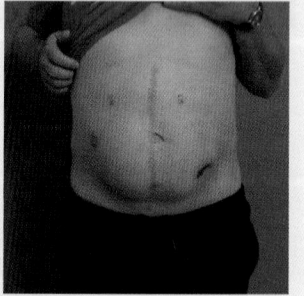

Photo credits: Umbilical hernia, image provided by Stedman's; epigastric hernia, reprinted with permission from Hawn, M. (2015). *Operative techniques in foregut surgery.* Fig. 38-3. Wolters Kluwer; incisional hernia, reprinted with permission from Dr. ML Corman, from Corman, M., Nicholls, R. J., Fazio, V. W., & Bergamaschi, R. (2013). *Corman's colon and rectal surgery* (6th ed., Fig. 19-61). Wolters Kluwer.

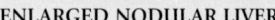

ABNORMAL FINDINGS | **19-4** | **Enlarged Abdominal Organs and Other Abnormalities**

ENLARGED LIVER

An enlarged liver (hepatomegaly) is defined as a span greater than 12 cm at the midclavicular line (MCL) and greater than 8 cm at the MSL. An enlarged nontender liver suggests cirrhosis. An enlarged tender liver suggests congestive heart failure, acute hepatitis, or abscess.

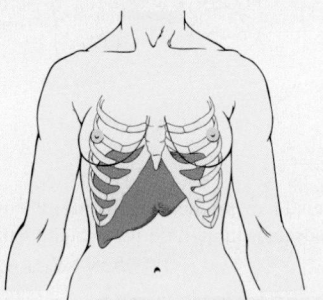

ENLARGED NODULAR LIVER

An enlarged, firm, hard, nodular liver suggests cancer. Other causes may be late cirrhosis or syphilis.

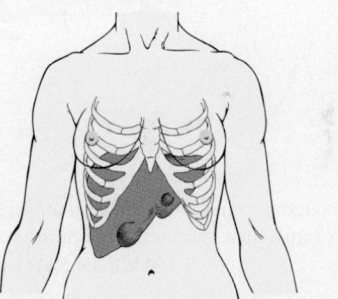

(*Continued on following page*)

ABNORMAL FINDINGS

ABNORMAL FINDINGS **19-4** **Enlarged Abdominal Organs and Other Abnormalities (*continued*)**

LIVER HIGHER THAN NORMAL
A liver that is in a higher position than normal span may be caused by an abdominal mass, ascites, or a paralyzed diaphragm.

LIVER LOWER THAN NORMAL
A liver in a lower position than normal with a normal span may be caused by emphysema because the diaphragm is low.

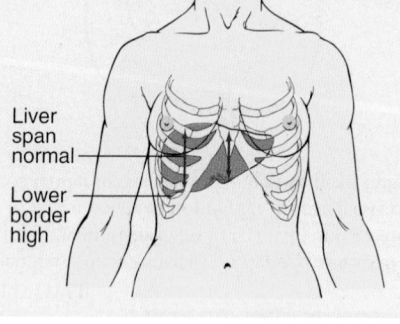

Liver span normal

Lower border high

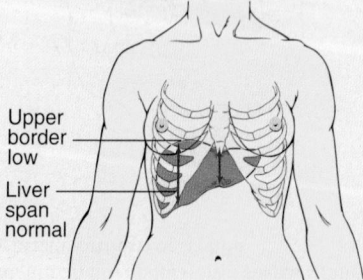

Upper border low

Liver span normal

| ABNORMAL FINDINGS | 19-4 | **Enlarged Abdominal Organs and Other Abnormalities (*continued*)** |

ENLARGED SPLEEN

An enlarged spleen (splenomegaly) is defined by an area of dullness exceeding 7 cm. When enlarged, the spleen progresses downward and toward the midline.

AORTIC ANEURYSM

A prominent, laterally pulsating mass above the umbilicus strongly suggests an aortic aneurysm. It is accompanied by a bruit and a wide, bounding pulse.

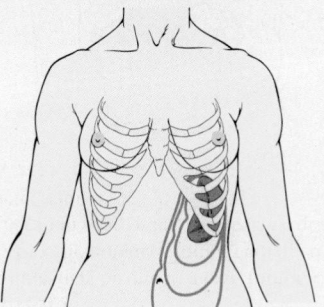
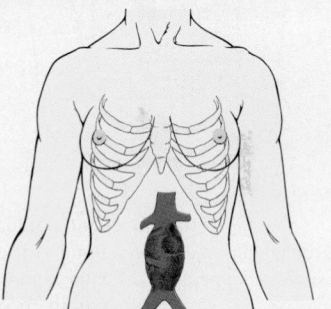

(*Continued on following page*)

ABNORMAL FINDINGS | **19-4** | **Enlarged Abdominal Organs and Other Abnormalities** (*continued*)

ENLARGED KIDNEY

An enlarged kidney may be due to a cyst, tumor, or hydrone-phrosis. It may be differentiated from an enlarged spleen by its smooth rather than sharp edge, the absence of a notch, and tympany on percussion.

ENLARGED GALLBLADDER

An extremely tender, enlarged gallbladder suggests acute cholecystitis. A positive finding is Murphy sign (sharp pain that causes the client to hold the breath).

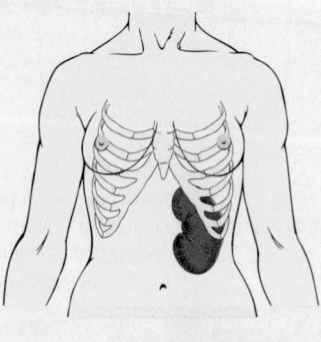

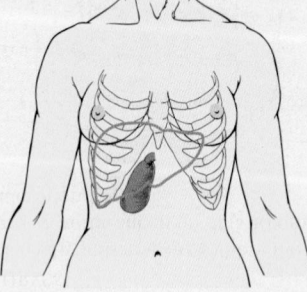

ASSESSMENT GUIDE 19-1   Liver and Spleen Palpation

Liver Palpation

1. Stand at client's right side and place your left hand under client's back at the 11th and 12th ribs.
2. Place right hand parallel to right costal margin.
3. Ask client to breathe deeply, and press upward with your right fingers with each inhalation.

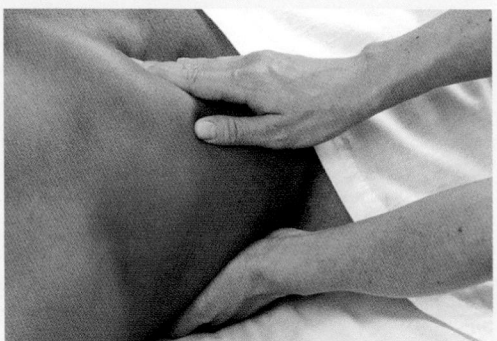

Spleen Palpation

1. Stand at client's right side; reach across client to place your left hand under client's posterior lower ribs, and push up.
2. Place your right hand below rib margin.
3. Ask client to breathe deeply.
4. Press hands together to palpate spleen on inhalation.

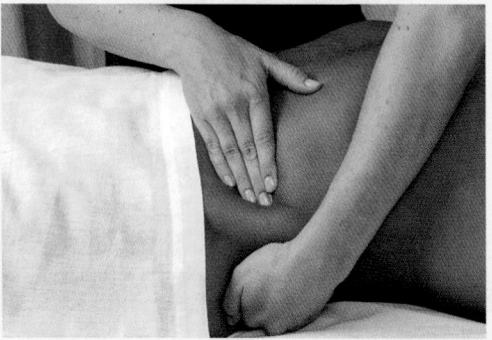

ASSESSMENT GUIDE 19-2   Kidney Palpation

1. Place one of your hands behind lower edge of rib cage and above iliac crest.
2. Place the other hand over corresponding anterior surface.
3. Instruct client to breathe deeply.
4. Lift up lower hand and push in with upper hand as client exhales.
5. Repeat on other side.

Note: The kidneys are rarely palpable.

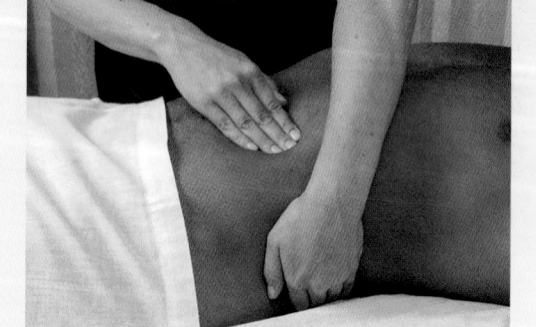

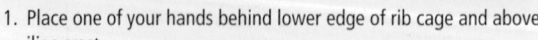 **PEDIATRIC VARIATIONS**

Questions to ask the parents when collecting *subjective data* include the following:
- Types of food, fluids, and formula?
- Bowel patterns?

- Frequent spitting up?
- Ability to feed self?
- Milk intake?
- Food intolerances?
- History of eating disorders?
- History of pica?

When collecting *objective data*, note the following:

ASSESSMENT PROCEDURE	NORMAL FINDINGS
Inspection	
Inspect **contour and size of abdomen.**	Prominent/cylindrical (protuberant) when erect, flat when supine. Superficial veins may be present in infants. An umbilical hernia is commonly seen in the infant and toddler, especially when the infant or toddler strains or cries. As the muscles in the abdomen grow and strengthen, this benign hernia will commonly resolve on its own. In adolescents, if piercing of the umbilicus is present, assess for signs of infection.
Inspect **abdominal movement** in children younger than 8 years.	Rises with inspiration in synchrony with chest; may have visible pulsations in epigastric region.
Palpation	
Palpate **liver border.**	Normal, shortened liver span on percussion. May not extend below costal margin. *Infants and young children:* Liver may be felt 1 to 3 cm below costal margin and may descend with inspiration.
Palpate **splenic border** (may have child roll on right side).	*Infants and young children:* Spleen may be felt 1 to 3 cm below costal margin.
Palpate for **abdominal tenderness.**	Extremely difficult to assess in young children, who may confuse pressure of palpation with pain. Distraction is important.
Palpate **kidney borders.**	Difficult to locate except in newborns.

GERIATRIC VARIATIONS

- May experience a decline in appetite from various factors such as altered metabolism, decreased taste sensation, decreased mobility, and, possibly, depression. If appetite declines, the client's risk for nutritional imbalance increases.
- Dilated superficial capillaries visible
- Abdomen is softer and organs more easily palpated owing to a decrease in tone of abdominal musculature.
- Decreased production of saliva, decreased peristalsis, decreased enzymes, and weaker gastric acid.
- Gastric mucosa and parietal cell degeneration result in a loss of intrinsic factor, which decreases absorption of vitamin B_{12}.
- Bowel sounds 5 to 30 sounds per minute
- Shortened liver span on percussion due to a decrease in liver size after the age of 50 years
- Liver border is more easily palpated.
- Decreased nerve sensation to lower bowel contributes to constipation.
- The U.S. Preventive Services Task Force (USPSTF, 2019) recommends one-time screening for AAA for men between 65 and 75 years of age who have ever smoked and only offer screening selectively to those in that age group who have never smoked. The USPSTF recommends against screening women who have never smoked and concludes that evidence is limited for screening women who have smoked.

CULTURAL VARIATIONS

- Black non-Hispanic, Hispanic, and Asian/Pacific Islanders had a 40% to 50% higher risk for gastric cancer than White people in a regional U.S. population (Dong et al., 2017).
- However, for the cardia region of the upper stomach, Gupta et al. (2019) found a different pattern; rates of cancer were lower for Blacks, Hispanics, Asians, Pacific Islanders, American Indians, and Alaska Natives than for non-Hispanic Whites.
- Stomach cancer incidence is highest in Asia (especially Korea, Mongolia, China, and Japan), Latin America, and the Caribbean, and lowest in North America and Africa (Ferlay et al., 2015; World Cancer Research Fund, 2018). The pattern may be related to *Helicobacter pylori* (which is higher in these locations and populations) because it is associated with both stomach ulcers and cancer.
- Esophageal cancers (adenocarcinomas and squamous cell cancers) show vast differences for Asians in Asia versus Asian Americans (Kim et al., 2016). The reasons for these differences are as yet unexplained.

- Gallbladder disease and gallbladder cancer vary by ethnic group in the United States, with Native Americans and Mexican Americans having higher rates of disease and cancer in this organ (American Cancer Society, 2018).
- Gallbladder disease cases included more women (57.9%) than men (42.1%), and the ethnicity breakdown was 35.2% Latinos, 23.3% Japanese, 19.4% Whites, 18.4% African Americans, and 3.8% Native Hawaiians (Figueiredo et al., 2017).

POSSIBLE COLLABORATIVE PROBLEMS—RISK OF

- Bowel strangulation
- Intestinal obstruction
- Peritonitis
- Ascites
- Paralytic ileus
- Malabsorption syndrome
- Metabolic acidosis/alkalosis
- Diverticulitis
- Pancreatitis
- GI bleeding
- Hepatic failure
- Stromal changes

- Gastric ulcer
- Evisceration
- Gallbladder disease (stones and cancer)

Teaching Tips for Selected Client Concerns

Client Concern: Obesity associated with intake greater than needed calories for activity level

Discuss essential components of a well-balanced diet in relation to client's level of physical development and energy expenditure (basal metabolic rate). Teach client how to keep a daily food diary in order to assess intake.

Discuss with client the following:

- Decreasing calories
- Increasing complex carbohydrates (whole grains and vegetables)
- Decreasing saturated fats
- Decreasing refined sugars
- Decreasing intake of cholesterol to 300 mg/day and salt to 5 g/day

Provide information on support groups such as Weight Watchers and TOPS (Take Off Pounds Sensibly).

Client Concern: *Risk for constipation*

Discuss bowel habits that are "normal" for client. Caution against overuse of laxatives. Discourage overuse of mineral oil as a laxative because it decreases absorption of vitamins A, D, E, and K. Explain the effects of nutrients, bulk, fluids, and exercise on elimination. The American Cancer Society (2020) recommends maintaining a healthy weight, engaging in 30 minutes of moderate to vigorous activity per day, eating five or more servings of vegetables and fruits each day, eating whole grains rather than processed (refined grains), limiting processed and red meats, and limiting alcohol consumption to no more than two drinks daily for men and one drink daily for women. Advise client to eat a varied diet, maintain a desirable weight, eliminate tobacco use, and be physically active. The American Cancer Society associated exercise with lowering risk of seven cancers.

 Client Concern: *Opportunity to enhance child's dietary health*

Teach parents nutritional needs of the child at various ages.

Infant: Exclusive breastfeeding is the ideal source of nutrition for the first 6 months. Gradually introduce iron-enriched solid food at 6 months to complement breastfeeding. When possible, continue breastfeeding for at least 1 year. Do not give cow's milk before 12 months of age. Introduce finger foods by 1 year. The American Academy of Pediatrics (2017) doubled the recommended intake of vitamin D in foods or as supplements for infants to 400 IU per day for infants less than 1 year of age and 600 IU for older children and adolescents.

Breastfed infants should get oral iron supplements. Fluoride supplements are required only if the water supply is severely deficient in fluoride.

Toddlers: Food fads are common. Accept this as long as child gets balanced diet over period of days versus every day.

 Client Concern: *Dehydration associated with vomiting or diarrhea*

Teach parents to give child small amounts of clear liquids (approximately 1 oz every hour for 8 hours) until symptoms subside. May recommend Pedialyte® for fluid and electrolyte replacement.

Client Concern: Risk for aspiration associated with improper feeding and small size of stomach in newborns

Explain size of infant's stomach to parents (holds 60 mL), and demonstrate proper burping technique to use after every ½ oz feeding.

References

Agency for Healthcare Research and Quality. (2018). *Abdominal aortic aneurysm screening.* https://psnet.ahrq.gov/web-mm/abdominal-aortic-aneurysm-screening

American Academy of Pediatrics. (2017). *Recommendations released on prevention, management of rickets.* https://www.aappublications.org/news/2017/02/10/Rickets021017

American Cancer Society. (2018). *Risk factors for gallbladder cancer.* https://www.cancer.org/cancer/gallbladder-cancer/causes-risks-prevention/risk-factors.html

American Cancer Society. (2020). *Study: Getting enough exercise lowers risk of 7 cancers.* https://www.cancer.org/latest-news/study-getting-enough-exercise-lowers-risk-of-7-cancers.html#:~:text=Exercise%20is%20a%20healthy%20habit,to%20get%20and%20stay%20active

Dong, E., Duan, L., & Wu, B. (2017). Racial and ethnic minorities at increased risk for gastric cancer in a regional US population study. *Clinical Gastroenterology and Hematology, 15*(4), 511–517. https://doi.org/10.1016/j.cgh.2016.11.033

Ferlay, J., Soerjomataram, I., Dikshit, R., Eser, S., Mathers, C., Rebelo, M., Parkin, D. M., Forman, D., & Bray, F. (2015). Cancer incidence and mortality worldwide: Sources, methods, and major patterns in GLOBSCAN 2012. *International Journal of Cancer, 136*(5), E359–E386. https://doi.org/10.1002/ijc.29210

Figueiredo, J. C., Haiman, C., Porcel, J., Boxman, J., Stram, D., Tambe, N., Cozen, W., Wilkens, L., Le Marchand, L., & Setiawan, V. W. (2017). Sex and ethnic/racial-specific risk factors for gallbladder disease. *BMC Gastroenterology, 17,* 153. https://doi.org/10.1186/s12876-017-0678-6

Gupta, S., Tao, L., Murphy, J. D., Camargo, M. C., Oren, E., Valseak, M. A., Gomez, S. L., & Martinez, M. E. (2019). Race/ethnicity-, socioeconomic status-, and anatomic subsite-specific risks for gastric cancer. *Gastroenterology, 156*(1), 59–62.E4. https://doi.org/10.1053/j.gastro.2018.09.045

Kim, J. Y., Winters, J., Kim, J., Bernstein, L., Raz, D., & Gomez, S. (2016). Birthplace and esophageal cancer incidence patterns among Asian-Americans. *Diseases of the Esophagus, 29*(1), 99–104. https://doi.org/10.1111/dote.12302

United States Preventive Services Task Force. (2019). *Abdominal aortic aneurysm: Screening: Final recommendation statement.* https://www.uspreventiveservicestaskforce.org/uspstf/recommendation/abdominal-aortic-aneurysm-screening

World Cancer Research Fund. (2018). *Stomach cancer statistics: Stomach cancer is the fifth most common cancer worldwide.* https://www.wcrf.org/dietandcancer/cancer-trends/stomach-cancer-statistics

20 ASSESSING MUSCULOSKELETAL SYSTEM

Structure and Function Overview

The body's bones, muscles, and joints compose the musculoskeletal system. Two hundred and six bones make up the axial skeleton (head and trunk) and the appendicular skeleton (extremities, shoulders, and hips; Fig. 20-1). There are varying shapes including short bones (e.g., carpals), long bones (e.g., humerus, femur), flat bones (e.g., sternum, ribs), and irregular shaped bones (e.g., hips, vertebrae). **Bones**, composed of osseous tissue, provide structure, give protection, serve as levers, store calcium, and produce blood cells. There are two types: **compact bone** (hard and dense) making up the bone shaft and outer layers; and **spongy bone** (numerous spaces) making up the bone ends and centers. Bone tissue is formed by **osteoblasts** and broken down by cells referred to as **osteoclasts.** The **periosteum** covers the bones and contains osteoblasts and blood vessels.

The body consists of three types of muscles: skeletal, smooth, and cardiac. The musculoskeletal system is made up of 650 skeletal (voluntary) muscles, which are under conscious control (Fig. 20-2). Skeletal muscles attach to bones by way of strong, fibrous cords called **tendons** and assist with posture, produce body heat, and allow the body to move.

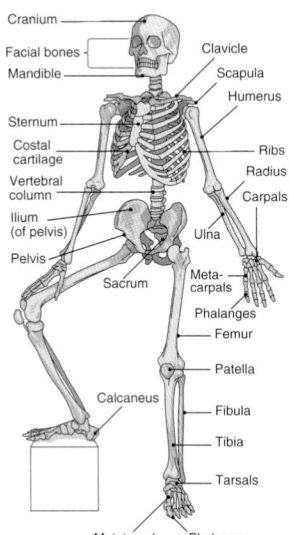

FIGURE 20-1 Major bones of the skeleton. The axial skeleton is shown in yellow and the appendicular in blue.

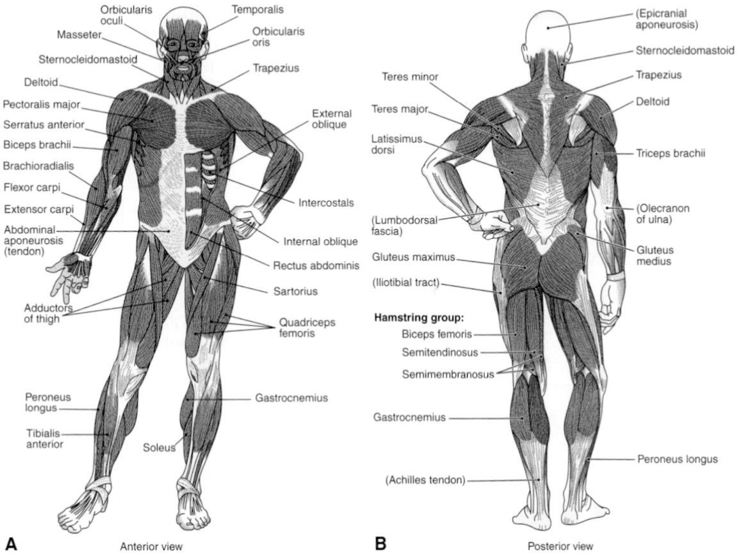

FIGURE 20-2 Muscles of the body. (A) Anterior. (B) Posterior.

The joint (or articulation) is the place where two or more bones meet and provide a variety of range of motion (ROM) for the body parts. There are three types of joints. **Fibrous joints** (e.g., sutures between skull bones) are joined by fibrous connective tissue and are immovable. **Cartilaginous joints** (e.g., joints between vertebrae) are joined by cartilage. **Synovial joints** (e.g., shoulders, wrists, hips, knees, ankles; Fig. 20-3) contain a space between the bones that is filled with synovial fluid, a lubricant that promotes a sliding movement of the ends of the bones. Bones in synovial joints are joined by ligaments, which are strong, dense bands of fibrous connective tissue. A fibrous capsule made of connective tissue and connected to the periosteum of the bone encloses synovial joints. Some synovial joints contain **bursae** (small sacs filled with synovial fluid) that cushion the joint.

Nursing Assessment

COLLECTING SUBJECTIVE DATA

Interview Questions

Pain in joints, muscles, or bones? At rest? With exercise? Changes in shape or size of an extremity? Changes in ability to carry out activities of daily living, sports, work? Stiffness? Time of day? Relation to weight bearing and exercise? Decreased, altered, or

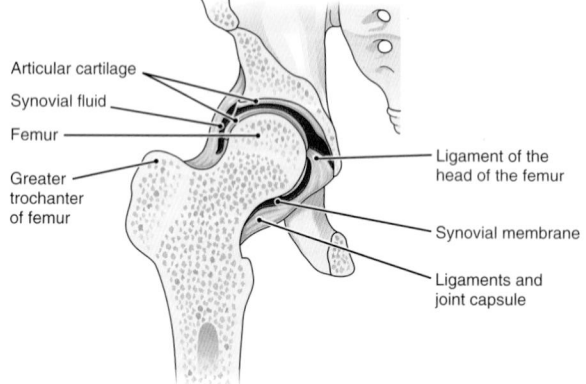

FIGURE 20-3 Components of synovial joints (right hip joint).

absent sensations? Redness or swelling of joints? History of past problems with bones, joints, muscles, fractures? Treatment? Orthopedic surgery? Last tetanus and polio immunizations? History of osteoporosis or osteomyelitis? Family history of rheumatoid arthritis, gout, osteoporosis, muscular dystrophy? Age of menopause, if applicable? Occupational and recreational history?

Self-care: exercise, weight lifting, weight reduction, diet, use of tobacco or alcohol? Last bone density screening?

Risk Factors

Risk for osteoporosis related to lack of exercise, low calcium intake, excessive caffeine or alcohol consumption, smoking, use of steroids, low estrogen levels in women or postmenopausal women not on estrogen replacement therapy. Risk for sports injury related to lack of wearing protective gear, poor physical fitness, lack of warm-up exercises, and overuse of joints.

COLLECTING OBJECTIVE DATA

Equipment Needed

- Tape measure
- Goniometer (measures angles of joints)
- Marking pen

Physical Assessment

See Figures 20-1 and 20-2 for diagrams of the bones and muscles of the body.

Inspection and palpation are performed while client is standing, sitting, and supine. ROM can be measured by degrees, using approximation or a goniometer. (Normal trunk ROM is given as an example—see Fig. 20-7.) In assessing muscle weakness or swelling, size is compared bilaterally by measuring circumference with a tape measure. Joints should not be forced into painful positions. Muscle strength can be estimated using a muscle strength scale (Table 20-1).

TABLE 20-1 **Scale for Muscle Strength**

Rating	Explanation	Strength Classification
5	Active motion against full resistance	Normal
4	Active motion against some resistance	Slight weakness
3	Active motion against gravity	Average weakness
2	Passive ROM (gravity removed and assisted by examiner)	Poor ROM
1	Slight flicker of contraction	Severe weakness
0	No muscular contraction	Paralysis

ROM, range of motion.

Inspection: Observe for ROM, swelling, deformity, atrophy, condition of surrounding tissues, and pain.

Palpation: Palpate for heat, strength, tone, edema, crepitus, and nodules. (***Note:*** Dominant side is normally stronger in muscle strength and tone.)

INSPECTION OF STANCE AND GAIT

Observe stance and gait as client enters and walks around the room.

ASSESSMENT PROCEDURE	NORMAL FINDINGS	ABNORMAL FINDINGS
Observe **posture.** With client standing with their feet together, noting alignment of the head, trunk, pelvis, and extremities, and with client sitting.	Posture is erect and comfortable for age (Fig. 20-4). 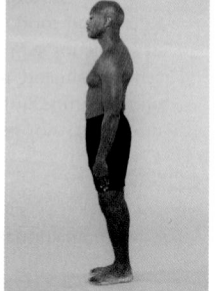	Slumped shoulders seen in poor posture, in which client may not be aware. Also seen in depression. See Abnormal Findings 20-1 for abnormal curvatures of the spine: lordosis, scoliosis, or kyphosis.

FIGURE 20-4 Normal spinal curves.

ASSESSMENT PROCEDURE	NORMAL FINDINGS	ABNORMAL FINDINGS
Observe **gait** as client enters and walks around the room. Note: • Base of support • Weight-bearing stability • Foot position • Stride and length and cadence of stride • Arm swing • Posture	Evenly distributed weight. Client able to stand on heels and toes. Toes point straight ahead. Equal on both sides. Posture erect, movements coordinated and rhythmic, arms swing in opposition, stride length appropriate.	Uneven weight bearing is evident. Client cannot stand on heels or toes. Toes point in or out. Client limps, shuffles, propels forward, or has wide-based gait (see Chapter 21, Assessing Neurologic System, for abnormal gait findings).
Assess for the risk of falling backward in the older or handicapped client by performing the **Nudge test.** Stand behind the client and put your arms around the client while you gently nudge the sternum. **Note:** *Some older clients have an impaired sense of position in space, which may contribute to the risk of falling.*	Client does not fall backward.	Falling backward easily is seen with cervical spondylosis and Parkinson disease.

(Continued on following page)

INSPECTION OF STANCE AND GAIT *(continued)*		
ASSESSMENT PROCEDURE	**NORMAL FINDINGS**	**ABNORMAL FINDINGS**
Temporomandibular Joint (TMJ)		
Inspection and Palpation		
Inspect and palpate the **TMJ**. With client sitting, put your index and middle fingers anterior to the external ear opening (Fig. 20-5). Ask the client to: • Open the mouth as widely as possible. (The tips of your fingers should drop into the joint spaces as the mouth opens.) • Move the jaw from side to side. • Protrude (push out) and retract (pull in) jaw.	Snapping and clicking may be felt and heard in the normal client. Mouth opens 1 to 2 in. (distance between upper and lower teeth). The client's mouth opens and closes smoothly. Jaw moves laterally 1 to 2 cm; protrudes and retracts easily. 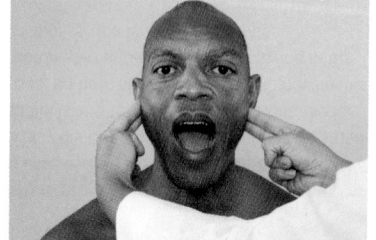	Decreased ROM, swelling, tenderness, or crepitus may be seen in arthritis. Decreased muscle strength with muscle and joint disease. Decreased ROM and a clicking, popping, or grating sound may be noted with TMJ dysfunction.

FIGURE 20-5 Palpating the temporomandibular joint.

ASSESSMENT PROCEDURE	NORMAL FINDINGS	ABNORMAL FINDINGS
Test **ROM.** Ask the client to open the mouth and move the jaw laterally against resistance. Next, as the client clenches the teeth, feel for the contraction of the temporal and masseter muscles to test the integrity of cranial nerve V (trigeminal nerve).	Jaw has full ROM against resistance. Contraction palpated with no pain or spasms.	Lack of full contraction with cranial nerve V lesion. Pain or spasms occur with myofascial pain syndrome.
Sternoclavicular Joint		
Inspection and Palpation		
With client sitting, inspect the **sternoclavicular joint** for location in midline, color, swelling, and masses. Then palpate for tenderness or pain.	There is no visible bony overgrowth, swelling, or redness; joint is nontender.	Swollen, red, or enlarged joint or tender, painful joint is seen with inflammation of the joint.
Cervical, Thoracic, and Lumbar Spine		
Inspection and Palpation		
Observe the **cervical, thoracic, and lumbar curves** from the side, then from behind. Have the client standing erect with the gown	Cervical and lumbar spines are concave; thoracic spine is convex. Spine is straight (when observed from behind).	Flattened lumbar curvature may be seen with herniated lumbar disc or ankylosing spondylitis. Lateral curvature of the thoracic spine with an

(Continued on following page)

INSPECTION OF STANCE AND GAIT (*continued*)

ASSESSMENT PROCEDURE	NORMAL FINDINGS	ABNORMAL FINDINGS
positioned to allow an adequate view of the spine (see Fig. 20-4). Observe for symmetry, noting differences in height of the shoulders, iliac crests, and buttock creases.		increase in the convexity on the curved side is seen in scoliosis. An exaggerated lumbar curve (lordosis) is often seen in pregnancy or obesity (Abnormal Findings 20-1). Unequal heights of the hips suggest unequal leg lengths.
Palpate the **spinous processes and the paravertebral muscles** on both sides of the spine for tenderness or pain.	Nontender spinous processes; well-developed, firm and smooth, nontender paravertebral muscles. No muscle spasm.	Compression fractures and lumbosacral muscle strain can cause pain and tenderness of the spinal processes and paravertebral muscles.
Test **ROM of the cervical spine.** Test ROM of the cervical spine by asking the client to touch the chin to the chest (flexion) and to look up at the ceiling (hyperextension) (Fig. 20-6A). *Note: Impaired ROM and neck pain associated with fever, chills, and headache could be indicative of a serious infection such as meningitis.*	Flexion of the cervical spine is 45 degrees. Extension of the cervical spine is 45 degrees.	Cervical strain is the most common cause of neck pain (characterized by impaired ROM and neck pain from abnormalities of the muscles, ligaments, and nerves, due to straining or injuring the neck). Causes of strains: sleeping in the wrong position, carrying heavy loads, or having an auto crash. Cervical disc degenerative disease and spinal cord tumors seen with impaired ROM and pain radiating to back, shoulder, or arms. Neck pain with a loss of leg sensation may occur with cervical spinal cord compression.

ASSESSMENT PROCEDURE	NORMAL FINDINGS	ABNORMAL FINDINGS

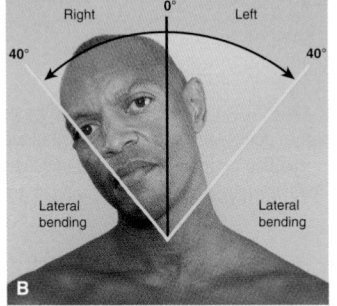 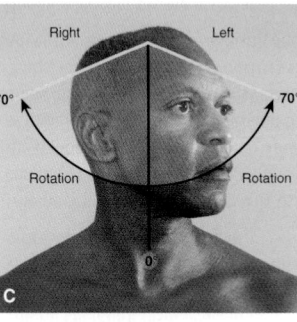

FIGURE 20-6 Normal range of motion of cervical spine. **(A)** Flexion–hyperextension. **(B)** Lateral bending. **(C)** Rotation.

ASSESSMENT PROCEDURE	NORMAL FINDINGS	ABNORMAL FINDINGS
Test lateral bending. Ask the client to touch each ear to the shoulder on that side (Fig. 20-6B).	Normally, the client can bend 40 degrees to the left side and 40 degrees to the right side.	Limited ROM is seen with neck injuries, osteoarthritis, spondylosis, or with disc degeneration.
Evaluate rotation. Ask the client to turn the head to the right and left (Fig. 20-6C).	About 70 degrees of rotation is normal.	Limited ROM is seen with neck injuries, osteoarthritis, spondylosis, or with disc degeneration.

(Continued on following page)

INSPECTION OF STANCE AND GAIT (continued)		
ASSESSMENT PROCEDURE	**NORMAL FINDINGS**	**ABNORMAL FINDINGS**
Ask the client to repeat the cervical ROM movements against resistance.	Client has full ROM against resistance. Strength 5/5.	Decreased ROM against resistance is seen with joint or muscle disease.
Test **ROM of the lumbar spine** (Fig. 20-7C). Ask the client to bend forward and touch the toes (flexion). Observe for symmetry of the shoulders, scapula, and hips.	Flexion of 75 to 90 degrees, smooth movement, lumbar concavity flattens out, and the spinal processes are in alignment.	Lateral curvature disappears in functional scoliosis; unilateral exaggerated thoracic convexity increases in structural scoliosis. Spinal processes are out of alignment.
Sit down behind the client, stabilize the client's pelvis with your hands, and ask the client to bend sideways (lateral bending), bend backward toward you (hyperextension), and twist the shoulders one way and then the other (rotation).	Lateral bending capacity of the thoracic and lumbar spines should be about 35 degrees; hyperextension about 30 degrees; and rotation about 30 degrees.	Low back strain from injury to soft tissues is a common cause of impaired ROM and pain in the lumbar and thoracic regions. Other causes of impaired ROM in the lumbar and thoracic areas include osteoarthritis, ankylosing spondylitis, and congenital abnormalities that may affect the spinal vertebral spacing and mobility.
Measure **leg length.** If you suspect that the client has one leg longer than the other, measure them. Ask the client to lie down with legs extended. With a measuring tape, measure the distance between the anterior superior iliac	Measurements are equal or within 1 cm. If the legs still look unequal, assess the apparent leg length by measuring from a nonfixed point (the umbilicus) to a fixed point (medial malleolus) on each leg.	Unequal leg lengths are associated with scoliosis. Equal true leg lengths but unequal apparent leg lengths are seen with abnormalities in the structure or position of the hips and pelvis.

ASSESSMENT PROCEDURE	NORMAL FINDINGS	ABNORMAL FINDINGS

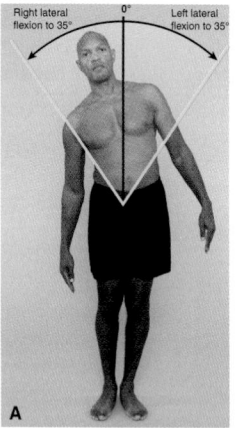 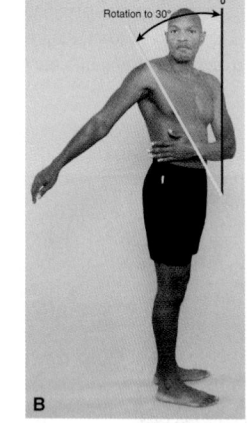 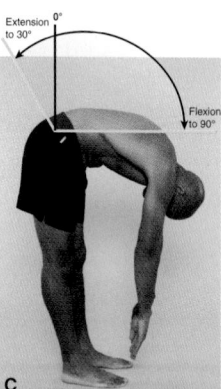

FIGURE 20-7 Range of motion of trunk. (**A**) Thoracic and lumbar spines: lateral bending. (**B**) Thoracic and lumbar spines: rotation. (**C**) Thoracic and lumbar spines: flexion.

(Continued on following page)

INSPECTION OF STANCE AND GAIT (*continued*)

ASSESSMENT PROCEDURE	NORMAL FINDINGS	ABNORMAL FINDINGS
spine and the medial malleolus, crossing the tape on the medial side of the knee (true leg length; Fig. 20-8).	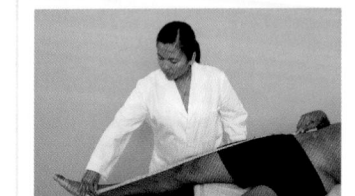 **FIGURE 20-8** Measuring true leg length.	

Shoulders, Arms, and Elbows

Inspection and Palpation

Inspect and palpate **shoulders and arms.** With the client standing or sitting, inspect anteriorly and posteriorly for symmetry, color, swelling, and masses. Palpate for tenderness, swelling, or heat. Anteriorly palpate the clavicle, acromioclavicular joint, subacromial area, and the biceps. Posteriorly palpate the glenohumeral joint, coracoid area, trapezius muscle, and the scapular area.	Shoulders are symmetrically round; no redness, swelling, deformity, or heat. Muscles are fully developed. Clavicles and scapulae are even and symmetric. The client reports no tenderness.	Flat, hollow, or less-rounded shoulders are seen with dislocation. Muscle atrophy is seen with nerve or muscle damage or lack of use. Tenderness, swelling, and heat may be noted with shoulder strains, sprains, arthritis, bursitis, and degenerative joint disease (DJD).

ASSESSMENT PROCEDURE	NORMAL FINDINGS	ABNORMAL FINDINGS
Test **ROM.** (See Table 20-2 for summary of ROM.) Explain to the client that you will be assessing ROM (consisting of flexion, extension, adduction, abduction, and motion against resistance). Ask client to stand with both arms straight down at the sides. Next, ask the client to move the arms forward (flexion), then backward with elbows straight (Fig. 20-9A).	Extent of forward flexion should be 180 degrees; hyperextension, 50 degrees; adduction, 50 degrees; and abduction 180 degrees.	Painful and limited abduction accompanied by muscle weakness and atrophy are seen with a rotator cuff tear. Client has sharp catches of pain when bringing hands overhead with rotator cuff tendinitis. Chronic pain and severe limitation of all shoulder motions are seen with calcified tendinitis.
Then have the client bring both hands together overhead, elbows straight, followed by moving both hands in front of the body past the midline with elbows straight (this tests adduction and abduction) (Fig. 20-9B).		
In a continuous motion, have the client bring the hands together behind the head with elbows flexed (this tests external rotation; Fig. 20-9D) and behind the back (internal rotation; Fig. 20-9C). Repeat these maneuvers against resistance.	Extent of external and internal rotation 90 degrees. Can flex, extend, adduct, abduct, rotate, and shrug shoulders against resistance.	Inability to shrug shoulders against resistance is seen with a lesion of cranial nerve XI (spinal accessory). Decreased muscle strength is seen with muscle or joint disease.

(Continued on following page)

INSPECTION OF STANCE AND GAIT (*continued*)

ASSESSMENT PROCEDURE	NORMAL FINDINGS	ABNORMAL FINDINGS

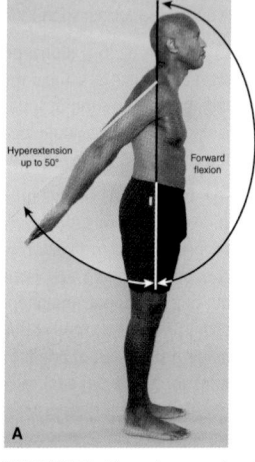

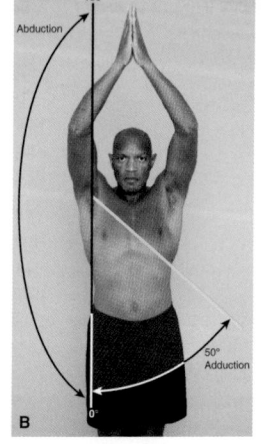

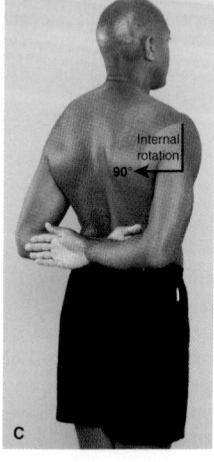

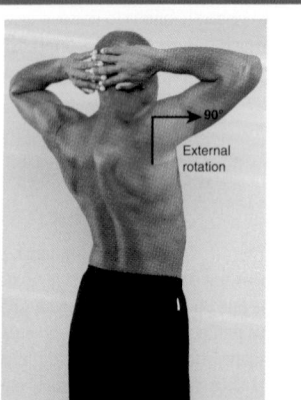

FIGURE 20-9 Normal range of motion of the shoulder. (**A**) Flexion–extension. (**B**) Adduction–abduction. (**C**) Internal rotation. (**D**) External rotation.

ASSESSMENT PROCEDURE	NORMAL FINDINGS	ABNORMAL FINDINGS
Elbows		
Inspection and Palpation		
Inspect for size, shape, deformities, redness, or swelling. Inspect elbows in both flexed and extended positions (Fig. 20-10A).	Elbows are symmetric, without deformities, redness, or swelling.	Redness, heat, and swelling may be seen with bursitis of the olecranon process due to trauma or arthritis.
With the elbow relaxed and flexed about 70 degrees, use your thumb and middle fingers to palpate the olecranon process and epicondyles.	Nontender; without nodules.	Firm, nontender, subcutaneous nodules may be palpated in rheumatoid arthritis or rheumatic fever. Tenderness or pain over the epicondyles may be palpated in epicondylitis (tennis elbow) due to repetitive movements.
Test ROM. (See Table 20-2 for summary of ROM.) Ask the client to perform the following movements to test ROM, flexion, extension, pronation, and supination (Fig. 20-10B). • Flex the elbow and bring the hand to the forehead (Fig. 20-10A). • Straighten the elbow. • Then the hold arm out, turn the palm down, then turn the palm up (Fig. 20-10B).	ROM: 160 degrees flexion, 180 degrees extension, 90 degrees pronation, and 90 degrees supination. May lack 5 to 10 degrees or have hyperextension.	Decreased ROM seen with joint or muscle disease or injury.

(Continued on following page)

INSPECTION OF STANCE AND GAIT (*continued*)		
ASSESSMENT PROCEDURE	**NORMAL FINDINGS**	**ABNORMAL FINDINGS**
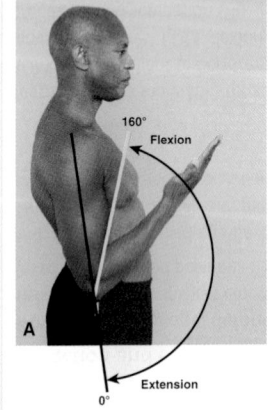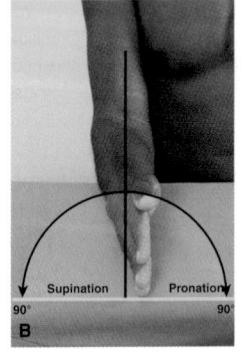 **FIGURE 20-10** Normal range of motion of the elbow. (A) Flexion–extension. (B) Pronation–supination.		
Lastly, have the client repeat the movements against your resistance.	The client should have full ROM against resistance.	Decreased ROM against resistance is seen with joint or muscle disease or injury.

ASSESSMENT PROCEDURE	NORMAL FINDINGS	ABNORMAL FINDINGS
Wrists		
Inspection and Palpation		
Inspect wrist size, shape, symmetry, color, and swelling. Then palpate for tenderness and nodules.	Wrists are symmetric, without redness, or swelling. They are nontender and free of nodules. 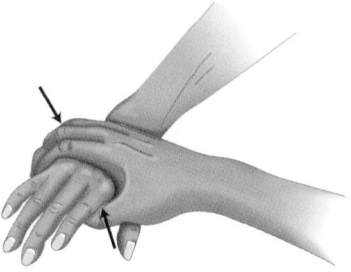 **FIGURE 20-11** Squeeze test (hand).	Swelling is seen with rheumatoid arthritis. Tenderness and nodules may be seen with rheumatoid arthritis. A nontender, round, enlarged, swollen, fluid-filled cyst (ganglion) may be noted on the wrists. Signs of a wrist fracture include pain, tenderness, swelling, and inability to hold a grip; as well as pain that goes away and then returns as a deep, dull ache. Extreme tenderness occurs when pressure is applied on the side of the hand between the two tendons leading to the thumb (UCSF Medical Center, 2016).
Perform the Squeeze test by squeezing the client's hand across the knuckle joints (Fig. 20-11).	Client tolerates without extreme pain.	Extreme pain may indicate rheumatoid arthritis and psoriatic arthritis of the hand (American Society for Surgery of the Hand, 2017; Delzell, 2019).

(Continued on following page)

INSPECTION OF STANCE AND GAIT (*continued*)

ASSESSMENT PROCEDURE	NORMAL FINDINGS	ABNORMAL FINDINGS
Palpate the anatomic snuffbox (the hollow area on the back of the wrist at the base of the fully extended thumb; Fig. 20-12).	No tenderness palpated in anatomic snuffbox.	Snuffbox tenderness may indicate a scaphoid fracture, which is often the result of falling on an outstretched hand.

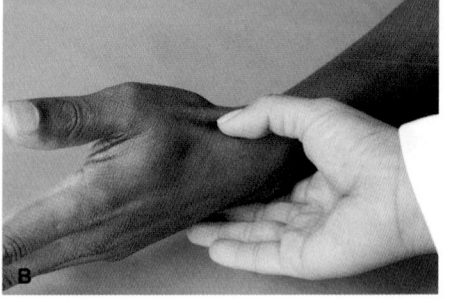

FIGURE 20-12 (A) Anatomic snuffbox. (B) Palpating anatomic snuffbox.

Test ROM. (See Table 20-2 for summary of ROM.) Ask the client to bend the wrist down and back (flexion and extension; Fig. 20-13A).	Normal ROM: 90 degrees of flexion, 70 degrees of hyperextension, 55 degrees of ulnar deviation, and 20 degrees of radial deviation. Client should have full ROM against resistance.	Ulnar deviation of the wrist and fingers with limited ROM is often seen in rheumatoid arthritis.

ASSESSMENT PROCEDURE	NORMAL FINDINGS	ABNORMAL FINDINGS
Next, have the client hold the wrist straight and move the hand outward and inward (deviation; Fig. 20-13B). Repeat these maneuvers against resistance.		Increased pain with extension of the wrist against resistance is seen in epicondylitis of the lateral side of the elbow. Increased pain with flexion of the wrist against resistance is seen in epicondylitis of the medial side of the elbow. Decreased muscle strength is noted with muscle and joint disease.

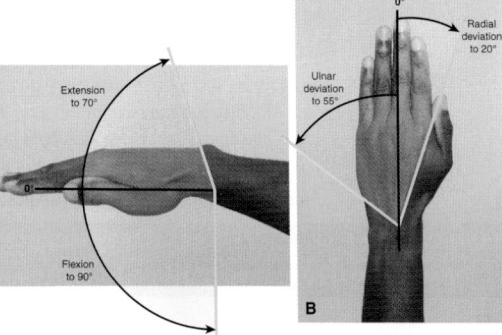

FIGURE 20-13 Range of motion of the wrists. (A) Flexion–hyperextension. (B) Radial–ulnar deviation.

(Continued on following page)

INSPECTION OF STANCE AND GAIT (*continued*)		
ASSESSMENT PROCEDURE	**NORMAL FINDINGS**	**ABNORMAL FINDINGS**
Assessment of Carpal Tunnel Syndrome. *Note: The following assessments for carpal tunnel syndrome vary in sensitivity and specificity. They can suggest but not diagnose the condition (University of Arkansas for Medical Sciences, 2018).*		
Client reports include:		
Pain and paresthesias along median nerve distribution (i.e., thumb, index finger, middle finger, or all fingers, but not in dorsum or palm of hand), may radiate to forearm, arm, and shoulder.	No reports of pain or paresthesias along median nerve distribution.	Pain and paresthesias along median nerve distribution (i.e., thumb, index finger, middle finger, or all fingers, but not in dorsum or palm of hand), may radiate to forearm, arm, and shoulder.
Note: These symptoms reported by client are the most reliable indicator of carpal tunnel syndrome.		

ASSESSMENT PROCEDURE	NORMAL FINDINGS	ABNORMAL FINDINGS
Physical assessment tests include: Test Thumb Strength and Muscle Weakness. Ask client to raise thumb perpendicular to palm against slight downward pressure applied by person completing assessment.	No weakness in thumb. Client will not shake or flick wrist when asked this question.	Muscle weakness in thumb in attempt to raise it against slight pressure. If the client responds with a motion that resembles shaking a thermometer (flick signal), carpal tunnel may be suspected.
Observe for the **flick signal.** Ask the client, "What do you do when your symptoms are worse?"		
Perform **Phalen test.** Ask client to hold the forearm vertically and allow the wrist to drop into 90 degrees of flexion under the influence of gravity for 1 minute. If stiffness of the wrist does not permit 90 degrees of flexion, then the wrist should be allowed to fall as far as possible. Avoid forced flexion, as this increases the number of false-positive tests. An important element of the test is that it is only positive if the symptoms elicited are essentially the same as the symptoms that the client reports.	Client reports no pain, numbness, or tingling with the 90 degrees flexion for 1 minute.	If symptoms develop within a minute with Phalen test, carpel tunnel syndrome is suspected. Client may report tingling, numbness, and pain with carpal tunnel syndrome. However, if the test lasts longer than a minute, pain and tingling may occur even in clients without carpel tunnel syndrome.

(Continued on following page)

INSPECTION OF STANCE AND GAIT (*continued*)

ASSESSMENT PROCEDURE	NORMAL FINDINGS	ABNORMAL FINDINGS
Ask the client to rest elbows on a table and place the back of both hands against each other while flexing the wrists 90 degrees with fingers pointed downward and wrists dangling (Fig. 20-14A). Have the client hold this position for 60 seconds. *Note*: *This test is no longer considered a reliable diagnosis for carpal tunnel syndrome but is still widely used.*	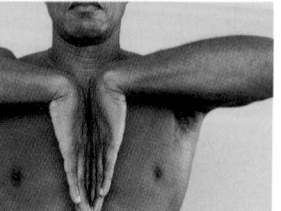	

FIGURE 20-14   Tests for carpal tunnel syndrome. (**A**) Phalen test. (**B**) Tinel test.

Perform test for **Tinel sign:** Use your finger to percuss lightly over the median nerve (located on the inner aspect of the wrist; Fig. 20-14B). *Note*: *This test has been found to be the least reliable of carpal tunnel syndrome tests but is still widely used.*	No tingling or shocking sensation experienced with test for Tinel sign.	Tingling or shocking sensation experienced with test for Tinel sign. Median nerve entrapped in the carpal tunnel results in pain, numbness, and impaired function of the hand and fingers (Fig. 20-15).

ASSESSMENT PROCEDURE	NORMAL FINDINGS	ABNORMAL FINDINGS

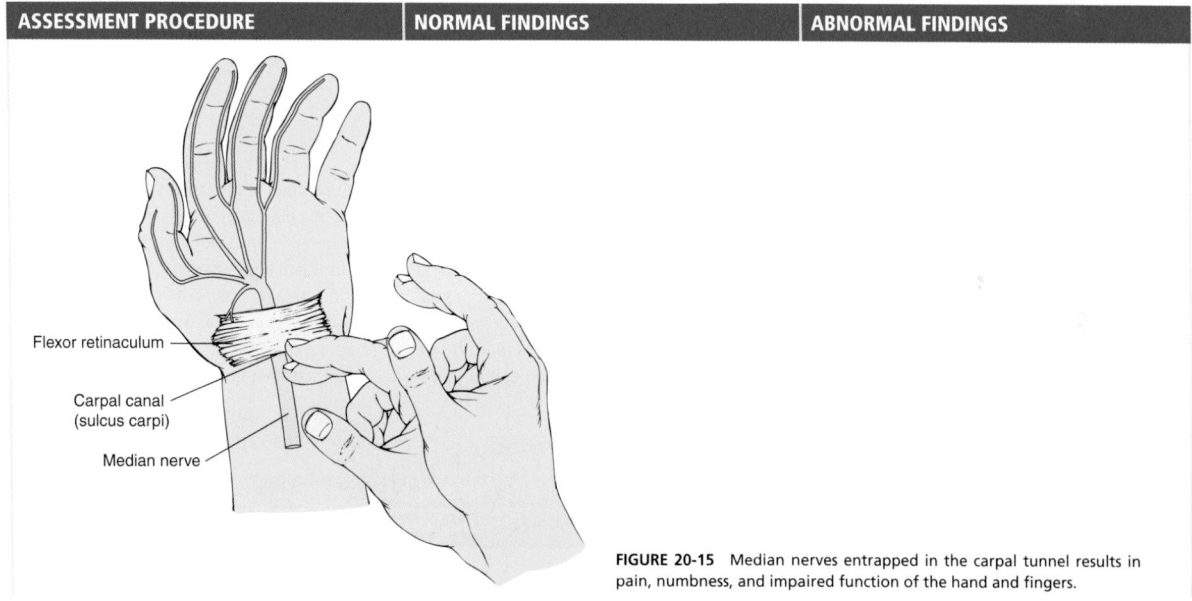

Flexor retinaculum

Carpal canal (sulcus carpi)

Median nerve

FIGURE 20-15 Median nerves entrapped in the carpal tunnel results in pain, numbness, and impaired function of the hand and fingers.

(Continued on following page)

INSPECTION OF STANCE AND GAIT (*continued*)

ASSESSMENT PROCEDURE	NORMAL FINDINGS	ABNORMAL FINDINGS
Hands and Fingers		
Inspection and Palpation		
Inspect size, shape, symmetry, swelling, and color. Palpate the fingers from the distal end proximally, noting tenderness, swelling, bony prominences, nodules, or crepitus of each interphalangeal joint. Assess the metacarpophalangeal joints by squeezing the hand from each side between your thumb and fingers. Palpate each metacarpal of the hand, noting tenderness and swelling.	Hands and fingers are symmetric, nontender, and without nodules. Fingers lie in straight line. No swelling or deformities. Rounded protuberance noted next to the thumb over the thenar prominence. Smaller protuberance seen adjacent to the small finger.	Pain, tenderness, swelling, shortened finger, depressed knuckle, finger crosses over adjacent finger when making a fist, and/or inability to move the finger are seen with finger fractures (UCSF Medical Center, 2016). Swollen, stiff, tender finger joints are seen in acute rheumatoid arthritis. Boutonnière deformity and swan-neck deformity are seen in long-term rheumatoid arthritis Atrophy of the thenar prominence may be evident in carpal tunnel syndrome. In osteoarthritis, hard, painless nodules may be seen over the distal interphalangeal joints (Heberden nodes) and over the proximal interphalangeal joints (Bouchard nodes); see Abnormal Findings 20-2.

ASSESSMENT PROCEDURE	NORMAL FINDINGS	ABNORMAL FINDINGS
Test ROM (Fig. 20-16). (See Table 20-2 for summary of ROM.) Ask the client to (A) spread the fingers apart (abduction), (B) make a fist (adduction), (C) bend the fingers down (flexion) and then up (hyperextension), (D) move the thumb away from other fingers, and then (E) touch the thumb to the base of the small finger. Repeat these maneuvers against resistance.	Normal ROM: 20 degrees abduction, full adduction of fingers (touching), 90 degrees of flexion, and 30 degrees of hyperextension. Thumb easily moves away from other fingers; 50 degrees of thumb flexion. Full ROM against resistance.	Inability to extend the ring and little fingers is seen in Dupuytren contracture. Painful extension of a finger may be seen in tenosynovitis (infection of the flexor tendon sheaths); decreased muscle strength against resistance is associated with muscle and joint disease.

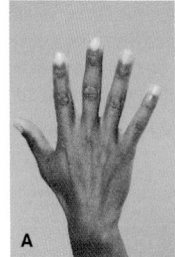 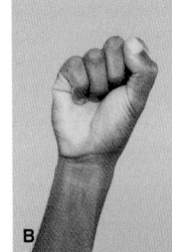 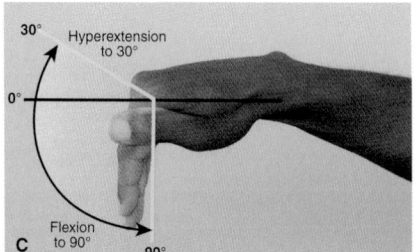 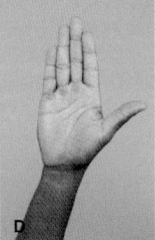 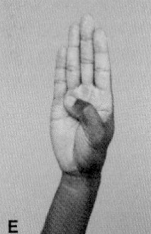

FIGURE 20-16 Normal range of motion of the fingers. (**A**) Abduction. (**B**) Adduction. (**C**) Flexion–hyperextension. (**D**) Thumb away from fingers. (**E**) Thumb touching base of small finger.

(Continued on following page)

INSPECTION OF STANCE AND GAIT (*continued*)		
ASSESSMENT PROCEDURE	**NORMAL FINDINGS**	**ABNORMAL FINDINGS**
Hips		
Inspection and Palpation		
With the client standing, inspect symmetry and shape of the hips (Fig. 20-17). Observe for convex thoracic curve and concave lumbar curve. Palpate for stability, tenderness, and crepitus.	Buttocks are equally sized; iliac crests are symmetric in height. Hips are stable, nontender, and without crepitus.	Instability, inability to stand, and/or a deformed hip area are indicative of a fractured hip. Tenderness, edema, decreased ROM, and crepitus are seen in hip inflammation and DJD.
		The most common injuries of the hip and groin region in athletes are adductor groin tears (Kerbel et al., 2018).
		Strains, a stretch or tear of muscle or tendons, often occur in the lower back and the hamstring muscle.
Test ROM. (See Table 20-2 for summary of ROM). ***Note:*** *If the client has had a total hip replacement, do not test ROM unless the physician gives permission to do so, due to the risk of dislocating the hip prosthesis.*	Normal ROM: 90 degrees of hip flexion with the knee straight and 120 degrees of hip flexion with the knee bent and the other leg remaining straight.	Inability to abduct the hip is a common sign of hip disease.
		Pain and a decrease in internal hip rotation may be a sign of osteoarthritis or femoral neck stress fracture. Pain on palpation of the greater trochanter and pain as the client moves from standing to lying down may indicate bursitis of the hip.

ASSESSMENT PROCEDURE	NORMAL FINDINGS	ABNORMAL FINDINGS

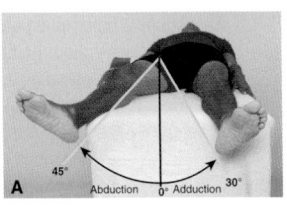
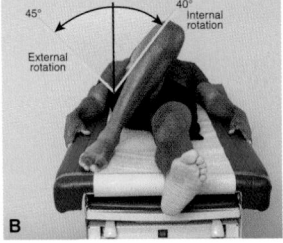
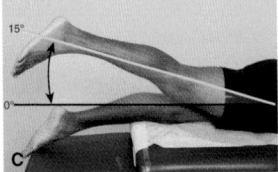
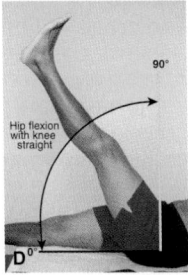
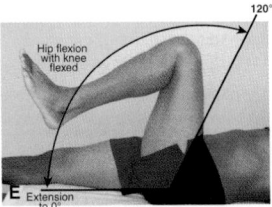

FIGURE 20-17 Normal range of hip motion. (**A**) Hip abduction and adduction. (**B**) Internal and external rotation. (**C**) Hyperextension. (**D**) Hip flexion with knee straight. (**E**) Hip flexion with knee flexed.

(Continued on following page)

INSPECTION OF STANCE AND GAIT (*continued*)

ASSESSMENT PROCEDURE	NORMAL FINDINGS	ABNORMAL FINDINGS
With the client supine, ask the client to: • Raise extended leg (Fig. 20-17D). • Flex knee up to chest while keeping other leg extended (Fig. 20-17E). • Move extended leg (Fig. 20-17A) away from midline of body as far as possible and then toward midline of body as far as possible (abduction and adduction). • Bend knee and turn leg (Fig. 20-17B) inward (rotation) and then outward (rotation). • Ask the client to lie prone (Fig. 20-17C) and lift extended leg off table. Alternatively, ask the client to stand and swing extended leg backward. • Repeat these maneuvers against resistance.	Normal ROM: • 45 to 50 degrees of abduction • 20 to 30 degrees of adduction • 40 degrees internal hip rotation • 45 degrees external hip rotation. • 15 degrees hip hyperextension. Full ROM against resistance. Strength 5/5.	Decreased muscle strength against resistance is seen in muscle and joint disease.

ASSESSMENT PROCEDURE	NORMAL FINDINGS	ABNORMAL FINDINGS
Knees		
Inspection and Palpation		
With the client supine and then sitting with knees dangling, inspect for size, shape, symmetry, swelling, deformities, and alignment. Observe for quadriceps muscle atrophy.	Knees symmetric, hollows present on both sides of the patella, no swelling or deformities. Lower leg in alignment with the upper leg.	Knees turn in with knock knees (genu valgum) and turn out with bowed legs (genu varum). Swelling above or next to the patella may indicate fluid in the knee joint or thickening of the synovial membrane.
Palpate for tenderness, warmth, consistency, and nodules. Begin palpation 10 cm above the patella, using your fingers and thumb to move downward toward the knee.	Nontender and cool. Muscles firm. No nodules.	Tenderness and warmth with a boggy consistency may be symptoms of synovitis. Asymmetric muscular development in the quadriceps may indicate atrophy.
Perform the **Bulge test** if swelling is present. If you notice swelling, perform Bulge test to determine whether cause is accumulation of fluid or soft-tissue swelling. The bulge will detect small amounts of fluid in the knee. With the client in a supine position, use the ball of your	No bulge of fluid appears on the medial side of knee.	Bulge of fluid appears on the medial side of knee, with a small amount of joint effusion.

(Continued on following page)

INSPECTION OF STANCE AND GAIT (*continued*)		
ASSESSMENT PROCEDURE	**NORMAL FINDINGS**	**ABNORMAL FINDINGS**
hand to firmly stroke the medial side of the knee upward, three to four times, to displace any accumulated fluid.		
Then press on the lateral side of the knee and look for a bulge on the medial side of the knee.		
Perform the **ballottement test.** This test helps to detect large amounts of fluid in the knee. With the client in a supine position, firmly press your nondominant thumb and index finger on each side of the patella. This displaces fluid in the suprapatellar bursa, located between the femur and the patella. Then, with your dominant fingers, push the patella down on the femur. Feel for a fluid wave or a click.	No movement of the patella is noted. Patella rests firmly over the femur.	Fluid wave or click palpated, with large amounts of joint effusion. A positive ballottement test may be present with meniscal tears.
Palpate the tibiofemoral space. As you compress the patella, slide it distally against the underlying femur. Note crepitus or pain.	There is no pain on examination. Crepitus may be present.	A patellofemoral disorder may be suspected if both crepitus and pain are present on examination.

ASSESSMENT PROCEDURE	NORMAL FINDINGS	ABNORMAL FINDINGS
Test **ROM.** (See Table 20-3 for summary of normal ROM.) Ask the client to: • Bend each knee up (flexion) toward buttocks or back. • Straighten the knee (extension/hyperextension). • Walk normally. Repeat these maneuvers against resistance.	Normal ROM (Fig. 20-18): 120 to 130 degrees of flexion; 0 degrees of extension to 15 degrees of hyperextension. Client should have full ROM against resistance. 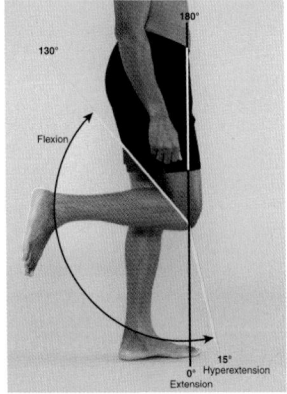 **FIGURE 20-18** Normal range of motion of knee.	Osteoarthritis is characterized by a decreased ROM with synovial thickening and crepitation. Flexion contractures of the knee are characterized by an inability to extend knee fully. Decreased muscle strength against resistance is seen in muscle and joint disease.

(*Continued on following page*)

INSPECTION OF STANCE AND GAIT (*continued*)		
ASSESSMENT PROCEDURE	**NORMAL FINDINGS**	**ABNORMAL FINDINGS**
Test for **pain and injury.** If the client complains of a "giving in" or "locking" of the knee, perform McMurray test. With client in supine position, ask client to flex one knee and hip. Then place your thumb and index finger of one hand on either side of the knee. Use your other hand to hold the heel of the foot up. Rotate the lower leg and foot laterally. Slowly extend the knee, noting pain or clicking. Repeat, rotating lower leg and foot medially. Again, note pain or clicking.	No pain or clicking noted.	Pain or clicking is indicative of a torn meniscus of the knee. There are a number of provocative knee tests for knee and ligament injuries that can be seen in Budoff and Nirschl (2013).
Ankles and Feet		
Inspection and Palpation		
With the client sitting, standing, and walking, inspect **position, alignment, shape, and skin.**	Toes usually point forward and lie flat; however, they may point in (pes varus) or point out (pes valgus). Toes and feet are in alignment with the lower leg. Smooth, rounded medial malleolar prominences with prominent heels and	A laterally deviated great toe with possible overlapping of the second toe and possible formation of an enlarged, painful, inflamed bursa (bunion) on the medial side is seen with hallux valgus. Common abnormalities include feet

ASSESSMENT PROCEDURE	NORMAL FINDINGS	ABNORMAL FINDINGS
	metatarsophalangeal joints. Skin is smooth and free of corns and calluses. Longitudinal arch; most of the weight bearing is on the foot midline.	with no arches (pes planus or "flat feet"), feet with high arches (pes cavus); painful thickening of the skin over bony prominences and at pressure points (corns); nonpainful thickened skin that occurs at pressure points (calluses); and painful warts (verruca vulgaris) that often occur under a callus (plantar warts; Abnormal Findings 20-2).
Palpate **ankles and feet for tenderness, heat, swelling, or nodules.** Palpate the toes from the distal end proximally, noting tenderness, swelling, bony prominences, nodules, or crepitus of each interphalangeal joint.	No pain, heat, swelling, or nodules are noted.	Ankles are the most common site of sprains, which occur with stretched or torn ligaments (tough bands of fibrous tissue connecting bones in a joint) (Rothman Orthopedics, 2019).
		Tender, painful, reddened, hot, and swollen metatarsophalangeal joint of the great toe is seen in gouty arthritis. Nodules of the posterior ankle may be palpated with rheumatoid arthritis.

(Continued on following page)

INSPECTION OF STANCE AND GAIT (continued)		
ASSESSMENT PROCEDURE	**NORMAL FINDINGS**	**ABNORMAL FINDINGS**
Assess the metatarsophalangeal joints by squeezing the foot from each side with your thumb and fingers. Palpate each metatarsal, noting swelling or tenderness. Palpate the plantar area (bottom) of the foot, noting pain or swelling.		Pain and tenderness of the metatarsophalangeal joints are seen in inflammation of the joints, rheumatoid arthritis, and DJD. Tenderness of the calcaneus of the bottom of the foot may indicate plantar fasciitis. Plantar fasciitis is the most common cause of heel pain, which occurs when the strong supportive band of tissue in the arch of the foot becomes irritated and inflamed (Mayo Clinic, 2019). Use the Ottawa ankle and foot rules (Box 20-1: Ottawa Ankle Rules for X-ray Referral) to determine need for x-ray referral (Gomes et al., 2020).
Perform the **Squeeze test** by squeezing the client's foot across the knuckle joints (Fig. 20-19).	Client tolerates without extreme pain.	Extreme pain may indicate rheumatoid arthritis and psoriatic arthritis of the hand.
Test **ROM**. (See Table 20-3 for summary of normal ROM.) Ask the client to: • Point toes upward (dorsiflexion) and then downward (plantar flexion, Fig. 20-20A). • Turn soles outward (eversion) and then inward (inversion, Fig. 20-20B).	Normal ROM: • 20 degrees dorsiflexion ankle and foot and 45 degrees plantar flexion ankle and foot.	Decreased strength against resistance is seen in muscle and joint disease.

ASSESSMENT PROCEDURE	NORMAL FINDINGS	ABNORMAL FINDINGS

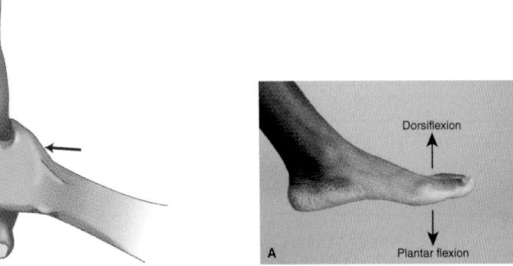

FIGURE 20-19 Squeeze test (foot).

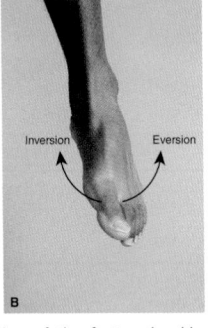 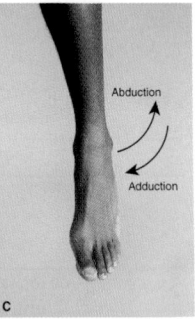

FIGURE 20-20 Normal range of motion of the feet and ankles. **(A)** Dorsiflexion–plantar flexion. **(B)** Eversion–inversion. **(C)** Abduction–adduction.

• Rotate foot outward (abduction) and then inward (adduction, Fig. 20-20C). • Turn toes under foot (flexion) and then upward (extension). Repeat these maneuvers against resistance.	• 20 degrees eversion and 30 degrees inversion. • 10 degrees abduction and 20 degrees adduction. • 40 degrees of flexion and 40 degrees of extension. Client has full ROM against resistance.	Hyperextension of the metatarsophalangeal joint and flexion of the proximal interphalangeal joint are apparent in hammer toe. Decreased strength against resistance is common in muscle and joint disease.

TABLE 20-2 **Normal Range of Motion for Joints of the Upper Extremities**

Shoulder	Elbow	Wrist	Fingers
Flexion	Flexion	Flexion	Flexion
Extension	Extension	Hyperextension	Hyperextension
Abduction	Supination	Deviation	Abduction
Adduction	Pronation	Radial	Adduction
Rotation (internal and external)		Ulnar	Thumb away from fingers
			Thumb to base of small finger

TABLE 20-3 **Normal Range of Motion for Joints of the Lower Extremities**

Hip	Knee	Ankle	Toes
Rotation (internal and external)	Flexion	Dorsiflexion	Flexion
Flexion	Extension	Plantar flexion	Extension
Extension		Inversion	
Abduction		Eversion	
Adduction			

ABNORMAL FINDINGS 20-1 Abnormal Spinal Curves

LORDOSIS KYPHOSIS SCOLIOSIS

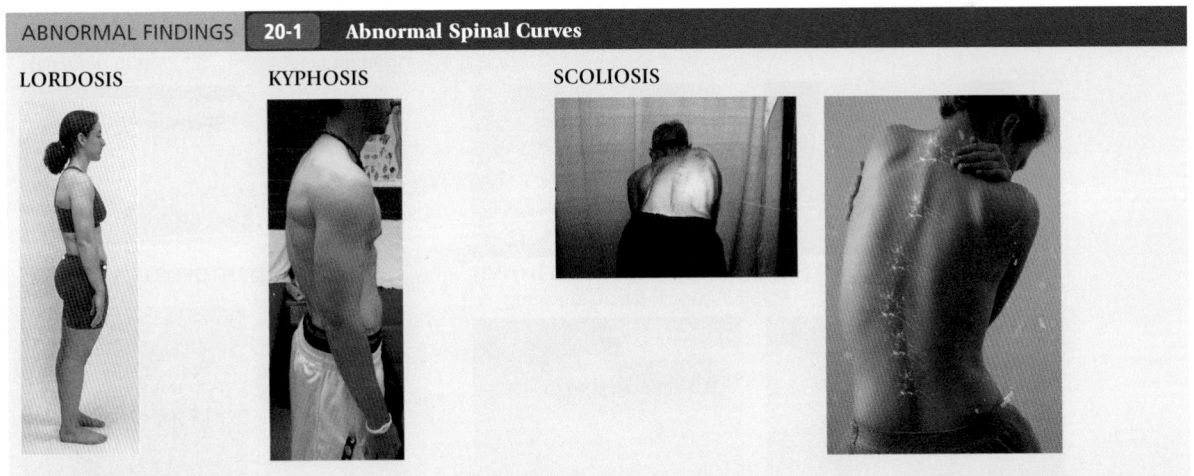

Photo credits: Lordosis, reprinted with permission from Oatis, C. A. (2004). *Kinesiology: The mechanics and pathomechanics of human movement.* Lippincott Williams & Wilkins; Kyphosis, courtesy of Martin Herman, MD.

ABNORMAL FINDINGS 20-2 Abnormal Upper and Lower Extremity Findings

ACUTE RHEUMATOID ARTHRITIS

CHRONIC RHEUMATOID ARTHRITIS

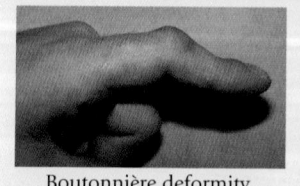
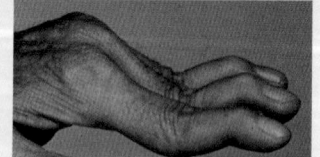

Boutonnière deformity.

Swan-neck deformity.

OSTEOARTHRITIS

HAMMER TOE

HALLUX VALGUS

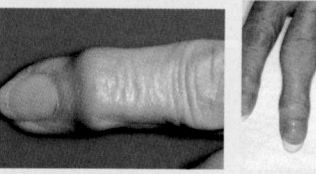
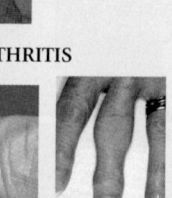
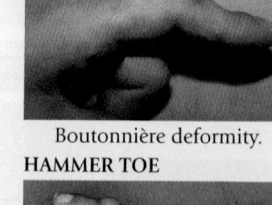

Heberden nodes.

Bouchard nodes.

Photo credits: Acute rheumatoid arthritis, reprinted with permission from Ballantyne, J. C., Fishman, S. M., & Rathmell, J. P. (2019). *Bonica's management of pain* (5th ed., Fig. 34-5). Wolters Kluwer; Boutonnière deformity, swan-neck deformity, reprinted with permission from Wiesel, S. W. (2016). *Operative techniques in orthopaedic surgery* (2nd ed., Fig. 6-105-2B, C). Lippincott Williams & Wilkins; Heberden nodes, reprinted with permission from Bickley, L. (2013). *Bates' guide to physical examination and history-taking* (11th ed., Fig. 16-73). Lippincott Williams & Wilkins; Bouchard nodes, Dr. P. Marazzi/Science Source.

BOX 20-1   OTTAWA ANKLE RULES FOR X-RAY REFERRAL

ANKLE X-RAY INDICATORS
Malleolar area pain and bone tenderness at the tips of 6-cm edges of the lateral malleolus or medial malleolus, or the inability to bear weight immediately or during examination, indicate the need for an ankle x-ray.

FOOT X-RAY INDICATORS
Pain in the midfoot area and bone tenderness at the base of the fifth metatarsal or the navicular bone area, or the inability to bear weight immediately or during examination, indicate the need for a foot x-ray.

From Gomes, Y. E., Chau, M., Banwell, H. A., Davies, J., & Causby, R. S. (2020). Adequacy of clinical information in X-ray referrals for traumatic ankle injury with reference to the Ottawa Ankle Rules—A retrospective clinical audit. *PeerJ, 8.* https://doi.org/10.7717/peerj.10152

 PEDIATRIC VARIATIONS

Questions to ask the parents when collecting *subjective data* include the following.
- Birth injuries?
- Alignment of hips?
- Trauma?
- Participation in sports or outdoor activities?
- Frequent pain in joints?
- Any previous injury or fracture?
- Any recent surgery?
- Any concerns from parent or client regarding mobility, strength, or movement of any joints, arms, legs?

When collecting *objective data,* note the following:

ASSESSMENT PROCEDURE	NORMAL FINDINGS
Infant: Inspect **lower extremities**.	A distinct bowlegged (Fig. 20-21A) growth pattern persists and begins to disappear at 18 months. At the age of 2 years, a knock-kneed pattern is common (Fig. 20-21B), persisting until the age of 6 to 10 years, when legs straighten.
	A greater ROM in joints is present in infants. Legs are wide set until the child begins walking; weight is borne on the inside of the feet.
Perform **Ortolani maneuver** to test for congenital hip dysplasia. With the infant supine, flex the knees while holding your thumbs on midthigh and your fingers over the greater trochanters; abduct the legs, moving the knees outward and down toward the table (Fig. 20-22A).	Positive Ortolani sign: A click heard along with feeling the head of the femur slip in or out of the hip.

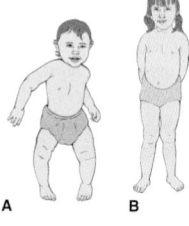

A   B

FIGURE 20-21 **(A)** Genu varum (bow legs). **(B)** Genu valgum (knock knees).

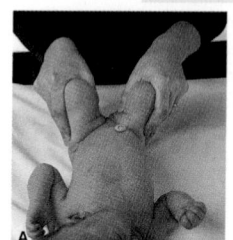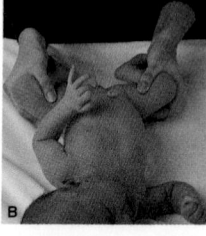

A   B

FIGURE 20-22 **(A)** Ortolani maneuver. **(B)** Barlow maneuver.

ASSESSMENT PROCEDURE	NORMAL FINDINGS
Perform **Barlow maneuver.** With the infant supine, flex the knees while holding your thumbs on midthigh and your fingers over the greater trochanters; adduct legs until thumbs touch (Fig. 20-22B).	Positive Barlow sign: A feeling of the head of the femur slipping out of the hip socket (acetabulum).
Greater than the age of 2 years: Inspect **gait.** Measure distance between knees with ankles together.	Wide-based gait common until the age of 2 years. Less than 5.1 cm (2 in.)
3 to 7 years of age: Measure distance between ankles with knees together. Longitudinal arch of foot is often obscured by adipose until the age of 3 years, and infant appears flat-footed.	Less than 7.6 cm (3 in.)
4 to 13 years of age: See also Appendix 5 for developmental milestones.	
INSPECT CURVATURE OF SPINE (FIG. 20-23):	
• Stand behind erect child and note asymmetry of shoulders and hips. • Have child bend forward at waist until back is parallel to floor; observe from side, looking for asymmetry or prominence of rib cage.	• Shoulders symmetrical, parallel with hips. • Shoulders, scapulae, iliac crests symmetrical.

(Continued on following page)

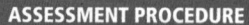

ASSESSMENT PROCEDURE	NORMAL FINDINGS

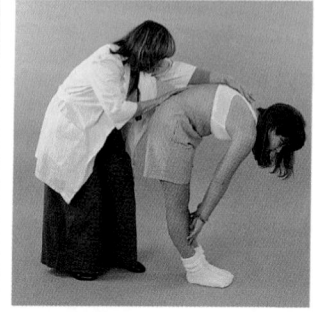

FIGURE 20-23 Assessing spinal curvature for scoliosis.

A preparticipation sports evaluation should be performed on all children and adolescents before participating in sports. Perform careful evaluation of the musculoskeletal system. This examination will assess mobility/motion of joints; strength of muscles; symmetry of hands, arms, legs, and shoulders; and motion of the spine and hips. Each state school program has its own form to be completed for the student athlete.

GERIATRIC VARIATIONS

- When assessing spinal mobility, you can ask an older client to bend forward, but do not insist that they touch toes unless the client is comfortable with the movement.
- Osteoporosis is more common as a person ages because that is when bone resorption increases, calcium absorption decreases, and production of osteoblasts decreases. Bones lose their density with age, putting the older client at risk for bone fractures, especially of the wrists, hips, and vertebrae. Older clients who have osteomalacia or osteoporosis are at an even higher risk for fractures.
- Slower gait with wide-based stance and smaller arm swing
- Exaggerated thoracic spinal curve (kyphosis)
- Loss of muscle bulk and tone
- Decreased ROM of spine, neck, and extremities
- Decrease in height (1.2 cm of height lost every 20 years)
- Shoulder width decreases; chest and pelvis widths increase
- May have bowlegged appearance due to decreased muscle control

 CULTURAL VARIATIONS

- Some variation in muscles and bones are seen in different racial/ethnic groups. A large gluteal prominence in some Blacks may be mistaken as lumbar lordosis; number of vertebrae may differ. Racial and sex variations from the usual 24 found in 85% to 93% of all people include 11% of African-American women with 23, and 12% of Eskimo and Native-American men with 25 (Andrews et al., 2020).
- Ulna and radius may have unequal lengths (e.g., Swedes and Chinese).
- Up to 90% of bone mass density (BMD) peaks by around 18 years in females and by age 20 in males (National Institutes of Health Osteoporosis and Related Bone Diseases National Resource Center, 2018). Bone mass in women remains stable until after menopause, when it begins to decrease. Bone mass decreases in both sexes with age and some specific conditions, including lack of weight-bearing exercise. BMD is higher in men and African Americans and lowest in Asians.

- Bone density (and osteoporosis) varies, with men having denser bones, Blacks having denser bones than Whites, and most East Asians having less dense bones than Whites (with some variation within population groups); however, the variation in bone density does not directly account for the variation in bone fracture rates (Zengin et al., 2015).
- American Indian/Native Alaskan and multirace non-Hispanics have a slightly higher rate of arthritis than African Americans and Whites; Hispanics have lower rates, and Asians have the lowest rates of arthritis (Centers for Disease Control and Prevention, 2018).
- Racial/ethnic trends in rheumatoid arthritis have shown Whites have the highest incidence and prevalence, followed by other races/ethnicities (Hispanic, Asian, African American), and in all groups more prevalent in females (Kawatkar et al., 2012).

Lactose intolerance (a deficiency of the lactase enzyme) affects up 70% of adult humans due to decreased production of the lactase enzyme at weaning. Between 80% and 95% of Asians and Native Americans are lactose intolerant, and between 18% and 26% of northern Europeans (Neville, 2017).

POSSIBLE COLLABORATIVE PROBLEMS—RISK OF

- Bone fractures
- Sprains
- Contractures of joints
- Osteoporosis
- Dislocation of joints
- Compartment syndrome
- Osteoarthritis
- Rheumatoid arthritis

Teaching Tips for Selected Client Concerns

Client Concern: *Opportunity to enhance musculoskeletal health associated with client request to be more mobile*

Teach client the importance of maintaining an ideal weight. Explain the importance of doing weight-bearing and muscle-toning exercises at least three times per week. Encourage client to wear seat belts in vehicles, to wear low, well-fitted shoes, and to use walking aids (e.g., cane) as needed to prevent injury. Caution client against the dangerous effects of excessive exercise. Teach proper body mechanics and correct posture.

Client Concern: *Chronic pain (muscles and joints) associated with rheumatoid arthritis)*

Discuss independent pain management measures the client may find useful (e.g., massage, relaxation, distraction). Weight loss may also reduce discomfort if obesity is straining the bones, muscles, and joints. Explain use and side effects of pain medications.

Rheumatoid arthritis pain and symptoms are varied and may include burning and/or throbbing on both sides of the body that may worsen after sitting for long periods; there may be an inconsistent pattern of worse and less pain, with a feeling of heat and soreness in joints, as well as weak muscles, feeling tired or depressed, weight loss, decreased appetite, slight elevated temperature, swollen glands, and significant stiffness in the morning that persists at least an hour (Rodriguez, 2021).

Client Concern: *Risk for injury (child) associated with parent's knowledge deficit of home safety measures to prevent child injuries*

Caution parents on home safety precautions (e.g., gates at stairways, removal of objects that may cause unnecessary falls, avoiding leaving child near water alone) based on child's level of musculoskeletal development. Develop home safety checklist with parents. Teach normal milestones of musculoskeletal development, and advise parent to encourage these skills as appropriate.

 Client Concern: *Risk for musculoskeletal injuries associated with unstable gait, decalcification of bones secondary to sedentary lifestyle and postmenopausal state*

Discuss importance of calcium supplements in diet for postmenopausal women. Explain effects of exercise on decreasing bone decalcification.

Explain the correct use of aids (e.g., crutches, canes, walkers) and other prostheses. Use referrals as necessary. Instruct client on measures to prevent falls (e.g., adequate lighting, avoidance of loose board ends and scatter rugs on floor). Discourage use of sleeping pills and suggest alternate methods of promoting sleep (e.g., watching TV, reading, warm bath, music, warm milk).

 Client Concerns: *Poor mobility, flexibility, and gait associated with sedentary lifestyle secondary to weakness and poor memory with aging process*

Instruct client on the hazards of immobility and methods to prevent complications (e.g., turning, coughing, deep breathing, repositioning, ROM, adequate diet, plentiful fluid intake, diversional activities). Encourage mild exercise to loosen joint stiffness.

Assess safe level of activity with the client, and teach methods to increase activity gradually to that level. Explore alternate self-help methods of maintaining self-care (e.g., feeding aids, wheelchairs, crutches, hygienic aids). Assist the client with identifying and utilizing services and groups to assist with activities of daily living (e.g., Meals on Wheels). Support and teach family caregivers.

References

American Society for Surgery of the Hand. (2017). *Rheumatoid arthritis*. https://www.assh.org/handcare/condition/rheumatoid-arthritis

Andrews, M., Boyle, J., & Collins, J. (2020). *Transcultural concepts in nursing care* (8th ed.). Wolters Kluwer.

Budoff, J., & Nirschl, R. (2013). Knee problems: Diagnostic tests for ligament injuries. *Consultant, 53*(9), 629–632. http://www.consultant360.com/articles/knee-problems-diagnostic-tests-ligament-injuries

Centers for Disease Control and Prevention. (2018). *Arthritis: Health disparity statistics*. https://www.cdc.gov/arthritis/data_statistics/disparities.htm

Delzell, E. (2019). *When psoriatic disease strikes the hands and feet*. https://www.psoriasis.org/advance/when-psoriatic-disease-strikes-the-hands-and-feet

Gomes, Y. E., Chau, M., Banwell, H. A., Davies, J., & Causby, R. S. (2020). Adequacy of clinical information in X-ray referrals for traumatic ankle injury with reference to the Ottawa Ankle Rules—A retrospective clinical audit. *PeerJ, 8*. https://doi.org/10.7717/peerj.10152

Kawatkar, A., Portugal, C., Chu, L.-H., & Iyer, R. (2012). *Racial/ethnic trends in incidence and prevalence of rheumatoid arthritis in a large multi-ethnic managed care population*. 2012 ACR/ACHP Annual Meeting, Abstract No 2514. https://acrabstracts.org/abstract/racialethnic-trends-in-incidence-and-prevalence-of-rheumatoid-arthritis-in-a-large-multi-ethnic-managed-care-population/#:~:text=Results%3A%20During%20the%20study%20period,the%20prevalent%20(64.2%25)%20cases

Kerbel, Y., Smith, C., Prodromo, J., Nzeogu, M., & Mulcahey, M. (2018). Epidemiology of hip and groin injuries in collegiate athletes in the United States. *Orthopedic Journal of Sports Medicine, 6*(5). https://doi.org/10.1177/2325967118771676

Mayo Clinic. (2019). *Plantar fasciitis*. https://www.mayoclinic.org/diseases-conditions/plantar-fasciitis/symptoms-causes/syc-20354846

National Institutes of Health Osteoporosis and Related Bone Diseases National Resource Center. (2018). *What people with diabetes need to know about osteoporosis*. https://www.bones.nih.gov/health-info/bone/osteoporosis/conditions-behaviors/diabetes

Neville, D. (2017). *Lactose intolerance: Millions of Americans don't know they have it*. https://intermountainhealthcare.org/blogs/topics/live-well/2017/07/lactose-intolerance/

Rodriguez, D. (2021). *What does arthritis pain feel like?* https://www.everydayhealth.com/arthritis/pain-and-stiffness.aspx

Rothman Orthopedics. (2019). *Five of the most common foot and ankle injuries*. https://rothmanortho.com/stories/blog/Common-Foot-And-Ankle-Injuries

UCSF Medical Center. (2016). *Hand and wrist fractures*. https://www.ucsfhealth.org/conditions/hand_and_wrist_fractures/

University of Arkansas for Medical Sciences. (2018). *Three tests for carpal tunnel syndrome*. https://familymedicine.uams.edu/three-tests-for-carpal-tunnel-syndrome/

Zengin, A., Prentice, A., & Ward, K. (2015). Ethnic differences in bone health. *Frontiers in Endocrinology, 6*, 24. https://doi.org/10.3389/fendo.2015.00024

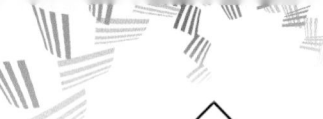

21 ASSESSING NEUROLOGIC SYSTEM

Structure and Function Overview

The very complex neurologic system is responsible for coordinating and regulating all body functions. It consists of two structural components: the central nervous system (CNS) and the peripheral nervous system.

CENTRAL NERVOUS SYSTEM

The CNS encompasses the brain and spinal cord, which are covered by three layers of protective meninges. The subarachnoid space surrounding the brain and spinal cord is filled with cerebrospinal fluid, which cushions the brain and spinal cord, nourishes the CNS, and removes waste materials. Electrical activity of the CNS is governed by neurons located in the sensory and motor neural pathways. The CNS contains upper motor neurons that influence lower motor neurons located mostly in the peripheral nervous system.

Located in the cranial cavity, the brain has four major divisions: the cerebrum, the diencephalon, the brainstem, and the cerebellum (Fig. 21-1).

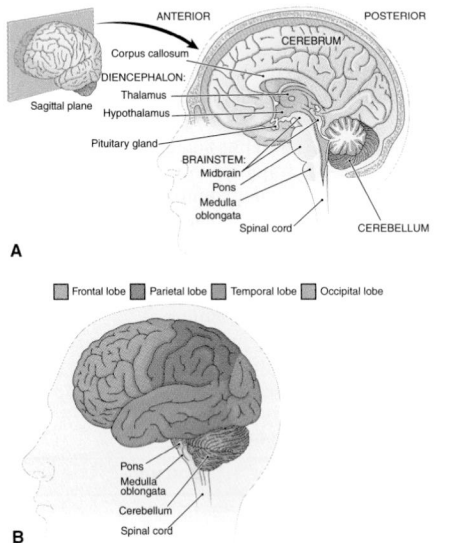

FIGURE 21-1 **(A)** Structures of the brain (sagittal section). **(B)** Lobes of the brain.

The cerebrum is divided into the right and left cerebral hemispheres, joined by the corpus callosum—a bundle of nerve fibers responsible for communication between the hemispheres. Each hemisphere sends and receives impulses from the opposite side of the body and consists of four lobes (frontal, parietal, temporal, and occipital), which mediate higher level functions (Table 21-1). Damage to a lobe impairs its specific function.

The diencephalon lies beneath the cerebral hemispheres and consists of the thalamus and hypothalamus. Most sensory impulses travel through the thalamus, which is responsible for screening and directing impulses to specific areas in the cerebral cortex. The hypothalamus (a part of the autonomic nervous system, which, in turn, is a part of the peripheral nervous system) is responsible for regulating many body functions, including water balance, appetite, vital signs (temperature, blood pressure, pulse, and respiratory rate), sleep cycles, pain perception, and emotional status.

Located between the cerebral cortex and the spinal cord, the brainstem consists of the midbrain, pons, and medulla oblongata. The midbrain serves as a relay center for ear and eye reflexes and relays impulses between the higher cerebral centers and the lower pons, medulla, cerebellum, and spinal cord. The pons links the cerebellum to the cerebrum and the midbrain to the medulla.

TABLE 21-1 **Lobes of the Cerebral Hemispheres and Their Function**

Lobe	Function
Frontal	Directs voluntary, skeletal actions (left side of lobe controls right side of body and right side of lobe controls left side of body). Also influences communication (talking and writing), emotions, intellect, reasoning ability, judgment, and behavior. Contains Broca area, which is responsible for speech.
Parietal	Interprets tactile sensations, including touch, pain, temperature, shapes, and two-point discrimination.
Occipital	Influences the ability to read with understanding and is the primary visual receptor center.
Temporal	Receives and interprets impulses from the ear. Contains Wernicke area, which is responsible for interpreting auditory stimuli.

It is responsible for various reflex actions. The medulla oblongata contains the nuclei for cranial nerves (CNs) and has centers that control and regulate respiratory function, heart rate and force, and blood pressure.

The cerebellum, located behind the brainstem and under the cerebrum, has two hemispheres and is responsible for coordination and smoothing of voluntary movements, maintenance of equilibrium, and maintenance of muscle tone.

The spinal cord (Fig. 21-2) is located in the vertebral canal and extends from the medulla oblongata to the first lumbar vertebra. The inner part of the cord has an H-shaped appearance and is made up of two pairs of columns (dorsal and ventral) consisting of gray matter. The outer part is made up of white matter and surrounds the gray matter. The spinal cord conducts sensory impulses up ascending tracts to the brain, conducts motor impulses down descending tracts to neurons that stimulate glands and muscles throughout the body, and is responsible for simple reflex activity. The simplest stretch reflex involves one sensory neuron (afferent), one motor neuron (efferent), and one synapse, such as the knee jerk, elicited by tapping the patellar tendon. More complex reflexes involve three or more neurons.

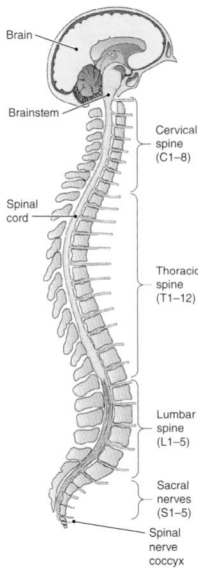

FIGURE 21-2 Spinal cord.

Neural Pathways

Sensory impulses travel to the brain by way of two ascending neural pathways (the spinothalamic tract and posterior columns) (Fig. 21-3). These impulses originate in the afferent fibers of the peripheral nerves and are carried through the posterior (dorsal) root into the spinal cord. Sensations of pain, temperature, and crude and light touch travel by way of the spinothalamic tract, whereas sensations of position, vibration, and fine touch travel by way of the posterior columns. Motor impulses are conducted to the muscles by two descending neural pathways: the pyramidal (corticospinal) tract and the extrapyramidal tract (Fig. 21-4). The motor neurons of the pyramidal tract originate in the motor cortex and travel down to the medulla where they cross over to the opposite side; then, they travel down to the spinal cord where they synapse with a lower motor neuron in the anterior horn of the spinal cord. These impulses are carried to muscles and produce voluntary movements that involve skill and purpose. The extrapyramidal tract motor neurons consist of those motor neurons that originate in the motor cortex, basal ganglia, brainstem, and spinal cord outside the pyramidal tract. They travel from the frontal lobe to the pons where they cross over to the opposite side and down the spinal cord where they connect with lower motor

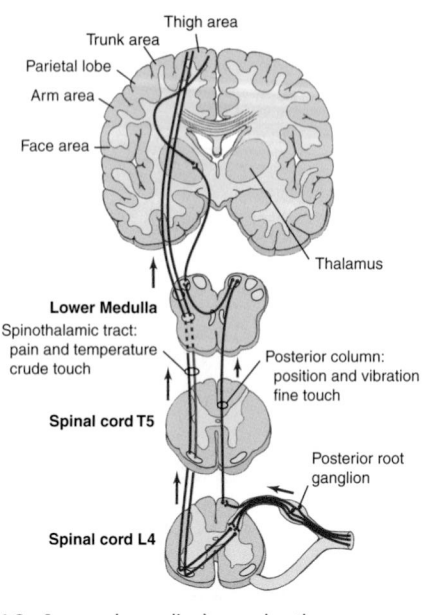

FIGURE 21-3 Sensory (ascending) neural pathways.

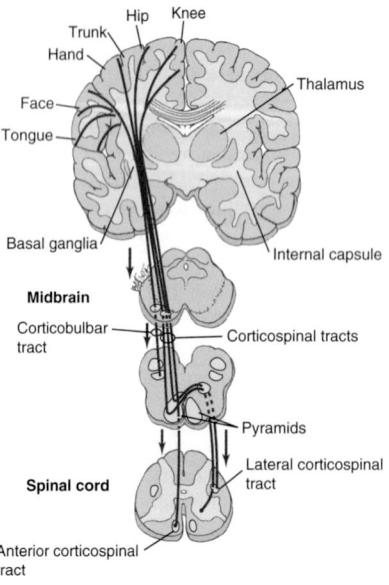

FIGURE 21-4 Motor (descending) neural pathways.

neurons that conduct impulses to the muscles. These neurons conduct impulses related to the maintenance of muscle tone and body control.

PERIPHERAL NERVOUS SYSTEM

Carrying information to and from the CNS, the peripheral nervous system consists of 12 pairs of CNs (Table 21-2) and 31 pairs

TABLE 21-2 **Cranial Nerves: Type and Function**

Cranial Nerve (Name)	Type of Impulse	Function
I (olfactory)	Sensory	Carries smell impulses from nasal mucous membrane to brain
II (optic)	Sensory	Carries visual impulses from eye to brain
III (oculomotor)	Motor	Contracts eye muscles to control eye movements (inferior lateral, medial, and superior), constricts pupils, and elevates eyelids
IV (trochlear)	Motor	Contracts one eye muscle to control inferomedial eye movement
V (trigeminal)	Sensory	Carries sensory impulses of pain, touch, and temperature from the face to the brain
	Motor	Influences clenching and lateral jaw movements (biting, chewing)
VI (abducens)	Motor	Controls lateral eye movements
VII (facial)	Sensory	Contains sensory fibers for taste on anterior two-thirds of tongue and stimulates secretions from salivary glands (submaxillary and sublingual) and tears from lacrimal glands
	Motor	Supplies the facial muscles and affects facial expressions (smiling, frowning, closing eyes)
VIII (acoustic, vestibulocochlear)	Sensory	Contains sensory fibers for hearing and balance
IX (glossopharyngeal)	Sensory	Contains sensory fibers for taste on posterior third of tongue and sensory fibers of the pharynx that result in the "gag reflex" when stimulated
	Motor	Provides secretory fibers to the parotid salivary glands; promotes swallowing movements

(*Continued on following page*)

TABLE 21-2 Cranial Nerves: Type and Function (*continued*)

Cranial Nerve (Name)	Type of Impulse	Function
X (vagus)	Sensory	Carries sensations from the throat, larynx, heart, lungs, bronchi, gastrointestinal tract, and abdominal viscera
	Motor	Promotes swallowing, talking, and production of digestive juices
XI (spinal accessory)	Motor	Innervates neck muscles (sternocleidomastoid and trapezius) that promote movement of the shoulders and head rotation. Also promotes some movement of the larynx
XII (hypoglossal)	Motor	Innervates tongue muscles that promote the movement of food and talking

of spinal nerves. Comprising 8 cervical, 12 thoracic, 5 lumbar, 5 sacral, and 1 coccygeal nerve, the 31 pairs of spinal nerves are named after the vertebrae below each one's exit point along the spinal cord (see Fig. 21-2). Each nerve is attached to the spinal cord by two nerve roots. The sensory (afferent) fiber enters through the dorsal (posterior) roots of the cord, whereas the motor (efferent) fiber exits through the ventral (anterior) roots of the cord. The sensory root of each spinal nerve innervates an area of the skin called a *dermatome* (Fig. 21-5). These nerves are categorized as two types of fibers: somatic and autonomic. Somatic fibers carry CNS impulses to voluntary skeletal muscles, whereas autonomic fibers carry CNS impulses to smooth, involuntary muscles (in the heart

and glands). The somatic nervous system mediates conscious, or voluntary, activities, whereas the autonomic nervous system mediates unconscious, or involuntary, activities.

Nursing Assessment

The neurologic assessment is performed last because several of its components may have been integrated into previous parts of the examination. For example, CN VIII may have been tested during the ear examination and, therefore, will not need to be tested again. A complete neurologic assessment consists of examining (1) mental status (see Chapter 5), (2) CN function, (3) motor

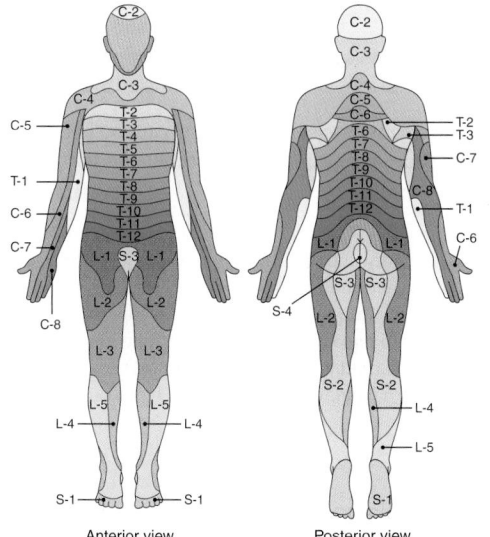

C-2
C-3
C-4
C-5
T-1
C-6
C-7
C-8
T-2
T-3
T-4
T-5
T-6
T-7
T-8
T-9
T-10
T-11
T-12
L-1 S-3 L-1
L-2   L-2
L-3   L-3
L-5   L-5
L-4   L-4
S-1   S-1

Anterior view

C-2
C-3
C-4
C-5
C-6
C-7
C-8
T-2
T-3
C-7
T-1
C-6
T-1
T-6
T-7
T-8
T-9
T-10
T-11
T-12
L-1 L-1 L-1
S-3 S-3
S-4
L-2   L-2
S-2   S-2
L-4
L-5
S-1

Posterior view

FIGURE 21-5 Anterior and posterior dermatomes (areas of the skin innervated by spinal nerves).

function (see Chapter 20), (4) cerebellar function, (5) sensory function, and (6) reflexes.

Perform the examinations in an order that moves from a level of higher cerebral integration (mental status) to a lower level (reflex activity).

COLLECTING SUBJECTIVE DATA

Interview Questions

Numbness? Paralysis? Tingling? Neuralgia? (Timing, duration, associated factors?) Seizures? Auras? Medications taken for seizures? Wear MedicAlert identification? Tremors? Headaches? (Frequency, duration, character, precipitating/relieving factors?) Loss of consciousness? Dizziness? Fainting? Loss of memory? Confusion? Visual loss, blurring, pain? Facial pain, weakness, twitching? Speech problems (aphasia—expressive/receptive)? Swallowing problems? Drooling? Neck weakness, spasms? Any muscle weakness or loss of bowel or urinary control? History of head injury? Meningitis? Encephalitis? Treatment? Family history of high blood pressure, stroke, Alzheimer disease, epilepsy, brain cancer, or Huntington chorea?

Self-care: Use of medications? Alcohol intake? Use of drugs such as marijuana, tranquilizers, barbiturates, or cocaine?

Smoking? Use of seat belt, head gear for sports? Daily diet and exercise? Prolonged exposure to lead, insecticides, pollutants, or other chemicals?

Risk Factors

Risk for cerebrovascular accident (stroke) related to age more than 60 years, male sex (slightly higher risk), hypertension, smoking, chronic alcohol intake, history of cardiovascular disease, sleep apnea, high levels of fibrinogen, diabetes mellitus, drug abuse, oral contraceptives, high estrogen levels, postmenopausal women not taking estrogen replacement, obesity, African-American ancestry, and newly industrialized environment.

◎ CLINICAL TIP

Stroke is an emergency. Recognize the signs and symptoms and act fast! (National Stroke Association, 2020).

Signs and symptoms

- Sudden numbness or weakness of face, arm, or leg, especially on one side of the body
- Sudden confusion, trouble speaking, or understanding speech
- Sudden trouble seeing in one or both eyes
- Sudden trouble walking, dizziness, loss of balance, or coordination
- Sudden severe headache with no known cause

Act FAST. Use FAST to remember the warning signs of a stroke:

- FACE: Ask the person to smile. Does one side of the face droop?
- ARMS: Ask the person to raise both arms. Does one arm drift downward?
- SPEECH: Ask the person to repeat a simple phrase. Is speech slurred or strange?
- TIME: If you observe any of these signs, call 9-1-1 immediately.

COLLECTING OBJECTIVE DATA

Equipment Needed

General

- Gloves

Equipment needed for a CN examination includes the following:

- Cotton-tipped applicators
- Newsprint to read
- Ophthalmoscope

- Paper clip
- Penlight
- Snellen chart
- Sterile cotton ball
- Substances to smell or taste such as soap, coffee, vanilla, salt, sugar, lemon juice
- Tongue depressor
- Tuning fork

Equipment needed for a motor and cerebellar examination includes the following:

- Tape measure

Equipment needed for a sensory examination includes the following:

- Cotton ball
- Objects to feel, such as a quarter or key
- Paper clip
- Test tubes containing hot and cold water
- Tuning fork (low pitched)

Equipment needed for a reflex examination includes the following:

- Cotton-tipped applicator
- Reflex (percussion) hammer

Physical Assessment

Ask the client to remove all clothing and jewelry and to put on an examination gown. Have the client sit on the examination table, but explain that several different position changes are needed throughout the examination. Explain the length of the examination and allow rest periods as needed. You may perform over two different time periods to avoid client fatigue. Explain some requests (e.g., counting backward or hopping on one foot) may seem unusual but that these activities are parts of a total neurologic evaluation. Demonstrate what you want the client to do, especially during the cerebellar examination, when the client will need to perform several movements.

See Chapter 5 for an examination of mental status.

CRANIAL NERVES

Assess CN I through CN XII.

ASSESSMENT PROCEDURE	NORMAL FINDINGS	ABNORMAL FINDINGS
Test **CN I (olfactory)**. With client sitting in comfortable position at your eye level, ask client to clear the nose to remove any mucus, then to close eyes (or to not look at the object), occlude one nostril, and identify a scented object that you are holding such as soap, coffee, or vanilla (Fig. 21-6). Repeat procedure for the other nostril.	Client correctly identifies scent presented to each nostril.	Inability to smell (neurogenic anosmia) or identify the correct scent may indicate olfactory tract lesion, tumor, or lesion of frontal lobe. Loss of smell may also be congenital, due to nasal or sinus problems, or nerve tissue at the top of the nose or the higher smell pathways in the brain due to viral upper respiratory infection. Smoking and cocaine use may also impair sense of smell.

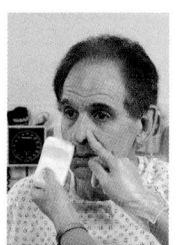

FIGURE 21-6   Testing cranial nerve I.

ASSESSMENT PROCEDURE	NORMAL FINDINGS	ABNORMAL FINDINGS
Test **CN II (optic).** Use a Snellen chart to assess vision in each eye (see Chapter 12 for additional information).	Client has 20/20 vision OD (right eye) and OS (left eye).	Abnormal findings include difficulty reading Snellen chart, missing letters, and squinting.
Ask the client to read a newspaper or magazine paragraph to assess near vision.	Client reads print at 14 in. without difficulty.	Client reads print by holding closer than 14 in. or holds print farther away as in presbyopia, which occurs with aging.
Assess visual fields of each eye by confrontation.	Full visual fields (see Chapter 12).	Loss of visual fields seen in retinal damage or detachment, lesions of optic nerve or parietal cortex (see Chapter 12).
Use an ophthalmoscope to view the retina and optic disc of each eye.	Round red reflex is present, optic disc is 1.5 mm, round or slightly oval, well-defined margins, creamy pink with paler physiologic cup. Retina is pink (see Chapter 12).	Papilledema (swelling of the optic nerve) results in blurred optic disc margins and dilated, pulsating veins; it occurs with increased intracranial pressure from intracranial hemorrhage or a brain tumor. Optic atrophy occurs with brain tumors (see Chapter 12).
Assess **CN III (oculomotor), CN IV (trochlear), and CN VI (abducens).** Inspect margins of the eyelids of each eye.	Eyelid covers about 2 mm of the iris.	Ptosis (drooping of the eyelid) is seen with weak eye muscles, such as in myasthenia gravis.

(Continued on following page)

CRANIAL NERVES (*continued*)

ASSESSMENT PROCEDURE	NORMAL FINDINGS	ABNORMAL FINDINGS
Assess extraocular movements. If nystagmus is noted, determine the direction of the fast and slow phases of movement (see Chapter 12).	Eyes move in a smooth, coordinated motion in all directions (the six cardinal fields).	Nystagmus (rhythmic oscillation of the eyes) seen in *cerebellar disorders.* Limited eye movement through the six cardinal fields of gaze seen in *increased intracranial pressure.* Paralytic strabismus seen with *paralysis of the oculomotor, trochlear, or abducens* nerves.
Assess pupillary response to light (direct and indirect) and accommodation in both eyes (see Chapter 12).	Bilateral illuminated pupils constrict simultaneously. Pupil opposite the one illuminated constricts simultaneously.	Dilated pupil (6–7 mm) seen in *oculomotor nerve paralysis.*
		Argyll Robertson pupils seen in *CNS syphilis, meningitis, brain tumor, alcoholism.*
		Constricted, fixed pupils seen in *narcotics abuse or damage to the pons.*
		Unilaterally dilated pupil unresponsive to light or accommodation seen with *damage to CN III* (oculomotor).
		Constricted pupil unresponsive to light or accommodation seen in *lesions of the sympathetic nervous system.*

ASSESSMENT PROCEDURE	NORMAL FINDINGS	ABNORMAL FINDINGS
Assess **CN V (trigeminal).** Test **sensory function.** Tell the client: "I am going to touch your forehead, cheeks, and chin with the sharp or dull side of this paper clip. Please close your eyes and tell me if you feel a sharp or dull sensation. Tell me where you feel it" (Fig. 21-7). Vary sharp and dull stimulus in facial areas comparing sides. Repeat for light touch with a wisp of cotton. *Note: To avoid transmitting infection, use a new object with each client. Avoid "stabbing" the client with the object's sharp side.*	Client correctly identifies sharp and dull stimuli and light touch to the forehead, cheeks, and chin. 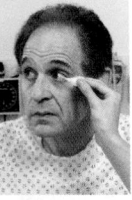 **FIGURE 21-7** Testing sensory function of cranial nerve V: dull stimulus using a paper clip.	Inability to feel and correctly identify facial stimuli occurs with lesions of the trigeminal nerve, lesions in the spinothalamic tract, or posterior columns.
Test **corneal reflex.** Ask the client to look away and up while you lightly touch the cornea with a fine wisp of cotton (Fig. 21-8). Repeat on the other side. *Note: This reflex may be absent or reduced in clients who wear contact lenses.*	Eyelids blink bilaterally. 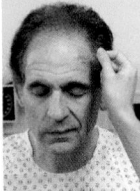 **FIGURE 21-8** Testing corneal reflex with wisp of cotton.	An absent corneal reflex may be noted with lesions of the trigeminal nerve or lesions of the motor part of CN VII (facial).

(Continued on following page)

CRANIAL NERVES (*continued*)

ASSESSMENT PROCEDURE	NORMAL FINDINGS	ABNORMAL FINDINGS
Test **motor function.** Ask the client to clench the teeth while you palpate the temporal and masseter muscles for contraction (Fig. 21-9). **Note:** *This test may be difficult to perform and evaluate in the client without teeth.*	Temporal and masseter muscles contract bilaterally. 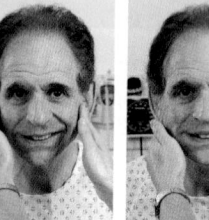 **FIGURE 21-9** Testing motor function of cranial nerve V. *Left:* Palpating temporal muscles. *Right:* Palpating masseter muscles.	Decreased contraction in one or both sides. Asymmetric strength in moving the jaw seen with lesion or injury of CN V. Pain occurs with clenching of the teeth. Bilateral muscle weakness is seen with peripheral nervous system or CNS dysfunction. Unilateral muscle weakness may indicate a lesion of CN V (trigeminal).
Test **CN VII (facial).** Test motor function. Ask the client to: • Smile • Frown and wrinkle forehead • Show teeth • Puff out cheeks • Purse lips • Raise eyebrows • Close eyes tightly against resistance	Client smiles, frowns, wrinkles forehead, shows teeth, puffs out cheeks, purses lips, raises eyebrows, and closes eyes against resistance. Movements are symmetric.	Inability to close eyes, wrinkle forehead, or raise forehead along with paralysis of the lower part of the face on the affected side is seen with Bell palsy (a peripheral injury to CN VII [facial]). Paralysis of the lower part of face on opposite side affected seen with central lesion that affects upper motor neurons, such as from stroke.

ASSESSMENT PROCEDURE	NORMAL FINDINGS	ABNORMAL FINDINGS
Sensory function of CN VII is not routinely tested. If testing is indicated, however, touch the anterior two-thirds of the tongue with a moistened applicator dipped in salt, sugar, or lemon juice. Ask the client to identify the flavor. If the client is unsuccessful, repeat the test using one of the other solutions. If needed, repeat the test using the remaining solution. *Note: Ask client to leave tongue protruded to identify flavor or the substance may move to posterior third of tongue (vagus nerve innervation). Posterior portion is tested similarly to assess CN IX and CN X function. Have client rinse mouth with water between each tasting.*	Client identifies correct flavor.	Inability to identify correct flavor on anterior two-thirds of the tongue suggests impairment of CN VII (facial).
Test **CN VIII (acoustic/vestibulocochlear).** Test the client's hearing ability in each ear. Perform Weber and Rinne tests to assess the cochlear (auditory) component of CN VIII (see Chapter 13).	Client hears whispered words from 1 to 2 feet. *Weber test:* Vibration heard equally well in both ears. *Rinne test:* AC > BC (air conduction [AC] is twice as long as bone conduction [BC]).	Vibratory sound lateralizes to good ear in sensorineural loss. AC is longer than BC, but not twice as long, in a sensorineural loss (see Chapter 13).

(Continued on following page)

CRANIAL NERVES (continued)

ASSESSMENT PROCEDURE	NORMAL FINDINGS	ABNORMAL FINDINGS
Note: The vestibular component, responsible for equilibrium, is not routinely tested. In comatose clients, the test is used to determine integrity of the vestibular system. (Refer to a neurology textbook for detailed testing procedures.)		
Test **CN IX (glossopharyngeal) and CN X (vagus).**		
Test **motor function.** Ask the client to open mouth wide and say "ah" while you use a tongue depressor on the client's tongue.	Uvula and soft palate rise bilaterally and symmetrically on phonation.	Soft palate does not rise with bilateral lesions of CN X (vagus). Unilateral rising of the soft palate and deviation of the uvula to the normal side are seen with a unilateral lesion of CN X (vagus).
Test **the gag reflex** by touching the posterior pharynx with the tongue depressor (Fig. 21-10). *Note: Warn client you are going to do this as it may feel uncomfortable.*	Gag reflex intact. Some normal clients may have a reduced or absent gag reflex.	An absent gag reflex may be seen with lesions of CN IX (glossopharyngeal) or CN X (vagus).

ASSESSMENT PROCEDURE	NORMAL FINDINGS	ABNORMAL FINDINGS
Check the client's **ability to swallow** by giving the client a drink of water. Also note the client's voice quality.	Client swallows without difficulty. No hoarseness noted.	Dysphagia or hoarseness may indicate a lesion of CN IX (glossopharyngeal) or CN X (vagus) or other neurologic disorder.
Test CN XI (spinal accessory). Ask the client to shrug the shoulders against resistance to assess the trapezius muscle (Fig. 21-11).	Symmetric, strong contraction of the trapezius muscles.	Asymmetric muscle contraction or drooping of the shoulder may be seen with paralysis or muscle weakness due to neck injury or torticollis.
Ask the client to turn the head against resistance, first to the right, then to the left, to assess the sternocleidomastoid muscle (Fig. 21-12).	Strong contraction of sternocleidomastoid muscle on the side opposite to the turned face.	Atrophy with fasciculations may be seen with peripheral nerve disease.

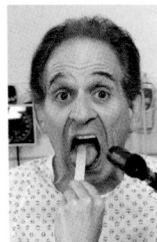

FIGURE 21-10 Testing cranial nerves IX and X: checking uvula rise and gag reflex.

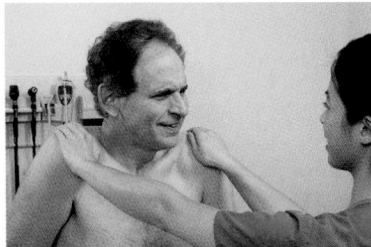

FIGURE 21-11 Testing cranial nerve XI: assessing strength of trapezius muscle.

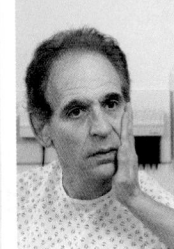

FIGURE 21-12 Testing cranial nerve XI: assessing strength of sternocleidomastoid muscle.

(Continued on following page)

CRANIAL NERVES (continued)

ASSESSMENT PROCEDURE	NORMAL FINDINGS	ABNORMAL FINDINGS
Test CN XII (hypoglossal). To assess strength and mobility of the tongue, ask the client to protrude tongue, move it to each side against the resistance of a tongue depressor, and then put it back in the mouth.	Tongue movement is symmetric and smooth, and bilateral strength is apparent.	Fasciculations and atrophy of the tongue often seen with peripheral nerve disease. Deviation to the affected side is seen with unilateral lesion.

CLINICAL TIP
Recognize the signs and symptoms of stroke. Act FAST! (National Stroke Association, 2020). Use FAST to recall stroke warning signs:
- **FACE drooping**: Ask the person to smile. Does one side of the face droop?
- **ARMS weakness**: Ask the person to raise both arms. Does one arm drift downward?
- **SPEECH**: Ask the person to repeat a simple phrase. Is speech slurred or strange?

If you observe any of these signs, call 9-1-1 immediately to avoid a lifelong disability.

If stroke is suspected, Act FAST! See Clinical Tip.

Additional symptoms of stroke include:
- Sudden numbness or weakness of face, arm, or leg, especially on one side of the body
- Sudden confusion, trouble speaking, or understanding speech
- Sudden trouble seeing in one or both eyes
- Sudden trouble walking, dizziness, loss of balance, or coordination
- Sudden severe headache with no known cause

MOTOR AND CEREBELLAR SYSTEMS		
ASSESSMENT PROCEDURE	**NORMAL FINDINGS**	**ABNORMAL FINDINGS**
Assess **condition and movement of muscles.** Assess the size and symmetry of all muscle groups (see Chapter 20).	Muscles fully developed and symmetric in size (bilateral sides may vary 1 cm from each other).	Muscle atrophy seen in lower motor neuron diseases or muscle disorders. Injury of central spinal cord seen with extremity weakness. Loss of motor function, pain, and temperature seen in anterior cord syndrome.
		Loss of proprioception seen in posterior cord syndrome. A loss of strength, proprioception, pain, and temperature seen in Brown-Séquard syndrome.
Assess the **strength and tone** of all muscle groups (see Chapter 20).	Relaxed muscles contract voluntarily and show mild, smooth resistance to passive movement. All muscle groups equally strong against resistance, without flaccidity, spasticity, or rigidity.	Soft, limp, flaccid muscles are seen with lower motor neuron involvement. Spastic muscle tone is noted with involvement of the corticospinal motor tract. Rigid muscles that resist passive movement are seen with abnormalities of the extrapyramidal tract.

(Continued on following page)

MOTOR AND CEREBELLAR SYSTEMS (*continued*)		
ASSESSMENT PROCEDURE	**NORMAL FINDINGS**	**ABNORMAL FINDINGS**
Note any unusual involuntary movements such as fasciculations, tics, or tremors.	No fasciculations, tics, or tremors are noted.	Fasciculation (rapid twitching of resting muscle) seen in lower motor neuron disease or fatigue. Tic (twitch of the face, head, or shoulder) from stress or neurologic disorder. Unusual, bizarre face, tongue, jaw, or lip movements from chronic psychosis or long-term use of psychotropic drugs. Tremors (rhythmic, oscillating movements) from Parkinson disease, cerebellar disease, multiple sclerosis (with movement), hyperthyroidism, or anxiety. Brief, rapid, irregular, jerky movements (at rest) from Huntington chorea. Slow, twisting movements in the extremities and face associated with spasticity (athetosis) seen with cerebral palsy.

ASSESSMENT PROCEDURE	NORMAL FINDINGS	ABNORMAL FINDINGS
Evaluate **gait and balance**. To assess gait and balance, ask the client to walk naturally across the room. Note posture, freedom of movement, symmetry, rhythm, and balance. **Note:** It is best to assess gait when the client is not aware that you are directly observing the gait. Ask the client to tandem walk (heel-to-toe manner) (Fig. 21-13). Demonstrate the walk to client, then stand close by in case the client loses balance.	Gait is steady; opposite arm swings. Client maintains balance with tandem walking. Walks on heels and toes with little difficulty. 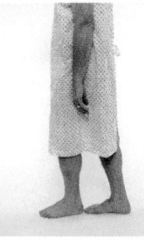 **FIGURE 21-13** Testing balance: tandem walking (heel to toe).	Gait and balance can be affected by disorders of the motor, sensory, vestibular, and cerebellar systems. Therefore, a thorough examination of all systems is necessary when an uneven or unsteady gait is noted. An uncoordinated or unsteady gait that did not appear with the client's normal walking may become apparent with tandem walking or when walking on heels and toes.
Perform the **Romberg test**. Ask the client to stand erect with arms at side and feet together. Note any unsteadiness or swaying. Then with the client in the same body position, ask the client to close the eyes for 20 seconds. Note imbalance or swaying. **Note:** Stand near the client to prevent a fall should the client lose balance.	Client stands erect with minimal swaying, with eyes both open and closed.	Positive Romberg test: Swaying and moving feet apart to prevent fall is seen with disease of the posterior columns, vestibular dysfunction, or cerebellar disorders.

(Continued on following page)

MOTOR AND CEREBELLAR SYSTEMS (*continued*)

ASSESSMENT PROCEDURE	NORMAL FINDINGS	ABNORMAL FINDINGS
Now ask the client to stand on one foot and to bend the knee of the leg the client is standing on. Then ask the client to hop on that foot. Repeat on the other foot (Fig. 21-14).	Bends knee while standing on one foot; hops on each foot without losing balance. 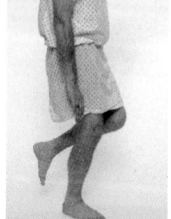 **FIGURE 21-14** Hop on one foot and then on the other foot.	Inability to stand or hop on one foot is seen with muscle weakness or disease of the cerebellum.
Assess **coordination.** Demonstrate the finger-to-nose test to assess accuracy of movements, then ask the client to extend and hold arms out to the side with eyes open. Next, say, "Touch the tip of your nose first with your right index finger, then with your left index finger. Repeat this three times" (Fig. 21-15). Next, ask the client to repeat these movements with eyes closed.	Client touches finger to nose with smooth, accurate movements, with little hesitation. *Note: When assessing coordination of movements, bear in mind that normally the client's dominant side may be more coordinated than the nondominant side.*	Uncoordinated, jerky movements and inability to touch the nose may be seen with cerebellar disease.

ASSESSMENT PROCEDURE	NORMAL FINDINGS	ABNORMAL FINDINGS
		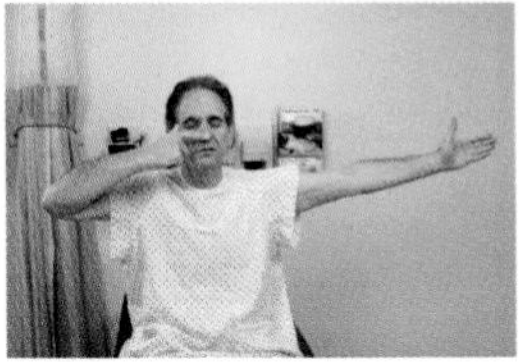 **FIGURE 21-15** Testing coordination: finger-to-nose test.
Assess **rapid alternating movements.** With client sitting, ask client to touch each finger to the thumb and to increase the speed as the client progresses. Repeat with the other side. Next, ask the client to put the palms of both hands down on both legs, then turn the palms up, then turn the palms down again (Fig. 21-16). Ask the client to increase the speed.	Client touches each finger to the thumb rapidly. *Note: For some older clients, rapid alternating movements are difficult because of decreased reaction time and flexibility.* Client rapidly turns palms up and down.	Inability to perform rapid alternating movements may be seen with cerebellar disease, upper motor neuron weakness, or extrapyramidal disease. Uncoordinated movements or tremors are abnormal findings. They are seen with cerebellar disease (dysdiadochokinesia).

(Continued on following page)

MOTOR AND CEREBELLAR SYSTEMS (*continued*)

ASSESSMENT PROCEDURE	NORMAL FINDINGS	ABNORMAL FINDINGS
Perform the heel-to-shin test. Ask the client to lie down (supine position) and to slide the heel of the right foot down the left shin (Fig. 21-17). Repeat with the other heel and shin.	Client is able to run each heel smoothly down each shin.	Deviation of heel to one side or the other may be seen in cerebellar disease.
If the client is unconscious, note his or her posture (Fig. 21-18, decorticate posture; and Fig. 21-19, decerebrate posture).		Clients with lesions of the corticospinal tract draw hands up to chest (decorticate posture). Clients with lesions of the diencephalon, midbrain, or pons have extended arms and legs with internal rotation and arched neck.

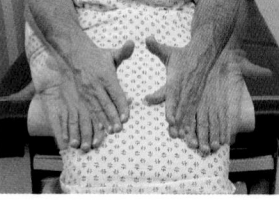

FIGURE 21-16 Testing rapid alternating movements of turning palms up and then down.

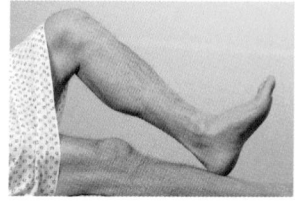

FIGURE 21-17 Performing heel-to-shin test.

ASSESSMENT PROCEDURE	NORMAL FINDINGS	ABNORMAL FINDINGS

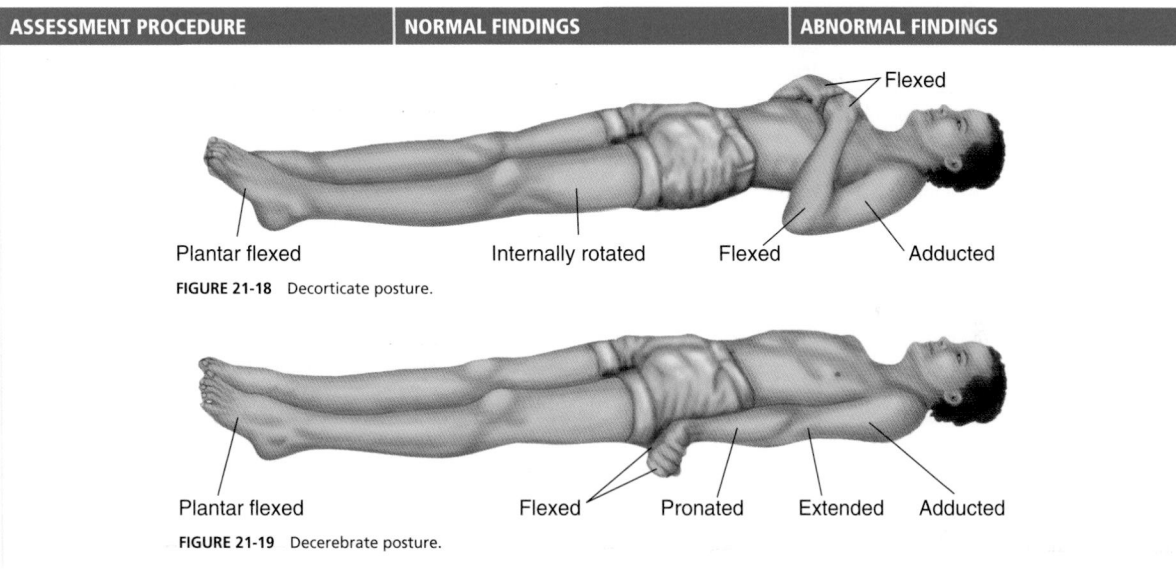

FIGURE 21-18   Decorticate posture.

FIGURE 21-19   Decerebrate posture.

(*Continued on following page*)

SENSORY SYSTEM

To test the client's ability to perceive various sensations over the extremities and abdomen, stimuli must be scattered to cover all dermatomes. The client is asked to close their eyes and identify the type of sensation perceived and the body area where it was felt. If a perceptual deficit is identified, the area is mapped out to determine the extent of impaired sensation.

ASSESSMENT PROCEDURE	NORMAL FINDINGS	ABNORMAL FINDINGS
Assess **light touch, pain, and temperature sensations.**	Client correctly identifies light touch.	Altered sensory perception may be seen in peripheral neuropathies (due to diabetes mellitus, folic acid deficiencies, and alcoholism) and lesions of the ascending spinal cord, brainstem, CNs, and cerebral cortex.
Test **light touch sensation** using wisp of cotton to touch the client. Test **pain sensation** using blunt and sharp end of safety pin/paper clip. Test **temperature sensation** using test tubes filled with hot and cold water **if abnormalities are found in the client's ability to perceive light touch and pain sensations.**	Client correctly differentiates between dull and sharp sensations and hot and cold temperatures over various body parts.	Client reports anesthesia (absence of touch sensation), hypesthesia (decreased sensitivity to touch), hyperesthesia (increased sensitivity to touch), analgesia (absence of pain sensation), hypalgesia (decreased sensitivity to pain), or hyperalgesia (increased sensitivity to pain).

ASSESSMENT PROCEDURE	NORMAL FINDINGS	ABNORMAL FINDINGS
Test **vibratory sensation.** Strike a low-pitched tuning fork on the heel of your hand and hold the base on the distal radius, forefinger tip, medial malleolus, and, last, the tip of the great toe. Ask client to indicate what they feel. Repeat on the other side. **Note:** *If vibratory sensation is intact distally, then it is intact proximally.*	Client correctly identifies sensation.	Inability to sense vibrations may be seen in posterior column disease or peripheral neuropathy (e.g., as seen with diabetes or chronic alcohol abuse).
Test **sensitivity to position.** Ask the client to close both eyes. Then hold the client's toe or a finger on the lateral sides and move it up or down (Fig. 21-20). Ask the client to tell you the direction it is moved. Repeat on the other side. **Note:** *If position sense is intact distally, then it is intact proximally.*	Client correctly identifies directions of movements. 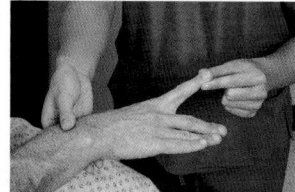 **FIGURE 21-20** Testing position sense (kinesthesia).	Inability to identify the directions of the movements may be seen in posterior column disease or peripheral neuropathy (e.g., as seen with diabetes or chronic alcohol abuse).

(*Continued on following page*)

SENSORY SYSTEM (*continued*)

ASSESSMENT PROCEDURE	NORMAL FINDINGS	ABNORMAL FINDINGS
Assess **tactile discrimination (fine touch).** Remember that the client should have eyes closed. To test stereognosis, place a familiar object such as a quarter, paper clip, or key in the client's hand and ask the client to identify it. Repeat with another object in the other hand.	Client correctly identifies object.	Inability to correctly identify objects (astereognosis), area touched, number written in hand; to discriminate between two points; or to identify areas simultaneously touched may be seen in lesions of the sensory cortex.
To test **point localization,** briefly touch the client and ask the client to identify the points touched.	Client correctly identifies area touched.	Same as above.
To test **graphesthesia,** use a blunt instrument to write a number, such as 2, 3, or 5, on the palm of the client's hand. Ask the client to identify the number. Repeat with another number on the other hand.	Client correctly identifies number written.	Same as above.
Two-point discrimination can be determined on the fingertips, forearm, dorsal hands, back, or thighs. Ask the client to identify the number of points (one or two) felt when touched with the electrocardiogram (EKG) calibers. Measure the distance between the two points when the client can no longer distinguish the two points as separate (client states only one point is felt) (Fig. 21-21)	Identifies two points on: • Fingertips at 2 to 5 mm apart • Forearm at 40 mm apart • Dorsal hands at 20 to 30 mm apart • Back at 40 mm apart • Thighs at 70 mm apart	Same as above.

ASSESSMENT PROCEDURE	NORMAL FINDINGS	ABNORMAL FINDINGS
	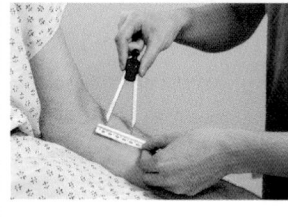 **FIGURE 21-21** Two-point discrimination.	
To test **extinction,** simultaneously touch the client in the same area on both sides of the body at the same point. Ask the client to identify the area touched.	Correctly identifies points touched. See Table 21-3 for normal two-point discrimination findings.	Same as above.

REFLEXES

The reflex (or percussion) hammer is used to elicit deep tendon reflexes (see Assessment Guide 21-1). To elicit superficial reflexes, lightly stroke the skin with a moderately sharp instrument (e.g., key, tongue blade). Follow specific maneuvers to elicit any pathologic reflexes.

(Continued on following page)

REFLEXES (*continued*)

ASSESSMENT PROCEDURE	NORMAL FINDINGS	ABNORMAL FINDINGS
Test **deep tendon reflexes.** Position client in a comfortable sitting position. Use the reflex hammer to elicit reflexes. *Note: If deep tendon reflexes are diminished or absent, two reinforcement techniques may be used to enhance their response. When testing the arm reflexes, have the client clench the teeth. When testing the leg reflexes, have the client interlock the hands.*	Normal reflex scores range from 1+ (present but decreased) to 2+ (normal) to 3+ (increased or brisk, but not pathologic).	Absent or markedly decreased (hyporeflexia) deep tendon reflexes (rated 0) occur when a component of the lower motor neurons or reflex arc is impaired; this may be seen with spinal cord injuries. Markedly hyperactive (hyperreflexia) deep tendon reflexes (rated 4+) may be seen with lesions of the upper motor neurons and when the higher cortical levels are impaired.
Test **biceps reflex.** Ask the client to partially bend arm at elbow with palm up. Place your thumb over the biceps tendon and strike your thumb with the pointed side of the reflex hammer (Fig. 21-22). Repeat on the other side. (This evaluates the function of spinal levels C5 and C6.)	Elbow flexes and contraction of the biceps muscle is seen or felt. Ranges from 1+ to 3+. Forearm flexes and supinates. Ranges from 1+ to 3+.	No response or an exaggerated response is abnormal. 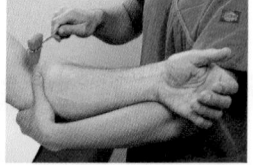 **FIGURE 21-22** Eliciting biceps reflex.

ASSESSMENT PROCEDURE	**NORMAL FINDINGS**	**ABNORMAL FINDINGS**
Assess **brachioradialis reflex.** Ask the client to flex elbow with palm down and hand resting on the abdomen or lap. Use the flat side of the reflex hammer to tap the tendon at the radius about 2 in. above the wrist (Fig. 21-23). Repeat on other side. (This evaluates the function of spinal levels C5 and C6.)	Flexion and supination of forearm. Ranges from 1+ to 3+. 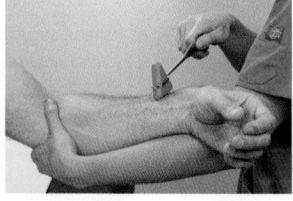 **FIGURE 21-23** Eliciting brachioradialis reflex.	No response or an exaggerated response is abnormal.
Test **triceps reflex.** Ask the client to hang the arm freely ("limp, like it is hanging from a clothesline to dry") while you support it with your nondominant hand. With the elbow flexed, use the flat side of the reflex hammer to tap the tendon above the olecranon process (Fig. 21-24). Repeat on the other side. This evaluates the function of spinal levels C6, C7, and C8.	Elbow extends, triceps contracts. 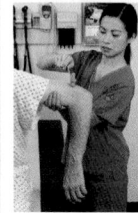 **FIGURE 21-24** Eliciting triceps reflex.	No response or exaggerated response.

(Continued on following page)

REFLEXES (*continued*)

ASSESSMENT PROCEDURE	NORMAL FINDINGS	ABNORMAL FINDINGS
Assess **patellar reflex.** Ask the client to let both legs hang freely off the side of the examination table. Using the flat side of the reflex hammer, tap the patellar tendon, which is located just below the patella (Fig. 21-25A). Repeat on the other side. For the client who cannot sit up, gently flex the knee and strike the patella (Fig. 21-25B). This evaluates the function of spinal levels L2, L3, and L4.	Knee extends, quadriceps muscle contracts. Ranges from 1+ to 3+. 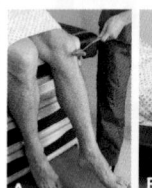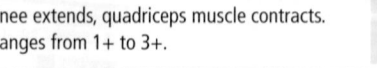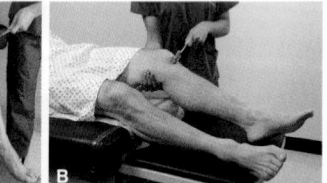 **FIGURE 21-25 (A)** Eliciting patellar reflex. **(B)** Eliciting patellar reflex (supine position).	No response or an exaggerated response is abnormal.
Test **Achilles reflex.** With the client's leg still hanging freely, dorsiflex the foot. Tap the Achilles tendon with the flat side of the reflex hammer (Fig. 21-26A). Repeat on the other side. For assessing the reflex in the client who cannot sit up, have the client flex one knee and support that leg against the other leg. Dorsiflex the foot and tap the tendon using the flat side of the reflex hammer (Fig. 21-26B). This evaluates the function of spinal levels S1 and S2.	Normal response is plantar flexion of the foot. Ranges from 1+ to 3+. 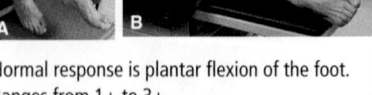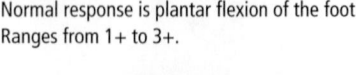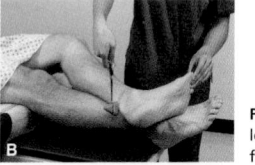 **FIGURE 21-26 (A)** Eliciting Achilles reflex. **(B)** Eliciting Achilles reflex (supine position).	No response or an exaggerated response is abnormal.

ASSESSMENT PROCEDURE	NORMAL FINDINGS	ABNORMAL FINDINGS
Test **ankle clonus** when the other reflexes tested have been hyperactive. Place one hand under the knee to support the leg, then briskly dorsiflex the foot toward the client's head. Repeat on the other side (Fig. 21-27). Test **superficial reflexes.** Use the handle end of the reflex hammer to elicit superficial reflexes, whose receptors are in the skin rather than the muscles.	No rapid contractions or oscillations (clonus) of the ankle are elicited. 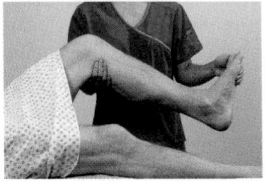 **FIGURE 21-27** Testing for ankle clonus.	Repeated rapid contractions or oscillations of the ankle and calf muscle are seen with lesions of the upper motor neurons.
Assess **plantar reflex.** With the end of the reflex hammer or tongue blade, stroke the lateral aspect of the sole from the heel to the ball of the foot, curving medially across the ball (Fig. 21-28A). Repeat on the other side. This evaluates the function of spinal levels L4, L5, S1, and S2.	Flexion of the toes occurs (plantar response; Fig. 21-28A with inversion and flexion of the forefoot).	Except in infancy, extension (dorsiflexion) of the big toe and fanning of all toes (positive Babinski response) are abnormal. Seen with lesions of upper motor neurons. Unconscious states resulting from drug and alcohol intoxication, brain injury, or subsequent to an epileptic seizure may also cause it (Fig. 21-28B).

(Continued on following page)

REFLEXES (*continued*)

ASSESSMENT PROCEDURE	NORMAL FINDINGS	ABNORMAL FINDINGS

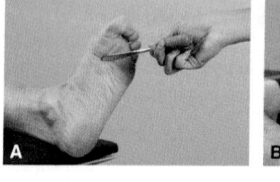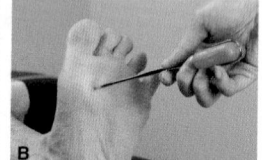

FIGURE 21-28 (**A**) Eliciting normal plantar reflex. (**B**) Eliciting abnormal positive Babinski.

Test abdominal reflex. Lightly stroke the abdomen on each side, above and below the umbilicus (Fig. 21-29). This evaluates the function of spinal levels T8, T9, and T10 with the upper abdominal reflex and spinal levels T10, T11, and T12 with the lower abdominal reflex.

Abdominal muscles contract; the umbilicus deviates toward the side being stimulated (Fig. 21-30).

Note: The abdominal reflex may be concealed because of obesity or muscular stretching from pregnancies. This is not an abnormality.

Superficial reflexes may be absent with lower or upper motor neuron lesions.

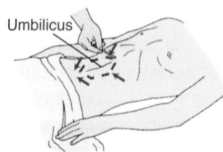

FIGURE 21-29 Abdominal reflex.

ASSESSMENT PROCEDURE	NORMAL FINDINGS	ABNORMAL FINDINGS
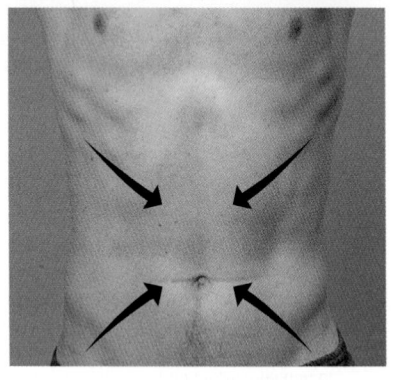 FIGURE 21-30 Abdominal and cremasteric reflexes.		
Test **cremasteric reflex** in male clients. Lightly stroke the inner aspect of the upper thigh. This evaluates the function of spinal levels T12, L1, and L2.	Scrotum elevates on stimulated side.	Absence of reflex may indicate motor neuron disorder.

(Continued on following page)

TESTS FOR MENINGEAL IRRITATION OR INFLAMMATION

ASSESSMENT PROCEDURE	NORMAL FINDINGS	ABNORMAL FINDINGS
If you suspect that the client has meningeal irritation or inflammation from infection or subarachnoid hemorrhage, assess **the client's neck mobility.** First, make sure that there is no injury to the cervical vertebrae or cervical cord. Then, with the client supine, place your hands behind the client's head and flex the neck forward until the chin touches the chest if possible.	Neck is supple; client can easily bend head and neck forward.	Pain in the neck and resistance to flexion can arise from meningeal inflammation, arthritis, or neck injury.
Test for Brudzinski sign. As you flex the neck, watch the hips and knees in reaction to your maneuver.	Hips and knees remain relaxed and motionless.	Pain and flexion of the hips and knees are positive Brudzinski signs, suggesting meningeal inflammation.
Test for Kernig sign. Flex the client's leg at both the hip and the knee, then straighten the knee.	No pain is felt. Discomfort behind the knee during full extension occurs in many normal people.	Pain and increased resistance to extending the knee are a positive Kernig sign. When Kernig sign is bilateral, the examiner suspects meningeal irritation.

TABLE 21-3 Two-Point Discrimination Findings

Two-Point Discrimination	Right	Left
Measurements in mm		
Fingertips	6	6
Dorsal hand	15	15
Chest	45	49
Forearm	39	35
Back	45	45
Upper arm	40	45
Reflexes		
Biceps	2+	2+
Triceps	2+	2+
Patellar	3+	3+
Achilles	2+	2+
Abdominal	1+	1+
Babinski	Negative	Negative

ASSESSMENT GUIDE 21-1 Eliciting Deep Tendon Reflexes

Proceed as follows to elicit a deep tendon reflex.
1. Encourage the client to relax and position the client properly.
2. Hold the handle of the reflex hammer between your thumb and index finger so it swings freely.

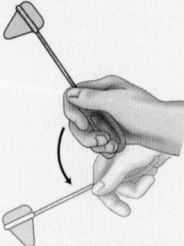

3. Palpate the tendon and use a rapid wrist movement to strike the tendon briskly. Observe the response.
4. Compare the response of one side with the other.
5. For arm reflexes, ask the client to clench their jaw or to squeeze one thigh with the opposite hand and then immediately strike the tendon. For leg reflexes, ask the client to lock the fingers of both

hands and pull them against each other and then immediately strike the tendon.
6. Rate and document reflexes using the following scale and figure.

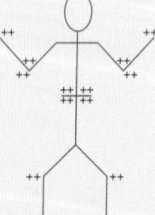

- Grade 4+: Hyperactive, very brisk, rhythmic oscillations (clonus); pathologic
- Grade 3+: Increased or brisk; more active than normal, but not pathologic
- Grade 2+: Normal, usual response
- Grade 1+: Present but decreased, less active than normal
- Grade 0: No response

CULTURAL VARIATIONS

- Cerebrovascular disease (CVD) has neurologic effects, but the cause is vascular. In the United States, the states of the "stroke belt" include North Carolina, South Carolina, Georgia, Alabama, Mississippi, Louisiana, Arkansas, and Tennessee.
- The highest incidence of stroke and vascular disease is found in the "stroke buckle" (North and South Carolina and Georgia); this is thought to be due to high percentages of older adults and African-American dietary factors (Grim, 2017).
- Children born and living in North Carolina, South Carolina, and Georgia during childhood show higher risk for stroke in adulthood (Howard et al., 2013).
- In the rural U.S. South, the symptoms described as "bad nerves" are the same as anxiety or worry. This may include "crying spells" but may refer to a serious emotional disorder or mental breakdown (Andrews et al., 2020, p. 230).
- A condition identified as a culture-bound syndrome, *ataque de nervios* (nerve attack), associated with Latin Americans, has various emotional expressions, including a sense of impending loss of control, chest tightness, a feeling of heat in the body, palpitations, shaking in the arms and legs, and feelings of imminent fainting. Clients may fear dying or engage in behaviors that result from loss of control, such as committing suicide or hurting others (Hoffman & Hinton, 2014).

PEDIATRIC VARIATIONS
Cranial Nerve Examination

The CNs are difficult to assess in the newborn and young child. Assessment of CNs may be performed in middle to later childhood and adolescence.

Motor and Cerebellar Examination

Cerebellar functioning may be assessed in older children and adolescents by performing Romberg test, finger-to-nose, finger-to-finger, heel-to-shin, and rapid alternating movements with hands and fingers.

Sensory Examination

Sensory nerve assessment may be assessed by asking the child to close their eyes and lightly touching the child in different places on the face, arm, hand, and lower legs.

Reflex Examination

Assess deep tendon reflexes in all children with the reflex hammer. The first finger may be used to assess infants if desired.

Average reflexes for children are 2+ to 3+. Newborns tend to have more brisk reflexes (3+).

INFANT REFLEXES (BIRTH TO AGE 1 YEAR; SEE APPENDIX 5 FOR DEVELOPMENTAL MILESTONES FOR AGES 1–3 YEARS)	NORMAL VARIATIONS
Cough	No cough reflex until 1 to 2 days of age; after 1 to 2 days, cough should be strong and present even during sleep throughout infancy.
Rooting: Infant turns head toward the side of face stroked.	Disappears at about age 3 to 12 months
Extension: When tongue is pressed or touched, infant forces tongue outward.	Disappears at about age 4 months

INFANT REFLEXES	NORMAL VARIATIONS
Palmar grasp: Touch to palm of hand or soles of feet causes flexion of hands/toes.	Palmar grasp should disappear at about age 3 months.
Plantar reflex: Stroking outer sole of foot from heel to toe causes big toe to rise (dorsiflexion) and other toes to fan out.	Disappears after 1 year
Moro: Sudden jarring or change in equilibrium causes sudden extension and abduction of extremities, with thumb forming "C" shape; crying.	Disappears at about age 3 to 4 months
Startle: Sudden noise causes abduction of arms, clenched hands.	Disappears at about age 4 months

INFANT REFLEXES	NORMAL VARIATIONS
Crawling: Infant on abdomen will make crawling movements with arms and legs.	Disappears at about age 6 weeks
Dance: Infant held on soles of feet touching table will simulate walking movements.	Disappears at about age 3 to 4 weeks
Neck righting: In supine infant, if head is turned to one side, shoulder and trunk will turn to that side.	Disappears around age 10 months
Asymmetrical tonic neck: Infant's head quickly turns to one side, arm and leg on that side will extend, and opposite leg and arm will flex.	Disappears at about age 3 to 4 months

 GERIATRIC VARIATIONS

Cranial Nerve Examination

- Decreased ability to see, hear, taste, and smell.

Motor and Cerebellar Examination

- May have reduced muscle mass from degeneration of muscle fibers
- Slowed coordination and voluntary movements
- Decreased fine motor coordination
- Older adults may experience intentional tremors (tremors that occur with intentional movements). This may be seen with extending the hands, head nodding for "yes or no," or extending one's tongue, which may protrude back and forth. Such tremors are not associated with disease, but they may cause embarrassment or emotional distress.
- May have slower and less certain gait; **tandem walking** may be very difficult for older client.

- It is not customary to perform the Tandem Walk Test or Hopping on One Foot Test with the older adult because it puts the client at risk.
- Hopping on one foot is often impossible because of decreased flexibility and strength; it is best to avoid this test with the older client because of risk for injury. The tandem walk may also be difficult, impossible, and dangerous for some older clients.

Sensory Examination

- Decreased taste and scent sensation occurs normally in older adults.
- Touch sensations may diminish normally with aging due to atrophy of peripheral nerve endings.
- Older adults are at increased risk for foot and ankle pathologies. A decrease or loss of vibratory sense is one of the earliest signs of sensory loss (Feilmeier & Dayton, 2015).
- There is a normal decrease in the older person's ability to see.
- Decreased light touch and pain perception
- Vibratory sensation at the ankles may decrease after age 70, but vibration sense is more likely to be absent at the great toe and preserved at the ankle bones (Feilmeier & Dayton, 2015).
- Sense of position of great toe may be reduced in some older adults.

Reflex Examination

- Usually have deep tendon reflexes intact, although a decrease in reaction time may slow the response (Chandrasekhar et al., 2013)
- May have decreased deep tendon reflexes and unstable balance due to peripheral neuropathy, which also causes disturbed proprioception and loss of vibratory sense, temperature sense, and possible pain, tingling, and distal weakness (Yeager, 2016)
- Achilles reflex may be absent or difficult to elicit.
- Flexion of the toes may be difficult to elicit and may be absent.

POSSIBLE COLLABORATIVE PROBLEMS—RISK OF

- Cranial nerve
  - CN impairment
  - Corneal ulceration
  - Increased intraocular pressure
- Motor/cerebellar
  - Increased intracranial pressure
  - Meningitis
  - Paralysis
  - Spinal cord compression
  - Seizures

- Sensory
  - Peripheral nerve impairment
  - Neuropathies

Teaching Tips for Selected Client Concerns

Client Concern: *Decreased sensation (visual, touch, taste, hearing) associated with physiological aging changes*

Explain to family the use and benefits of sensory therapy. Refer for hearing/visual aids as necessary. Teach client slowly and concisely. Speak clearly and demonstrate instructions from client's best side for hearing and seeing. Teach client how to prevent thermal injuries.

Client Concern: *Risk for Injury related to seizure activity*

Teach appropriate precautions and care, including the following:
- The CDC (and EFMK) states to not put anything into a person's mouth while they are having a seizure. https://www.cdc.gov/epilepsy/about/first-aid.htm
- Protection of client from harm during seizures
- Positioning on side after seizure
- Significance of drug maintenance

Client Concern: *Risk for injury associated with decreased tactile sensations*

Instruct on proper inspection and protective care of extremities. Caution client on dangers of exposure to extreme hot and cold temperatures, contact with sharp objects, and wearing tight-fitting shoes or garments.

Client Concern: *Opportunity to promote health associated with client request to learn ways to prevent stroke and concerns regarding history of stroke in family*

Teach clients to:
- Avoid smoking or to quit if they already smoke.
- Control cholesterol through diet, exercise, and medicines, if needed.
- Control high blood pressure and/or diabetes through diet, exercise, and medicines, if needed.
- Exercise at least 30 minutes a day.
- Maintain a healthy weight by eating healthy foods, eating less, and joining a weight loss program, if needed.
  - Choose a diet rich in fruits, vegetables, and whole grains.

- Choose lean proteins, such as chicken, fish, beans, and legumes.
- Choose low-fat dairy products, such as 1% milk and other low-fat items.
- Avoid sodium (salt) and fats found in fried foods, processed foods, and baked goods.
- Eat fewer animal products and foods that contain cheese, cream, or eggs.
- Read labels, and stay away from saturated fat and anything that contains partially hydrogenated or hydrogenated fats. These products are usually loaded with unhealthy fats.
- Limit alcohol (to 1 drink a day for women and 2 a day for men).
- Avoid cocaine and other illegal drugs.
- Talk to doctor about the risk of taking birth control pills.
- Teach clients to recognize the following symptoms of stroke (National Stroke Association, 2020):
  - Sudden numbness or weakness of face, arm, or leg (especially on one side of body)
  - Sudden confusion, trouble speaking, or understanding speech
  - Sudden trouble seeing in one or both eyes
  - Sudden trouble walking, dizziness, loss of balance, or coordination
  - Sudden severe headache with no known cause

References

Andrews, M., Boyle, J., & Collins, J. (2020). *Transcultural concepts in nursing care* (8th ed.). Wolters Kluwer.

Chandrasekhar, A., Abu Osman, N., Tham, L., Lim, K., & Abas, W. (2013). Influence of age on patellar tendon reflex response. PLoS One. 2013; 8(11): e80799. https://journals.plos.org/plosone/article?id=10.1371/journal.pone.0080799

Feilmeier, M., & Dayton, P. (2015). Identifying foot and ankle pathologies. *Today's Geriatric Medicine*, 8(3), 22. https://www.todaysgeriatricmedicine.com/archive/0515p22.shtml

Grim, C. (2017). Abstract P396: The stroke belt: Forged in the heat of the buckle? A hypothesis. *Hypertension*, 70(1). https://www.ahajournals.org/doi/10.1161/hyp.70.suppl_1.p396

Hoffman, S., & Hinton, D. (2014). Cross-cultural aspects of anxiety disorders. *Current Psychiatry Reports*, 16(6). https://doi.org/10.1007/s11920-014-0450-3

Howard, V. J., McClure, L. A., Glymour, M. M., Cunningham, S. A., Kleindorfer, D. O., Crowe, M., Wadley, V. G., Peace, F., Howard, G., & Lackland, D. T. (2013). Effect of duration and age of exposure to the Stroke Belt on incident stroke in adulthood. *Neurology*, 80(18), 1655–1661. https://doi.org/10.1212/WNL.0b013e3182904d59

National Stroke Association. (2020). *Stroke symptoms*. https://www.stroke.org/en/about-stroke/stroke-symptoms

Yeager, D. (2016). Diagnosing peripheral neuropathy. *Aging Well*, 5(4),14. http://www.todaysgeriatricmedicine.com/archive/070912p14.shtml

22 ASSESSING MALE GENITALIA, ANUS, AND RECTUM

Structure and Function Overview

EXTERNAL GENITALIA

The penis is the male reproductive organ (Fig. 22-1). The penile shaft is composed of three masses of vascular erectile tissue bound by fibrous tissue—two corpora cavernosa on the dorsal side and the corpus spongiosum on the ventral side, which forms the acorn-shaped glans. The urethra is located in the center of the corpus spongiosum and opens at the glans tip as the urethral meatus. The frenulum, a fold of foreskin, extends ventrally from the urethral meatus. The scrotum, a thin-walled sac suspended below the pubic bone posterior to the penis, contains sweat and sebaceous glands and consists of skinfolds (rugae) and the cremaster muscle. The scrotum protects the testes, epididymis, and vas deferens and maintains a temperature ($<37°C$) required for sperm production.

INTERNAL GENITALIA

The internal genitalia consists of the testes, a pair of ovoid-shaped organs located in the scrotal sac that produce spermatozoa and testosterone (see Fig. 22-1). The testes are covered by the tunica vaginalis, a serous membrane

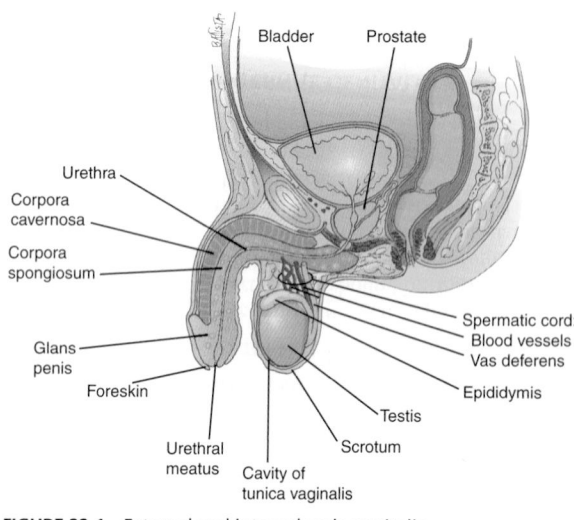

FIGURE 22-1 External and internal male genitalia.

that protects the testes. The testes are suspended by a spermatic cord that contains blood vessels, lymphatic vessels, nerves, and the vas deferens, which transports spermatozoa away from the testes. The left side of the spermatic cord is usually longer; thus, the left testis hangs lower than the right testis. The epididymis, a comma-shaped, coiled tubular structure, curves up over the upper and posterior surfaces of the testis. It is here that the spermatozoa mature. The vas deferens is a firm, muscular tube continuous with the lower portion of the epididymis, which travels up within the spermatic cord through the inguinal canal into the abdominal cavity. It joins with the duct of the seminal vesicle to form the ejaculatory duct, which empties into the urethra. The vas deferens transports sperm from the testes to the urethra for ejaculation. Along the way, secretions from the vas deferens, seminal vesicles, prostate gland, and Cowper, or bulbourethral, glands mix with the sperm to form semen.

INGUINAL AREA

The inguinal (groin) area, located between the anterior superior iliac spine and the symphysis pubis, is a common area for hernias (Fig. 22-2). Located within this area is the inguinal canal, a tube-like structure through which the vas deferens travels as it passes

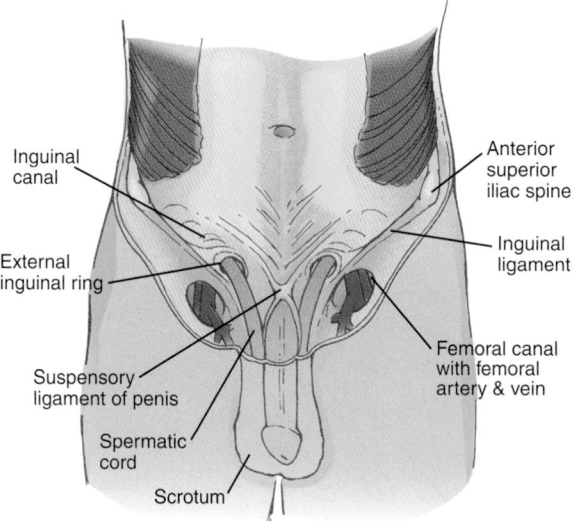

FIGURE 22-2 Inguinal area.

Labels: Inguinal canal; External inguinal ring; Suspensory ligament of penis; Spermatic cord; Scrotum; Anterior superior iliac spine; Inguinal ligament; Femoral canal with femoral artery & vein.

through the lower abdomen. The external inguinal ring can be palpated above and lateral to the symphysis pubis. The internal inguinal ring cannot be palpated. The femoral canal, located posterior to the inguinal canal and medial to the femoral artery and vein, is another area in which hernias may occur.

ANUS AND RECTUM

The **anal canal**, 2.5 to 4 cm long, begins at the anal sphincter and ends at the anorectal junction (Fig. 22-3). It is lined with somatic sensory nerves, making it susceptible to painful stimuli. The **anal opening** is hairless and overlies the external anal sphincter. Within the anus are the two sphincters that hold the anal canal closed, except when passing gas and feces. The **external sphincter**, composed of skeletal muscle, is under voluntary control. The **internal sphincter**, composed of smooth muscle, is under involuntary control by the autonomic nervous system. Just above the internal sphincter is the **anorectal junction**, the dividing point of the anal canal and the rectum. The rectum is lined with mucosal folds (columns of Morgagni) that contain arteries, veins, and visceral nerves. These tissues may engorge from chronic pressure and form hemorrhoids. The **rectum** (12 cm long) extends from the **sigmoid colon** to the anorectal junction. It enlarges above

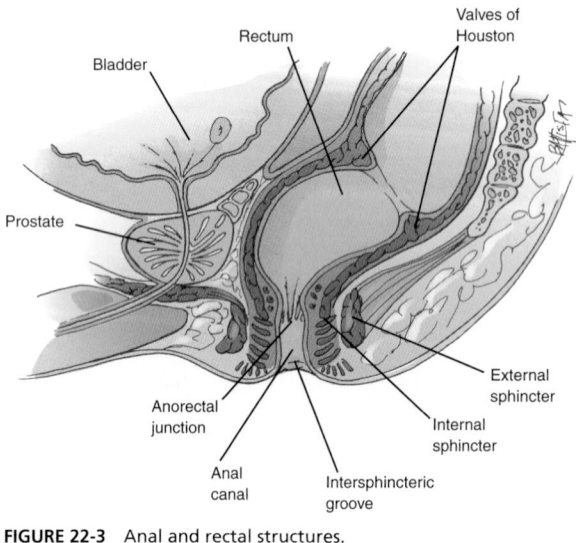

FIGURE 22-3 Anal and rectal structures.

the anorectal junction and proceeds toward the hollow of the sacrum and coccyx, forming the rectal ampulla. The inside of the rectum contains three foldings (valves of Houston).

PROSTATE

The **prostate gland** (2.5–4 cm in diameter) surrounds the bladder neck and urethra and lies between these structures and the rectum. It has two lobes separated by a shallow groove (median sulcus). It secretes a milky substance that promotes sperm motility and neutralizes acidic vaginal secretions. This organ can be palpated through the anterior wall of the rectum. The **seminal vesicles**, located on the sides and above the prostate, produce the ejaculate that nourishes and protects sperm. The **Cowper**, or bulbourethral, glands are pea-sized glands located posterior to the prostate; these glands produce mucus.

Health Assessment

COLLECTING SUBJECTIVE DATA

Interview Questions

Pain in penis, scrotum, testes, or groin? Itching in pubic hair area? Lesions in penis or genital area? Discharge from penis? Color?

Odor? Lumps, masses, or swelling in scrotum, groin, or genital area? Heavy, draggy feeling in scrotum? Difficulty voiding—hesitancy, frequency, difficulty starting or maintaining stream? Change in color, odor, or amount of urine? Pain or burning when urinating? Incontinence or dribbling? Change in sexual activities? Difficulty with maintaining an erection? Problem with ejaculation? Trouble with fertility? Any bulges or pain when straining or lifting heavy objects? History of inguinal or genitalia surgery? History of sexually transmitted infection (STI)? Self-care: last testicular examination? Testicular self-examination (TSE) (Box 22-1)? Tested for human immunodeficiency virus (HIV)? Result? History of cancer in family? Number of sexual partners? Contraceptive form? Exposure to chemical or radiation? Fertility concerns? Comfort with communicating with sexual partner?

Usual bowel pattern? Changes? Diarrhea? Constipation? Color of stools? Mucus in stools? Stools oily or greasy, bulky or float? Pain? Itching? Bleeding after stools? History of rectal or anal surgery? Proctosigmoidoscopy? Family history of polyps, colon, rectal, or prostate cancer? Self-care: use of laxatives? Engage in anal sex? Amount of roughage, fat, and water in diet? Last digital rectal examination (DRE) by a physician or health care provider?

Risk Factors

- Risk for colorectal cancer related to age greater than 40 years; history of rectal or colon polyps; inflammatory bowel disease; history of colorectal cancer; and diet high in fat, protein, and beef and low in fiber.
- Risk for prostate cancer related to dietary fat intake; age greater than 60 years; African-American or Hispanic origin; exposure to cadmium, dioxin, or agent orange; high-risk occupations (e.g., tire and rubber manufacturers, farmers, mechanics, sheet metal workers); lack of circumcision; brother or father with prostate cancer; high testosterone levels may be a factor; excessive alcohol consumption; and lack of sleep or sleeping with light on.
- Risk for HIV/AIDS related to having unprotected sex (especially male-on-male anal intercourse); having multiple sexual partners, bisexual partners, or a partner who uses intravenous drugs; having another STI; using intravenous drugs, especially sharing needles; being an uncircumcised male; being the fetus of an HIV-positive mother (mother–infant transmission during pregnancy or delivery); exchanging blood or body fluids through blood transfusions or needlesticks; being breastfed by HIV-infected mother; and having body piercings with nonsterilized instruments (Centers for Disease Control and Prevention [CDC], 2019a, b, c).

BOX 22-1 SELF-ASSESSMENT: TESTICULAR SELF-EXAMINATION

TSE is to be performed once a month; it is neither difficult nor time-consuming. A convenient time is often after a warm bath or shower when the scrotum is more relaxed.

1. Stand in front of a mirror and check for scrotal swelling.
2. Use both hands to palpate the testis; the normal testicle is smooth and uniform in consistency.
3. With the index and middle fingers under the testis and the thumb on top, roll the testis gently in a horizontal plane between the thumb and fingers **(A)**.
4. Feel for any evidence of a small lump or abnormality.
5. Follow the same procedure and palpate upward along the testis **(B)**.
6. Locate the epididymis **(C)**, a cord-like structure on the top and back of the testicle that stores and transports sperm.
7. Repeat the examination for the other testis. It is normal to find that one testis is larger than the other.
8. If you find any evidence of a small, pea-like lump, consult your physician. It may be due to an infection or a tumor growth.

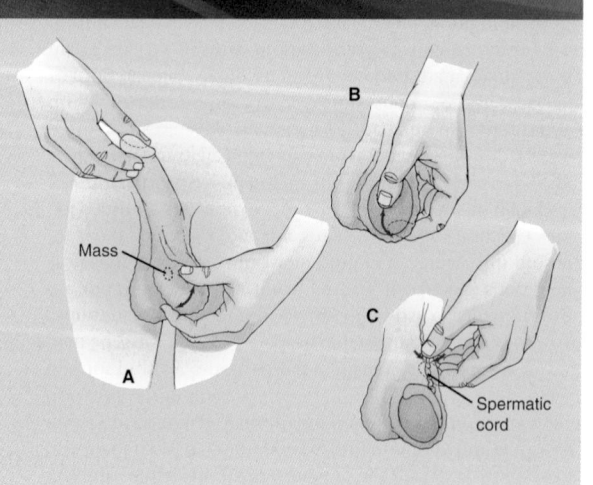

COLLECTING OBJECTIVE DATA

Equipment Needed

- Stool to sit on
- Gown
- Disposable nonlatex gloves
- Flashlight (for possible transillumination)
- Stethoscope (for possible auscultation)
- Drape
- Pillow
- Water-soluble lubricant for rectal examination

Physical Assessment

Review Figures 22-1 to 22-3 for anatomy of the external and internal genital structures, the inguinal area, and the anus and rectal area. Explain the purpose of the examination and procedure to put client at ease. Preserve the client's modesty and privacy. Teach client the importance of TSE and explain how to perform the examination as you are performing it. Ask a third person to be present to protect the client and examiner from false allegations. Wear gloves for every step of this examination to ensure safety for the nurse and the client.

ASSESSMENT PROCEDURE	NORMAL FINDINGS	ABNORMAL FINDINGS
Observe for **sexual maturity**.	See norms in Table 22-1.	Underdevelopment or excessive development noted in relation to Table 22-1.
PENIS		
Inspect the **base of the penis and pubic hair.** Sit on a stool with the client facing you and standing. Ask the client to raise his gown or drape. Note pubic hair growth pattern and any excoriation, erythema, or infestation at the base of the penis and within the pubic hair.	Pubic hair is coarser than scalp hair. The normal pubic hair pattern in adults is hair covering the entire groin area, extending to the medial thighs and up the abdomen toward the umbilicus.	Absence or scarcity of pubic hair may be seen in clients receiving chemotherapy. Lice or nit (eggs) infestation at the base of the penis or pubic hair is known as pediculosis pubis. This is commonly referred to as "crabs."

(Continued on following page)

PENIS (*continued*)

ASSESSMENT PROCEDURE	NORMAL FINDINGS	ABNORMAL FINDINGS
	The base of the penis and the pubic hair are free of excoriation, erythema, and infestation.	
Inspect **the skin of the shaft**. Observe for rashes, lesions, or lumps.	The skin of the penis is wrinkled and hairless and is normally free of rashes, lesions, or lumps. Genital piercing is becoming more common, and nurses may see male clients with one or more piercings of the penis.	Rashes, lesions, or lumps may indicate STI or cancer (see Abnormal Findings 22-1). Drainage around piercings indicates infection.
Palpate **the shaft**. Palpate any abnormalities noted during inspection. Also note any hardened or tender areas.	The penis in a nonerect state is usually soft, flaccid, and nontender.	Tenderness may indicate inflammation or infection.
Inspect **the foreskin** for color, location, and integrity in uncircumcised men.	The foreskin, which covers the glans in an uncircumcised male client, is intact and uniform in color with the penis.	Discoloration of the foreskin may indicate scarring or infection.
Inspect **the glans** for size, shape, lesions, or redness.	The glans size and shape vary, appearing rounded, broad, or even pointed. The surface of the glans is normally smooth, free of lesions and redness.	Chancres (red, oval ulcerations) from syphilis, genital warts, and pimple-like lesions from herpes are sometimes detected on the glans.

ASSESSMENT PROCEDURE	NORMAL FINDINGS	ABNORMAL FINDINGS
If the client is not circumcised, ask him to retract his foreskin (if the client is unable to do so, the nurse may retract it) to allow observation of the glans. This may be painful.	The foreskin retracts easily. A small amount of whitish material, called smegma, normally accumulates under the foreskin.	A tight foreskin that cannot be retracted is called *phimosis*. A foreskin that, once retracted, cannot be returned to cover the glans is called *paraphimosis*. Chancres (red, oval ulcerations) from syphilis and genital warts are sometimes detected under the foreskin (see Abnormal Findings 22-1).
Note the location of the urinary meatus on the glans.	The urinary meatus is slitlike and normally found in the center of the glans.	*Hypospadias* is displacement of the urinary meatus to the ventral surface of the penis. *Epispadias* is displacement of the urinary meatus to the dorsal surface of the penis.
Palpate for urethral discharge. Gently squeeze the glans between your index finger and thumb (Fig. 22-4).	The urinary meatus is normally free of discharge. 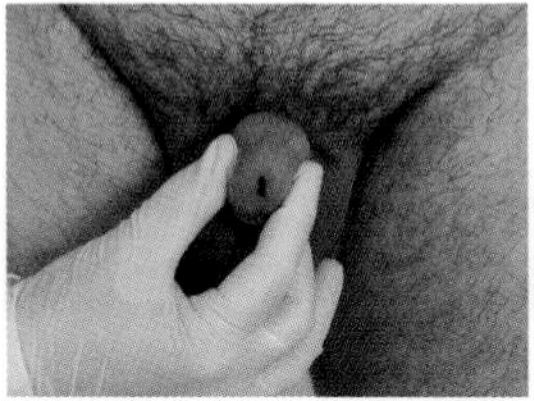 **FIGURE 22-4** Palpating for urethral discharge. (Photo by B. Proud.)	A yellow discharge is usually associated with gonorrhea. A clear or white discharge is usually associated with urethritis. Any discharge should be cultured.

(Continued on following page)

SCROTUM

ASSESSMENT PROCEDURE	NORMAL FINDINGS	ABNORMAL FINDINGS
Inspect **the size, shape, and position of the scrotum.** Ask the client to hold his penis out of the way. Observe for swelling, lumps, or bulges.	The scrotum varies in size (according to temperature) and shape. The scrotal sac hangs below or at the level of the penis. The left side of the scrotal sac usually hangs lower than the right side.	Hydrocele (enlarged scrotal sac) may result from fluid, blood (hematocele), bowel (hernia), or tumor (cancer). A varicocele (VAR-ih-koe-seel) is an enlargement of the **veins** within the scrotum, which may cause low sperm production and decreased sperm quality, which can cause infertility.
Inspect **the scrotal skin.** Observe color, integrity, and lesions or rashes. To perform an accurate inspection, you must spread out the scrotal folds (rugae) of skin. Lift the scrotal sac to inspect the posterior skin.	Scrotal skin is thin and rugated (crinkled) with little hair dispersion. Its color is slightly darker than that of the penis. Lesions and rashes are not normally present. However, sebaceous cysts (small, yellowish, firm, nontender, benign nodules) are a normal finding.	Rashes, lesions, and inflammation are abnormal findings.
Palpation		
Palpate the scrotal contents. Palpate each *testis* and *epididymis* between your thumb and first two fingers. Note size, shape, consistency, nodules, masses, and tenderness (Fig. 22-5). *Note: Do not apply too much pressure to the testes because this will cause pain.*	Testes are ovoid, approximately 3.5 to 5 cm long, 2.5 cm wide, and 2.5 cm deep, and equal bilaterally in size and shape. They are smooth, firm, rubbery, mobile, free of nodules, and rather tender to pressure. The epididymis is nontender, smooth, and softer than the testes.	Absence of a testis suggests *cryptorchidism* (an undescended testicle). Painless nodules may indicate cancer. Tenderness and swelling may indicate acute orchitis, torsion of the spermatic cord, a strangulated hernia, or epididymitis. If the client has epididymitis, passive elevation of the testes may relieve the scrotal pain (Prehn sign).

ASSESSMENT PROCEDURE	NORMAL FINDINGS	ABNORMAL FINDINGS

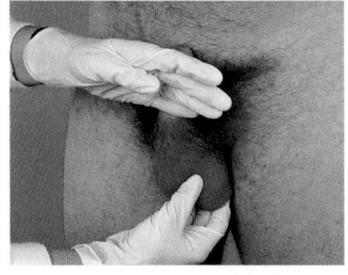

FIGURE 22-5 Palpating the scrotal contents. (Photo by B. Proud.)

Palpate each *spermatic cord* and vas deferens from the epididymis to the inguinal ring. The spermatic cord will lie between your thumb and finger. Note nodules, swelling, or tenderness. See Box 22-1 to teach client TSE.	The spermatic cord and vas deferens should feel uniform on both sides. The cord is smooth, nontender, and rope like.	• Palpable, tortuous veins suggest varicocele. A beaded or thickened cord indicates infection or cysts. A cyst suggests hydrocele of the spermatic cord.

(Continued on following page)

SCROTUM (*continued*)		
ASSESSMENT PROCEDURE	**NORMAL FINDINGS**	**ABNORMAL FINDINGS**
Assessment of Scrotal Mass Found During Examination		
If an abnormal mass or swelling was noted during inspection and palpation of the scrotum, perform transillumination. Darken the room and shine a light from the back of the scrotum through the mass. Look for a red glow.	Normally, scrotal contents do not transilluminate.	Swellings or masses that contain serous fluid—hydrocele, spermatocele—light up with a red glow. Swellings or masses that are solid or filled with blood—tumor, hernias, or varicocele—do not light up with a red glow.
If during inspection and palpation of the scrotal contents, you palpated a scrotal mass, ask the client to lie down. Note whether the mass disappears. If it remains, **auscultate it for bowel sounds.** Finally, **gently palpate the mass and try to push it upward into the abdomen.** *Note: If the client complains of extreme tenderness or nausea, do not try to push the mass up into the abdomen.*	Normal findings are not expected.	• If bulge disappears, no scrotal hernia is present, but mass may result from something else. Refer for further evaluation. Mass on or around scrotum should be considered malignant until further testing. If mass remains, place your fingers above scrotal mass. If you can get fingers above mass, suspect hydrocele. Bowel sounds auscultated over mass indicate the presence of bowel and, thus, a scrotal hernia. Bowel sounds will not be heard over a hydrocele.

ASSESSMENT PROCEDURE	NORMAL FINDINGS	ABNORMAL FINDINGS
		If you cannot push the mass into the abdomen, suspect an *incarcerated hernia*. A hernia is *strangulated* when its blood supply is cut off. Client typically complains of extreme tenderness and nausea. If strangulated hernia is suspected, refer immediately to physician.
INGUINAL AREA		
Inspection		
Inspect for **inguinal and femoral hernia.** Inspect the inguinal and femoral areas for bulges. Ask the client to turn head and cough or to bear down as if having a bowel movement, and continue to inspect the areas.	The inguinal and femoral areas are normally free from bulges.	Bulges that appear at the external inguinal ring or at the femoral canal when the client bears down may signal a hernia.
Palpation		
Palpate for **inguinal hernia and inguinal nodes.** Ask client to shift his weight to the left for palpation of the right inguinal canal and vice versa. Place your right index finger into the client's right	Bulging or masses are not normally palpated.	A bulge or mass may indicate a hernia.

(Continued on following page)

INGUINAL AREA (continued)

ASSESSMENT PROCEDURE	NORMAL FINDINGS	ABNORMAL FINDINGS
scrotum and press upward, invaginating the loose folds of skin. Palpate up spermatic cord until you reach triangular-shaped, slit-like opening of external inguinal ring. Try to push your finger through opening. If possible, continue palpating up inguinal canal. When your finger is in canal or at external inguinal ring, ask client to bear down or cough. Feel any bulges against your finger. Repeat procedure on the opposite side (Fig. 22-6).	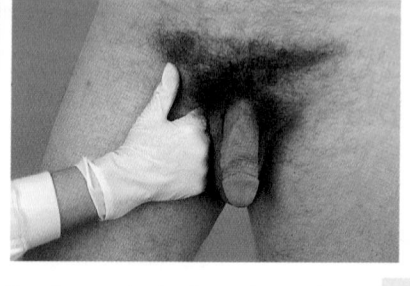 **FIGURE 22-6** Palpating for an inguinal hernia. (Photo by B. Proud.)	
Palpate inguinal lymph nodes. If nodes are palpable, note size, consistency, mobility or tenderness.	No enlargement or tenderness is normal.	Enlarged or tender lymph nodes may indicate an inflammatory process or infection of the penis or scrotum.
Palpate for femoral hernia. Palpate on front of thigh in femoral canal area. Ask client to bear down or cough. Feel for bulges. Repeat on opposite thigh.	Bulges or masses are not normally palpated.	Bulge or mass palpated as client bears down or coughs.

ASSESSMENT PROCEDURE	NORMAL FINDINGS	ABNORMAL FINDINGS

(See Fig. 22-7 for selected positions for anorectal examination.)

Standing

Left lateral

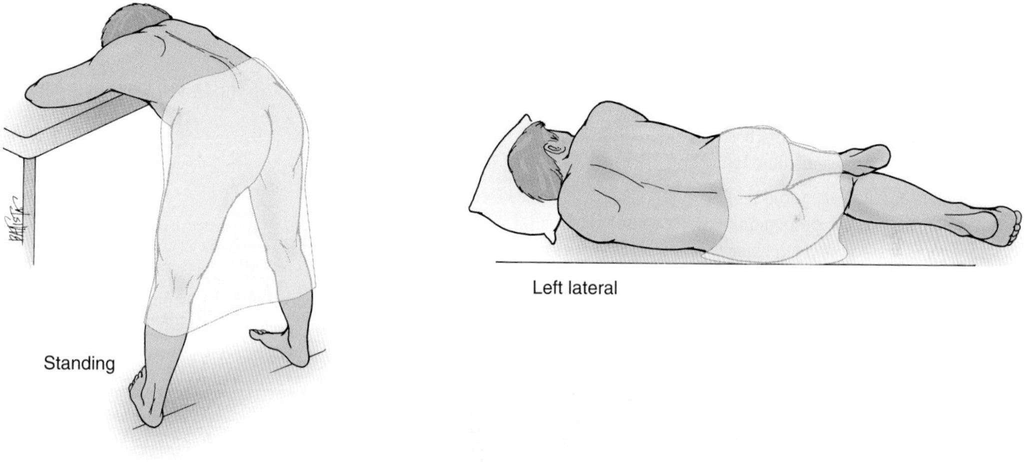

FIGURE 22-7 Selected positions for anorectal examination.

(Continued on following page)

INGUINAL AREA (*continued*)		
ASSESSMENT PROCEDURE	**NORMAL FINDINGS**	**ABNORMAL FINDINGS**
Inspection		
Inspect the perianal area. Spread client's buttocks and inspect anal opening and surrounding area for: • Lumps • Ulcers • Lesions • Rashes • Redness • Fissures Thickening of the epithelium (Fig. 22-8)	The anal opening should appear hairless, moist, and tightly closed. The skin around the anal opening is coarser and more darkly pigmented. The surrounding perianal area should be free of redness, lumps, ulcers, lesions, and rashes. 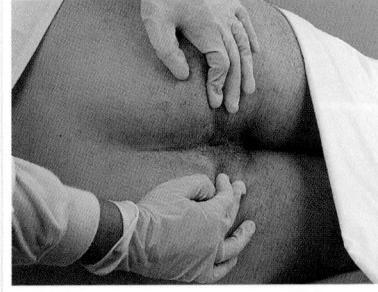 **FIGURE 22-8** Inspecting the perianal area. (Photo by B. Proud.)	Lesions may indicate STIs, cancer, or hemorrhoids. A thrombosed external hemorrhoid appears swollen. It is itchy, painful, and bleeds when the client passes stool. A previously thrombosed hemorrhoid appears as a skin tag that protrudes from the anus. A painful mass that is hardened and reddened suggests a perianal abscess. A swollen skin tag on anal margin may indicate fissure in anal canal. Redness and excoriation may be from scratching an area infected by fungi or pinworms. A small opening in the skin that surrounds the anal opening may be an anorectal fistula. Thickening of epithelium suggests repeated trauma from anal intercourse.

ASSESSMENT PROCEDURE	NORMAL FINDINGS	ABNORMAL FINDINGS
Ask the client to perform Valsalva maneuver by straining or bearing down. Inspect the anal opening for any bulges or lesions.	No bulging or lesions appear.	Bulges of red mucous membrane may indicate a rectal prolapse. Hemorrhoids or an anal fissure may also be seen.
Inspect the **sacrococcygeal area.** Inspect this area for any signs of swelling, redness, dimpling, or hair.	Area is normally smooth and free of redness and hair.	Reddened, swollen, or dimpled area covered by a small tuft of hair located midline on the lower sacrum suggests a pilonidal cyst.
Palpation		
Palpate anus. Inform client you are going to perform the internal examination at this point. Explain it may feel like his bowels are going to move, but this will not happen. Lubricate gloved index finger; ask client to bear down. As client bears down, place pad of your index finger (not fingertip as it causes sphincter to tighten) on anal opening and apply slight pressure causing sphincter to relax (Fig. 22-9). **Note:** *Do not force examination if severe pain occurs on entrance to the anus.*	Client's sphincter relaxes, permitting entry. 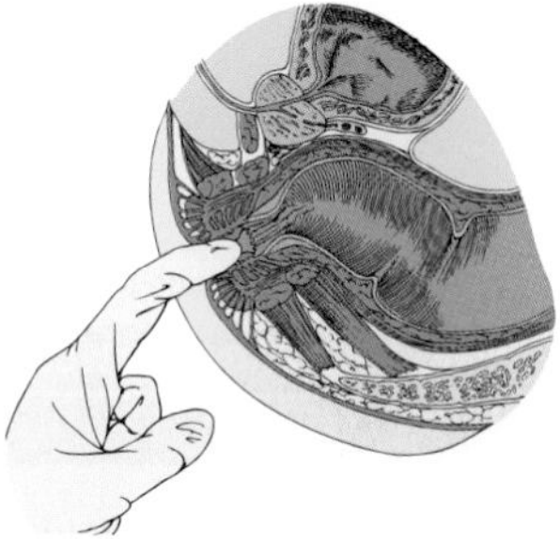 **FIGURE 22-9** Palpating the anus.	Sphincter tightens, making further examination unrealistic.

(Continued on following page)

INGUINAL AREA (*continued*)

ASSESSMENT PROCEDURE	NORMAL FINDINGS	ABNORMAL FINDINGS
When you feel sphincter relax, insert finger gently with pad facing down. If sphincter does not relax and client reports severe pain, spread gluteal folds with your hands close to anus to try to visualize any lesion that may be causing pain. If tension is maintained on gluteal folds for 60 seconds, the anus usually dilates.	Examination finger enters anus.	Examination finger cannot enter the anus.
Ask the client to tighten the external sphincter; note the tone.	The client can normally close the sphincter around the gloved finger.	Poor sphincter tone may be the result of a spinal cord injury, previous surgery, trauma, or a prolapsed rectum. Tightened sphincter tone may indicate anxiety, scarring, or inflammation.
Rotate finger to examine the muscular anal ring. Palpate for tenderness, nodules, and hardness.	The anus is normally smooth, nontender, and free of nodules and hardness.	Tenderness may indicate hemorrhoids, fistula, or fissure. Nodules may indicate polyps or cancer. Hardness may indicate scarring or cancer.

ASSESSMENT PROCEDURE	NORMAL FINDINGS	ABNORMAL FINDINGS
Palpate the rectum. Insert your finger further into the rectum as far as possible. Next, turn your hand clockwise, then counterclockwise. This allows palpation of as much rectal surface as possible. Note tenderness, irregularities, nodules, and hardness.	The rectal mucosa is normally soft, smooth, nontender, and free of nodules.	Hardness and irregularities may be from scarring or cancer. Nodules may indicate polyps or cancer.
Palpate the peritoneal cavity. This area may be palpated in men above the prostate gland in the area of the seminal vesicles on the anterior surface of the rectum. Note tenderness or nodules.	This area is normally smooth and nontender.	A peritoneal protrusion into the rectum, called a *rectal shelf,* may indicate a cancerous lesion or peritoneal metastasis. Tenderness may indicate peritoneal inflammation.

PROSTATE GLAND

Palpation

The prostate can be palpated on anterior surface of the rectum by turning hand fully counterclockwise so that pad of your index finger faces toward client's umbilicus. Tell client he may feel urge to urinate but he will not. Move pad of your index finger over prostate gland, try to feel sulcus between lateral lobes. Note size, shape, and consistency of prostate, and any nodules or tenderness (Fig. 22-10).	The prostate is normally nontender and rubbery. It has two lateral lobes that are divided by a median sulcus. The lobes are normally smooth, 2.5 cm long, and heart shaped.	A swollen, tender prostate may indicate acute prostatitis. An enlarged smooth, firm, slightly elastic prostate that may not have a median sulcus suggests benign prostatic hypertrophy (BPH). A hard area on the prostate or hard, fixed, irregular nodules on the prostate suggest cancer (see Abnormal Findings 22-2).

(Continued on following page)

PROSTATE GLAND (*continued*)		
ASSESSMENT PROCEDURE	**NORMAL FINDINGS**	**ABNORMAL FINDINGS**
Note: Palpating prostate gland prior to drawing prostate-specific antigen (PSA) may raise PSA level. Move your body away from client for proper examination angle.	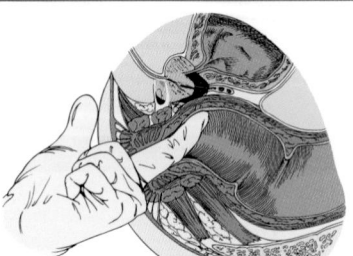 **FIGURE 22-10** Palpating the prostate gland.	
Check Stool		
Inspect the stool. Withdraw your gloved finger. Inspect any fecal matter on your glove. Assess the color, and test the feces for occult blood. Provide the client with a towel to wipe the anorectal area.	Stool is normally semisolid, brown, and free of blood.	Black stool may indicate upper gastrointestinal bleeding, gray or tan stool results from lack of bile pigment, and yellow stool suggests steatorrhea (increased fat content). Blood detected in stool may indicate cancer of rectum or colon. Refer client for examination of the colon.

TABLE 22-1 **Tanner Sexual Maturity Rating: Male Genitalia Development and Pubic Hair Growth**

Developmental Stage		Genitalia	Pubic Hair
Stage 1		Prepubertal	Prepubertal: No pubic hair; fine vellus hair
Stage 2		Initial enlargement of scrotum and testes with rugation and reddening of the scrotum	Sparse, long, straight, downy hair
Stage 3		Elongation of the penis; testes and scrotum further enlarge	Darker, coarser, curly; sparse over entire pubis

(*Continued on following page*)

TABLE 22-1   Tanner Sexual Maturity Rating: Male Genitalia Development and Pubic Hair Growth (*continued*)

Developmental Stage		Genitalia	Pubic Hair
Stage 4		Increase in size and width of penis and the development of the glans; scrotum darkens	Dark, curly, and abundant in pubic area; no growth on thighs or up toward umbilicus
Stage 5		Adult configuration	Adult pattern (growth up toward umbilicus may not be seen); growth continues until mid-20s

Reprinted with permission from Tanner, J. M. (1962). *Growth at adolescence* (2nd ed.). Blackwell Scientific Publications.

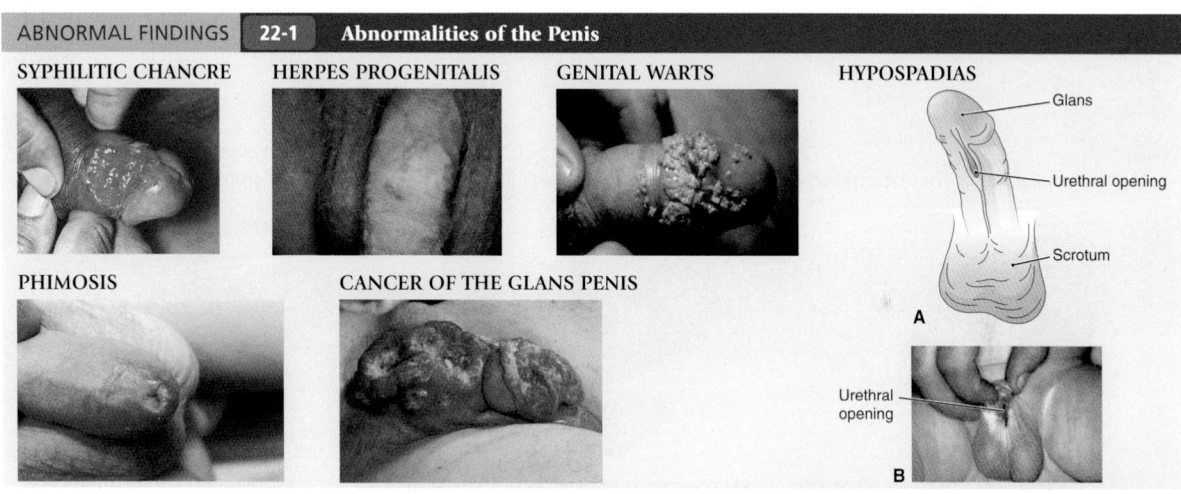

ABNORMAL FINDINGS 22-1 Abnormalities of the Penis

SYPHILITIC CHANCRE

HERPES PROGENITALIS

GENITAL WARTS

HYPOSPADIAS
- Glans
- Urethral opening
- Scrotum

A

PHIMOSIS

CANCER OF THE GLANS PENIS

Urethral opening

B

Photo credits: Syphilitic chancre, reprinted with permission from Nath, J. (2019). *Programmed learning approach to medical terminology* (3rd ed., Fig. 13-11). Wolters Kluwer; Genital warts, reprinted with permission from Goodheart, H., & Gonzalez, M. (2016). *Goodheart's photoguide to common pediatric and adult skin disorders* (4th ed., 53rd figure in 1st appendix). Wolters Kluwer; Cancer of the glans penis, CNRI/Science Source.

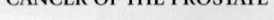

| ABNORMAL FINDINGS | 22-2 | **Abnormalities of the Prostate Gland** |

ACUTE PROSTATITIS

BENIGN PROSTATIC HYPERTROPHY

CANCER OF THE PROSTATE

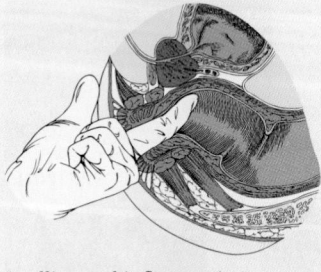

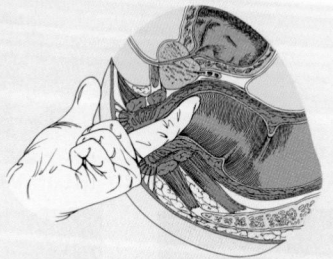

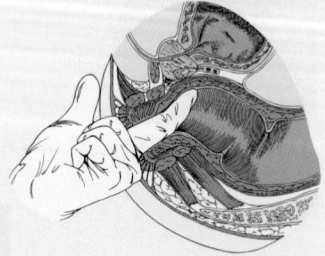

Swelling and inflammation characteristic of acute prostatitis.

Enlargement characteristic of BPH.

Mass characteristic of prostate cancer.

PEDIATRIC VARIATIONS

Questions to ask the parents or the adolescent when collecting *subjective data* include the following.
- Development of secondary sexual characteristics?
- Previous education on sexual development and activities?
- Use of contraceptives? Type?

    When collecting *objective data*, note the following.

    Inspection and palpation of external genitalia constitute the *total* genitourinary assessment until puberty. Assessment of the level of sexual development usually begins at approximately the age of 11 years. This determination involves assessment of secondary characteristics associated with sexual maturity. Refer to Table 22-1 for a summary of the timing of sexual development for boys.

 GERIATRIC VARIATIONS

- Pubic hair may be gray and sparse.
- Penis becomes smaller, and the testes hang lower in the scrotum.
- Decrease in size and firmness of testicles
- Loss of tone in musculature of scrotum
- The skin of the scrotal sac has fewer rugae.
- Slowed erections and less forceful ejaculations
- Enlargement of medial lobe of prostate

 CULTURAL VARIATIONS

- Pubertal rites in some cultures include (among many genital mutilations) slitting the penile shaft (penile subincision), leaving an opening that may extend the entire length of the shaft (Jewell, 2018).
- If pubertal mutilation has occurred, actual discharge of urine and semen will occur at the location of the shaft opening.
- Modern circumcision is linked especially to Abrahamic faiths, Judaism, Christianity, and Islam (rates vary from 80% to 100% in North Africa, Middle East, Whites, and Southeast Asia to near 0% in South and Central America; Martin, 2018).

POSSIBLE COLLABORATIVE PROBLEMS—RISK OF

Bladder perforation	Obstruction of	Renal calculi
Urinary tract infection	urethra	Hormonal
Genitalia ulcers or	Hemorrhage	imbalances
lesions	Renal failure	Hemorrhoids
BPH	Sexually transmitted	
	diseases (STDs)	

Teaching Tips for Selected Client Concerns and Collaborative Problems

Client Concern: Opportunity to promote urinary, bowel, and reproductive health associated with asking questions regarding urination and male health

Explain the importance of drinking eight glasses of fluid per day (unless contraindicated in certain medical conditions) and to limit intake of alcohol, caffeine, and carbonated beverages.

Instruct client on proper method of TSE, performed once a month after a warm bath or shower. Instruct the client to roll each testicle gently between the thumb and the fingers of both hands, feeling for lumps or nodules (see Box 22-1). Have client demonstrate. Begin at puberty, because testicular cancer is one of the most common cancers in men between 15 and 34 years old.

Teach alternate forms of birth control, proper use of methods, and advantages and disadvantages of each.

The American Cancer Society (ACS, 2018) recommends a stool test every year to detect occult blood beginning at age 45, and for persons with a life expectancy of at least 10 years. Tests should be continued to age 75. For ages 76 to 85, screening depends on current health, life expectancy, prior history, and personal preference. Colonoscopy is recommended every 10 years, or a computed tomography (CT) virtual colonoscopy every 5 years, or a flexible sigmoidoscopy every 5 years (ACS, 2018).

The DRE may also be done as a part of screening for prostate cancer. It is less effective than the PSA blood test, which also has a lack of specificity to detect prostate cancer, but it may find cancers in men with normal PSA levels (National Cancer Institute, 2019; U.S. Preventive Services Task Force [USPSTF], 2019).

Client Concern: Fear of testicular cancer associated with existing risk factors

Prostate cancer is one of the leading causes of cancer death in men in the United States (lung cancer is first) (CDC, 2019e). There is no sure way to prevent prostate cancer, but diet and lifestyle behaviors are thought to help with prevention. In almost all aging men, the prostate enlarges (BPH).

The decision to screen for prostate cancer for men aged 55 to 69 years should be an individual one, based on discussion of benefits and harms with their health care provider. For men 70 years and above, the USPSTF recommends against screening for prostate cancer (USPSTF, 2019).

Teach clients behaviors found to lower risk of prostate cancer:
- Frequent ejaculation, especially early in adulthood (Harvard Medical School, 2019)
- Eating a diet high in fruits and vegetables (at least 2½ cups of a variety of vegetables and fruits daily), staying physically active (exercise most days of the week), and maintaining a healthy weight (ACS, 2019)
- Taking vitamin E and selenium (ambivalent study results)
- Possible preventive effect from medications for BPH; aspirin (unclear results)
- Sleeping in a completely dark room
- Avoiding shift work that requires daytime sleep
- Drink green tea daily (Moffitt Cancer Center, 2019, is undertaking one study of the possible relation of green tea to prostate cancer)

Observe for the following symptoms (which may or may not be present, but are likely in more advanced stages of prostate cancer and report to health care provider; Mayo Clinic, 2020):
- Trouble urinating
- Decreased force in the stream of urine
- Blood in the semen
- Discomfort in the pelvic area
- Bone pain
- Erectile dysfunction

Client Concern: *Risk for acquiring STD associated with frequent unprotected intercourse with multiple partners*

Teach early warning signs and symptoms of STD. Discuss methods of prevention (limit to one uninfected partner and use of condoms) and modes of transmission. Routine screening for infection is recommended during pelvic examination (Healthy People 2030).

Because HIV is preventable, knowing risks and practicing risk-reducing behaviors will help to stem the epidemic of this infection. The World Health Organization (WHO, 2019) lists the following risks for HIV:
- Having unprotected anal or vaginal sex
- Having another STI, such as syphilis, herpes, chlamydia, gonorrhea, or bacterial vaginosis
- Sharing contaminated needles, syringes, other injecting equipment, and drug solutions when injecting drugs
- Receiving unsafe injections, blood transfusions and tissue transplantation, and medical procedures that involve unsterile cutting or piercing
- Experiencing accidental needlestick injuries, especially among health care workers

Teach clients to use precautions to decrease transfer of body fluids:

- Avoid unprotected sex (condom use, if used throughout the sexual act, used 100% of the time for every sexual encounter, and used correctly, has been shown to lower risk of HIV transmission to below 8%) (CDC, 2019d).
- Avoid having multiple sex partners.
- Avoid anal sex.
- Avoid intravenous drug use.
- Avoid mixing sex and alcohol or drugs.
- If you take medications requiring needle use, use a new, sterile needle each time.
- Consider circumcision, if uncircumcised and lifestyle is risky (WHO, 2020).
- Follow CDC guidelines for handling body secretions, objects that touch bodily secretions, or contaminated items.
- Openly discuss HIV risk behavior history with partner and use above precautions.
  If client already has HIV/AIDS, teach client to:
- Eat healthy, well-rounded diet.
- Avoid food and drink that may easily transmit foodborne illness (e.g., raw eggs, unpasteurized dairy products, raw seafood, undercooked meat [cook well done]).

- Get immunizations against other illnesses if allowed by physician.
- Be aware that companion animals may harbor parasites that can cause infections.
- Tell your sex partner right away if you are HIV positive.
- Seek support from support group to deal with your emotions.
- Obtain and stay on antiretroviral protocol, if available.

Client Concern: *Impaired sexual functioning associated with impotence related to unknown etiology and/or poor partner communication and deficient knowledge of psychological and physical health and sexual performance*

Explore possible etiologies and alternate forms of sexual satisfaction. Refer to urologist for information on penile implants, surgery, and other alternatives.

Teach effects and benefits of exercise. Explore communication with partner. Refer to counselor (psychiatric, sexual, marriage) as needed. Provide adequate literature on sex and health teaching for client.

Client Concern: *Impaired sexual functioning associated with loss of body part or physiologic limitations*

Explore prior sexual patterns. Explore alternatives. Provide resource material on self-help groups (e.g., Ostomy Association). Suggest use of foreplay and lubricants to increase secretions as necessary. Provide literature and referrals.

 Client Concern: *Poor bowel and bladder control related to lack of routine elimination pattern associated with lack of parental knowledge of healthy toilet-training techniques*

Teach parents the importance of physiologic and psychological readiness in toilet training. Explain use of "potty chairs" and that bowel control precedes bladder control. Inform parents of the benefits of positive reinforcement and that nocturnal enuresis may persist up to the age of 4 to 5 years.

 Client Concern: *Opportunity to promote sexual education associated with parent requesting advice for answering sexuality questions from child*

Sexual education is recommended in the early school years. Assess what child already knows and what they are ready to know.

Fourth to fifth grades: Interested in conception and birth

Fifth to sixth grades: Interested in their bodies and opposite sex changes. Education on birth control may be appropriate because of early experimentation. Discuss normal development of secondary sexual characteristics and the normal psychological changes associated with puberty. The CDC now recommends administering the human papillomavirus (HPV) vaccine at 11 to 12 years of age for boys and girls to prevent the HPV; and for anyone up to age 26 if not previously vaccinated (CDC, 2020a).

Adolescent: Teach the importance of abstinence or use of condoms if currently sexually active. Explain that there is a higher risk of HIV infection if you have another STD. Risks include anal, vaginal, or oral sex without a condom, having multiple sex partners, especially if anonymous partners, and having sex while under the influence of drugs or alcohol (CDC, 2020b).

 Client Concern: *Potential complication: Prostate hypertrophy*

Teach client about effects of normal enlargement of prostate on urination (frequency, dribbling, and nocturia). Men over 50 years of age should discuss with their health care provider the benefits and risks of having prostate cancer screening, including yearly DREs and PSA testing.

References

American Cancer Society. (2018). *American Cancer Society guideline for colorectal screening.* https://www.cancer.org/cancer/colon-rectal-cancer/detection-diagnosis-staging/acs-recommendations.html

American Cancer Society. (2019). *Prostate cancer risk factors.* https://www.cancer.org/cancer/prostate-cancer/causes-risks-prevention/risk-factors.html

Centers for Disease Control and Prevention. (2019a). *About HIV.* https://www.cdc.gov/hiv/basics/whatishiv.html

Centers for Disease Control and Prevention. (2019b). *AIDS and opportunistic infections.* https://www.cdc.gov/hiv/basics/livingwithhiv/opportunisticinfections.html

Centers for Disease Control and Prevention (CDC). (2021). Ways HIV can be transmitted. Available at https://www.cdc.gov/hiv/basics/hiv-transmission/ways-people-get-hiv.html

Centers for Disease Control and Prevention. (2019d). *Condom use.* https://www.cdc.gov/hiv/clinicians/prevention/condoms.html

Centers for Disease Control and Prevention. (2019e) *New CDC report: STDs continue to rise in the U.S.* https://www.cdc.gov/nchhstp/newsroom/2019/2018-STD-surveillance-report-press-release.html

Centers for Disease Control and Prevention. (2020a). *HPV vaccine recommendations.* https://www.cdc.gov/vaccines/vpd/hpv/hcp/recommendations.html

Centers for Disease Control and Prevention. (2020b). *STDs and HIV—CDC Fact Sheet.* https://www.cdc.gov/std/hiv/stdfact-std-hiv.htm

Centers for Disease Control and Prevention. (2021). *Ways HIV can be transmitted.* https://www.cdc.gov/hiv/basics/hiv-transmission/ways-people-get-hiv.html

Harvard Medical School. (2019). *Ejaculation frequency and prostate cancer.* https://www.health.harvard.edu/mens-health/ejaculation_frequency_and_prostate_cancer

Healthy People 2030. (2020). *Sexually transmitted infections.* https://health.gov/healthypeople/objectives-and-data/browse-objectives/sexually-transmitted-infections

Jewell, T. (2018). *11 things to know about penile bisection (penis splitting).* https://www.healthline.com/health/penis-splitting

Martin, R. (2018). *Rites of circumcision.* https://www.psychologytoday.com/us/blog/how-we-do-it/201810/rites-circumcision

Mayo Clinic. (2020). *Prostate cancer.* https://www.mayoclinic.org/diseases-conditions/prostate-cancer/symptoms-causes/syc-20353087

Moffitt Cancer Center. (2019). *Is green tea beneficial to prostate health?* https://moffitt.org/endeavor/archive/is-green-tea-beneficial-to-prostate-health/

National Cancer Institute. (2019). *Prostate cancer screening (PDQ®)-Patient version.* https://www.cancer.gov/types/prostate/patient/prostate-screening-pdq

U.S. Preventive Services Task Force. (2019). *Final recommendation statement: Human immunodeficiency virus (HIV) infection: Screening.* https://www.uspreventiveservicestaskforce.org/uspstf/recommendation/human-immunodeficiency-virus-hiv-infection-screening

World Health Organization. (2019). *HIV/AIDS.* https://www.who.int/news-room/fact-sheets/detail/hiv-aids

World Health Organization. (2020). *HIV/AIDS: Male circumcision for HIV prevention.* https://www.who.int/hiv/topics/malecircumcision/fact_sheet/en/

23 ASSESSING FEMALE GENITALIA, ANUS, AND RECTUM

Structure and Function Overview

EXTERNAL GENITALIA

The external genitalia include the *vulva* that extends from the mons pubis to the anal opening. The *mons pubis*, a fat pad located over the symphysis pubis covered with pubic hair, protects the symphysis pubis during sexual intercourse. The *labia majora*, the two folds of skin that are composed of adipose tissue, sebaceous glands, and sweat glands, extend from the mons pubis to the perineum. The inner surface of the labia majora is pink, smooth, and moist.

Inside the labia majora are the *labia minora*, folds that join anteriorly at the clitoris and form a *prepuce*, or hood, and join posteriorly to form the *frenulum*. The labia minora contain sebaceous glands that produce lubrication for the vaginal area. The *clitoris*, located at the anterior end of the labia minora, is a small, cylindrical mass of erectile tissue and nerves. The skinfolds of the labia majora and labia minora form a boat-shaped area or fossa called the *vestibule*. Located between the clitoris and the vaginal orifice is the *urethral meatus*. The openings of *Skene glands*, usually not visible, are on either side of the urethral opening and secrete mucus.

Below the urethral meatus is the *vaginal orifice*, covered by the hymen, a fold of membranous tissue that covers a part of the vagina. The *Bartholin glands*, located on both sides of the vagina and not visible to the eye, secrete mucus (Fig. 23-1).

INTERNAL GENITALIA

The internal genital reproductive organs (Fig. 23-2) are the vagina, the uterus, the cervix, the fallopian tubes, and the ovaries. The *vagina*, about 10 cm long, extends up and slightly back toward the rectum from the vaginal orifice to the cervix. It allows the passage of menstrual flow, receives the penis during sexual intercourse, and serves as the birth canal during delivery. The *cervix* (or neck of the uterus) separates the upper end of the vagina from the isthmus of the uterus. The junction of the isthmus and the cervix forms the *internal os*, and the junction of the cervix and the vagina forms the *external os*. The cervix allows the entrance of sperm into the uterus, allows the passage of menstrual flow, and secretes mucus and prevents the entrance of vaginal bacteria. During childbirth, the cervix can stretch to allow the passage of the fetus. The *uterus*, a pear-shaped organ, has two components: the *corpus* and the *cervix*. The corpus is divided into the fundus (upper portion), the body (central portion), and the isthmus

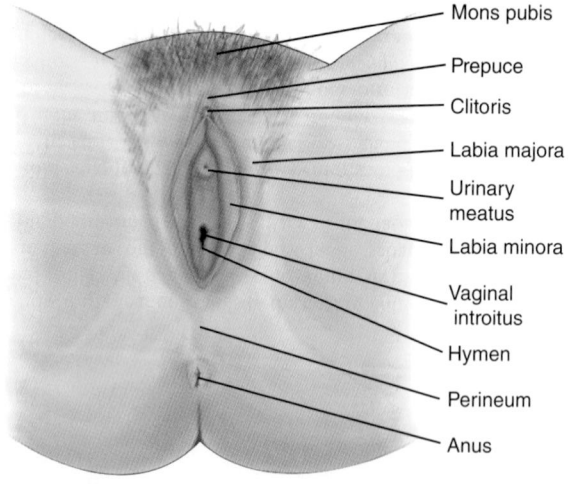

FIGURE 23-1 External female genitalia. (Reprinted with permission from Jensen, S. [2019]. *Nursing health assessment: A best practices approach* [3rd ed., Fig. 24-1]. Wolters Kluwer.)

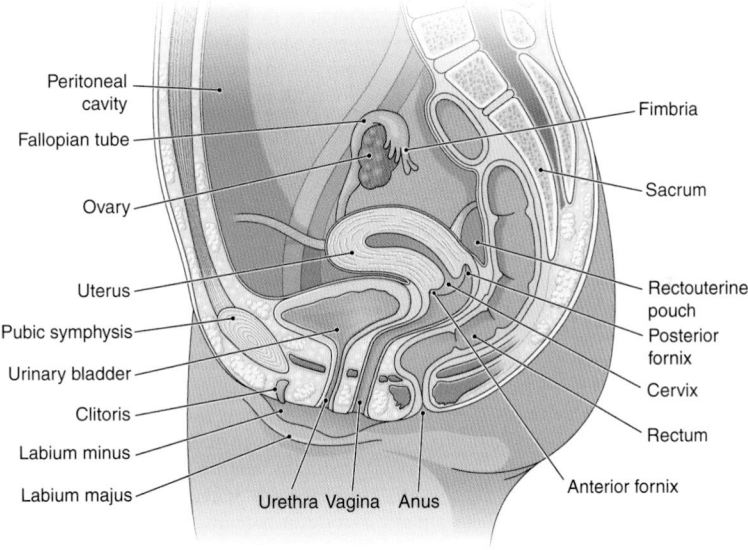

FIGURE 23-2 Internal female reproductive system and relationship to other pelvic structures including the rectum and anus.

(narrow lower portion). The uterus is usually situated in a forward position above the bladder at approximately a 45-degree angle to the vagina when standing. The *endometrium*, the myometrium, and the *peritoneum* are the three layers of the uterine wall. The endometrium, the inner mucosal layer, has glands that secrete an alkaline substance to keep the uterine cavity moist. A portion of the endometrium sheds during menses and childbirth. The myometrium is the middle layer that functions to expel the products of conception. The peritoneum is the outer uterine layer that covers the uterus and separates it from the abdominal cavity. The *ovaries*, small oval-shaped organs, are on the lateral sides of the pelvic cavity and produce ova, estrogen, progesterone, and testosterone. The ovum travels from the ovary to the uterus through the fallopian tubes.

ANUS AND RECTUM

The *anal canal* begins at the anal sphincter and ends at the anorectal junction. It is 2.5 to 4 cm long. Within the anus are the two sphincters that hold the anal canal closed, except when passing gas and feces. The *external sphincter* is composed of skeletal muscle and is under voluntary control. The *internal sphincter* is composed of smooth muscle and is under involuntary control by the autonomic nervous system. Just above the internal sphincter

is the *anorectal junction*, the dividing point of the anal canal and the rectum. The rectum is lined with folds of mucosa, known as the columns of Morgagni, which contain arteries, veins, and visceral nerves. The *rectum* is the lowest portion of the large intestine and is approximately 12 cm long, extending from the end of the *sigmoid colon* to the anorectal junction. It enlarges above the anorectal junction and proceeds in a posterior direction toward the hollow of the sacrum and coccyx, forming the rectal ampulla. The inside of the rectum contains three inward foldings called the valves of Houston. The *peritoneum* lines the upper two-thirds of the anterior rectum and dips down so that it may be palpated where it forms the *rectouterine pouch* in women.

Nursing Assessment

COLLECTING SUBJECTIVE DATA

Interview Questions

Last menstrual period? Length of cycle? Amount of blood flow? Associated symptoms? Age of menarche? Unpleasant odor? Knowledge about toxic shock syndrome? Age of menopause if applicable? Hormone replacement therapy? Vaginal discharge? Pain, itching, or lumps in inguinal/groin area?

Pain with intercourse? Difficulty urinating? Color or odor of urine? Difficulty controlling urine? Stress incontinence? Sexual performance? Activity? Change in libido? Fertility problems/concerns? History of gynecologic problems or sexually transmitted infections (STIs)? Pregnancies? Number of children? Chance of pregnancy now? Family history of reproductive or genital cancer? Self-care: Monthly genital self-examinations? Cotton underwear? Wiping pattern after bowel movement? Douching—how often? Use of contraceptives? Number of sexual partners? Comfort level with talking with sexual partner? Fears related to sex? Tested for human immunodeficiency virus (HIV)? Tested for human papillomavirus (HPV)? Last Pap test? Received HPV vaccine?

Bowel pattern? Constipation? Diarrhea? Character of stools? Rectal itching or pain? Hemorrhoids? Rectal surgery? Last stool test for blood detection? Proctosigmoidoscopy? Last digital rectal examination by a primary care provider? History of polyps, colon, or rectal cancer? Use of laxatives, engagement in anal sex? Usual diet? Amount of fiber? Exercise? Use of calcium supplements? Anal or rectal problems that have affected activities of daily living?

Risk Factors

Risk for cervical cancer related to sexually active female, HPV infection, the first and frequent intercourse at young age, multiple sexual partners, history of STI, multiple births, history of no prior Pap examinations, lower socioeconomic status, low level of education, poor hygiene especially with uncircumcised partner.

COLLECTING OBJECTIVE DATA

Equipment Needed

Some of the following equipment is depicted in Figure 23-3.

- Stool
- Light
- Speculum
- Water-soluble lubricant
- Cotton-tipped applicators
- *Chlamydia* culture tube
- Culturette
- Test tube with water
- Sterile disposable gloves
- Ayre spatula (plastic)

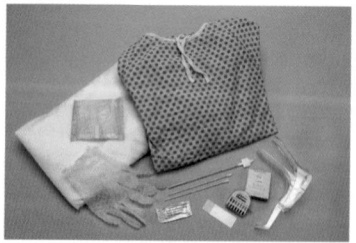

FIGURE 23-3 Some of the equipment needed for female genitalia examination.

- Endocervical cytobroom
- pH paper
- Feminine napkins
- Mirror

Physical Assessment

See Figures 23-1 and 23-2 for a review of the structures and the function of the female genitalia and anorectal structures. Maintain client privacy with a chaperone in the room. Wash hands, wear gloves, and make sure the equipment is between room and body temperatures.

ASSESSMENT PROCEDURE	NORMAL FINDINGS	ABNORMAL FINDINGS
Inspect the **mons pubis.** Wash your hands and put on gloves. As you begin the examination, note the distribution of pubic hair. Also be alert for signs of infestation.	Pubic hair is distributed in an inverted triangular pattern, and there are no signs of infestation. Some clients may remove or trim pubic hair and may have piercing of the genitals.	Lice or nits (eggs) at the base of the pubic hairs indicate infestation with pediculosis pubis, referred to as "crabs," which is most often transmitted by sexual contact.
Observe and palpate **inguinal lymph nodes.**	No enlargement or swelling of the lymph nodes.	Enlarged inguinal nodes may indicate a vaginal infection or irritation from hair removal.

ASSESSMENT PROCEDURE	NORMAL FINDINGS	ABNORMAL FINDINGS
Inspect the **labia majora and perineum.** Observe the labia majora and perineum for lesions, swelling, and excoriation.	Labia majora equal in size and free of lesions, swelling, and excoriation. A healed tear or episiotomy scar may be visible on the perineum if the client has given birth. Perineum smooth. Labia of a woman who has not delivered offspring vaginally will meet in the middle. The labia of a woman who has delivered vaginally will not meet in the middle and may appear shriveled. It is increasingly common to find piercings of female genitalia.	Lesions may be from an infectious disease, such as herpes or syphilis (see Abnormal Findings 23-1). Excoriation and swelling may be from scratching or self-treatment of the lesions. Evaluate all lesions and refer the client to a primary care provider for further diagnoses and treatment.
Inspect the **labia minora, clitoris, urethral meatus, and vaginal opening.** Use your gloved hand to separate the labia majora and inspect for lesions, excoriation, swelling, and/or discharge (Fig. 23-4).	Labia minora symmetric, dark pink, and moist. Clitoris is small mound of erectile tissue, sensitive to touch with variation in size. Urethral meatus is small and slitlike. Vaginal opening is positioned below urethral meatus. Size depends on sexual activity or vaginal delivery. A hymen may cover the vaginal opening partially or completely.	Asymmetric labia may indicate abscess. Lesions, swelling, bulging in the vaginal opening, and discharge are abnormal findings. Excoriation may result from the client scratching or self-treating a perineal irritation.

(Continued on following page)

ASSESSMENT PROCEDURE	NORMAL FINDINGS	ABNORMAL FINDINGS
Palpate **Bartholin glands.** If the client has labial swelling or a history of it, palpate Bartholin glands for swelling, tenderness, and discharge. Place index finger in the vaginal opening and thumb on the labia majora. With gentle pinching motion, palpate from the inferior portion of posterior labia majora to the anterior portion. Repeat on the opposite side (Fig. 23-5).	Bartholin glands are usually soft, nontender, and drainage free. 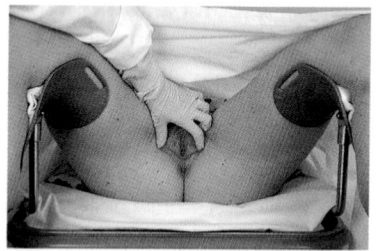 **FIGURE 23-4** Inspecting the labia minora, clitoris, urethral meatus, and vaginal opening.	Swelling, pain, and discharge may result from infection and abscess. If you detect a discharge, obtain and send specimen to laboratory for culture. 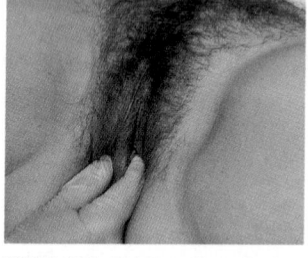 **FIGURE 23-5** Technique for palpating Bartholin gland.
Palpate the urethra. If client reports urethral symptoms or urethritis, or you suspect Skene gland inflammation, insert gloved index finger into superior portion of vagina; push up and out to milk urethra from inside.	No drainage noted from the urethral meatus. Area is soft and nontender.	Drainage from the urethra indicates possible urethritis. Culture any discharge. Urethritis may occur with infection with *Neisseria gonorrhoeae* or *Chlamydia trachomatis.*

ASSESSMENT PROCEDURE	NORMAL FINDINGS	ABNORMAL FINDINGS
Inspect the **size of the vaginal opening and the angle of the vagina** (see Fig. 23-7). Insert gloved index finger into vagina; note size of opening and for thinning or dryness of vaginal lining. Attempt to touch cervix to establish size of the speculum needed for examination and the angle to insert it. Next, while maintaining tension, gently pull the labia majora outward. Note hymenal configuration and transections or injury.	Vaginal opening varies in size according to client's age, sexual history, and whether she has given birth vaginally. Vagina is typically tilted posteriorly at a 45-degree angle and should feel moist.	Vagina becomes thinner and dryer in vaginal atrophy, occurring with lack of estrogen caused by menopause, breastfeeding, surgical removal of ovaries, radiation or chemotherapy, breast cancer hormone treatment, smoking, not having had a vaginal birth, or engaging rarely in sexual activity (Mayo Clinic, 2019).
Inspect the **vaginal musculature.** Keep index finger inserted in the client's vaginal opening. Ask the client to squeeze around your finger.	Client can squeeze around the examiner's finger. Typically, the nulliparous woman can squeeze tighter than the multiparous woman.	Absent or decreased ability to squeeze examiner's finger indicates decreased muscle tone, which may decrease sexual satisfaction.
Use middle and index fingers to separate labia minora. Ask client to bear down.	No bulging and no urinary discharge.	Bulging of anterior wall may indicate cystocele. Bulging of posterior wall may indicate rectocele. If cervix or uterus protrudes down, client may have uterine prolapse (see Abnormal Findings 23-1). Urine leakage may indicate stress incontinence.

(Continued on following page)

ASSESSMENT PROCEDURE	NORMAL FINDINGS	ABNORMAL FINDINGS
Inspect the **cervix.** (Follow the guidelines for using a speculum in Assessment Guide 23-1.) With the speculum inserted in position to visualize the cervix, observe cervical color, size, and position and surface and appearance of the os (Fig. 23-6). Observe discharge or lesions.	Cervix smooth, pink, and even, in midline position, projects 1 to 3 cm into vagina. In pregnant clients, the cervix appears blue (Chadwick sign). Cervical os is small, round opening in nulliparous women and appears slitlike in parous women.	In nonpregnant woman, bluish cervix may indicate cyanosis; in nonmenopausal woman, pale cervix may indicate anemia. Redness seen in inflammation. Asymmetric, reddened areas, strawberry spots, and white patches. Cervical lesions may result from polyps, cancer, or infection. Cervical enlargement or projection into the vagina more than 3 cm may be from prolapse or tumor. Refer for further evaluation.
After inspecting the cervix, obtain specimens for Pap smear and specimens for culture and sensitivity if needed to identify possible STIs. (Follow procedure in Assessment Guide 23-2.)	Cervical secretions clear or white without unpleasant odor. Secretions vary according to timing within menstrual cycle.	Colored, malodorous, or irritating discharge. Specimen should be obtained for culture.
Inspect the **vagina.** Unlock speculum; slowly rotate and remove it noting vaginal color, surface, consistency, and discharge.	The vagina pink, moist, smooth, and free of lesions and irritation. Also free of any colored or malodorous discharge.	Reddened areas, lesions, and colored, malodorous discharge may indicate vaginal infections, STIs, or cancer. Altered pH may indicate infection.

ASSESSMENT PROCEDURE	NORMAL FINDINGS	ABNORMAL FINDINGS

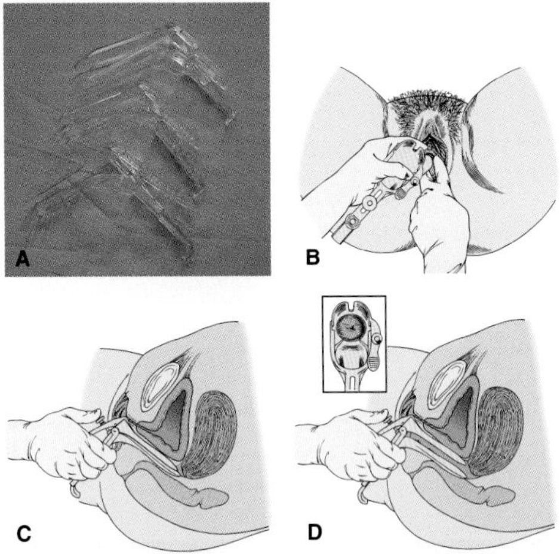

FIGURE 23-6 Speculum insertion for inspection of cervix. **(A)** Select proper size speculum. **(B)** Use right, middle, and index fingers to push the introitus down and open to relax muscle, while inserting the speculum blades downward at a 45-degree angle. **(C)** Withdraw fingers once the blades pass fingers and switch to holding speculum with right hand. **(D)** After the blades are fully inserted, open them by squeezing the handles together to view the full cervix.

(Continued on following page)

ASSESSMENT PROCEDURE	NORMAL FINDINGS	ABNORMAL FINDINGS
If preparing wet mount slide, use cotton swab to collect vaginal secretion specimen from anterior vaginal fornix or lateral vaginal walls before collecting Pap or other specimens. Avoid posterior fornix, contaminated with cervical secretions. Use part of wet mount sample to test vaginal secretion pH.		
BIMANUAL EXAMINATION		
Palpate **vaginal wall** (Fig. 23-7). Tell client you are going to do manual examination; explain purpose. Apply water-soluble lubricant to gloved index and middle fingers of dominant hand. Stand and approach client at correct angle; placing nondominant hand on client's lower abdomen, insert index and middle fingers into vaginal opening. Apply pressure to posterior wall; wait for vaginal opening to relax before palpating vaginal walls for texture and tenderness.	The vaginal wall should feel smooth, and the client should not report any tenderness.	Tenderness or lesions may indicate infection.

ASSESSMENT PROCEDURE	NORMAL FINDINGS	ABNORMAL FINDINGS

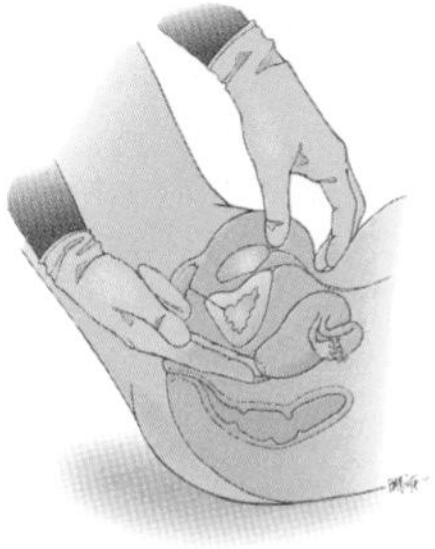

FIGURE 23-7 Palpating the vaginal walls.

Palpate **cervix**. Advance fingers until they touch cervix and run fingers around circumference palpating for: • Contour • Consistency • Mobility • Tenderness	Cervix firm and soft (like the tip of your nose). Rounded and can be moved somewhat from side to side without causing tenderness.	A hard, immobile cervix may indicate cancer. Pain with movement of the cervix (cervical motion tenderness [CMT]) may indicate infection (Chandelier sign).

(Continued on following page)

BIMANUAL EXAMINATION (*continued*)

ASSESSMENT PROCEDURE	NORMAL FINDINGS	ABNORMAL FINDINGS
Palpate the **uterus.** Move fingers intravaginally into opening above cervix and gently press hand resting on abdomen downward, squeezing uterus between two hands (Fig. 23-8). Note uterine size, position, shape, and consistency.	Fundus, the large, upper end of the uterus, is round, firm, and smooth. In most women, it is at the level of pubis; cervix is aimed posteriorly (anteverted position) with variation of other positions.	Enlarged uterus above level of the pubis is abnormal; an irregular shape suggests abnormalities such as myomas (fibroid tumors) or endometriosis.

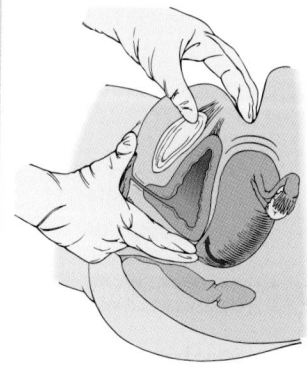

FIGURE 23-8 Palpating the uterus.

ASSESSMENT PROCEDURE	NORMAL FINDINGS	ABNORMAL FINDINGS
Attempt to bounce the uterus between your two hands to assess mobility and tenderness.	The normal uterus moves freely and is not tender.	A fixed or tender uterus may indicate fibroids, infection, or masses.
Palpate the **ovaries.** Slide intravaginal fingers toward left ovary in left lateral fornix; place abdominal hand on left lower abdominal quadrant. Press abdominal hand toward your intravaginal fingers and attempt to palpate ovary (Fig. 23-9).	Ovaries approximately 3 cm × 2 cm × 1 cm (or the size of a walnut) and almond shaped.	Enlarged size, masses, immobility, and extreme tenderness are abnormal and should be evaluated.

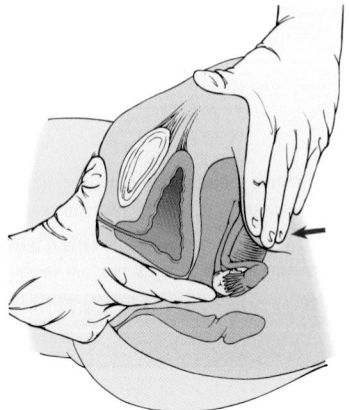

FIGURE 23-9 Palpating the ovaries.

(Continued on following page)

BIMANUAL EXAMINATION (*continued*)

ASSESSMENT PROCEDURE	NORMAL FINDINGS	ABNORMAL FINDINGS
Slide your intravaginal fingers to right lateral fornix, attempting to palpate right ovary. Note size, shape, consistency, mobility, and tenderness. Withdraw your intravaginal hand and inspect glove for secretions. **Note:** *It is normal for ovaries to be difficult or impossible to palpate in obese women, in postmenopausal women because ovaries atrophy, or in women who are tense during examination.*	Ovaries are firm, smooth, mobile, and somewhat tender on palpation. A clear, minimal amount of drainage appearing on the glove from the vagina is normal.	Large amounts of colorful, frothy, or malodorous secretions are abnormal. Ovaries that are palpable 3 to 5 years after menopause are also abnormal.

RECTOVAGINAL EXAMINATION

Explain procedure and purpose. Warn client of possible discomfort as if she wants to move bowels but she will not. Encourage her to relax. **Change the glove** on your dominant hand and lubricate index and middle fingers with water-soluble lubricant.		

ASSESSMENT PROCEDURE	NORMAL FINDINGS	ABNORMAL FINDINGS
Ask client to bear down to relax sphincter and insert your index finger into vaginal orifice and middle finger into the rectum (Fig. 23-10). Push down on abdominal wall with other hand, palpate internal reproductive structures through the anterior rectal wall. Note area behind cervix, rectovaginal septum, the cul-de-sac, and posterior uterine wall. Withdraw vaginal finger and continue with rectal examination.	The rectovaginal septum is normally smooth, thin, movable, and firm. The posterior uterine wall is normally smooth, firm, round, movable, and nontender.	Masses, thickened structures, immobility, and tenderness are abnormal.

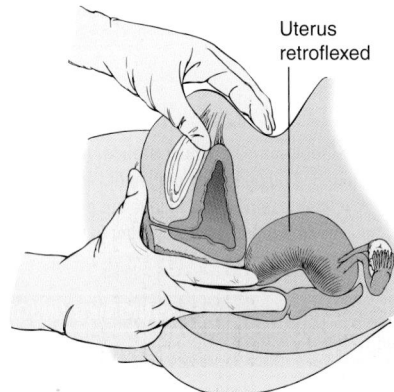

Uterus retroflexed

FIGURE 23-10 Hands positioned for rectovaginal examination.

(*Continued on following page*)

ANUS AND RECTUM		
ASSESSMENT PROCEDURE	**NORMAL FINDINGS**	**ABNORMAL FINDINGS**
Inspection		
Inspect the **perianal area.** Spread the client's buttocks and inspect the anal opening and surrounding area for: • Lumps • Ulcers • Lesions • Rashes • Redness • Fissures • Thickening of the epithelium	Anal opening hairless, moist, and tightly closed. Skin around the anal opening coarser and more darkly pigmented. Surrounding perianal area free of redness, lumps, ulcers, lesions, and rashes.	Lesions may indicate STIs, cancer, or hemorrhoids. A thrombosed external hemorrhoid appears swollen, is itchy, painful, and bleeds when passing stool. Previously thrombosed hemorrhoid appears as skin tag protruding from anus. A painful, hardened, red mass suggests perianal abscess. A swollen skin tag on anal margin may indicate anal canal fissure. Redness and excoriation seen with scratching areas infected by fungi or pinworms. Small opening in skin surrounding anal opening may be an anorectal fistula. Thickened epithelium seen in repeated anal intercourse trauma.
Ask the client to perform Valsalva maneuver by straining or bearing down. Inspect anal opening for any bulges or lesions.	No bulging or lesions appear.	Bulges of red mucous membrane may indicate a rectal prolapse. Hemorrhoids or an anal fissure may also be seen.

ASSESSMENT PROCEDURE	NORMAL FINDINGS	ABNORMAL FINDINGS
Inspect the sacrococcygeal area for swelling, redness, dimpling, or hair.	Area is smooth and free of redness and hair.	Reddened, swollen, or dimpled area covered by a small tuft of hair located midline on lower sacrum suggests a pilonidal cyst.
Palpation		
Palpate the **anus.** Explain procedure and that it may feel like her bowels are going to move but will not. Lubricate gloved index finger; ask client to bear down and place pad of index finger on anal opening and apply slight pressure to relax sphincter. ***Note:*** *Never use fingertip as this causes sphincter to tighten and, if forced into the rectum, may cause pain.*	Sphincter relaxes, permitting entry.	Sphincter tightens preventing further examination.
When you feel sphincter relax, insert finger gently with pad facing down. ***Note:*** *If severe pain prevents your entrance to the anus, do not force the examination.*	Examination finger enters anus.	Examination finger cannot enter the anus.

(Continued on following page)

ANUS AND RECTUM (*continued*)

ASSESSMENT PROCEDURE	NORMAL FINDINGS	ABNORMAL FINDINGS
If sphincter does not relax and client reports severe pain, spread gluteal folds with hands close to anus and attempt to visualize a lesion that may be causing the pain. If tension is maintained on gluteal folds for 60 seconds, the anus will dilate normally.		
Ask client to tighten the external sphincter; note the tone.	Client can close the sphincter around the gloved finger.	Poor sphincter tone may be due to spinal cord injury, previous surgery, trauma, or prolapsed rectum. Tightened sphincter tone may indicate anxiety, scarring, or inflammation.
Rotate finger to examine muscular anal ring. Palpate for tenderness, nodules, and hardness.	Anus smooth, nontender, and free of nodules and hardness.	Tenderness may indicate hemorrhoids, fistula, or fissure. Nodules may indicate polyps or cancer. Hardness may indicate scarring or cancer.
Palpate the **rectum:** Insert finger further into rectum as far as possible. Next, turn hand clockwise and then counterclockwise to allow palpation of as much rectal surface as possible. Note tenderness, irregularities, nodules, and hardness.	Rectal mucosa soft, smooth, nontender, and free of nodules.	Hardness and irregularities may be from scarring or cancer. Nodules may indicate polyps or cancer.

ASSESSMENT PROCEDURE	NORMAL FINDINGS	ABNORMAL FINDINGS
Palpate the cervix through the anterior rectal wall.	Cervix palpated as small round mass. May also palpate tampon or retroverted uterus. No blood noted on gloved finger when removed.	Bright red blood on gloved finger when removed. Large mass palpated. Do not mistake tampon for mass.
Check Stool		
Inspect stool on withdrawn gloved finger for color and test feces for occult blood. Provide client with a towel to wipe the anorectal area.	Stool is semisolid, brown, and free of blood.	Black stool may indicate upper gastrointestinal bleeding, gray or tan stool results from lack of bile pigment, and yellow stool suggests steatorrhea (increased fat content). Blood detected in stool may indicate rectal or colon cancer. Refer client for colon endoscopic examination.

ASSESSMENT GUIDE 23-1 Using a Speculum

1. Before using the speculum, choose the instrument that is the correct size for the client. Vaginal speculums come in two basic types:
   • *Graves speculum*—appropriate for most adult women and available in various lengths and widths.

• *Pederson speculum*—appropriate for virgins and some postmenopausal women who have a narrow vaginal orifice. Speculums can be metal, with a thumbscrew that is tightened to lock the blades in place, or plastic, with a clip that is locked to keep the blades in place. (Plastic speculums are shown in Fig. A.)

(Continued on following page)

ASSESSMENT GUIDE 23-1   Using a Speculum (*continued*)

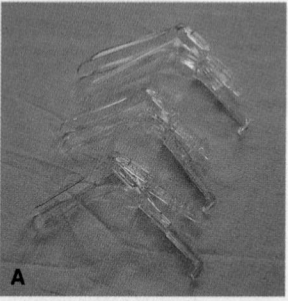

A

2. Encourage the client to take deep breaths and to maintain her feet in the stirrups with her knees resting in an open, relaxed manner.
3. Place two fingers of your gloved, nondominant hand against the posterior vaginal wall and wait for relaxation to occur.
4. Insert the fingers of your gloved nondominant hand about 2.5 cm into the vagina and spread them slightly while pushing down against the posterior vagina (Fig. B).

5. Lubricate the blades of the speculum with vaginal secretions from the client. Do not use commercial lubricants on the speculum. Lubricants are typically bacteriostatic and will alter vaginal pH and the cell specimens collected for cytologic, bacterial, and viral analysis.
6. Hold the speculum with two fingers around the blades and the thumb under the screw or lock. This is important for keeping the blades closed. Position the speculum so that the blades are vertical.
7. Insert the speculum between your fingers into the posterior portion of the vaginal orifice at a 45-degree angle downward. When the blades pass your fingers inside the vagina, rotate the closed speculum so that the blades are in a horizontal position.

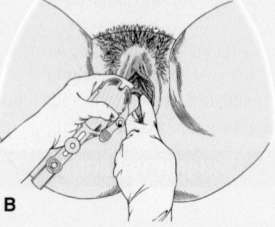

B

⊚ **CLINICAL TIP**
Be careful during the speculum insertion not to pinch the labia or pull the pubic hair. If the vaginal orifice seems tight or you are having trouble inserting the speculum, ask the client to bear down. This may help relax the muscles of the perineum and promote opening of the orifice.

8. Continue inserting the speculum until the base touches the fingertips inside the vagina.

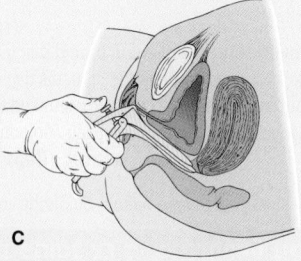

C

9. Remove the fingers of your gloved nondominant hand from the client's posterior vagina (Fig. C).
10. Press handles together (Fig. D) to open blades and allow visualization of the cervix.
11. Secure the speculum in place by tightening the thumbscrew or locking the plastic clip (Fig. D).

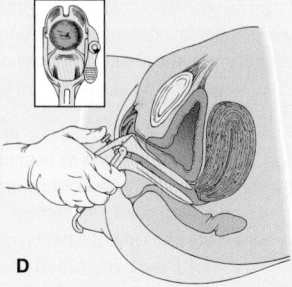

D

ASSESSMENT GUIDE 23-2   Obtaining Tissue Specimens for Analysis

Some methods for obtaining female tissue specimens follow.

Papanicolaou (Pap) Smear

Liquid-based technology has improved the accuracy of findings to test for human papillomavirus (HPV) and determine the HPV type. The specimen for the Pap smear is obtained using a wooden spatula, cotton swab, or brush and placed in the preservative solution slide (Lab Tests Online, 2021).

Obtaining an Ectocervical and Endocervical Specimen

This procedure is performed on nonpregnant clients. This combined procedure uses a special cytobroom to collect *both* endocervical and ectocervical cells. (1) Insert cytobroom into the cervical os rotating cytobroom in a full circle five times, collecting cells from squamocolumnar junction and cervical surface. (2) Withdraw cytobroom. (3) Swish cytobroom in the preservative solution by pushing cytobroom into the bottom of the vial 10 times, forcing the bristles apart. Swirl cytobroom vigorously to further release material. (4) Discard the cytobroom. (5) Tighten cap on preservative and send to laboratory.

Obtaining an Ectocervical Specimen

(1) Insert one end of plastic spatula into the cervical os. (2) Press down rotating spatula, scraping cervix and transformation zone (squamocolumnar junction) in a full circle. (3) Withdraw spatula. (4) Rinse spatula in preservative solution by swishing spatula vigorously in vial 10 times. (5) Discard spatula.

Obtaining an Endocervical Specimen

(1) Insert endocervical brush into cervical os rotating brush one half turn in one direction gently to minimize possible bleeding. (2) Withdraw brush. (3) Rinse brush in preservative solution by rotating device in solution 10 times while pushing against vial wall. Swirl brush vigorously to further release material. (4) Discard brush. (5) Tighten cap on solution. (6) Record client's name and date on vial to send to laboratory.

Vaginal Specimen

1. Select appropriate-sized, warmed speculum, testing on client's leg for comfortable temperature.
2. Insert speculum at 45-degree angle, rotate, and open when completely inserted.

3. Obtain a specimen of vaginal fluid from the posterior fornix.
4. On a glass slide, place a drop of sodium chloride (NaCl) and a drop of potassium hydroxide (KOH) on separate ends of the slide.
5. Mix small amount of vaginal fluid with each solution and apply cover-slip (Association of Professors of Gynecology and Obstetrics, 2008).

Culture Specimens: Gonorrhea and Chlamydia
Specimens for gonorrhea or *Chlamydia* cultures are obtained if you suspect the client has these sexually transmitted diseases. The exact procedures for gathering and preparing the specimens vary according to each laboratory's policy.

ABNORMAL FINDINGS | **23-1** | **Abnormalities of the External Genitalia and Vaginal Opening**

When assessing the female genitalia, the nurse will see various abnormal lesions on the external genitalia as well as abnormal bulging in the vaginal opening. Some common findings that appear are as follows.

SYPHILITIC CHANCRE
Syphilitic chancres often first appear on the perianal area as silvery-white papules that become superficial red ulcers. Syphilitic chancres are painless. They are sexually transmitted and usually develop at the site of initial contact with the infecting organism.

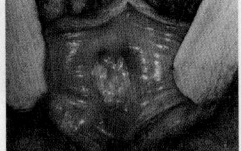

GENITAL WARTS
Genital warts, caused by the HPV, are moist, fleshy lesions on the labia and within the vestibule. They are painless and believed to be sexually transmitted.

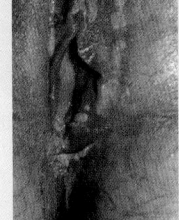

(Continued on following page)

ABNORMAL FINDINGS   **23-1**   **Abnormalities of the External Genitalia and Vaginal Opening (*continued*)**

GENITAL HERPES SIMPLEX

The initial outbreak of herpes may have many small, painful ulcers with erythematous base. Recurrent herpes lesions are usually not as extensive.

CYSTOCELE

A cystocele is a bulging in the anterior vaginal wall caused by thickening of the pelvic musculature. As a result, the bladder, covered by vaginal mucosa, prolapses into the vagina.

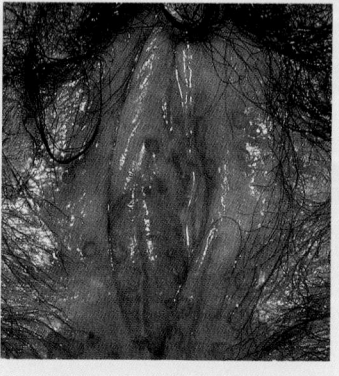
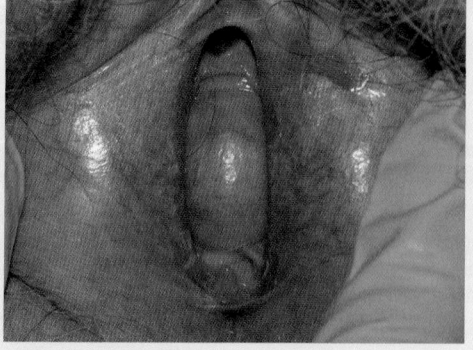

RECTOCELE

A rectocele is a bulging in the posterior vaginal wall caused by weakening of the pelvic musculature. Part of the rectum covered by the vaginal mucosa protrudes into the vagina.

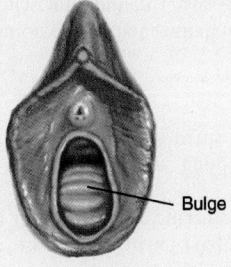

Bulge

UTERINE PROLAPSE

Uterine prolapse occurs when the uterus protrudes into the vagina. It is graded according to how far it protrudes into the vagina. In first-degree prolapse, the cervix is seen at the vaginal opening; in second-degree prolapse, the uterus bulges outside the vaginal opening in third-degree prolapse, the uterus bulges completely out of the vagina.

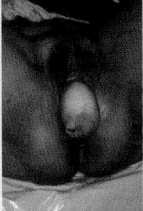

Photo credits: Syphilitic chancre, CNRI/Science Source; Genital warts and Cystocele, Reprinted with permission from Edwards, L., & Lynch, P. (2018). *Genital dermatology Atlas and manual* (3rd ed., Figs. 8-43 and 16-31). Wolters Kluwer; Genital herpes simplex, Reprinted with permission from Nath, J. (2019). *Programmed learning approach to medical terminology* (3rd ed., Fig. 14-9). Wolters Kluwer; Prolapsed uterus, Scott Camazine/Sue Trainor/Science Source.

PEDIATRIC VARIATIONS

Interview Questions

During puberty: Development of secondary sexual characteristics? Previous education on sexual development and activities? Use of contraceptives? Type? Age of menarche? Frequency of menstrual periods? Amount of flow? Pain? Irregularities? Attitude toward menstrual cycle?

Loss of hymenal tissue between the 3 and 9 o'clock position indicates trauma (penetration by digits, penis, or foreign objects) in children.

Physical Assessment

Inspection and palpation of external genitalia constitute the *total* genitourinary assessment until puberty. Assessment of the level of sexual development usually begins at approximately age 11 years. This determination involves the assessment of secondary characteristics associated with sexual maturity. Table 23-1 summarizes the timing of sexual development for girls.

GERIATRIC VARIATIONS

- Due to decreased natural vaginal lubrication, make sure that instruments are well lubricated. If there is vaginal stenosis, only one gloved finger may be needed for the bimanual examination. If the older person has arthritis, a mild analgesic or anti-inflammatory medicine may be taken to ease comfort for examination positioning.
- Bladder capacity decreases to 250 mL owing to periurethral atrophy.
- Pubic hair may become gray, thin, and sparse.
- Mons pubis is smaller with flatter labia due to thinner skin and decreased fat deposits.
- Clitoris decreases in size.
- Estrogen production decreases, causing atrophy of the vaginal mucosa.
- Decrease in size and elasticity of labia; constriction of vaginal opening.
- Diminished vaginal secretions and decreased elasticity of vaginal walls.
- Shortened and narrowed vaginal vault.
- Cervix appears pale after menopause.
- Uterus is smaller and firmer.
- Nonpalpable ovaries.
- Women over age 65 years who have had regular cervical cancer testing in the past 10 years with normal results should not be tested for cervical cancer. Once testing is stopped, it should

TABLE 23-1   Tanner Sexual Maturity Rating: Female Pubic Hair Growth and Breast Development

Developmental Stage	Pubic Hair	Breast
Stage 1	Prepubertal: no pubic hair; fine vellus hair	Prepubertal: elevation of nipple only
Stage 2	Sparse, long, straight, downy hair	Breast bud stage; elevation of breast and nipple as small mound, enlargement of areolar diameter

(*Continued on following page*)

TABLE 23-1 **Tanner Sexual Maturity Rating: Female Pubic Hair Growth and Breast Development** (*continued*)

Developmental Stage	Pubic Hair	Breast
Stage 3	Darker, coarser, curly; sparse over mons pubis	Enlargement of the breasts and areola with no separation of contours
Stage 4	Dark, curly, and abundant on mons pubis; no growth on medial thighs	Projection of areola and nipple to form secondary mound above the level of breast

Developmental Stage	Pubic Hair	Breast
Stage 5	Adult pattern of inverse triangle; growth on medial thighs	Adult configuration; projection of nipple only, areola receded into contour of breast

not be started again. Women who have had a total hysterectomy for any reason other than cervical precancer should stop texting. If done for precancer, then testinng should continue. People vaccinated for HPV should still follow guidelines for screening (CDC, 2021).

CULTURAL VARIATIONS

- In pubertal rites in some cultures, the clitoris is surgically removed and the labia are sutured, leaving only a small opening for menstrual flow. Once married, the woman undergoes surgery to reopen the labia (World Health Organization, 2020).

- Menarche (beginning of menstruation) tends to occur earlier in women living in developed countries and later in women who live in undeveloped countries.
- Women living in resource-poor countries have earlier menopause (Isaac, 2016).

POSSIBLE COLLABORATIVE PROBLEMS—RISK OF

- Bladder perforation
- Urinary tract infection
- Pelvic inflammatory disease
- Genitalia ulcers or lesions
- Obstruction of urethra
- Hemorrhage
- Hormonal imbalances
- Renal failure
- Renal calculi
- Hypermenorrhea
- Polymenorrhea

Teaching Tips for Selected Client Concerns and Collaborative Problems

Client Concern: *Opportunity to enhance female reproductive and urinary health as client requested information regarding urinary health and prevention of cervical cancer*

Teach client to drink eight glasses of fluid per day and to limit intake of alcohol, caffeine, and carbonated beverages. Teach client to avoid bubble baths and scented tissue that may irritate urethra. Teach female client to wear cotton underwear and to wipe perineum from front to back when cleansing.

Teach client ways to prevent cervical cancer as follows:

- Avoid risky sexual practices: Do not have multiple partners; avoid high-risk sexual activities and partners who participate in these. Avoid sex before the age of 13 because this has been associated with increased sexual risk behaviors among teens and young adults, including STIs, alcohol use, delinquency, violence, and unintended pregnancies (*Life Course Indicator: Early Sexual Intercourse*, 2014; Magnusson et al., 2019).
- Consult with a health care professional about having an HPV vaccination for boys and girls as early as 9 years old and up to 26 years old, but especially between the ages of 10 and 11 years (American Congress of Obstetricians and Gynecologists [ACOG], 2019).
- Follow the U.S. Preventive Services Task Force (USPSTF) guidelines for routine Pap smears (USPSTF, 2018).
- If your mother took diethylstilbestrol (DES) to prevent miscarriage, maintain a careful preventive screening schedule.
- Eat nutritious food and have routine care for illnesses that weaken your immune system.
- Talk to your partner about your expectations of sexual health before becoming intimate.

Teach alternate forms of birth control, proper use of methods, and advantages and disadvantages of each. Discuss the importance of increasing vitamin B_6 and folic acid in the diet because of malabsorption of these vitamins while taking birth control pills. Instruct on use of alternate birth control for 3 months after discontinuing the pill to reestablish menstrual cycle before attempting to conceive.

Approach sexuality as a normal part of activities of daily living. The ACS (2020b) recommends that an annual Pap test and pelvic examination should be done at age 21 (not before). The Pap test may be performed less frequently at the discretion of the health care provider.

Note: There is much controversy over pelvic examinations, when they should begin, when they should no longer be done, and how extensive the examination should be (bimanual palpation or not). The ACS (2020b) dropped pelvic examination from early detection recommendations for cancer screening of persons without symptoms. The ACOG (2018) suggested that pelvic examination is still important, but only with consultation of provider and for persons with symptoms. The USPSTF (2017) found that there is insufficient evidence to determine the benefits or harms of performing screening pelvic examinations in asymptomatic, nonpregnant adult women (does not apply to pelvic examinations performed for the purposes of screening for specific disorders for which the USPSTF has already issued a recommendation; i.e., cervical cancer, gonorrhea, and chlamydia). The USPSTF (2014) recommended that all women aged 24 years or younger who are sexually active, or older women at risk for infection, be screened for STIs.

Women at high risk for endometrial cancer (major risk factors: weak immune system, estrogen replacement therapy, tamoxifen, early menarche, late menopause, never having children, and history of failure to ovulate; other risk factors: infertility, diabetes, gallbladder disease, hypertension, obesity, or having hereditary nonpolyposis colorectal cancer [HNPCC]) should have an endometrial biopsy at menopause and thereafter at the physician's discretion; or a yearly biopsy starting at age 35 for those with HNPCC (ACS, 2020a).

Note: **The Centers for Disease Control and Prevention (CDC, 2019c) changed its recommendation regarding offering serologic testing for Zika virus to asymptomatic pregnant women. This testing is no longer recommended as the antibodies for Zika may remain for long periods of time and may not indicate disease.**

Client Concern: Opportunity to improve health maintenance during menopause

Inform client that pregnancy may still occur during early menopausal years. Instruct to consume calcium 1,200 mg/day along with a well-balanced diet (NIH, 2021). Explain that water-soluble lubricant may be used for vaginal dryness if intercourse is painful. Explain ways to help client cope with hot flashes (e.g., use of cool clothing, fans, showers, cool drinks; avoidance of red wine, aged cheeses, and chocolate—these contain tyramine, which can trigger hot flashes).

Client Concern: Opportunity to improve bowel health associated with request to improve bowel health and current lack of exercise regimen and poor dietary habits

Teach the importance of balanced diet high in fiber, regular exercise pattern, and adequate water/fluid intake.

The ACS (2018) updated recommendation for colorectal cancer screening, moving to an earlier age for initial screening, from age 50 to age 45. For those at increased risk (genetics, history of cancer or polyps, or prior abdominal radiation), screening should begin at age 40. Screening can be with either a high-sensitivity stool-based test or a visual examination, such as colonoscopy (in which any polyps found can be removed during the examination).

Client Concern: Poor sexual functioning and relationships associated with ineffective partner communication, deficient knowledge of psychological and physical health and sexual performance, loss of body part, or physiologic limitations (e.g., dyspareunia with aging)

Teach effects and benefits of exercise. Explore communication with partner. Refer to counselor (psychiatric, sexual, marriage) as needed. Provide adequate literature on sex and health teaching for client.

Explore prior sexual patterns. Explore alternatives. Provide resource material on self-help groups (e.g., Ostomy Association, Reach for Recovery). Suggest use of foreplay and lubricants to increase secretions as necessary. Provide literature and referrals.

 Client Concern: Risk for impaired elimination pattern related to parental knowledge deficit of toilet-training techniques

Teach parents the importance of physiologic and psychological readiness in toilet training. Explain the use of "potty chairs" and that bowel control precedes bladder control. Inform parents of the benefits of positive reinforcement and that nocturnal enuresis may persist up to age 4 to 5 years.

 Client Concern: *Opportunity to enhance sexual function*

Sexual education is recommended in the early school years. Assess what child already knows and what they are ready to know.

Fourth to fifth grades: Interested in conception and birth.

Fifth to sixth grades: Interested in their bodies and opposite sex changes. Education on birth control may be appropriate because of early experimentation. Discuss normal development of secondary sexual characteristics and the normal psychological changes associated with puberty. The CDC (2020b) now recommends administering the HPV vaccine at 11 to 12 years of age for boys and girls to prevent the HPV and can begin as early as 9 years of age, and for anyone up to age 26 who has not yet been vaccinated. It is a three-dose series. The first dose is given, with the second and the third doses administered 2 and 6 months following the first dose.

Adolescent: Teach the importance of abstinence or use of condoms and/or methods of birth control if sexually active. Explain that incidence of STIs (chlamydia, syphilis [primary, secondary, and congenital], and gonorrhea) has increased significantly, especially in young adults from 15 to 24 years of age, even between 2017 and 2018 (CDC, 2019b). As for HIV, the annual number of newly diagnosed cases has declined by 7% overall but has increased in Native-American, Alaskan, and Hawaiian groups; the number of people who have had HIV is 1.2 million (CDC, 2020a).

In 2017, a total of 194,377 babies were born to women aged 15 to 19 years, for a **birth rate** of 18.8 per 1,000 women in this age group; this is another record low for **U.S. teens** and a drop of 7% from 2016 (CDC, 2019a). Advise that teens who are pregnant are at higher risk for complications during pregnancy and after delivery. Some of these complications include elevated blood pressure, STIs, preterm labor, premature birth, low birth weight, delivery complications, postpartum depression, and feelings of loneliness and isolation.

 Client Concern: *Poor control of urination: functional, reflex, or stress incontinence*

Explain to family how to decrease environmental barriers (offer bedpan frequently, provide proper lighting, ensure availability and proximity of commode) for functional incontinence. Teach client cutaneous triggering mechanisms for reflex incontinence. Teach client Kegel exercises to strengthen pelvic floor muscles (i.e., tightening of buttocks and practicing starting and stopping stream) for stress incontinence.

References

American Cancer Society. (2018). *Earlier ACS screening guidelines for colorectal cancer.* https://cancercarenews.com/ccn-blog/earlier-acs-screening-guidelines-for-colorectal-cancer/

American Cancer Society. (2020a). *Can endometrial cancer be found early?* https://www.cancer.org/cancer/endometrial-cancer/detection-diagnosis-staging/detection.html

American Cancer Society. (2020b). *History of ACS recommendations for the early detection of cancer in people without symptoms.* https://www.cancer.org/health-care-professionals/american-cancer-society-prevention-early-detection-guidelines/overview/chronological-history-of-acs-recommendations.html

American Congress of Obstetricians and Gynecologists. (2018). *The utility of and indications for routine pelvic examination.* https://www.acog.org/-/media/project/acog/acogorg/clinical/files/committee-opinion/articles/2018/10/the-utility-of-and-indications-for-routine-pelvic-examination.pdf

American Congress of Obstetricians and Gynecologists. (2019). *ACOG statement on HPV vaccination.* https://www.acog.org/news/news-releases/2019/06/acog-statement-on-hpv-vaccination

Association of Professors of Gynecology and Obstetrics. (2008, reviewed 2017). *Cervical cytology.* https://tools.apgo.org/basic-clinical-skills/cervical-cytology-2017/

Centers for Disease Control and Prevention. (2019a). *About teen pregnancy.* https://www.cdc.gov/teenpregnancy/about/index.htm#:~:text=In%202017%2C%20a%20total%20of,drop%20of%207%25%20from%202016

Centers for Disease Control and Prevention. (2019b). *New CDC report: STDs continue to rise in the U.S.* https://www.cdc.gov/nchhstp/newsroom/2019/2018-STD-surveillance-report-press-release.html#:~:text=New%20CDC%20Report%3A%20STDs%20Continue%20to%20Rise%20in%20the%20U.S.&text=Combined%20cases%20of%20syphilis%2C%20gonorrhea,Control%20and%20Prevention%20(CDC)

Centers for Disease Control and Prevention. (2019c). *Testing guidance: New Zika and Dengue testing guidance (Updated November 2019).* https://www.cdc.gov/zika/hc-providers/testing-guidance.html#:~:text=Asymptomatic%20pregnant%20women%3A&text=Zika%20virus%20serologic%20testing%20is,not%20indicate%20a%20recent%20infection

Centers for Disease Control and Prevention. (2020a). Estimated HIV incidence and prevalence in the United States 2014–2018. *HIV Surveillance*

Supplemental Report, 25(1). https://www.cdc.gov/hiv/pdf/library/reports/surveillance/cdc-hiv-surveillance-supplemental-report-vol-25-1.pdf

Centers for Disease Control and Prevention. (2020b). *HPV vaccine recommendations.* https://www.cdc.gov/vaccines/vpd/hpv/hcp/recommendations.html

Centers for Disease Control and Prevention. (2021). *The American Cancer Society guidelines for the prevention and early detection of cervical cancer.* https://www.cancer.org/cancer/cervical-cancer/detection-diagnosis-staging/cervical-cancer-screening-guidelines.html

Isaac, R. (2016). Early natural menopause—A marker of adverse life situations in women across the world: Not unique in Indian women. *Indian Journal of Medical Research, 144*(3), 317–318. https://www.ncbi.nlm.nih.gov/pmc/articles/PMC5320836/

Lab Tests Online. (2021). *Pap smear (Pap test).* http://labtestsonline.org/understanding/analytes/pap/tab/sample

Life course indicator: Early sexual intercourse. (2014). http://www.amchp.org/programsandtopics/data-assessment/LifeCourseIndicatorDocuments/LC-50%20Early%20Sexual%20Intercourse_Final_9-15-2014.pdf

Magnusson, B., Crandall, A., & Evans, K. (2019). Early sexual debut and risky sex in young adults: The role of low self-control. *BMC Public Health, 19,* 1483. https://bmcpublichealth.biomedcentral.com/articles/10.1186/s12889-019-7734-9

Mayo Clinic. (2019). *Vaginal atrophy.* https://www.mayoclinic.org/diseases-conditions/vaginal-atrophy/symptoms-causes/syc-20352288

National Institutes of Health. (2021). *Calcium: Fact sheet for health professionals.* https://ods.od.nih.gov/factsheets/Calcium-Health Professional/#h2

U.S. Preventive Services Task Force. (2014). *Screening for chlamydia and gonorrhea: U.S. Preventive Services Task Force recommendation statement.* https://www.uspreventiveservicestaskforce.org/uspstf/document/RecommendationStatementFinal/chlamydia-and-gonorrhea-screening

U.S. Preventive Services Task Force. (2017). *Screening for gynecological conditions with pelvic examination.* https://www.uspreventiveservicestaskforce.org/uspstf/recommendation/gynecological-conditions-screening-with-the-pelvic-examination#:~:text=The%20USPSTF%20recommends%20screening%20in,HPV)%20testing%20every%205%20years.

U.S. Preventive Services Task Force. (2018). *Final recommendation statement: Screening for cervical cancer.* https://www.uspreventiveservicestaskforce.org/uspstf/announcements/final-recommendation-statement-screening-cervical-cancer

World Health Organization. (2020). *Female genital mutilation.* https://www.who.int/news-room/fact-sheets/detail/female-genital-mutilation

Nursing Assessment of Special Groups

24 ASSESSING CHILDBEARING WOMEN

Improving the well-being of mothers, infants, and children is an important public health goal for the United States, as their well-being determines the health of the next generation and can help predict future public health challenges for families, communities, and the health care system. In addition, pregnancy can provide an opportunity to identify existing health risks in women and thereby prevent future health problems for the women and their children.

The body experiences many physiologic and anatomic changes during pregnancy. Most of these changes are influenced by the hormones of pregnancy, primarily estrogen and progesterone. Normal physiologic and anatomic changes during pregnancy are discussed in this chapter. Changes that are not a result of pregnancy, or that represent an abnormal state during pregnancy, are identified as deviations from normal. Refer to a maternal text—or to Weber and Kelley, *Health Assessment in Nursing*, Seventh Edition, copyright 2022—for a detailed description of physiologic changes that occur within each body system during pregnancy.

This chapter is divided into three sections: Prenatal Maternal and Fetal Assessment, Intrapartum Maternal and Fetal Assessment, and Postpartum Maternal Assessment.

Prenatal Maternal and Fetal Assessment

COLLECTING SUBJECTIVE DATA

Ask the following *interview questions*.

Past pregnancies: Age in years of pregnancy? Outcome of each pregnancy? Number of living children? Complications? Length of labor? Type of delivery? Years since last pregnancy? Current pregnancy: First day of last menstrual period (LMP)? Estimated due date? Confirmed by ultrasound? Problems during pregnancy? Nausea? Vomiting? Cramping or bleeding? Planned pregnancy? Date of first prenatal visit? Prenatal education? Concurrent medical conditions? Current medications? Date of initial fetal movement? Has the fetus been active?

COLLECTING OBJECTIVE DATA

Equipment Needed

See Chapters 10 to 23 for the equipment needed for the specific body system to be assessed for the maternal assessment. The following equipment are needed for the prenatal fetal assessment:

- Bed or examination table
- Drape
- Pillow
- Paper centimeter tape measure
- Fetoscope or Doppler

Physical Assessment

PRENATAL MATERNAL AND FETAL ASSESSMENT		
ASSESSMENT PROCEDURE	**NORMAL FINDINGS**	**ABNORMAL FINDINGS**
Assess the following:		
• Age	• Ideal childbearing years: 18 to 35	• Younger than 18 or older than 35; advanced maternal age increases risk of genetic abnormalities such as Down syndrome; increased risk of complications to mother and baby with age extremes.
• Maternal history	• Uncomplicated maternal/neonatal history. Determine gravida/para status (see Box 24-1).	• Premature labor and/or delivery; pregnancy-induced hypertension (PIH); previous abortion or tubal pregnancy
• Weight	• Prenatal weight gain: Determine weight gain by the prepregnancy body mass index (BMI). Underweight women (BMI < 19.8): 12.7 to 18.1 kg (28–40 lb); women of normal weight (BMI 19.8–26): 11.3 to 15.9 kg (25–35 lb); overweight women (BMI > 26–29): 6.8 to 11.3 kg (15–25 lb); obese women (BMI > 29): 6.8 kg (15 lb) (Fig. 24-1).	• Prepregnancy weight less than 45.4 or greater than 90.7 kg (<100 or >200 lb); sudden gain of more than 0.91 kg (2 lb) per week may be seen in PIH; weight loss or failure to gain weight.

(Continued on following page)

PRENATAL MATERNAL AND FETAL ASSESSMENT (*continued*)		
ASSESSMENT PROCEDURE	**NORMAL FINDINGS**	**ABNORMAL FINDINGS**

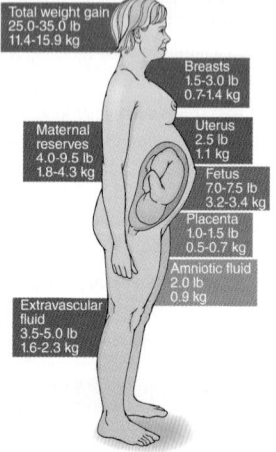

Total weight gain
25.0–35.0 lb
11.4–15.9 kg

Breasts
1.5–3.0 lb
0.7–1.4 kg

Maternal reserves
4.0–9.5 lb
1.8–4.3 kg

Uterus
2.5 lb
1.1 kg

Fetus
7.0–7.5 lb
3.2–3.4 kg

Placenta
1.0–1.5 lb
0.5–0.7 kg

Amniotic fluid
2.0 lb
0.9 kg

Extravascular fluid
3.5–5.0 lb
1.6–2.3 kg

FIGURE 24-1 Distribution of weight gain during pregnancy.

ASSESSMENT PROCEDURE	NORMAL FINDINGS	ABNORMAL FINDINGS
	First trimester: 0.91 to 1.81 kg (2–4 lb)	
	Second trimester: 4.99 kg (11 lb) (0.45 kg [1 lb] per week)	
	Third trimester: 4.99 kg (11 lb) (0.45 kg [1 lb] per week)	
• Blood pressure (BP)	• Range of 90 to 139/60 to 89 mmHg; falls during the second trimester, prepregnancy level in the first and third trimesters	• Greater than or equal to 140/90 mmHg or increase in 30 mmHg above baseline systolic or 15 mmHg above baseline diastolic taken with client in side-lying position; increased levels are seen with PIH.
• Pulse	• 60 to 90 beats/min; may increase 10 to 15 beats/min higher than prepregnancy levels	• Irregularities; persistently less than 60 or greater than 100 beats/min at rest
• Behavior	• *First trimester:* Tired, ambivalent. *Second trimester:* Introspective, energetic. *Third trimester:* Restless, preparing for baby, labile moods (the father may experience some of these same behaviors)	• Denial of pregnancy, withdrawal, depression, psychosis

(Continued on following page)

PRENATAL MATERNAL AND FETAL ASSESSMENT (*continued*)

ASSESSMENT PROCEDURE	NORMAL FINDINGS	ABNORMAL FINDINGS
Observe **skin color**.	Linea nigra, striae gravidarum (see Fig. 24-2); chloasma (Fig. 24-3); spider nevi	Pale, yellowing changes of the skin as seen with liver diseases

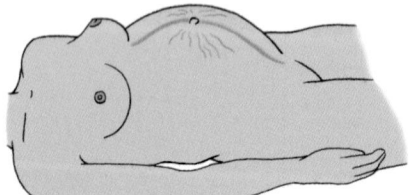

FIGURE 24-2 Pregnancy pigmentation: Abdominal midline (linea nigra) and striae gravidarum. Dark-haired, brown-skinned women are more prone to pregnancy pigmentation.

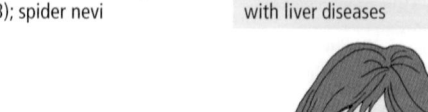

FIGURE 24-3 Marked chloasma of pregnancy.

Assess **head and neck**.		Facial edema, headache
• Nose	• Nasal stuffiness, nosebleeds	• Ulceration of mucosa, yellow, or green drainage
• Eyes	• No changes in examination or vision	• Blurred vision and visual spots are symptoms of PIH.
• Neck	• Slight enlargement of thyroid	• Nodules or marked enlargement, asymmetry of thyroid gland as seen with thyroid disease

ASSESSMENT PROCEDURE	NORMAL FINDINGS	ABNORMAL FINDINGS
Assess **cardiovascular system**.		
• Heart	• Short systolic blowing murmurs	• Progressive dyspnea, palpitations, markedly decreased activity tolerance may be seen with cardiac diseases
• Blood volume	• Increases throughout pregnancy; peaks at 32 to 34 weeks, reaching 30% to 50% above prepregnancy levels	Monitor women with heart disease closely due to the high cardiac demands during pregnancy. Shortness of breath, chest pain, heart failure, etc.
Assess **peripheral vascular system**.	Late pregnancy: Dependent edema, varicose veins, supine hypotension	Perineal varicosities; calf pain may be related to deep vein thrombosis; generalized edema; diminished pedal pulses
Assess **respiratory system**.	Increased anteroposterior diameter, thoracic breathing, slight hyperventilation, shortness of breath in late pregnancy, especially with activity/walking	Dyspnea may be seen in clients with cardiac disease and/or lung diseases such as asthma
Assess **breasts**.	Increased size and nodularity, tenderness, prominent vascularization, darkening of nipples and areola, colostrum in the third trimester (Fig. 24-4)	Localized redness; localized pain and warmth; erythemic streaks are commonly seen with mastitis; inverted nipples may cause difficulty for breastfeeding infants.

(Continued on following page)

PRENATAL MATERNAL AND FETAL ASSESSMENT (*continued*)

ASSESSMENT PROCEDURE	NORMAL FINDINGS	ABNORMAL FINDINGS

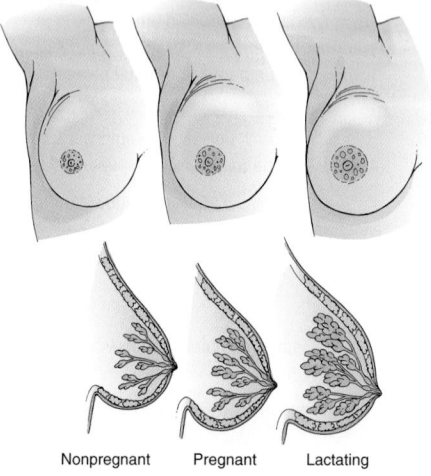

Nonpregnant Pregnant Lactating

FIGURE 24-4 Breast changes during pregnancy.

ASSESSMENT PROCEDURE	NORMAL FINDINGS	ABNORMAL FINDINGS
Assess **gastrointestinal system**.	Nausea and vomiting, increased saliva, heartburn, bloating, constipation	Severe epigastric pain is seen with PIH; severe nausea and vomiting may be seen during the first trimester with hyperemesis gravidarum.
Assess **genitourinary reproductive system**.	Urinary frequency in the first and third trimesters, increased pigmentation of vulva and vagina, increased vaginal discharge	Flank pain, dysuria, oliguria, proteinuria, purulent vaginal discharge, vaginal bleeding
Assess **musculoskeletal system**.	Relaxation of pelvic joints: "Waddling" gait; increased lumbar curve, backache, diastasis recti, leg cramps	Generalized weakness, back pain, difficulty walking, joint pain
Assess **neurologic system**.	Cranial nerves II to XII intact	Hyperactive reflexes, positive clonus seen with PIH
Assess **prenatal labs/immunizations**.	Lab work within normal limits; recent influenza immunization for women who are pregnant during influenza season	Hepatitis positive, rubella nonimmune, HIV positive, anemia, positive drug screen, positive testing for sexually transmitted infections, gestational diabetes, positive antibody screen for Rh-negative antibody screen

(Continued on following page)

PRENATAL MATERNAL AND FETAL ASSESSMENT (*continued*)		
ASSESSMENT PROCEDURE	**NORMAL FINDINGS**	**ABNORMAL FINDINGS**
Palpate and measure the uterine fundal height. Using both hands, gently palpate the outline of the fetus and the top of the uterus (fundus). Using the centimeter tape, measure from the top of the symphysis pubis to the top of the uterine fundus (Fig. 24-5). Take fundal height measurement and multiply by 8/7 (this equals weeks of gestation; McDonald rule: Fundal height (cm) × 8/7 = gestation of pregnancy in weeks). Auscultate **fetal heart rate (FHR).** With Doppler or fetoscope, listen for fetal heartbeat. Locate fundus; begin listening halfway between the fundus and the pubis. Work outward in widening circles until a beating sound is heard. Compare with the maternal pulse. If different, count FHR for 1 full minute.	Accurate within 2 weeks until 36 weeks (Fig. 24-6). Obesity or extremes in height may alter findings. Fundal height measures greater than dates with multiple gestations (twins, triplets, etc.) 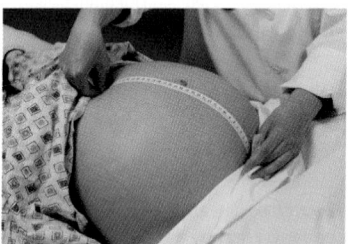 **FIGURE 24-5** Measuring the fundal height.	Lag in progression may indicate problems with fetal development and/or oligohydramnios commonly seen with congenital abnormalities. Sudden increase in fundal height size may also indicate fetal abnormalities. 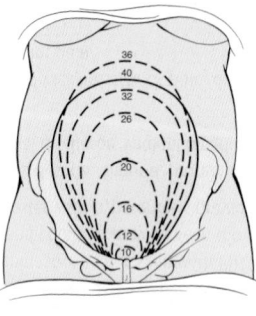 **FIGURE 24-6** Approximate height of fundus at various weeks of gestation.

ASSESSMENT PROCEDURE	NORMAL FINDINGS	ABNORMAL FINDINGS
Assess for the following: • Presence	• Audible at 10 to 12 weeks' gestation with fetal Doppler; audible at 15 to 20 weeks' gestation with fetoscope	• Absence of fetal heart tones after the 20th week of gestation indicates intrauterine fetal demise
• Rate	• Very rapid initially; gradually slows to 120 to 160 beats/min at term; increased rate with fetal movement; during fetal sleep cycle, FHR may be in the 110 to 120 range	• Less than 120 beats/min with activity and not in sleep cycle; no change or decrease in FHR with movement may indicate fetal distress
• Rhythm	• Regular	• A marked variance or variance of less than 5 beats/min may indicate fetal distress
Inspect abdomen for shape and contour of the fetus. With the client supine and head slightly elevated on a pillow, inspect abdomen for shape and contour of the fetus. *Note: During the second and third trimesters, time spent in the supine position should be minimal. This position puts the weight of the fetus and uterus on the aorta and obstructs blood flow.*	*First trimester:* Unable to palpate fetal parts. *Second trimester:* In early trimester, may be difficult to palpate body parts. *Third trimester:* Lower abdomen/distal—palpate to identify fetal head (feels firm with palpation), buttocks (feels soft with palpation). Palpate lateral sides of abdomen—fetal back (palpates as smooth, no bony prominences palpated), fetal parts (arms, fists, legs, and feet may be palpated as small, firm bony prominences).	Abdomen: (distal) Should palpate as firm, bony prominence, fetal head, vertex presentation. Palpation of soft prominence, high probability of breech presentation.

(Continued on following page)

BOX 24-1 GRAVIDA/PARA STATUS

Determine client's gravida/para status.

- **Gravida:** Total number of pregnancies
- **Para:** Number of pregnancies that have delivered at 20 weeks' gestation or greater
- **Term gestation:** Delivery of pregnancy 38 to 42 weeks
- **Preterm gestation:** Delivery of pregnancy after 20 weeks and before the start of 38 weeks' gestation
- **Abortion:** Termination of pregnancy (miscarriage) prior to the 20th week of gestation
- **Living:** Number of living children

Example:

G # P T Pt Ab L

G 4 P 2 1 1 3

This represents a client who has been pregnant four times: two term deliveries, one preterm delivery, one miscarriage, and three children living.

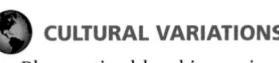

CULTURAL VARIATIONS

- Rh-negative blood is rare in non-White groups.

- Certain inherited disorders occur more often in particular ethnic groups such as Tay–Sachs disease in Ashkenazi Jews, Eastern Europeans, and certain French Canadians and Louisiana Cajuns (National Institute of Neurological Disorders and Stroke, 2019).

POSSIBLE COLLABORATIVE PROBLEMS—RISK OF

- Bleeding disorder of pregnancy
- Hyperemesis gravidarum
- Spontaneous abortion
- Ectopic pregnancy
- Placenta previa
- Abruptio placentae
- PIH
- Gestational diabetes
- Preexisting medical conditions
- Hyperglycemia/hypoglycemia
- Hypertension
- Dehydration
- Renal disease
- Cardiac conditions

Teaching Tips for Selected Client Concerns

Client Concern: Opportunity to enhance healthy practices during pregnancy

Inform client of normal variations during the prenatal period. Also inform the client of those abnormal symptoms to be reported immediately. Encourage the client to write down questions; provide time to discuss them. Instruct the client on methods to cope with normal variations (e.g., nausea and vomiting). Encourage attendance at prenatal classes and appropriate reading material. Prenatal health care should begin in the first trimester of pregnancy.

Diet should be selected from basic five food groups, with an additional 300 calories per day over recommended daily allowances. A balanced diet should provide all essential nutrients during pregnancy, except folic acid and iron. These should be supplemented throughout pregnancy, because adequate amounts are closely related to fetal well-being and pregnancy outcome.

Client Concern: *Poor body image associated with effects of physical changes during pregnancy*

An exercise program started early in pregnancy and continued throughout will help maintain muscle tone and facilitate a return to prepregnancy size after delivery. Exercise has the added benefit of creating a feeling of well-being and satisfaction. Exercise programs should be approved by the obstetrician prior to initiation.

In general, those activities practiced prior to pregnancy can be continued unless they have a potential of causing physical harm to mother and baby.

Allow the client to express her feelings about body changes, and reassure her that most changes are reversible or minimized after delivery. Emphasize positive changes.

Client Concern: *Opportunity to enhance parenting and infant care skills*

Beginning education on growth and development of fetus and infant early in pregnancy can provide an opportunity for prospective parents to anticipate and understand development and expected patterns of developmental skill mastery.

Intrapartum Maternal and Fetal Assessment

During the intrapartum period, an initial physical assessment should be done on admission to the labor room, and findings should be compared with those of the prenatal period. The order of the assessment will vary based on the presenting signs of labor.

COLLECTING SUBJECTIVE DATA

History of prenatal care? Gravida? Para? Age? Estimated date of confinement (EDC)? Are contractions occurring? If so, when did contractions begin? Rupture of membranes? Color of vaginal fluid? Vaginal bleeding and amount? Frequency and duration of contractions? Is fetal movement present? Has there been a decrease in fetal movement? If so, when was fetal movement last noted? Problems with this pregnancy? Duration and outcome of previous labors? Childbirth preparation? Blood type and Rh status? Concurrent disease?

COLLECTING OBJECTIVE DATA

Equipment Needed

- Bed with pillow
- Sterile examination glove
- Lubricant
- Electronic fetal monitor or Doppler
- Nitrazine paper
- Reflex hammer

Physical Assessment

INTRAPARTUM MATERNAL AND FETAL ASSESSMENT		
ASSESSMENT PROCEDURE	**NORMAL FINDINGS**	**ABNORMAL FINDINGS**
Abdomen		
Have the client completely undress, except for gown. Place the client in a supine position with head slightly elevated. Knees and hips should be flexed, with feet resting on mattress. **Note:** *Examination with the client in this position should be performed as rapidly as possible to prevent supine hypotension or fetal compromise.*		

ASSESSMENT PROCEDURE	NORMAL FINDINGS	ABNORMAL FINDINGS
With the client on back and head slightly elevated, place fingertips on fundus. During a contraction, the fundus becomes firm. The client should relate when she feels a contraction begins and when it ends. Time seconds from beginning to end of contractions (duration). Calculate elapsed time from beginning of one contraction to beginning of another (frequency). Do this for several contractions in sequence to determine regularity. During contraction, gently push in on uterus with fingertips and note the degree to which uterus indents (intensity). A large amount of subcutaneous tissue over the uterus may interfere with accurate assessment of intensity. Palpate several contractions in a row. To palpate bladder, gently push in on abdomen directly above symphysis pubis and release. Note the degree of resistance met.		

Inspect **abdomen** for the following:

• Uterine size (see Fig. 24-6)	• Large variation; fundus just below xiphoid process	• Uterus small or large for gestational age may indicate fetal malformations.
• Uterine shape	• Fetal outline longitudinal	• Fetal outline horizontal indicates the presentation of the baby may be transverse or breech.

Palpate **uterus** for the following:

• Frequency of contractions	• As labor progresses, contractions gradually get closer together, in a regular pattern progressing to every 2 to 3 minutes; may be less frequent during the second stage.	• Irregular pattern; more frequent than every 2 minutes may cause placental insufficiency for the fetus to get sufficient oxygenation during labor.

(Continued on following page)

INTRAPARTUM MATERNAL AND FETAL ASSESSMENT (*continued*)		
ASSESSMENT PROCEDURE	**NORMAL FINDINGS**	**ABNORMAL FINDINGS**
• Duration of contractions	• Gradually increases to 60 to 90 seconds as labor progresses	• No increase; duration greater than 90 seconds may deplete fetal oxygenation reserves.
• Intensity of contractions	• Gradually become stronger, uterus feels firm (rock-like); internal pressure monitor 40 to 60 mmHg	• No increase; pressure greater than 60 mmHg is seen with hypertonic contractions.

Note: Contraction frequency and duration may be monitored with an electronic fetal monitor tocodynamometer. Initial assessment of contraction frequency and duration may be performed by palpation. Accurate intensity can only be determined, however, with an intrauterine pressure catheter.

Palpate **above symphysis pubis** for the bladder	Soft, spongy	Bouncy, full, distended is seen with overdistention of the bladder.

FHR

Locate FHR (see "Prenatal Maternal and Fetal Assessment" section) and apply external fetal monitor ultrasound transducer or Doppler. Monitor FHR every 5 minutes during the second stage of labor. Monitor high-risk pregnancies with ruptured amniotic fluid membranes with internal electrodes to assess fetal well-being accurately.

ASSESSMENT PROCEDURE	NORMAL FINDINGS	ABNORMAL FINDINGS
Monitor **FHR** for the following:		
• Baseline rate (must be determined by a 10-minute strip)	• 120 to 160 beats/min	• Less than 120 or greater than 160 beats/min for a 10-minute period may indicate fetal distress.
• Baseline variability (measurable only with internal fetal electrode)	• 5 to 25 beats/min	• Less than 5 beats/min for longer than 20 minutes and not associated with maternal medication
• Periodic changes	• Periodic acceleration (increased FHR with fetal movement, stimulation, or contractions); early-onset deceleration (mirrors contraction and occurs in late first stage and second stage of labor)	• Periodic deceleration; decreased FHR occurs with contractions; repetitive variable decelerations are seen with cord compression; late decelerations are seen in fetal distress; prolonged or slow return to baseline and associated loss of variability may be seen in fetal distress.

Perineum

With the client supine, have her rest her feet on the bed with knees and hips flexed. Instruct the client to relax and separate knees. If discharge is noted, obtain specimen to assess for ruptured membranes with nitrazine paper.

Observe **perineum** for the following:		
• Lesions	• None	• Vesicles could indicate genital herpes; genital warts or open sores may be seen with sexually transmitted infections.

(Continued on following page)

INTRAPARTUM MATERNAL AND FETAL ASSESSMENT (*continued*)

ASSESSMENT PROCEDURE	NORMAL FINDINGS	ABNORMAL FINDINGS
• Discharge	• Bloody mucus; clear or milky fluid; amniotic fluid will turn nitrazine paper blue	• Bright red blood is seen with placenta previa; purulent fluid; green or brown fluid may indicate meconium stool in utero, which puts the fetus at risk for meconium aspiration at delivery. Lubricant or blood may give a false-positive result with nitrazine paper.
• Swelling	• May be present in the second stage of labor	• Present before the second stage of labor
• Shape	• As fetal head descends, perineum flattens and bulges	
• Fetal parts	• Occiput becomes visible during the second stage of labor	• Fetal hand or foot visible with the presenting part indicates a compound presentation, which may occur with the occiput or breech presentation; loop of umbilical cord visible on the perineum puts the fetus at high risk for prolapse cord and requires immediate cesarean section.

ASSESSMENT PROCEDURE	NORMAL FINDINGS	ABNORMAL FINDINGS
Cervix and Fetal Presenting Part		

Have the client separate knees, and instruct her to relax perineum. Put on sterile examination glove, and lubricate index and middle fingers. Gently insert fingers into vagina and palpate cervix and fetal presenting part. Insert finger between cervix and the presenting part, and rotate entire circumference of cervix. This examination should be performed on admission and thereafter only when behavior and contraction pattern indicate progression of labor.

Palpate **cervix** for the following:

ASSESSMENT PROCEDURE	NORMAL FINDINGS	ABNORMAL FINDINGS
• Position	• In early labor, cervix may be in posterior vaginal vault; it becomes more anterior as labor progresses.	
• Effacement	• *Primipara:* Effacement before dilatation • *Multipara:* Effacement and dilatation simultaneous	• Swelling of part or all of cervix occurs when the client begins pushing before the cervix is completely dilated.
• Dilatation (in cm)	• *Primipara:* Average 1 cm per hour; may be slower in early phase • *Multipara:* Average 1.5 cm per hour	• Failure to progress with active labor longer than 24 hours; complete dilatation in less than 3 hours of labor.
Palpate **presenting part of the fetus** for the following:		
• Amniotic membrane	• If intact, can be felt over presenting part; may rupture prior to or during labor	

(Continued on following page)

INTRAPARTUM MATERNAL AND FETAL ASSESSMENT (*continued*)		
ASSESSMENT PROCEDURE	**NORMAL FINDINGS**	**ABNORMAL FINDINGS**
• Presentation	• Cephalic; should feel skull, suture lines, and one or both fontanelles (Fig. 24-7); caput succedaneum may mask landmarks.	• Breech: Soft tissue, anus, or testicles; other small parts such as hands and feet

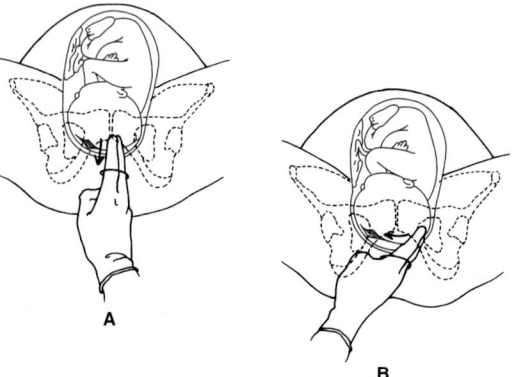

FIGURE 24-7 Assessment of fetal position and station. (**A**) Palpate the sagittal suture and assess station. (**B**) Identify posterior fontanelle. (**C**) Identify anterior fontanelle.

ASSESSMENT PROCEDURE	NORMAL FINDINGS	ABNORMAL FINDINGS
• Position	• Cephalic; posterior fontanelle felt in anterior position, anterior fontanelle in posterior position	• Anterior fontanelle in anterior position; fontanelles in transverse position
• Station (Fig. 24-8)	• *Primipara:* 0 station; gradually descends during the second stage • *Multipara:* Maybe −1 station or higher at onset of labor	• Failure to descend to 0 station during the first stage of labor; failure to descend during the second stage with pushing longer than 2 hours is seen in failure to progress, which requires cesarean section.

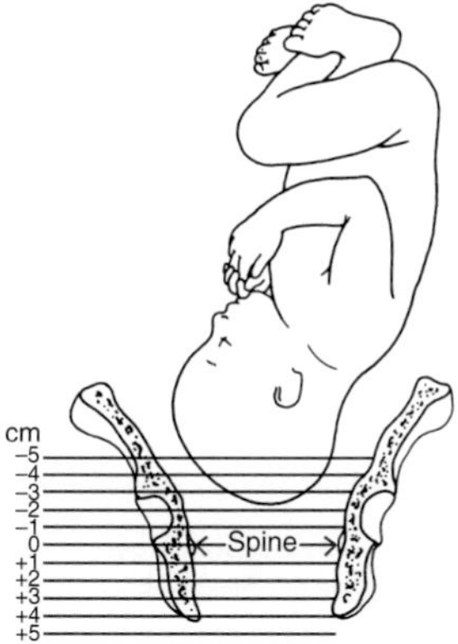

FIGURE 24-8 Measuring station of the fetal head while it is descending.

(Continued on following page)

INTRAPARTUM MATERNAL AND FETAL ASSESSMENT (*continued*)		
ASSESSMENT PROCEDURE	**NORMAL FINDINGS**	**ABNORMAL FINDINGS**
• Umbilical cord	• Not palpable	• May feel loop or pulsations in the umbilical cord, which requires immediate cesarean section

Note: If painless, bright red vaginal bleeding occurs, vaginal examination should be omitted. If fetal gestational age is less than 34 weeks and membranes have ruptured with no evidence of labor, vaginal examination should be omitted.

Face, Extremities, and Behavior

With client in semi-Fowler position, observe face, hands, legs, and feet. Also assess client's mood.

Observe **client's face** for the following:		
• Color	• Pink	• Red, pale
• Edema	• None	• Periorbital edema
Observe **extremities** for the following:		
• Color	• Pink	• Pale, blue seen with cyanosis
• Swelling	• Dependent in ankles	• Swelling in the tibia or hands, not relieved by elevating
Percuss **extremities** for reflexes and clonus.	See Chapter 21 for normal findings.	Hyperreflexia or clonus seen in PIH.

ASSESSMENT PROCEDURE	NORMAL FINDINGS	ABNORMAL FINDINGS
Auscultate **BP** every hour or more often as indicated. With the client in a side-lying position, auscultate BP between contractions.	BP less than 140/90 mmHg. May see BP increase during contractions.	BP greater than or equal to 140/90 mmHg or increase in 30 mmHg systolic or 15 mmHg diastolic over prenatal baseline seen in PIH.
Observe **for behavior changes**:		
• Early labor (1–4 cm) • Active labor (4–7 cm) • Transition (7–10 cm)	• Excited, happy • Cooperative; increased dependence on support person • Irritable, inner focused, hopeless	• Irrational • Uncooperative, psychotic • Confused

 CULTURAL VARIATIONS

- The National Center for Health Statistics (2018) reported that 7.2% of women who gave birth in 2016 smoked. Non-Hispanic American Indian and Alaska Natives had the highest rates, and non-Hispanic Asians the lowest rate, of smoking in pregnancy.
- Exploration of the partner's social or cultural habits may identify needs of the family unit.

- Approximately 200 million girls and women alive today have been subjected to female genital mutilation/cutting (FGM/C; also referred to as *female circumcision*). FGM/C is against the law, and it is a crime to perform FGM/C on a girl younger than 18 or to take, or attempt to take, a girl out of the United States for FGM/C. Girls and women who have experienced FGM/C are not at fault and have not broken any U.S. laws. Often, the vaginal opening has been sutured almost closed (infibulation). Deinfibulation (cutting open this vaginal opening) is needed for childbirth. Performing reinfibulation is discouraged, as there is no medical benefit, but if a client insists upon the procedure and the provider is agreeable, a repair may legally be performed. The provider who agrees to do this is protected under the Federal Prohibition of Female Genital Mutilation Act of 1996, under which the initial mutilation is prohibited, but not the repair (Lee & Strong, 2015).

POSSIBLE COLLABORATIVE PROBLEMS—RISK OF

- Preeclampsia/eclampsia
- Bleeding disorders
- Placenta previa
- Abruptio placentae
- Uterine rupture
- Fetal malpresentation
- Fetal distress
- Labor dystocia
- Cephalopelvic disproportion
- Premature labor
- Fetal malposition

Teaching Tips for Selected Client Concerns

Client Concern: Pain associated with intense uterine contractions

Instruct and demonstrate relaxation techniques. Provide feedback on muscle relaxation. Offer encouragement and support. Provide comfort measures such as gentle massage; temperature control; clean, dry, and wrinkle-free linens; or ice chips or lip lubricant. The laboring woman should be encouraged to assume varying positions of comfort and to ambulate unless complications contraindicate this. Provide analgesics as needed.

Client Concern: Fear associated with unfamiliar environment and concern for fetal well-being

Orient to surroundings. Provide short and simple explanation for all procedures and encourage questions.

Provide evidence of fetal well-being (monitor data). Encourage support person to stay with the client. The client should not be left alone during active labor.

Postpartum Maternal Assessment

The postpartum period begins with the delivery of the placenta and lasts an average of 6 weeks, during which time all body systems return to prepregnancy levels. Some changes are rapid, and others occur over time. During the first 24 hours, many changes occur and frequent assessment is essential.

Changes occurring as an expected part of postpartum recovery are identified as *Normal Findings.* See Chapter 2 for a more detailed description of technique for assessing various body systems. See Chapter 25 for assessment of the newborn.

COLLECTING SUBJECTIVE DATA

Problems during pregnancy? Labor—induction, augmentation, length of labor? Gravida, para? Method of delivery? Size of baby? Anesthesia/analgesia? Concurrent disease and/or chronic conditions?

COLLECTING OBJECTIVE DATA

POSTPARTUM MATERNAL ASSESSMENT		
ASSESSMENT PROCEDURE	**NORMAL FINDINGS**	**ABNORMAL FINDINGS**
Monitor the following:		
• Temperature	• 38°C (100.4°F) in the first 24 hours	• Higher than 38°C (100.4°F) in the first 24 hours or 38°C (100.4°F) and above on any 2 of the first 10 days postpartum seen in puerperal infection.
• BP	• No change from prepregnancy levels	• PIH can occur up to 48 hours postpartum; persistent elevation of BP from PIH beyond 48 hours.

(Continued on following page)

POSTPARTUM MATERNAL ASSESSMENT		
ASSESSMENT PROCEDURE	**NORMAL FINDINGS**	**ABNORMAL FINDINGS**
• Pulse	• Bradycardia (50–70 beats/min) for 6 to 10 days	• Tachycardia; preexisting hypertension may be difficult to control; postural hypotension may occur when assuming the upright position after delivery.
• Weight	• Initial 4.53 to 5.44 kg (10–12 lb) loss; 4.53 to 9.07 kg (10–20 lb) loss in next 6 to 8 weeks	
• Behavior	• *First 2 to 3 days postpartum:* Preoccupied with food and sleep; passive and dependent	• Psychosis is noted when client is unable to care for herself and newborn.
	• *After 2 to 3 days postpartum:* Increased interest in control of body functions, mothering skills; gradually includes others in social circle; transient depression, let-down feeling, cries easily	• Failure to assume maternal role; prolonged depression; unrealistic expectations of newborn

Breasts

With client in supine or semi-Fowler position, inspect breasts. Gently palpate all quadrants of each breast.

Inspect and palpate the **breasts** in non-nursing mothers for the following:		
• Size	• May be enlarged initially; will gradually return to prepregnancy size	• Full, engorged breasts

ASSESSMENT PROCEDURE	NORMAL FINDINGS	ABNORMAL FINDINGS
• Shape	• May sag	
• Color	• May have striae	• Localized redness, tenderness, and pain may be seen with mastitis.
• Tenderness	• Soft	• Full, tender
• Texture	• Nodular	• Lumps, masses may be seen with clogged breast ducts.
Inspect and palpate the **breasts in nursing mothers** for the following:		
• Size	• Enlarged	• Heat, localized pain
• Texture	• Increased nodularity	• Blisters, cracked, bleeding
• Nipples	• Everted, tender	• Purulent, bloody discharge may indicate infection.
• Discharge	• Colostrum, thin milk, may leak between feedings	
• Tenderness	• Full, slightly tender	• Painful breasts are seen with mastitis.
• Texture	• Small lumps	
• Hardened area, most often in upper, outer quadrant, indicates clogged milk ducts and/or mastitis		

(Continued on following page)

POSTPARTUM MATERNAL ASSESSMENT (*continued*)		
ASSESSMENT PROCEDURE	**NORMAL FINDINGS**	**ABNORMAL FINDINGS**

Abdomen

Place client in a supine position with knees extended and head slightly elevated on a pillow. For palpation, have the client empty bladder and assume supine position. Place one hand over lower abdomen above symphysis pubis to support uterus. With the fingertips of the other hand, locate the fundus. Start in the midline, slightly above the umbilicus, and press in and down. Work fingers gradually down toward the symphysis pubis until the fundus of the uterus is located. It should feel like a firm, round ball, similar to a grapefruit. Measure the distance above or below the umbilicus in fingerbreadths (Figs. 24-9 and 24-10). If the uterus is not firm, gently massage until firm, and then gently push down on fundus and observe for expression of clots from the vagina.

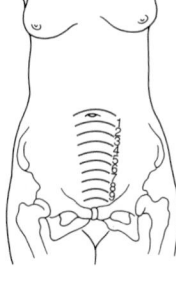

FIGURE 24-9 Involution of the uterus. The height of the fundus decreases about 1 fingerbreadth (~1 cm) each day.

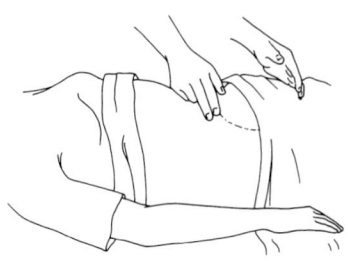

FIGURE 24-10 Measurement of the descent of the fundus. The fundus is located 2 fingerbreadths below the umbilicus.

ASSESSMENT PROCEDURE	NORMAL FINDINGS	ABNORMAL FINDINGS
Inspect **abdomen** for the following:		
• Size	• Uterus visible, outlined unless obese; gradually recedes to prepregnancy size with exercise	• Distention seen when client is unable to void and bladder becomes distended.
• Color	• Striae dark red or purple; recede to silvery or white and become smaller	• Yellow, pale
• Texture	• Loose and flabby	• Dry, cracked
Palpate **uterine fundus** for the following:		
• Location	• Midline	• Deviated to the left or right could indicate a distended bladder.
• Consistency	• Firm; boggy to firm with massage; smooth surface	• Boggy; does not stay firm after massage; may indicate uterine atony and/or retained placental fragments
• Height	• Halfway between umbilicus and symphysis immediately after delivery; within 12 hours, at the umbilicus or 1 cm above; descends 1 cm per day	• More than 1 cm above umbilicus; failure to descend
• Expression of clots	• Small clots or increased flow with massage	• Large clots; continuous trickle of bright red blood with firm fundus indicates an unrepaired laceration.

(Continued on following page)

POSTPARTUM MATERNAL ASSESSMENT (*continued*)		
ASSESSMENT PROCEDURE	**NORMAL FINDINGS**	**ABNORMAL FINDINGS**
Face and Extremities		
To inspect the face and extremities, the supine position is preferred. Adequate light must be available. With legs extended, gently palpate calves. Place one hand on knee, and gently dorsiflex each foot. Pregnancy-related seizures can occur for up to 48 hours postpartum. Reflexes should be assessed for hyperreflexia and clonus during this time. See Chapter 21 for technique.		
Inspect **face** for the following:		
• Color	• Petechiae after prolonged second stage of labor	• Paleness may be seen with anemia.
• Edema	• None	• Periorbital
Inspect **extremities** for the following.		
• Color	• Pink; red tones visible under dark pigmentation	• Dusky, mottled color indicates decreased oxygenation.
• Edema	• Slight pedal edema	• Pitting edema, edema of hands seen with PIH.
• Tenderness	• Calves may have generalized muscle tenderness	• Calf with localized tenderness or pain seen with deep vein thrombosis.
• Texture	• Smooth	• Knots or lumps in calf
• Homan sign	• Negative (no pain in calf)	• Positive (pain in calf) may indicate deep vein thrombosis.

ASSESSMENT PROCEDURE	NORMAL FINDINGS	ABNORMAL FINDINGS
Bladder		
Have the client void within 4 hours after delivery or sooner if there are bleeding problems during the immediate postpartum period. To palpate the bladder, have the client empty bladder and assume supine position. Palpate for bladder above the symphysis pubis. If unable to void within 4 hours after delivery, or if the bladder is full, empty the bladder with a catheter.		
Inspect **voiding** for the following:		
• Amount	• 200 mL or more each voiding; diuresis of greater than 2,000 mL in the first 24 hours	• Less than 100 mL per voiding; unable to void
• Color	• Yellow, clear; may be mixed with lochia	• Dark, cloudy, bloody urine may indicate urinary tract infection.
Palpate **bladder**	Nonpalpable	Spongy mass in lower abdomen
Perineum		
Have the client turn to side and flex upper leg. Place one hand on upper buttock and gently separate so that perineum is visible.		
Inspect **perineum** for the following:		
• Approximation of episiotomy	• Skin edges meet	• Skin edges gape
• Color	• Pink to red	• Purple, mottled
• Swelling	• Generalized swelling for 12 to 24 hours	• Localized swelling with increased pain indicates hematoma.

(Continued on following page)

POSTPARTUM MATERNAL ASSESSMENT (*continued*)		
ASSESSMENT PROCEDURE	**NORMAL FINDINGS**	**ABNORMAL FINDINGS**
• Lochia	• *Color: Days 1 to 3:* Rubra (dark red); small clots may also be expelled *Days 4 to 10:* Serosa (pinkish red) *Days 11 to 20:* Alba (creamy yellow) *Amount: Days 1 to 10:* Vaginal discharge requires 6 to 10 pads per day (moderate flow). *Days 11 to 20:* Decreased amount of vaginal discharge still requires pad change (<6–8 pads per day).	• More than eight peripads per day or saturated pad in 1 hour seen in postpartum hemorrhage; purulent, large clots; return to dark red after several days.
• Odor • Hemorrhoids	• None; musky scent • Small, nontender	• Foul odor with bacterial infections • Swollen, painful

POSSIBLE COLLABORATIVE PROBLEMS—RISK OF

- Urinary retention
- Breast engorgement/abscess
- Preeclampsia/eclampsia
- Hemorrhage

- Infections
- Exacerbation of preexisting medical conditions
- Heart conditions

- Uterine atony
- Hematoma
- Cervical/vaginal lacerations
- Retained placenta

- Hypertension
- Hyperglycemia
- Hypoglycemia

Teaching Tips for Selected Client Concerns

***Client Concern:** Poor, interrupted sleep associated with post-partum fatigue and increased need for sleep*

All teaching sessions should be brief and reinforced with written information about infant care and self-care (e.g., care of breasts). Encourage mother to sleep when baby sleeps. Advise mother to avoid strenuous activities until 6-week postpartum physical examination. Enlist help of other family members.

***Client Concern:** Opportunity to enhance infant care and self-care*

Demonstrate infant care and allow time for mother to practice. A follow-up phone call or home visit can assist in evaluation and reinforcement of information taught. Include father whenever possible.

Discuss normal growth and development of infant; emphasize things infant can do. Provide early and continued contact of infant and parents to maximize bonding. Teach parents the skills needed to meet infant's physical and psychological needs.

***Client Concern:** Opportunity to enhance family adjustment to newborn and role changes within family*

Discuss plans for incorporating new member into family. Offer suggestions to decrease sibling jealousy. Explore plans for infant care, division of labor, and changes in activities of daily living.

Be aware of risk factors for child abuse/neglect that may be evident during postpartum period. Explore resources available to parents, and make appropriate referrals for follow-up or support groups.

***Client Concern:** Opportunity to enhance breastfeeding associated with request for assistance and information on breast-feeding process and technique*

The decision to breastfeed or bottle-feed the infant is usually made prior to or during pregnancy. Providing factual information with an opportunity for questions and answers early in pregnancy will facilitate a decision best suited to the client's needs and lifestyle.

Clarify misconceptions, and provide instructions or proper technique. Assist with first feedings and problems such as soreness or difficulty latching on to breasts.

Breast milk is the most desirable the first 6 months of a child's life. However, commercially prepared, iron-fortified formula is an acceptable alternative. Formula intake varies, but most infants take 100 cal/kg body weight/day. This amount of formula should be offered to the infant every 3 to 4 hours, approximately four to six times a day. For exclusively breastfed infants, the American Academy of Pediatrics (AAP) recommended in 2008/2016 a daily intake of vitamin D of 400 IU/day for all infants and children beginning in the first few days of life (AAP, 2020; Centers for Disease Control and Prevention, 2020). Human milk typically contains a vitamin D concentration of 25 IU per liter or less. Therefore, a supplement of 400 IU per day of vitamin D meets the requirement for all breastfed infants.

To continue breast milk supply, mother should pump breasts at intervals similar to infant feeding patterns. Milk letdown is optimal immediately after infant contact. Mother should be relaxed and have privacy. If possible, both breasts should be emptied at each feeding. Increased fluid consumption is needed for milk production. Discuss methods to enhance milk production if deficient. To terminate breastfeeding, mother should avoid any stimulation of breasts. Encourage use of good support bra. Painful engorgement may be alleviated with analgesics and intermittent ice packs to breasts.

Client Concern: *Poor infant bottle feeding associated with sluggish sucking and difficulty latching onto nipple*

May use nipple with larger hole. Hold infant in upright position during feeding. Burp infant often (after every 14.8–29.6 mL [0.5–1 oz]). Infant needs frequent feedings with careful monitoring of intake and weight gain. May need to teach parents gavage feedings. If so, infant will attempt to nurse at each feeding and be gavage-fed remaining formula/breast milk.

References

American Academy of Pediatrics. (2020). *Adherence to vitamin D intake guidelines in the United States.* https://pediatrics.aappublications.org/content/145/6/e20193574

Centers for Disease Control and Prevention. (2020). *Vitamin D.* https://www.cdc.gov/breastfeeding/breastfeeding-special-circumstances/diet-and-micronutrients/vitamin-d.html

Lee, M. J., & Strong, N. (2015). *Female genital mutilation: What ob/gyns need to know.* https://www.contemporaryobgyn.net/view/female-genital-mutilation-what-obgyns-need-know

National Center for Health Statistics. (2018). *Cigarette smoking during pregnancy: United States, 2016.* https://www.cdc.gov/nchs/products/databriefs/db305.htm

National Institute of Neurological Disorders and Stroke. (2019). *Tay-Sachs disease information page.* https://www.ninds.nih.gov/Disorders/All-Disorders/Tay-Sachs-Disease-Information-Page

ASSESSING NEWBORNS AND INFANTS

A newborn, or neonate, is the term used to describe a child from birth to 28 days old. An *infant* refers to a child between the ages of 28 days and 1 year. Refer to a pediatric or maternity nursing text to review the physical, cognitive, motor, sensory, moral, psychosocial, and psychosexual growth and development of newborns and infants.

Nursing Assessment of the Newborn and Infant

Nursing assessment of the newborn and infant consists of collecting subjective and objective data. The nurse interviews the parents or primary caretaker of the newborn or infant to collect subjective data. The nurse will perform an initial newborn physical assessment right at the time of birth; subsequent physical assessments of the newborn and infant are performed at regular intervals throughout the first year of life.

COLLECTING SUBJECTIVE DATA

- *Prenatal history:* Planned pregnancy? Gravida? Para? Estimated date of confinement (EDC)? Gestational age? Maternal health history? Prenatal care? Problems, illnesses, or accidents during pregnancy? Risk factors? Prenatal exposure to tobacco, alcohol, medications, illegal or recreational drugs? Complications? Blood type? Maternal testing?

- *Labor and delivery history:* Date, time, type of delivery? Prolonged labor? Where was the infant born? What type of delivery (vaginal or C-section) did you have? Any anesthesia? Type? Complications? Time of rupture of membranes? Induction? Duration of labor, late decelerations? Shoulder dystocia? Hip dysplasia? Meconium? RhoGAM? Mother positive for sepsis such as group B strep (GBS)?
- *Postdelivery history:* Infant's Apgar scores? Respiratory effort? Resuscitation efforts? Weight, length, and head circumference (HC)? What immunizations has the infant received thus far? Any reactions to immunizations? Any problems after birth (e.g., feeding, jaundice)? Allergies? Hospitalizations, major illnesses? Medications? Procedures performed? Evidence of injury? Voiding? Stool?
- *Social parental history:* Are parents married, single, divorced, LGBTQ (lesbian, gay, bisexual, transgender, queer)? Who else lives in this residence? What are the parents' ages? Is the infant adopted, foster, or natural? Parental occupation? Parental religion? Parental interaction? Significant others? Cultural variations? Male circumcision requested? Family history of diseases?
- *Current history:* Is the infant being breastfed or bottle-fed? What foods and fluids does the infant eat and drink? Sleep patterns? Skin rashes? Hair texture, scalp scaling? Bruising? Birthmarks? Fontanelle closure? Head injuries? Eye movements? Follows voice with head? Any teeth? Any grunting, nasal flaring, chest retractions during the day, at night, or during feedings? Shortness of breath with feedings? Urination and bowel movement patterns? Limited range of motion (ROM)? Seizures? Motor coordination?

COLLECTING OBJECTIVE DATA

Equipment

- Denver Development Kit
- Measuring tape
- Ophthalmoscope
- Otoscope
- Scale
- Stethoscope
- Thermometer

Physical Assessment

At birth, the newborn will undergo an *initial assessment.* This special assessment is performed to evaluate the following:

- Apgar score
- Vital signs

- Measurements
- Gestational age
- Newborn reflexes

These assessments are performed in order to evaluate the newborn's transition from intrauterine to extrauterine life and to detect any health concerns that may require prompt intervention.

The *initial assessment* is performed immediately after birth, while the infant is supine under a radiant warmer with the temperature probe attached to the abdomen.

Subsequent physical assessments of the infant are performed using the guide provided below. Physical assessment of the infant is a complete head-to-toe examination that also includes developmental screening.

INITIAL NEWBORN ASSESSMENT		
ASSESSMENT PROCEDURE	**NORMAL FINDINGS**	**ABNORMAL FINDINGS**
Apgar Score		
Assign Apgar scores at 1 and 5 minutes after delivery. The Apgar score is an assessment of infant's ability to adapt to extrauterine life. Assess the following:	The score is 8 to 10. See Table 25-1 for Apgar scoring.	Less than 8 points may indicate poor transition from intrauterine to extrauterine life.
Auscultate **apical pulse.**	Greater than 100 beats/min	Less than 100 beats/min indicates bradycardia; absent heart beat indicates fetal demise.
Inspect chest and abdomen for **respiratory effort.**	Crying	Absent, slow, irregular respirations

(Continued on following page)

INITIAL NEWBORN ASSESSMENT (*continued*)

ASSESSMENT PROCEDURE	NORMAL FINDINGS	ABNORMAL FINDINGS
Stroke **back or soles of feet**.	Crying	Delayed neurologic function may be seen in grimace, no response.
Inspect **muscle tone** by extending legs and arms. Observe degree of flexion and resistance in extremities.	Extremities flexed, active movement	Moderate degree of flexion, limp may indicate neurologic deficits.
Inspect body and extremities for **skin color**.	Full body pink, acrocyanosis	Cyanosis, pale
Vital Signs		
Monitor **axillary temperature**.	36.38°C to 37.2°C (97.5°F–99°F)	Less than 36.38°C (<97.5°F): hypothermia, which may indicate sepsis Greater than 37.2°C (>99°F): hyperthermia (consider infection or improper monitoring of temperature probe)
Inspect and auscultate **lung sounds**.	Easy, nonlabored, clear lungs bilaterally	Labored breathing, nasal flaring, rhonchi, rales, retractions, grunting
Monitor **respiratory rate**.	Rate: 30 to 60 breaths/min	Rate less than 30 or greater than 60 breaths/min is seen with respiratory distress.

ASSESSMENT PROCEDURE	NORMAL FINDINGS	ABNORMAL FINDINGS
Auscultate **apical pulse.**	Regular 120 to 160 beats/min (100 sleeping, 180 crying)	Irregular less than 100 or greater than 180 beats/min may indicate cardiac abnormalities.
Measurements		
Weigh newborn unclothed using a newborn scale (Fig. 25-1).	2,500 to 4,000 g	Less than 2,500 g Greater than 4,000 g
	 FIGURE 25-1 Weighing the newborn.	
Measure **length.**	44 to 55 cm	Less than 44 cm Greater than 55 cm
Measure **HC.**	33 to 35.5 cm	Less than 33 cm Greater than 35.5 cm
Measure **chest circumference.**	30 to 33 cm (1–2 cm < head)	Less than 30 cm Greater than 33 cm

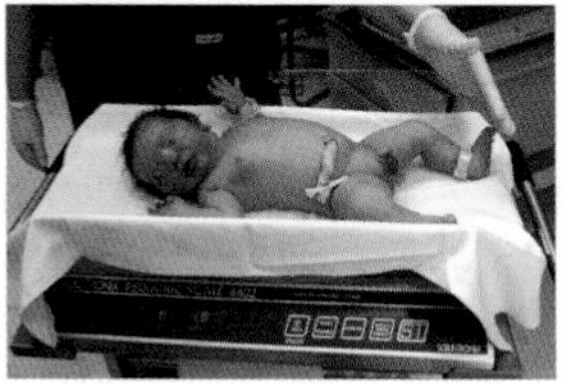

(*Continued on following page*)

INITIAL NEWBORN ASSESSMENT (*continued*)

ASSESSMENT PROCEDURE	NORMAL FINDINGS	ABNORMAL FINDINGS

Gestational Age

Assess the newborn's gestational age within 4 hours after birth to identify any potential age-related problems that may occur within the next few hours. Examine the newborn's neuromuscular and physical maturity. After examination, use the Ballard scale to rate the gestational age (Figs. 25-2 and 25-3).

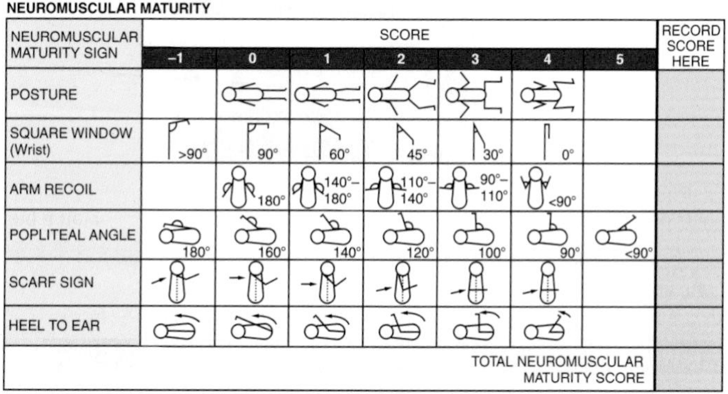

NEUROMUSCULAR MATURITY

NEUROMUSCULAR MATURITY SIGN	SCORE							RECORD SCORE HERE
	−1	0	1	2	3	4	5	
POSTURE								
SQUARE WINDOW (Wrist)	>90°	90°	60°	45°	30°	0°		
ARM RECOIL		180°	140°–180°	110°–140°	90°–110°	<90°		
POPLITEAL ANGLE	180°	160°	140°	120°	100°	90°	<90°	
SCARF SIGN								
HEEL TO EAR								
						TOTAL NEUROMUSCULAR MATURITY SCORE		

FIGURE 25-2 New Ballard scale. Used to rate neuromuscular maturity of gestational age.

| ASSESSMENT PROCEDURE | NORMAL FINDINGS | ABNORMAL FINDINGS |

PHYSICAL MATURITY

PHYSICAL MATURITY SIGN	SCORE							RECORD SCORE HERE
	−1	0	1	2	3	4	5	
SKIN	sticky, friable, transparent	gelatinous, red, translucent	smooth, pink, visible veins	superficial peeling and/or rash, few veins	cracking pale areas, rare veins	parchment, deep cracking, no vessels	leathery, cracked, wrinkled	
LANUGO	none	sparse	abundant	thinning	bald areas	mostly bald		
PLANTAR SURFACE	heel-toe 40–50 mm: −1 <40 mm: −2	>50 mm no crease	faint red marks	anterior transverse crease only	creases ant. 2/3	creases over entire sole		
BREAST	impercep- tible	barely perceptible	flat areola no bud	stippled areola 1–2 mm bud	raised areola 3–4 mm bud	full areola 5–10 mm bud		
EYE-EAR	lids fused loosely: −1 tightly: −2	lids open pinna flat stays folded	sl. curved pinna; soft; slow recoil	well-curved pinna; soft but ready recoil	formed and firm instant recoil	thick cartilage, ear stiff		
GENITALS (Male)	scrotum flat, smooth	scrotum empty, faint rugae	testes in upper canal, rare rugae	testes descending, few rugae	testes down, good rugae	testes pendulous, deep rugae		
GENITALS (Female)	clitoris prominent and labia flat	prominent clitoris and small labia minora	prominent clitoris and enlarging minora	majora and minora equally prominent	majora large, minora small	majora cover clitoris and minora		
						TOTAL PHYSICAL MATURITY SCORE		

SCORE

Neuromuscular ____
Physical ____
Total ____

MATURITY RATING

Score	Weeks
−10	20
−5	22
0	24
5	26
10	28
15	30
20	32
25	34
30	36
35	38
40	40
45	42
50	44

GESTATIONAL AGE (weeks)

By dates _____
By ultrasound _____
By exam _____

FIGURE 25-3 New Ballard scale. Used to rate physical maturity of gestational age.

(Continued on following page)

INITIAL NEWBORN ASSESSMENT (continued)		
ASSESSMENT PROCEDURE	**NORMAL FINDINGS**	**ABNORMAL FINDINGS**
Assess **neuromuscular maturity** (see Fig. 25-2) by performing each of the following with the newborn in the supine position:		
Inspect **posture** (with newborn undisturbed)	• Arms and legs flexed	• Arms and legs limp, extended away from body seen in premature infants.
Assess for **square window.** Bend wrist toward ventral forearm until resistance is met. Measure angle (Fig. 25-4).	• 0 to 30 degrees • Premature infants may have square window measurement greater than 30 degrees.	

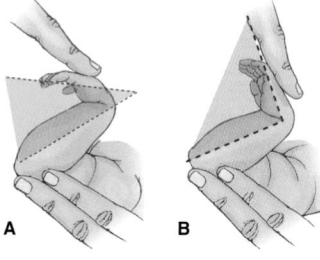

FIGURE 25-4 Square window sign. (**A**) Term infant. (**B**) Preterm infant.

ASSESSMENT PROCEDURE	NORMAL FINDINGS	ABNORMAL FINDINGS
Test **arm recoil.** Bilaterally flex elbows up with hands next to shoulders and hold approximately 5 seconds; extend arms down next to side, release; observe elbow angle and recoil.	• Elbow angle less than 90 degrees, rapid recoil to flexed state	• Elbow angle greater than 110 degrees, delayed recoil seen in premature infants.
Assess **popliteal angle.** Flex thigh on top of abdomen; push behind ankle and extend lower leg up toward head until resistance is met; measure angle behind knee.	• Less than 100 degrees	• Greater than 100 degrees
Assess for **scarf sign.** Lift arm across chest toward opposite shoulder until resistance is met; note location of elbow in relation to middle of chest (Fig. 25-5).	• Elbow position less than midline of chest	• Elbow position midline of chest or greater, toward opposite shoulder seen in premature infants.

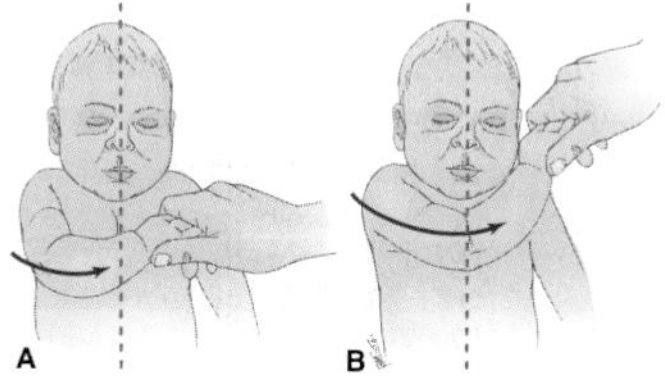

FIGURE 25-5 Scarf sign. **(A)** Term infant. **(B)** Preterm infant.

(Continued on following page)

INITIAL NEWBORN ASSESSMENT (*continued*)

ASSESSMENT PROCEDURE	NORMAL FINDINGS	ABNORMAL FINDINGS
Perform **heel-to-ear test.** Pull leg toward ear on same side, keeping buttocks flat on bed; inspect popliteal angle and proximity of heel to ear.	• Popliteal angle less than 90 degrees, heel distal from ear	• Popliteal angle greater than 90 degrees, heel proximal to ear seen in premature infants.
Assess **physical maturity** (see Fig. 25-3) by performing the following:		
• Inspect skin. • Inspect for lanugo. • Inspect plantar surface of feet for creases. • Inspect and palpate breast bud tissue with middle finger and forefinger; measure bud in millimeters. • Observe ear cartilage in upper pinna for curving. Fold pinna down toward the side of head and release; observe recoil of ear.	• Parchment, few or no vessels on abdomen, cracking in ankle area • Thinning, balding on back, shoulders, knees • Creases on anterior two-thirds or entire sole • Raised areola, full areola • Pinna well curved, cartilage formed, instant recoil	• Translucent, visible veins; rash; leathery, wrinkled skin seen in postmature infants. • Abundant amount of fine hair on face seen in premature infants. • Anterior transverse crease on sole only, no creases; fewer creases indicate prematurity. • Absence of bud tissue, bud less than 3 mm seen in premature infants. • Pinna slightly curved, slow recoil seen in premature infants.

ASSESSMENT PROCEDURE	NORMAL FINDINGS	ABNORMAL FINDINGS
		Note: If there is an ear anatomical anomaly, the neonate should be examined for renal anomalies, as the ears and kidneys develop at the same embryologic stage (D'Alessandro, 2015).
• Inspect genitals.		
Male: Observe scrotum for rugae and palpate position of testes.	*Male:* Deep rugae; testes positioned down in scrotal sac	*Male:* Decreased presence of rugae; testes positioned in upper inguinal canal.
Female: Observe labia majora, labia minora, and clitoris.	*Female:* Labia majora cover labia minora and clitoris.	*Female:* Labia majora and labia minora equally prominent, clitoris prominent seen with premature infants.
Determine **score rating:** Use Figures 25-2 and 25-3. Mark the boxes that most closely represent each observation.		
• Add the total scores from both tables.	• Total score: 35 to 45 points	• Total score: less than 35 points or greater than 45 points
• Using Figure 25-2, plot total score in column on right-hand side of page; this score corresponds to the number in weeks on the maturity rating scale; circle the number of weeks.	• Gestational age: 38 to 42 weeks	• Gestational age: less than 38 or greater than 42 weeks

(Continued on following page)

INITIAL NEWBORN ASSESSMENT (*continued*)

ASSESSMENT PROCEDURE	NORMAL FINDINGS	ABNORMAL FINDINGS
• Using gestational weeks assessed, plot weight, length, and HC on the growth charts found at http://www.cdc.gov/growthcharts and record **classification** of infant for gestational age in Figure 25-6.	• 10th to 90th percentile is appropriate for gestational age (AGA).	• Less than the 10th percentile (small for gestational age); greater than the 90th percentile (large for gestational age [LGA])

CLASSIFICATION OF INFANT*	Weight	Length	Head Circ.
Large for Gestational Age (LGA) (>90th percentile)			
Appropriate for Gestational Age (AGA) (10th to 90th percentile)			
Small for Gestational Age (SGA) (<10th percentile)			

*Place an "X" in the appropriate box (LGA, AGA, or SGA) for weight, for length, and for head circumference.

FIGURE 25-6 Classification of infant for gestational age.

Newborn Reflexes

Assess **newborn reflexes.** See Box 25-1.	Infantile reflexes are present when appropriate and are symmetrical. See Box 25-1.	Presence of newborn reflexes beyond the time they are expected to disappear. See Box 25-1.

TABLE 25-1 **Apgar Scoring System**

	0 Points	1 Point	2 Points
Activity and muscle tone	Absent	Flexion of arms and legs	Active movement
Pulse	Absent	Below 100 bpm	Over 100 bpm
Grimace (reflex) with stimulation, such as suctioning of the nares	No response, floppy	Some extremity flexion or cry	Pulls away, sneezes, or coughs
Skin color (appearance)	Pale, blue body and extremities	Body pink, extremities blue	Body and extremities pink
Respirations	Absent	Slow and irregular	Robust cry

Done at 1 and 5 minutes after birth, Apgar scoring is used to assess if an infant needs immediate medical care; it does not predict long-term outcomes.

APGAR Interpretation
- 0–3: Severely depressed: prompt resuscitation indicated
- 4–6: Moderately depressed: some assistance for breathing indicated
- 7–10: Excellent condition

Reprinted with permission from O'Meara, A. M. (2019). *Maternity, newborn, and women's health nursing: A case-based approach* (Table 1.4). Wolters Kluwer.

BOX 25-1 NEWBORN REFLEXES: DIFFERENTIATING NORMAL AND ABNORMAL FINDINGS

The reflexes illustrated and described are the most commonly tested newborn reflexes. These reflexes are present in all normal newborns, and most disappear within a few months after birth. Therefore, absence of a reflex at birth or persistence of a reflex past a certain age may indicate a problem with CNS function.

ROOTING REFLEX

To elicit the rooting reflex, touch the newborn's upper or lower lip or cheek with a gloved finger or sterile nipple. The newborn will move the head toward the stimulated area and open the mouth.

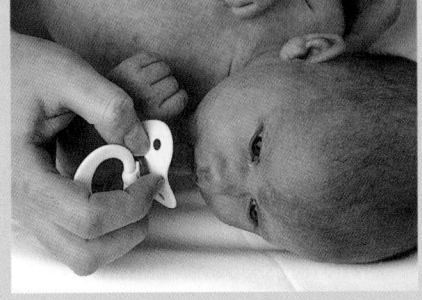

Disappearance of Reflex
The rooting reflex disappears by 3 to 4 months.

Abnormal Findings
Absence of a rooting indicates serious CNS disease.

SUCKING REFLEX

Place a gloved finger or nipple in the newborn's mouth, and note the strength of the sucking response. (A diminished response is normal in a recently fed newborn.)

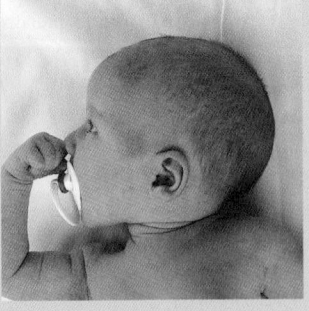

Disappearance of Reflex
This reflex disappears at 10 to 12 months.

Abnormal Findings
A weak or absent sucking reflex may indicate a neurologic disorder, prematurity, or CNS depression caused by maternal drug use or medication during pregnancy.

PALMAR GRASP REFLEX
Press your fingers against the palmar surface of the newborn's hand from the ulnar side. The grasp should be strong—you may even be able to pull the newborn to a sitting position.

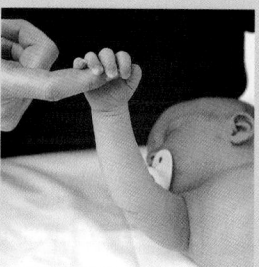

Disappearance of Reflex
This reflex disappears at 3 to 4 months.

Abnormal Findings
A diminished response usually indicates prematurity; no response suggests neurologic deficit; asymmetric grasp suggests fracture of the humerus or peripheral nerve damage. If this reflex persists past 4 months, cerebral dysfunction may be present.

PLANTAR GRASP REFLEX
Touch the ball of the newborn's foot. The toes should curl downward tightly.

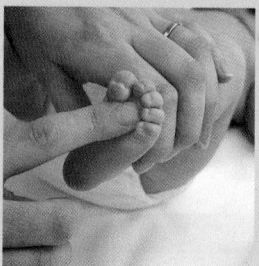

(Continued on following page)

BOX 25-1 NEWBORN REFLEXES: DIFFERENTIATING NORMAL AND ABNORMAL FINDINGS (*continued*)

Disappearance of Reflex
This reflex disappears at 8 to 10 months.

Abnormal Findings
A diminished response usually indicates prematurity; no response suggests neurologic deficit.

TONIC NECK REFLEX
The newborn should be supine. Turn the head to one side, with newborn's jaw at the shoulder. The tonic neck reflex is present when the arm and leg on the side to which the head is turned extend and the opposite arm and leg flex. This reflex usually does not appear until 2 months of age.

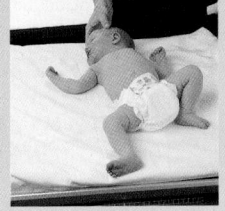

Disappearance of Reflex
This reflex disappears by 4 to 6 months. The reflex may not occur every time that the examiner tries to elicit it, in which case, repeat stimulus of turning head to one side to re-elicit the response.

Abnormal Findings
If this reflex persists until later in infancy, brain damage is usually present.

MORO (OR STARTLE) REFLEX
The Moro reflex is a response to sudden stimulation or an abrupt change in position. This reflex can be elicited by using either one of the following two methods:

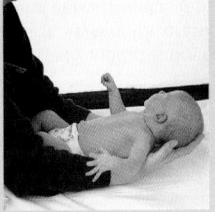

1. Hold the infant with the head supported and rapidly lower the whole body a few inches.
2. Place the infant in the supine position on a flat, soft surface. Hit the surface with your hand or startle the infant in some way.

The reflex is manifested by the infant slightly flexing and abducting the legs, laterally extending and abducting the arms, forming a "C" with thumb and forefinger, and fanning the other fingers. This is immediately followed by anterior flexion and adduction of the arms. All movements should be symmetric.

Disappearance of Reflex
This reflex disappears by 3 months.

Abnormal Findings
An asymmetric response suggests injury of the part that responds more slowly. Absence of a response suggests CNS injury. If the reflex was elicited at birth and disappears later, cerebral edema or intracranial hemorrhage is suspected. Persistence of the response after 4 months suggests CNS injury.

BABINSKI REFLEX
Hold the newborn's foot and stroke up the lateral edge and across the ball. A positive Babinski reflex is fanning of the toes. Many normal newborns will not exhibit a positive Babinski reflex; instead, they will exhibit the normal adult response, which is flexion of the toes. Response should always be symmetric bilaterally.

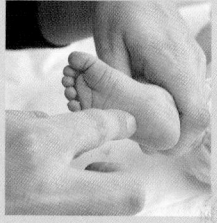

Disappearance of Reflex
This reflex disappears within 2 years.

Abnormal Findings
A positive response after 2 years suggests pyramidal tract disease.

(Continued on following page)

BOX 25-1 NEWBORN REFLEXES: DIFFERENTIATING NORMAL AND ABNORMAL FINDINGS (*continued*)

STEPPING REFLEX

Hold the newborn upright from behind, provide support under the arms, and let the newborn's feet touch a surface. The reflex response is manifested by the newborn stepping with one foot and then the other in a walking motion.

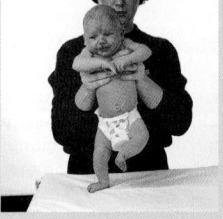

Disappearance of Reflex

This reflex usually disappears within 2 months.

Abnormal Findings

An asymmetric response may indicate injury of the leg, CNS damage, or peripheral nerve injury.

SUBSEQUENT INFANT PHYSICAL ASSESSMENT		
ASSESSMENT PROCEDURE	**NORMAL FINDINGS**	**ABNORMAL FINDINGS**
General Appearance and Behavior		
Observe **general appearance.** Observe hygiene. Note interaction with parents and yourself (and siblings if present). Note also facies (facial expressions) and posture.	Child appears stated age; is clean, has no unusual body odor, and clothing is in good condition and appropriate for climate. Child is alert, active, responds appropriately to stress of the situation. Child is appropriately interactive for age, seeks comfort from parent; appears happy. Newborn's arms and legs are in flexed position.	Note any facies that indicate acute illness, respiratory distress. Flaccidity or rigidity in newborn may be from neurologic damage, sepsis, or pain. Poor hygiene and clothes may indicate neglect, poverty. Infant does not appear stated age (mental retardation, abuse, neglect).
Developmental Assessment		
Screen for **cognitive, language, social, and gross and fine motor developmental delays** in the beginning of the physical assessment in infants.	Infant meets normal parameters for age, see Appendix 5. Gross and fine motor skills should be appropriate for the child's developmental age.	Child lags in earlier stages. Gross and fine motor skills that are inappropriate for developmental age and lack of head control by age 6 months may indicate cerebral palsy.

(Continued on following page)

SUBSEQUENT INFANT PHYSICAL ASSESSMENT (*continued*)		
ASSESSMENT PROCEDURE	**NORMAL FINDINGS**	**ABNORMAL FINDINGS**
Growth and development of the newborn/infant may be assessed using the Denver Developmental Screening Test. This test is used to guide the nurse to the appropriate developmental milestones for the child's gross motor, language, fine motor, and personal social development.		
Vital Signs		
Assess **temperature.** Use rectal or axillary routes in infants less than 6 months of age. The tympanic and temporal arterial routes may be used in infants older than 6 months (see Chapter 6 for detailed information on measuring temperature in infants).	Normal axillary temperature ranges from 36.3°C to 37.3°C (97.4°F–99.3°F). Normal rectal, tympanic and temporal arterial temperature is 37.8°C (100.2°F) or less.	Temperature may be altered by exercise, stress, crying, environment, diurnal variation (highest between 4 and 6 PM). Both hyperthermic and hypothermic conditions are noted in infants.

ASSESSMENT PROCEDURE	NORMAL FINDINGS	ABNORMAL FINDINGS
Note **apical pulse rate.** Count the pulse for a full minute.	Awake and resting rates vary with the age of the child (see Chapter 6). For a newborn to 1-month-old child, it should be 120 to 160 beats/min. When crying, the heart rate may increase up to 180 beats/min. Rate decreases gradually with age. At 6 months to 1 year, rate is approximately 110 beats/min.	Pulse may be altered by medications, activity, and pain as well as pathologic conditions. Bradycardia (<100 beats/min) in an infant is usually an ominous finding. Tachycardia may also indicate cardiac/respiratory problems or sepsis.
Assess **respiratory rate and character.** Measure respiratory rate and character in infants by observing abdominal movements.	In newborns up to 3 months of age, rate is 30 to 50 breaths/min. In infants greater than 3 months of age, rate is 20 to 30 breaths/min. Breathing is unlabored; lung sounds clear. Newborns are obligatory nose breathers.	Respiratory rate and character may be altered by medications, positioning, fever, activity as well as pathologic conditions. Retractions, seesaw respirations, apnea greater than 15 seconds, grunting, nasal flaring, stridor, rale, tachypnea greater than 60 breaths/min should be further evaluated for respiratory distress.

(Continued on following page)

SUBSEQUENT INFANT PHYSICAL ASSESSMENT (*continued*)

ASSESSMENT PROCEDURE	NORMAL FINDINGS	ABNORMAL FINDINGS
Measure **length.** Determine infant's height by measuring the recumbent length. Fully extend the body, holding the head in midline and gently grasping the knees and pushing them downward until the legs are fully extended and touching the table. If using a measuring board, place the head at the top of the board and the heels firmly at the bottom. Without a board, use paper under the infant and mark the paper at the top of the head and bottom of the heels. Then measure the distance between the two points. Plot height measurement on an appropriate age- and gender-specific growth chart.	See the growth charts at http://www.cdc.gov/growthcharts for normal findings.	Significant deviation from normal in the growth charts would be considered abnormal.
Measure **weight.** Measure weight on an appropriately sized beam scale with nondetectable weights. Weigh an infant lying or sitting on a scale that measures to the nearest 14.1 g (0.5 oz) or 10 g. Weigh an infant naked. Plot weight measurement on age- and gender-appropriate growth chart.	See the growth charts in http://www.cdc.gov/growthcharts for normal findings.	Deviation from the wide range of normal weights is abnormal. See http://www.cdc.gov/growthcharts and compare differences.

ASSESSMENT PROCEDURE	NORMAL FINDINGS	ABNORMAL FINDINGS
Determine HC/**chest circumference.** Measure **HC** or occipital frontal circumference (OFC) at every physical examination for infants and toddlers up to 2 years of age.	HC (OFC) measurement should fall between the 5th and 95th percentiles and should be comparable to the child's height and weight percentiles.	Abnormal circumference of head includes less than 29 and greater than 34 cm. HC (OFC) not within the normal percentiles may indicate pathology. Those greater than 95% may indicate macrocephaly. Those under the 5th percentile may indicate microcephaly.
Skin, Hair, and Nails		
Assess for **skin color, odor, and lesions.**	Skin color ranges from pale white with pink, yellow, brown, or olive tones to dark brown or black. Skin is without strong odor and lesion free. Common variations: acrocyanosis (sluggish perfusion of peripheral circulation); harlequin sign (one side of the body turns red; the other side is pale); mottling (general red/white discoloration of skin caused by chilling); Mongolian spots (Fig. 25-7); petechiae or bruising on the presenting part (due to rapid pressure and release with delivery); physiologic jaundice;	Yellow skin may indicate jaundice or passage of meconium in utero secondary to fetal distress. Jaundice within 24 hours after birth is pathologic and may indicate hemolytic disease of the newborn. Blue skin suggests cyanosis, pallor suggests anemia, and redness suggests fever, irritation.
		Ecchymoses in various stages or in unusual locations or circular burn areas suggest child abuse. Petechiae, lesions, or rashes may indicate blood disorders or neurologic disorders.

(Continued on following page)

SUBSEQUENT INFANT PHYSICAL ASSESSMENT (*continued*)

ASSESSMENT PROCEDURE	NORMAL FINDINGS	ABNORMAL FINDINGS
	birthmarks; milia; erythema toxicum; telangi-ectatic nevi (stork bites) (Fig. 25-8); café au lait less than 1.5 cm; benign hemangioma (including port wine stain, strawberry mark).	Abnormal skin lesions include: café au lait spots (six or more hyperpigmented macules, >1.5 cm diameter, may indicate neurofibromatosis, an inherited neurocutaneous disease).

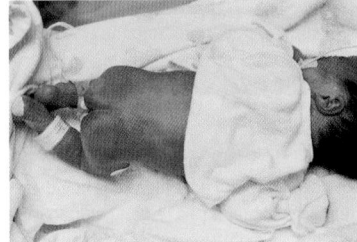

FIGURE 25-7 Mongolian spots.

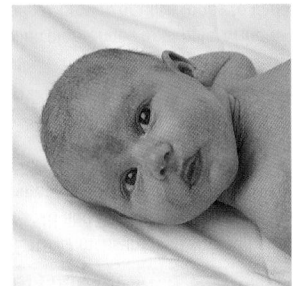

FIGURE 25-8 Stork bites.

ASSESSMENT PROCEDURE	NORMAL FINDINGS	ABNORMAL FINDINGS
Palpate for **texture, temperature, moisture, turgor, and edema.**	Skin soft, warm, and slightly moist. Vernix caseosa (cheesy, white substance that is found on the skin, especially in skinfolds) is a common finding; it eventually absorbs into the skin. Skin turgor should have quick recoil. Edema may be present around the eyes and genitalia of the newborn.	Pallor, ruddy complexion, and jaundice should be further evaluated for cardiac anomalies, blood disorders.
Inspect and palpate **hair.** Observe for distribution, characteristics, and the presence of any unusual hair on body.	Hair is normally lustrous, silky, strong, and elastic. Lanugo, fine, downy hair that covers parts of the body, such as the shoulders, back and sacral areas, may be seen in the newborn or young infant.	Dirty, matted hair may indicate neglect. Tufts of hair over spine may indicate spina bifida occulta.
Inspect and palpate **nails.** Note color, texture, shape, and condition of nails.	Nails extend to the end of fingers or beyond; are well formed.	Blue nail beds indicate cyanosis. Yellow nail beds indicate jaundice. Blue-black nail beds suggest a nail bed hemorrhage.

(Continued on following page)

SUBSEQUENT INFANT PHYSICAL ASSESSMENT (*continued*)

ASSESSMENT PROCEDURE	NORMAL FINDINGS	ABNORMAL FINDINGS

Head, Neck, and Cervical Lymph Nodes

Inspect and palpate the **head.** Note shape and symmetry. In newborns, inspect and palpate the condition of fontanelles and sutures (Fig. 25-9).

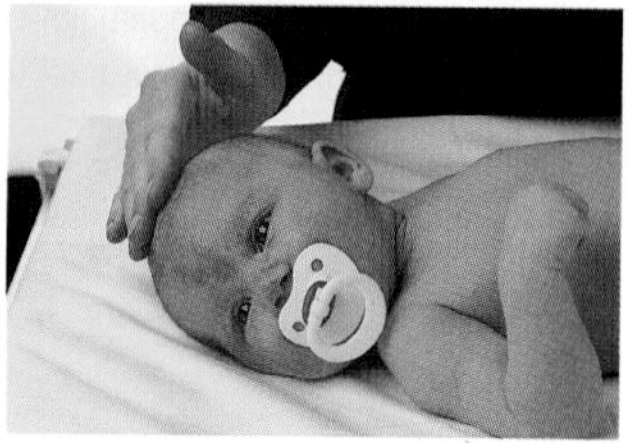

FIGURE 25-9 Palpating the anterior fontanelle. (Photo by B. Proud.)

Head is normocephalic and symmetric. In newborns, the head may be oddly shaped from molding (overriding of the sutures) during vaginal birth. The diamond-shaped anterior fontanelle measures about 4 to 5 cm at its widest part; it usually closes by 12 to 18 months. The triangular posterior fontanelle measures about 0.5 to 1 cm at its widest part, and it should close at 2 months of age (Fig. 25-10).

A common variation is caput succedaneum (Fig. 25-11A).

A very large head is found with hydrocephalus.

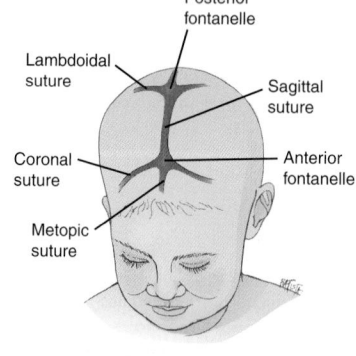

FIGURE 25-10 The infant head.

ASSESSMENT PROCEDURE	NORMAL FINDINGS	ABNORMAL FINDINGS
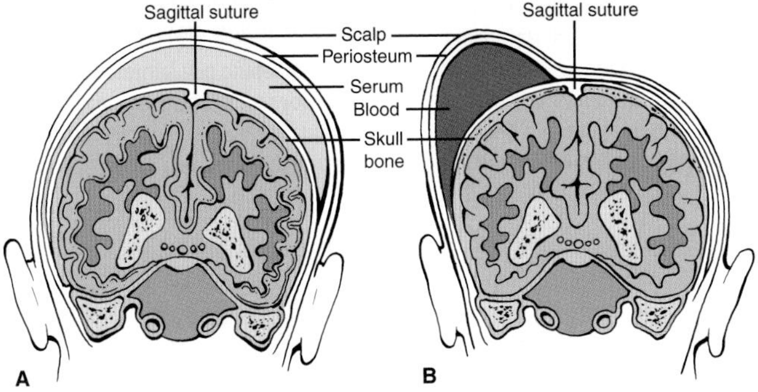 FIGURE 25-11 **(A)** Caput succedaneum. **(B)** Cephalohematoma.		An oddly shaped head is found with premature closure of sutures (possibly genetic). One-sided flattening of the head suggests prolonged positioning on one side. A third fontanelle between the anterior and posterior fontanelle is seen with Down syndrome. Bulging fontanelle indicates increased cranial pressure. Microcephaly is seen with infants who have been exposed to congenital infections. Premature closure of sutures (craniosynostosis) may result in caput succedaneum (edema from trauma), which crosses the suture line, and cephalohematoma (bleeding into the periosteal space), which does not extend across the suture line (Fig. 25-11B).
Test **head control, head posture, and ROM.**	Full ROM—up, down, and sideways—is normal. Infants should have head control by 4 months of age.	Hyperextension is seen with opisthotonos or significant meningeal irritation. Limited ROM may indicate torticollis (wryneck).

(Continued on following page)

SUBSEQUENT INFANT PHYSICAL ASSESSMENT (continued)

ASSESSMENT PROCEDURE	NORMAL FINDINGS	ABNORMAL FINDINGS
Inspect and palpate the **face**. Note appearance, symmetry, and movement. Palpate the parotid glands for swelling.	Face is normally proportionate and symmetric. Movements are equal bilaterally. Parotid glands are normal size.	Unusual proportions (short palpebral fissures, thin lips, and wide and flat philtrum, which is the groove above the upper lip) may be hereditary, or they may indicate specific syndromes such as Down syndrome and fetal alcohol syndrome. Unequal movement may indicate facial nerve paralysis. Abnormal facies may indicate chromosomal anomaly.
Inspect and palpate **the neck**. Palpate the thyroid gland and the trachea. Also inspect and palpate the cervical lymph nodes for swelling, mobility, temperature, and tenderness. *Note: The thyroid is very difficult to palpate in an infant because of the short, thick neck.*	The neck is usually short with skinfolds between the head and the shoulder during infancy. The isthmus is the only portion of the thyroid that should be palpable. The trachea is midline. Lymph nodes are usually nonpalpable in infants. Clavicles are symmetrical and intact.	Implications of some abnormal findings include the following: • Short, webbed neck suggests anomalies or syndromes such as Down syndrome. • Distended neck veins may indicate difficulty breathing. • Enlarged thyroid or palpable masses suggest a pathologic process.

ASSESSMENT PROCEDURE	NORMAL FINDINGS	ABNORMAL FINDINGS
		• Shift in tracheal position from midline suggests a serious lung problem (e.g., foreign body or tumor).
		• Crepitus when clavicle palpated along with decreased movement in arm of that side may indicate fractured clavicle.
Eyes		
Inspect the **external eye.** Note the position, slant, and epicanthal folds of the external eye.	Inner canthus distance approximately 2.5 cm, horizontal slant, nonepicanthal folds. Outer canthus aligns with tips of the pinnae.	Wide-set position (hypertelorism), upward slant, and thick epicanthal folds suggest Down syndrome. "Sun-setting" appearance (upper lid covers part of the iris) suggests hydrocephalus.
Observe **eyelid placement, swelling, discharge, and lesions.** Lacrimal duct obstruction is common in the newborn and leads to increased discharge from the affected eye.	Eyelids have transient edema, absence of tears. Lacrimal ducts unobstructed.	Eyelid inflammation may result from infection. Swelling, erythema, or purulent discharge may indicate infection or blocked tear ducts.
		Purulent discharge seen with sexually transmitted infections (gonorrhea, chlamydia). Increased discharge from the affected eye.

(Continued on following page)

SUBSEQUENT INFANT PHYSICAL ASSESSMENT (continued)

ASSESSMENT PROCEDURE	NORMAL FINDINGS	ABNORMAL FINDINGS
Inspect the **sclera and conjunctiva** for color, discharge, lesions, redness, and lacerations.	Sclera and conjunctiva are clear and free of discharge, lesions, redness, or lacerations. Small subconjunctival hemorrhages may be seen in newborns.	Yellow sclera suggests jaundice; blue sclera may indicate osteogenesis imperfecta ("brittle bone disease").
Observe **the iris and pupils.**	Typically, the iris is blue in light-skinned infants and brown in dark-skinned infants; permanent color develops within 9 months. Brushfield spots (white flecks on the periphery of the iris) may be normal in some infants. Pupils are equal, round, and reactive to light and accommodation (PERRLA).	Brushfield spots may indicate Down syndrome. Sluggish pupils indicate a neurologic problem. Miosis (constriction) indicates iritis or narcotic use or abuse. Mydriasis (pupillary dilation) indicates emotional factors (fear), trauma, or certain drug use.
Inspect the **eyebrows and eyelashes.**	Eyebrows should be symmetric in shape and movement. They should not meet midline. Eyelashes should be evenly distributed and curled outward.	Sparseness of eyebrows or lashes could indicate skin disease.

ASSESSMENT PROCEDURE	NORMAL FINDINGS	ABNORMAL FINDINGS
Perform **visual acuity tests.** Assess visual acuity by observing infant's ability to gaze at an object.	Visual acuity is difficult to test in infants; test by observing the infant's ability to fix on and follow objects. Normal visual acuity is as follows: • Birth: 20/100 to 20/400 • 1 year: 20/200 By 4 weeks of age, the infant should be able to fixate on objects. By 6 to 8 weeks, eyes should follow a moving object. By 3 months, the infant is able to follow and reach for an object.	Children with a one-line difference between eyes should be referred for ophthalmology examination.
Perform **extraocular muscle tests.** Hirschberg test: Shine light directly at the cornea while the infant looks straight ahead.	In the Hirschberg test, the light reflects symmetrically in the center of both pupils. Light causes pupils to vasoconstrict bilaterally and blink reflex occurs. Blink reflex also occurs as an object is brought toward the eyes. By 10 days of age, when turning the head, the infant's eyes should follow the position of the head.	Unequal alignment of light on the pupils in the Hirschberg test signals strabismus. Doll's-eye reflex is an abnormal reflex that occurs when the eyes do not follow or adjust to movement of head. Hirschsprung disease could also be considered, especially with a rigid abdomen. The most common finding is failure to have a bowel movement within 48 hours after birth.

(Continued on following page)

SUBSEQUENT INFANT PHYSICAL ASSESSMENT (*continued*)

ASSESSMENT PROCEDURE	NORMAL FINDINGS	ABNORMAL FINDINGS
Perform **ophthalmoscopic examination.** The procedure is the same as for adults. Distraction is preferred over the use of restraint, which is likely to result in crying and closed eyes. Careful ophthalmoscopic examination of newborns is difficult without the use of mydriatic medications.	Red reflex is present. This reflex rules out most serious defects of the cornea, aqueous chamber, lens, and vitreous humor. When visualized, the optic disc appears similar to an adult's. A newborn's optic discs are pale; peripheral vessels are not well developed.	Absence of the red reflex indicates cataracts. Papilledema is unusual in children of this age owing to the ability of the fontanelles and sutures to open during increased intracranial pressure. Disc blurring and hemorrhages should be reported immediately. Abnormal findings include congenital defects, such as cataracts.
Ears		
Inspect **external ears.** Note placement, discharge, or lesions of the ears.	Top of pinna should cross the eye-occiput line and be within a 10-degree angle of a perpendicular line drawn from the eye-occiput line to the lobe. No unusual structure or markings should appear on the pinna.	Low-set ears with an alignment greater than a 10-degree angle suggest retardation or congenital syndromes, such as Down syndrome. Abnormal shape may suggest renal disease process, which may be hereditary. Preauricular skin tags or sinuses suggest other anomalies of ears, or the renal system.

ASSESSMENT PROCEDURE	NORMAL FINDINGS	ABNORMAL FINDINGS
Inspect **internal ear.** The internal ear examination requires using an otoscope. The nurse should always hold the otoscope in a manner that allows for rapid removal if the child moves. Have the caregiver hold and restrain the infant. Because an infant's external canal is short and straight, pull the pinna down and back.	No excessive cerumen, discharge, lesions, excoriations, or foreign body in external canal. Amniotic fluid/vernix may be present in canal of the ear of newborn. Tympanic membrane is pearly gray to light pink with normal landmarks. Tympanic membranes redden bilaterally when child is crying or febrile.	Presence of foreign bodies or cerumen impaction. Purulent discharge may indicate otitis externa or the presence of foreign body. Purulent, serous discharge suggests otitis media. Bloody discharge suggests trauma, and clear discharge may indicate cerebrospinal fluid leak. Perforated tympanic membrane may also be noted.
Hearing acuity. Routine newborn hearing screening is performed in most newborn nurseries 24 to 48 hours after birth or prior to discharge. In the infant, test hearing acuity by noting the reaction to noise. Stand approximately 30.48 cm (12 in.) from the infant and create a loud noise (e.g., clap hands, shake/squeeze a noisy toy).	A newborn will exhibit the startle (Moro) reflex and blink eyes (acoustic blink reflex) in response to noise. Older infant will turn head. Infants normally attend to the human voice. Therefore, question parents as to whether their child turns their head toward the spoken voice or loud noises.	Audiometry results outside normal range suggest hearing deficit. No reactions to noise may indicate a hearing deficit.

(Continued on following page)

SUBSEQUENT INFANT PHYSICAL ASSESSMENT (*continued*)

ASSESSMENT PROCEDURE	NORMAL FINDINGS	ABNORMAL FINDINGS
Mouth, Throat, Nose, and Sinuses		
Inspect **mouth and throat**. Note the condition of the lips, palates, tongue, and buccal mucosa.	Epstein pearls, small, yellow-white retention cysts on the hard palate and gums, are common in newborns and usually disappear in the first weeks of life. In infants, a sucking tubercle (pad), from the friction of sucking, may be evident in the middle of the upper lip.	White discharge noted on the tongue or buccal mucosa is thrush. Cleft lip and/or palate are congenital abnormalities. Excessive salivation, unable to tolerate feedings may indicate esophageal atresia.
Observe the **condition of the gums**. When teeth appear, count teeth and note location.	Gums appear pink and moist. Teeth may begin erupting at 4 to 6 months. Teeth develop in sequential order. By 10 months, most infants have two upper and two lower central incisors.	Abnormal findings include lesion and edema.
Inspect **nose and sinuses**. To inspect the nose and sinuses in infants, push up the tip of the nose and shine a light into each nostril. Observe the structure and patency of the nares, discharge, tenderness, and any color or swelling of the turbinates.	Nose is midline in face, septum is straight, and nares are patent. No discharge or tenderness is present. Turbinates are pink and free of edema.	Choanal atresia is blockage of the posterior nares in the newborn. If the blockage is bilateral, the newborn is at risk for acute respiratory distress. Immediate referral is necessary. Deviated septum may be congenital or caused by injury. Foul discharge from one nostril may indicate a foreign body.

ASSESSMENT PROCEDURE	NORMAL FINDINGS	ABNORMAL FINDINGS
Note: The maxillary and ethmoid sinuses begin to develop in the 10th week and are present at birth. However, they are small and cannot be examined until they develop further.		
Note: Infants are obligatory nose breathers. Consequently, obstructed nasal passages may precipitate serious health conditions, making it very important to assess the patency of the nares in the newborn. If, after suctioning fluid and mucus from the nares, you suspect obstruction, insert a small-lumen catheter into each nostril to assess patency.		
Thorax		
Inspect the **shape of the thorax**.	Infant's thorax is smooth, rounded, and symmetric.	Abnormal shapes of the thorax include pectus excavatum and pectus carinatum.

(Continued on following page)

SUBSEQUENT INFANT PHYSICAL ASSESSMENT (*continued*)

ASSESSMENT PROCEDURE	NORMAL FINDINGS	ABNORMAL FINDINGS
Observe **respiratory effort,** keeping in mind that newborns and young infants are obligatory nose breathers.	Respirations should be unlabored and regular in all ages, except for immediate newborn period when respirations are irregular (see "Vital Signs" section). Some newborns, especially the premature, have periodic irregular breathing, sometimes with apnea (episodes when breathing stops) lasting a few seconds. This is a normal finding if bradycardia does not accompany irregular breathing.	Retractions (suprasternal, sternal, substernal, intercostal) and grunting suggest increased inspiratory effort, which may be due to airway obstruction. Periods of apnea that last longer than 15 seconds and are accompanied by bradycardia may be a sign of a cardiovascular or central nervous system (CNS) disease. Nasal flaring, tachypnea, and seesaw movement of chest indicate respiratory distress.
Auscultate for **breath sounds and adventitious sounds.** If a newborn's lung sounds seem noisy, auscultate the upper nostrils.	Breath sounds may seem louder and harsher in young children because of their thin chest walls. No adventitious sounds should be heard, although transmitted upper airway sounds may be heard on auscultation of thorax.	Diminished breath sounds suggest respiratory disorders such as pneumonia or atelectasis. Stridor (inspiratory wheeze) is a high-pitched, piercing sound that indicates a narrowing of the upper tracheobronchial tree. Expiratory wheezes indicate narrowing in the lower tracheobronchial tree. Rhonchi and rales (crackles) may indicate a number of respiratory diseases such as pneumonia, bronchitis, or bronchiolitis.

ASSESSMENT PROCEDURE	NORMAL FINDINGS	ABNORMAL FINDINGS
Breasts		
Inspect and palpate **breasts.** Note shape, symmetry, color, tenderness, discharge, lesions, and masses.	Newborns may have enlarged and engorged breasts with a white liquid discharge resulting from the influence of maternal hormones. This condition resolves spontaneously within days.	A palpable mass of the breast is abnormal. The newborn or infant may have extra nipples noted on the chest or abdomen called *supernumerary nipples.*
Heart		
Inspect and palpate the **precordium.** Note lifts, heaves, apical impulse.	The apical pulse is at the fourth intercostal space (ICS) until the age of 7 years, when it drops to the fifth. It is to the left of the midclavicular line (MCL) until age 4.	A systolic heave may indicate right ventricular enlargement. Apical impulse that is not in proper location for age may indicate cardiomyopathy, pneumothorax, or diaphragmatic hernia.
Auscultate **heart sounds.** Listen to the heart. Note rate and rhythm of apical impulse, S_1, S_2, extra heart sounds, and murmurs. Keep in mind that sinus arrhythmia is normal in infants. Heart sounds are louder, higher pitched, and of shorter duration in infants. A split S_2 at the apex occurs normally in some infants and S_3 is a normal heart sound in some children. A venous hum also may be normally heard in children.	Normal heart rates are cited in the "Vital Signs" section. Innocent murmurs, which are common throughout childhood, are classified as systolic; short duration; no transmission to other areas; grade III or less; loudest in pulmonic area (base of heart); low-pitched, musical, or groaning quality that varies in intensity in relation to position, respiration, activity, fever, and anemia. No other associated signs of heart disease should be found.	Murmurs that do not fit the criteria for innocent murmurs may indicate a disease or disorder. Extra heart sounds and variations in pulse rate and rhythm also suggest pathologic processes.

(Continued on following page)

SUBSEQUENT INFANT PHYSICAL ASSESSMENT (*continued*)

ASSESSMENT PROCEDURE	NORMAL FINDINGS	ABNORMAL FINDINGS
Abdomen		
Inspect the **shape of the abdomen**.	In infants, the abdomen shape is cylindrical, round, soft.	A scaphoid (boat-shaped; i.e., sunken with prominent rib cage) abdomen may result from malnutrition or dehydration. Distended abdomen may indicate pyloric stenosis.
Inspect **umbilicus.** Note color, discharge, and evident herniation of the umbilicus.	Umbilicus is pink, no discharge, odor, redness, or herniation. Cord should demonstrate three vessels (two arteries and one vein). Remnant of cord should appear dried 24 to 48 hours after birth.	Inflammation, discharge, and redness of umbilicus suggest infection. Diastasis recti (separation of the abdominal muscles) is seen as midline protrusion from the xiphoid to the umbilicus or pubis symphysis. This condition is secondary to immature musculature of abdominal muscles and usually has little significance. As the muscles strengthen, the separation resolves on its own.

ASSESSMENT PROCEDURE	NORMAL FINDINGS	ABNORMAL FINDINGS
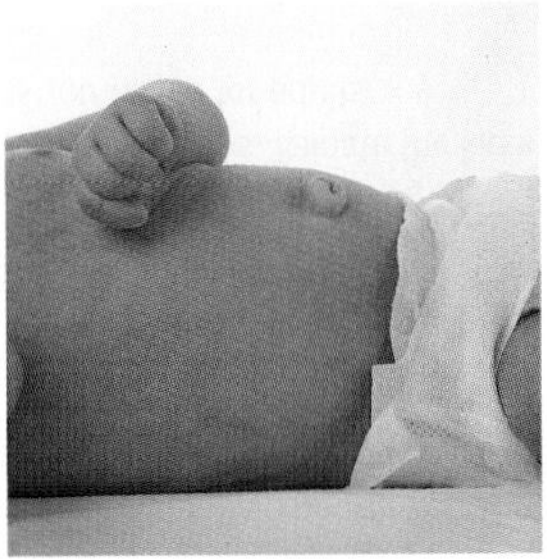 FIGURE 25-12 Umbilical hernia.		A bulge at the umbilicus suggests an umbilical hernia, which may be seen in newborns; many disappear by the age of 1 year (Fig. 25-12). Abnormal insertion of cord, discolored cord, or two-vessel cord could indicate genetic abnormalities; however, these are also seen in newborns without abnormalities.
Observe **abdomen**.	The infant's abdomen is cylindrical, and no peristaltic waves are visible.	Peristaltic waves may be visible in infants up to 3 months of age and may be indicative of a disease or disorder such as pyloric stenosis (Mayo Clinic, 2018).
Auscultate **bowel sounds**. Follow auscultation guidelines for adult clients provided in Chapter 19.	Bowel sounds present 30 to 60 minutes after birth. Normal bowel sounds occur every 10 to 30 seconds. They sound like clicks, gurgles, or growls.	See Chapter 19.

(Continued on following page)

SUBSEQUENT INFANT PHYSICAL ASSESSMENT (*continued*)

ASSESSMENT PROCEDURE	NORMAL FINDINGS	ABNORMAL FINDINGS
Palpate for **masses and tenderness.** Palpate abdomen for softness or hardness.	Abdomen is soft to palpation and without masses or tenderness.	A rigid abdomen is almost always an emergent problem. Masses or tenderness warrant further investigation. Hirschsprung disease may be considered, with rigid abdomen and no bowel movement within 48 hours after birth.
Palpate **liver.** Palpate the liver the same as you would for adults (see Chapter 19).	Liver is usually palpable 1 to 2 cm below the right costal margin. ***Note:*** *It is difficult to palpate the liver in the newborn.*	An enlarged liver with a firm edge that is palpated more than 2 cm below the right costal margin usually indicates a pathologic process.
Palpate **spleen.** Palpate the spleen the same as you would for adults.	Spleen tip may be palpable during inspiration. The spleen is difficult to palpate in the newborn.	Enlarged spleen is usually indicative of a pathologic process.
Palpate **kidneys.** Palpate the kidneys the same as you would for adults.	The tip of the right kidney may be palpable during inspiration. The newborn voids within first 24 hours after birth.	Enlarged kidneys are usually indicative of a pathologic process. No urinary output beyond 48 hours after birth may indicate kidney problems.
Palpate **bladder.** Palpate the bladder the same as you would for adults.	Bladder may be slightly palpable in infants and small children.	An enlarged bladder is usually due to urinary retention but may be due to a mass.

ASSESSMENT PROCEDURE	NORMAL FINDINGS	ABNORMAL FINDINGS
Male Genitalia		
Inspect **penis and urinary meatus.** Inspect the genitalia, observing size for age and any lesions. *Note: Circumcision is a topic of discussion due to increased anticircumcision activism (Strobbe, 2014). It is a personal decision often based on cultural or religious beliefs; studies in Africa suggest circumcision may reduce spread of HIV-AIDS; benefits of circumcision have become more clear over the past 10 years; acceptance of circumcision has swung wildly in the United States from about 25% of males in 1900, to high acceptance and back to 58% in 2010. Stobbe lists the Centers for Disease Control and Prevention (CDC) conclusions that male circumcision can:* • *Cut a man's risk by 50% to 60% of becoming infected with HIV from an infected female partner*	Penis is normal size for age, and no lesions are seen; however, diaper rash is a common finding in infants. The foreskin is retractable in an uncircumcised child. Urinary meatus is at tip of glans penis and has no discharge or redness. Penis may appear small in LGA boys because of overlapping skinfolds. For circumcised boys, the site is dry with minimal swelling and drainage.	An unretractable foreskin in a child older than 3 months suggests phimosis. Paraphimosis is indicated when the foreskin is tightened around the glans penis in a retracted position. Hypospadias, urinary meatus on ventral surface of glans, and epispadias, urinary meatus on dorsal surface of glans, are congenital disorders.

(Continued on following page)

SUBSEQUENT INFANT PHYSICAL ASSESSMENT (*continued*)		
ASSESSMENT PROCEDURE	**NORMAL FINDINGS**	**ABNORMAL FINDINGS**
• *Reduce risk by 30% of becoming infected with genital herpes or human papillomavirus* • *Lower the risk of urinary tract infection (UTI) in infancy and of cancer of penis in adulthood* • *There is no support that circumcision stops the spread of AIDS to women or same sex partners*		
Inspect and palpate **scrotum and testes.** To rule out cryptorchidism, it is important to palpate for testes in the scrotum in infants.	Scrotum is free of lesions. Testes are palpable in scrotum, with the left testicle usually lower than the right. Testes are equal in size, smooth, mobile, and free of masses. If a testicle is missing from the scrotal sac but the scrotal sac appears well developed, suspect physiologic cryptorchidism. The testis has originally descended into the scrotum but has moved back up into the inguinal canal because of the cremasteric reflex and the small size of the testis. You should be able to milk the testis down into the scrotum from the inguinal canal. This normal condition subsides at puberty.	Absent testicle(s) and atrophic scrotum suggest true cryptorchidism (undescended testicles). This suggests that the testicle(s) never descended. This condition occurs more frequently in preterm than term infants because testes descend at 8 months of gestation. It can lead to testicular atrophy and infertility and increases the risk for testicular cancer.

ASSESSMENT PROCEDURE	NORMAL FINDINGS	ABNORMAL FINDINGS
		Hydroceles are common in infants. They are a collection of fluid along the spermatic cord within the scrotum that can be transilluminated. They usually resolve spontaneously.
		A scrotal hernia is most often caused by an indirect inguinal hernia that has descended into the scrotum. It can usually be pushed back into the inguinal canal. This mass will not transilluminate.
Inspect and palpate **inguinal area for hernias.** Observe for any bulge in the inguinal area. Using your pinky finger, palpate up the inguinal canal to the external inguinal ring if a hernia is suspected.	No inguinal hernias are present.	A bulge in the inguinal area or palpation of a mass in the inguinal canal suggests an inguinal hernia. Indirect inguinal hernias occur most frequently in children.

(Continued on following page)

SUBSEQUENT INFANT PHYSICAL ASSESSMENT (*continued*)

ASSESSMENT PROCEDURE	NORMAL FINDINGS	ABNORMAL FINDINGS
Female Genitalia		
Inspect **external genitalia**. Note labia majora, labia minora, vaginal orifice, urinary meatus, and clitoris.	Labia majora and minora are pink and moist. Newborn's genitalia may appear prominent because of influence of maternal hormones. Bruises and swelling may be caused by breech vaginal delivery. Pseudomenstruation (blood-tinged discharge) and smegma (cheesy, white discharge) of the sebaceous gland. Reddish, orange, pink-tinged urine or stain on diaper may also be normal due to uric acid crystals.	Enlarged clitoris in newborn combined with fusion of the posterior labia majora suggests ambiguous genitalia.
Anus and Rectum		
Inspect the **anus**. The anus should be inspected in infants. Spread the buttocks with gloved hands; note patency of anal opening, the presence of any lesions and fissures, and condition and color of perianal skin.	The anal opening should be visible and moist. Meconium is passed within 24 to 48 hours after birth. Perianal skin should be smooth and free of lesions. Perianal skin tags may be noted.	Imperforate anus (no anal opening) should be referred. No passage of meconium stool could indicate no patency of anus or cystic fibrosis. Pustules may indicate secondary infection of diaper rash.

ASSESSMENT PROCEDURE	NORMAL FINDINGS	ABNORMAL FINDINGS
Musculoskeletal		
Assess **arms, hands, feet, and legs.** Note symmetry, shape, movement, and positioning of the feet and legs. Perform neurovascular assessment.	Five fingers and toes on each extremity, no webbing, normal palmar creases. Bilateral movement with full ROM in arms and legs. Legs have equal length, normal position of feet.	Short, broad extremities, hyperextensible joints, and palmar simian crease may indicate Down syndrome. Polydactyly (extra digits) and syndactyly (webbing) are sometimes found in children with mental retardation.
		Fixed-position (true) deformities do not return to normal position with manipulation. Metatarsus varus is inversion (a turning inward that elevates the medial margin) and adduction of the forefoot.
		Talipes varus is adduction of the forefoot and inversion of the entire foot.
		Talipes equinovarus (clubfoot) is indicated if foot is fixed in the following position: adduction of forefoot, inversion of entire foot, and equinus (pointing downward) position of entire foot.

(Continued on following page)

SUBSEQUENT INFANT PHYSICAL ASSESSMENT (*continued*)		
ASSESSMENT PROCEDURE	**NORMAL FINDINGS**	**ABNORMAL FINDINGS**
Assess for **congenital hip dysplasia**. Assessing for hip dysplasia is an important aspect of the physical examination for infants. The assessment should be performed at each visit until the child is about 1 year old. (Several tests are described below.)	Symmetrical bilateral gluteal folds and full hip abduction are normal findings.	Unequal gluteal folds and limited hip abduction are signs of congenital hip dysplasia.
Begin by assessing the symmetry of the gluteal folds. Also assess hip abduction using the maneuvers below.		
Perform Ortolani maneuver to test for congenital hip dysplasia. With the infant supine, flex infant's knees while holding your thumbs on midthigh and your fingers over the greater trochanters; abduct the legs, moving the knees outward and down toward the table.	Negative Ortolani sign is normal.	Positive Ortolani sign: A click heard along with feeling the head of the femur slip in or out of the hip.
Perform Barlow maneuvers. With the infant supine, flex the infant's knees while holding your thumbs on midthigh and your fingers over the greater trochanters; adduct legs until thumbs touch.	Negative Barlow sign is normal.	Positive Barlow sign: A feeling of the head of the femur slipping out of the hip socket (acetabulum).

ASSESSMENT PROCEDURE	NORMAL FINDINGS	ABNORMAL FINDINGS
Assess **spinal alignment.** Observe spine and posture.	No spinal openings. In newborns, the spine is flexible and rounded in infants younger than 3 months (Fig. 25-13).	Opening in spinal column, pilonidal dimple could indicate spina bifida or other spinal abnormalities. In newborns, flaccid or rigid posture is considered abnormal. In older infants, abnormal posture suggests neuromuscular disorders such as cerebral palsy.

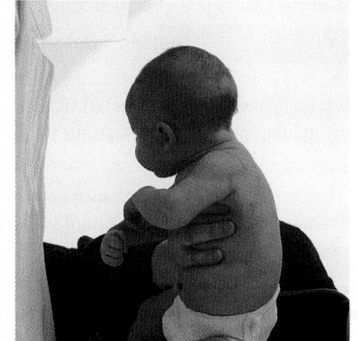

FIGURE 25-13 The spine is rounded in infants less than 3 months.

(Continued on following page)

SUBSEQUENT INFANT PHYSICAL ASSESSMENT (*continued*)		
ASSESSMENT PROCEDURE	**NORMAL FINDINGS**	**ABNORMAL FINDINGS**
Assess **joints.** Note ROM, swelling, redness, and tenderness.	Full ROM and no swelling, redness, or tenderness.	Limited ROM, swelling, redness, and tenderness indicate problems ranging from mild injuries to serious disorders.
Assess **muscles.** Note size and strength. (For example, can the infant bear weight on their legs?)	Muscle size and strength should be adequate for the particular age and should be equal bilaterally.	Inadequate muscle size and strength for the particular age indicate neuromuscular disorders such as muscular dystrophy.
Neurologic System		
Assess the newborn's and infant's **cry, responsiveness, and adaptation.**	The newborn's and infant's cries are lusty and strong; responds appropriately to stimuli and quiets to soothing when held in the en face position.	Inappropriate response to stimuli suggests CNS disorders or problems. An inability to quiet to soothing and gaze aversion is seen in "cocaine babies." Infantile reflexes present when inappropriate, absent, or asymmetric may indicate a CNS problem.
Test **deep tendon and superficial reflexes** (see Chapter 21).	Infantile reflexes are present when appropriate and are symmetric.	Absence or marked intensity of these reflexes, asymmetry may demonstrate pathology.
Test **motor function.** See "Developmental Assessment" section in the beginning of the subsequent infant physical assessment.		

POSSIBLE COLLABORATIVE PROBLEMS—RISK OF

- Elevated bilirubin levels
- Infection
  - Circumcision
  - Nosocomial
  - Bacterial

Teaching Tips for Selected Client Concerns

Client Concern: *Opportunity to enhance healthy feeding pattern for infant*

Solid foods are not recommended before 4 to 6 months, at which time the baby stops using the tongue to push food out of mouth and develops coordination to move food from the front of mouth to the back for swallowing. The baby can also hold head in steady, upright position; sit with support; and is mouthing hands or toys. Now the baby shows a desire for food by leaning forward and opening mouth (Mayo Clinic, 2019). For most infants, it does not matter what the first solid foods are, but Mayo Clinic provides the following guidelines: Start with single-ingredient salt- and sugar-free foods. Offer this chosen food for 3 to 5 days to see if diarrhea occurs. If tolerated, another single-ingredient food can be added. Next begin adding fruits and vegetables one at a time. By 8 to 10 months, finely chopped finger foods can be added. Essential ingredients that must be added by 4 months are iron and zinc, which are found in pureed meats and single-grain iron-fortified cereal (cultural variation using beans and lentils is also acceptable). Verify with a health care provider the recommended iron supplementation for the infant, which is based on prematurity, term, and whether the infant is breastfed or formula-fed (with variations depending on the formula).

Client Concern: *Risk for sudden death of infant associated with suffocation and mother's lack of knowledge of safe infant positioning in bed*

Because of the possibility of sudden infant death syndrome (SIDS), caution parents to place their young infants to sleep in the supine or side-lying position.

Healthy infants should be placed on their back, using a firm sleep surface, when putting them to sleep (Colson et al., 2017).

Client Concern: *Ineffective thermoregulation related to newborn decrease in body fat and cool environment*

Assess temperature every 30 minutes $\times$ 4, then per protocol. Maintain temperature at 36.4°C to 37.3°C (97.6°F–99.2°F). Keep infant temperature probe attached properly to skin to ensure reading probe accurately. Monitor for signs and symptoms of cold stress. Keep infant warm and dry. Postpone bath until temperature is stable. Apply cap to head and extra blankets to infant if temperature less than 36.4°C (97.6°F). Teach parents the mechanisms of heat loss: radiation, convection, conduction, and evaporation. Teach techniques used to prevent cold stress and to maintain or increase infant temperature (e.g., dress, cap, blanket wrap, cuddle). Teach parents correct procedure in taking newborn axillary temperature, reading thermometer, and interpreting results.

***Client Concern:** Opportunity to enhance understanding of circumcision practices associated with parental questions regarding circumcision*

Circumcision has become a topic of discussion due to increased anticircumcision activism (Strobbe, 2014). However, the CDC (Morris et al., 2017) concluded that the benefits greatly outweigh the risks; the scientific evidence shows that, in addition to benefits that are found in both poor and wealthy countries (such as cost-savings over the long term and protection against numerous conditions and infections), male circumcision "has no adverse effect on sexual function, sensitivity, or pleasure, nor is there reliable evidence for any long-term adverse psychological effect" (p. 22).

References

Colson, E., Geller, N., Heeren, T., & Corwin, M. (2017). Factors associated with choice of infant sleep position. *Pediatrics, 140*(3). https://doi.org/10.1542/peds.2017-0596

D'Alessandro, D. (2015). *With an isolated ear tag, does the baby need to have a renal ultrasound?* https://pediatriceducation.org/2015/08/17/with-an-isolated-ear-tag-does-the-baby-need-to-have-a-renal-ultrasound/

Mayo Clinic. (2018). *Pyloric stenosis.* https://www.mayoclinic.org/diseases conditions/pyloric-stenosis/symptoms-causes/syc-20351416

Mayo Clinic. (2019). *Solid foods: How to get your baby started.* https://www.mayoclinic.org/healthy-lifestyle/infant-and-toddler-health/in-depth/healthy-baby/art-20046200

Morris, B., Krieger, J., & Klausner, J. (2017). CDC's male circumcision recommendations represent a key public health measure. *Global Health, Science and Practice, 5*(1), 15–27. https://doi.org/10.9745/GHSP-D-16-00390

Strobbe, M. (2014, December 2). *CDC: Circumcision outweighs risks.* https://www.yahoo.com/news/cdc-circumcision-benefits-outweigh-risks-134651002.html?ref=gs

26 ASSESSING OLDER ADULTS

Common physical findings in older adult clients have been identified throughout the preceding body system chapters. Advancing age places a person at higher risk for chronic illness and disability. It is not, however, the physiologic changes of aging alone that warrant a special approach to assessment of the older adult client. Many older adults are healthy, active, and independent despite these normal physical changes in their bodies. It is, rather, that advancing age has a tendency to place a person at higher risk for chronic illness and disability. The term "frail elderly" describes the vulnerability of the "old-old" (generally mid-80s, 90s, and centenarians) to be in poorer health, to have more chronic disabilities, and to function less independently. Loss of physiologic reserve is the main reason that older adults are more likely to be sick and disabled.

Older Adult Nursing Assessment

Some type of disability (e.g., difficulty in hearing, vision, cognition, ambulation, self-care, or independent living) was reported by 35% of people aged 65 years and over in 2017, and many with more severe disabilities need assistance to meet daily needs (Administration on Aging, 2018). Additional aspects of frailty include cognitive impairment, depression, and decline in mobility, strength, endurance, nutrition, and physical activity. Weakness and fatigue are central to almost all definitions of frailty. Sarcopenia (skeletal muscle mass decrease) and sarcopenic obesity (muscle mass decrease with excessive body fat), common in aging, are related to functional impairments in older adults (Batsis et al., 2015). Although frailty is associated with increasing age, aging itself is independent of frailty. Frailty involves multisystem dysfunction. DNA damage also occurs throughout the body, causing changes in cells, enzymes, ion, and nutrient production and much more, including decreases in metabolism (National Institute on Aging [NIH], 2021). Cellular aging affects organ function.

When the physiology of advanced age is combined with comorbidity, assessment is complicated. In fact, the signs and symptoms of illness often present differently in the oldest-old. Adverse drug effects (ADEs) in this population include falls, confusion, incontinence, generalized weakness, and lethargy. These responses are associated with common geriatric syndromes, which are conditions with potential multiple causes found in the elderly. The most common geriatric syndromes are urinary incontinence, cognitive impairment, pressure injury, falls, polypharmacy, delirium, and weight loss (Kim & Miller, 2017). Other issues related to the syndromes include malnutrition, eating and feeding problems, sleeping problems, dizziness and syncope, and self-neglect. Knowing the older person's usual level-of-functioning baseline is essential to compare new assessment data collected. Clearly, the key to recognizing pathology and illness in the very old is in knowing the person's baseline functional status and recognizing a deviation from it.

Symptoms of disease in the very old frequently manifest as incontinence, falls, weakness and lethargy, confusion, changes in sleep or level of alertness, and loss of appetite or weight loss. These syndromes describe the common and most recognizable ways in which disease often presents itself in the frail elderly and result from the consequences of physiologic stress. For example, incontinence and confusion are often signs of infection in the frail older adult. The incontinence and confusion can easily lead to a fall when the older person attempts to walk to the bathroom. This cascading of unfortunate events often leads a frail but independent older adult living at home to disability and dependence on others.

COLLECTING SUBJECTIVE DATA

Be sensitive to the older person's need to be respected and acknowledged. Always begin the interview by addressing an older person as "Mr.," "Mrs.," or "Ms.," or with an appropriate title such as "Reverend" or "Doctor." If the older person is too lethargic, agitated, or medically unstable to respond, family or professional caregivers should be queried with regard to how current cognition and behavior compares with the client's prior level of function.

Mental status: History of falls, weakness, incontinence, confusion, sleep difficulties, or loss of appetite? Social and economic resources? Current living environment including isolation, physical barriers, or neglect? Changes in memory? Anger or inability to control frustrations?

Falls: Use of assistive devices to walk or for balance? Lightheaded or dizzy when getting up from chair or bed? Difficulty getting up out of bed or sitting in a chair? Stiffness and soreness inhibit ability to move about? Feel like legs are weak or going to "give way"?

Weakness: fatigue and dyspnea: Daily activities and exercise? Leg pain, cramping, aching, fatigue, or weakness in the calf? Change in energy level and effects on daily activities? Shortness of breath and relationship to activities? Sweating, cough, and sputum production?

Weakness: nutrition and hydration: Daily nutrition and habits? Change in weight or appetite? A screening tool (36-hour food diary or Mini-Nutritional Assessment) may be helpful in identifying those at risk for being malnourished. Anorexia? Choking? Amount of fluid intake? Pneumococcal vaccine?

Urinary incontinence: Leakage, difficulty starting stream, dribbling, nighttime medications? (Male) Do you have difficulty starting a stream of urine? Frequency? Nighttime frequency? Dribbling?

Bowel elimination: Problems with bowel elimination? Change in bowel habits? Blood in stools? Narcotics?

Pain: Pain, discomfort, aching, or soreness? Relieved by rest or aggravated with activity? If the older adult is nonverbal and demented, routinely evaluate behaviors such as grimacing, striking out, moaning, and agitation to identify pain as well as to evaluate the degree to which the pain is being relieved (Box 26-1).

Activities of daily living: Assess the client's abilities to perform activities of daily living using the Katz Activities of Daily Living (Box 26-2) and the Lawton Scale for Instrumental Activities of Daily Living (IADL) (Box 26-3).

BOX 26-1 ASSESSMENT OF PAIN IN OLDER ADULT CLIENTS WITH OR WITHOUT COGNITIVE IMPAIRMENT

Hulla et al. (2019) reported that an NIH study found that 53% of persons over age 65 years had some level of persistent pain and 75% of those had pain in more than one site. Such pain limits physical capacity, which tends to limit physical activity, leading to greater pain and disability, possible weight gain and obesity, which again contribute to further pain of weight-bearing joints. Sleep and social isolation may also result. Banicek (2010) lists tools and behaviors for assessing pain in older adults with and without cognitive impairment.

To assess pain in the *cognitively impaired older adult*, consider the following indicators of pain:

- Medical diagnoses known to commonly cause pain such as arthritis, osteoporosis, fractures, cancer, and history of back pain
- Pain history and use of analgesics
- Family or professional caregiver reports of possible pain
- Behavioral patterns of aggressiveness or resisting care
- Rubbing on specific areas of body
- Vocalizations, such as moaning (yelling, or increases in the loudness of existing vocalizations)

In addition, observe behaviors that may indicate pain, such as facial expressions (frowning, grimacing); vocalization (crying, groaning); change in body language (rocking, guarding); rubbing on specific areas of body; behavioral change (refusing to eat, alteration in usual patterns); physiologic change (blood pressure, heart rate); and physical change (skin tears, pressure areas). A good pain assessment scale to use for the older adult with cognitive impairment is the Faces Pain Scale – Revised (FPS-R) (International Association for the Study of Pain, 2001) (see Chapter 7).

To assess pain in the older adult *without* cognitive impairment, use one of the three following pain assessment tools: Visual Analog Scale (VAS), the Verbal Numerical Rating Scale (VNRS), or the categorical rating scale using words such as "none (0)," "mild (1)," "moderate (2)," or "severe (3)." The VNRS has been shown to be the best scale for assessing pain in older adults with no cognitive impairment.

See Chapter 7 for more details of pain assessment scales.

BOX 26-2	KATZ ACTIVITIES OF DAILY LIVING	
Activities	**Independence**	**Dependence**
Points (1 or 0)	(1 Point) NO supervision, direction, or personal assistance	(0 Points) WITH supervision, direction, personal assistance, or total care
Bathing Points: _____	(1 POINT) Bathes self completely or needs help in bathing only a single part of the body such as the back, genital area, or disabled extremity.	(0 POINTS) Needs help with bathing more than one part of the body or help getting in or out of the tub or shower. Requires total bathing.
Dressing Points: _____	(1 POINT) Gets clothes from closets and drawers, and puts on clothes and outer garments complete with fasteners. May have help tying shoes.	(0 POINTS) Needs help with dressing self or needs to be completely dressed.
Toileting Points: _____	(1 POINT) Goes to toilet, gets on and off, arranges clothes, cleans genital area without help.	(0 POINTS) Needs help transferring to the toilet, cleaning self, or uses bedpan or commode.
Transferring Points _____	(1 POINT) Moves in and out of bed or chair unassisted. Mechanical transferring aides are acceptable.	(0 POINTS) Needs help in moving from bed to chair or requires a complete transfer.
Continence Points: _____	(1 POINT) Exercises complete self-control over urination and defecation.	(0 POINTS) Is partially or totally incontinent of bowel or bladder.
Feeding Points: _____	(1 POINT) Gets food from plate into mouth without help. Preparation of food may be done by another person.	(0 POINTS) Needs partial or total help with feeding or requires parenteral feeding.
Total Points = _____	6 = High (patient independent)	0 = Low (patient very dependent)

Adapted with permission from Gerontological Society of America; Katz, S., Down, T. D., Cash, H. R., & Grotz, R. C. (1970). Progress in development of the index of ADL. *Gerontologist, 10*, 20–30. https://doi.org/10.1093/geront/10.1_Part_1.20, with permission.

BOX 26-3 LAWTON SCALE FOR INSTRUMENTAL ACTIVITIES OF DAILY LIVING (IADL)

Instructions: Start by asking the client to describe their functioning in each category; then complement the description with specific questions as needed.

ABILITY TO TELEPHONE
1. Operates telephone on own initiative: looks up and dials numbers, and so on.
2. Answers telephone and dials a few well-known numbers.
3. Answers telephone but does not dial.
4. Does not use telephone at all.

SHOPPING
1. Takes care of all shopping needs independently.
2. Shops independently for small purchases.
3. Needs to be accompanied on any shopping trip.
4. Completely unable to shop.

FOOD PREPARATION
1. Plans, prepares, and serves adequate meals independently.
2. Prepares adequate meals if supplied with ingredients.
3. Heats and serves prepared meals, or prepares meals but does not maintain adequate diet.
4. Needs to have meals prepared and served.

HOUSEKEEPING
1. Maintains house alone or with occasional assistance (e.g., heavy work done by domestic help).
2. Performs light daily tasks such as dishwashing and bed making.
3. Performs light daily tasks but cannot maintain acceptable level of cleanliness.
4. Needs help with all home maintenance tasks.
5. Does not participate in any housekeeping tasks.

LAUNDRY
1. Does personal laundry completely.
2. Launders small items; rinses socks, stockings, and so on.
3. All laundry must be done by others.

MODE OF TRANSPORTATION
1. Travels independently on public transportation, or drives own car.
2. Arranges own travel via taxi, but does not otherwise use public transportation.
3. Travels on public transportation when assisted or accompanied by another.

4. Travel is limited to taxi, automobile, or ambulette, with assistance.
5. Does not travel at all.

RESPONSIBILITY FOR OWN MEDICATION
1. Is responsible for taking medication in correct dosages at correct time.
2. Takes responsibility if medication is prepared in advance, in separated dosages.
3. Is not capable of dispensing own medication.

ABILITY TO HANDLE FINANCES
1. Manages financial matters independently (budgets, writes checks, pays rent and bills, goes to bank); collects and keeps track of income.
2. Manages day-to-day purchases but needs help with banking, major purchases, controlled spending, and so on.
3. Incapable of handling money.

Scoring: Circle one number for each domain. Total the numbers circled. Total score can range from 8 to 28. The lower the score, the more independence. Scores are only good for individual patients. Useful to see score comparison over time.

Reprinted with permission from Lawton, M. P. (1971). The functional assessment of elderly people. *Journal of the American Geriatrics Society, 19*(6), 465–481. https://doi.org/10.1111/j.1532-5415.1971.tb01206.x. Reprinted by permission of Blackwell Science, Inc.

COLLECTING OBJECTIVE DATA

Equipment Needed

The following items will be needed for assessing the functional capacity of the frail elderly adult:

- Newspaper or book and lamplight for vision testing
- Lemon slice or mint for sense of smell test
- Pudding, or food of pudding consistency, and spoon for swallowing examination. A teacup may also be used.
- Food and fluid diary sheets or forms
- Two or three pillows for client comfort and positioning
- Straight-backed chair for "Timed Up and Go" (TUG) test (see Box 26-6)

Physical Assessment

ASSESSMENT PROCEDURE	NORMAL FINDINGS/VARIATIONS	ABNORMAL FINDINGS
Measure **client's height and weight**, noting weight changes, appetite changes, and problems with swallowing or chewing. Review **laboratory values** (complete blood count and levels of vitamin B_{12}, cholesterol, albumin, and prealbumin). *Note: Suspect drug toxicity in clients taking medications such as digoxin, theophylline, quinidine, or antibiotics if client reports nausea, diarrhea, or sudden and severe appetite loss.*	Antral cells and intestinal villi atrophy, and gastric production of hydrochloric acid decreases with age. Chronic diseases such as cancer and arthritis are associated with increases in inflammatory chemicals that can cause anorexia and fatigue. A certain degree of anorexia also always accompanies pain—especially chronic pain.	Indicators of malnutrition include the following: • Client weighs less than 80% of ideal body weight. • Client has had 10% loss in body weight over past 6 months or 5% loss in body weight over past month. Hemoglobin level is less than 12 g/dL. Hematocrit is less than 35%. Vitamin B_{12} level is less than 100 µg/mL. Indicators of poor nutritional status include serum cholesterol level less than 160 mg/dL; serum albumin level less than 3.5 g/dL; prealbumin level less than 19.5 g/dL.
Evaluate **hydration status** as you would nutritional status. Begin with accurate serial measurements of weight, careful review of laboratory test findings (serial serum sodium level, hematocrit, osmolality, blood urea nitrogen [BUN] level, and urine-specific gravity), and a 2- to 3-day diary of fluid intake and output.	Normal findings include stable weight and stable mental status. *Note: Increases over time in laboratory values may be indicators of deteriorating hydration (even though values may be within normal limits).*	Sudden weight loss; fever; dry, warm skin; furrowed, swollen, and red tongue; decreased urine output; lethargy and weakness are all signs of dehydration. Acute changes in mental status (particularly confusion), tachycardia, and hypotension may indicate severe dehydration, which may be precipitated by certain medications (e.g., diuretics,

SKIN AND HAIR

ASSESSMENT PROCEDURE	NORMAL FINDINGS/VARIATIONS	ABNORMAL FINDINGS
Inspect and palpate **skin lesions.** Wear gloves while palpating lesions (flat, raised, palpable or nonpalpable, color, size, and exudates).	Despite decrease in total number of melanocytes, hyperpigmentation occurs in sun-exposed skin (neck, face, and arms). Environmental exposure and diminished immunity increase risk of skin cancer and cutaneous infections such as ringworm and *Candida* infections of mouth, vagina, and nail beds. This risk is increased in diabetes mellitus, malnutrition, and steroid or antibiotic use.	Abnormal findings include the following: • Irregularly shaped lesion or scaly, elevated lesion (squamous cell carcinoma). • Actinic keratoses, round or irregularly shaped tan, scaly lesions that may bleed or be inflamed (premalignancy). • Waxy or raised lesion, especially on sun-exposed areas (basal cell carcinoma).
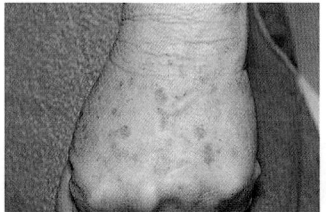 **FIGURE 26-1** Solar lentigines are very common on aging skin.	Normal variations include the following: • Lentigines: Hyperpigmentation in sun-exposed areas appears as brown, pigmented, round, or rectangular patches, often called *liver spots* (Fig. 26-1). • Venous lakes: Reddish vascular lesions on ears or other facial areas resulting from dilation of small, red blood vessels. • Skin tags: Acrochordons, flesh-colored pedunculated lesions.	• Herpes zoster vesicles (shingles) draining clear fluid or pustules atop an erythematous base following a clear linear pattern and accompanied by pain. More than half of elderly with shingles will have neuralgia that persists after resolution of the skin lesions. • Pinpoint-sized, red-purple, nonblanchable petechiae (common sign of platelet deficiency).

(Continued on following page)

SKIN AND HAIR (*continued*)

ASSESSMENT PROCEDURE	NORMAL FINDINGS/VARIATIONS	ABNORMAL FINDINGS
	• Seborrheic keratoses: Tan, brown, or reddish, flat lesions commonly found on fair-skinned people in sun-exposed areas. • Cherry angiomas: Small, round, red spots. • Senile purpura: Vivid purple patches (lesion should not blanch to touch).	• Large bruises may result from anticoagulant therapy, a fall, renal or liver failure, or elder abuse.
Note **color, texture, integrity, and moisture of skin and sensitivity to heat or cold.** *Note*: Pinching skin is not an accurate test of turgor in older adults. *Note*: Room humidifiers, avoidance of harsh deodorants or soaps, and use of lanolin-containing products after bathing (while skin is still moist) may help relieve effects of dry skin.	Somewhat transparent, pale skin with an overall decrease in body hair on lower extremities. Dry skin is common. Elastic collagen is gradually replaced with more fibrous tissue and loss of subcutaneous tissue. Skin may wrinkle and tent when pinched.	Torn skin (possibly the result of abrasive tape used to hold bandages or tubes in place). Extremely thin, fragile skin (friable skin) with excessive purpura (possibly from corticosteroid use). Dry, warm skin; furrowed tongue; and sunken eyes due to dehydration (especially with decreased urinary output; increased serum sodium, BUN, and creatinine levels; increased osmolality, and hematocrit values; tachycardia; and mental confusion).

ASSESSMENT PROCEDURE	NORMAL FINDINGS/VARIATIONS	ABNORMAL FINDINGS
		Sudden heat or cold intolerance could be signs of thyroid dysfunction.
		Decreased vascularity and diminished neurologic response to temperature changes and atrophy of eccrine sweat glands increase the risk of hyperthermia and hypothermia.
Inspect and palpate **hair, scalp, and nails.**	Loss of pigmentation causes graying of scalp, axillary, and pubic hair.	Patchy or asymmetric hair loss is abnormal.
	Mild hair growth on upper lip of women may appear as a result of decreased estrogen-to-testosterone ratio. Toenails usually thicken, while fingernails often become thinner. Both usually become yellowish and dull.	

(Continued on following page)

HEAD AND NECK

ASSESSMENT PROCEDURE	NORMAL FINDINGS/VARIATIONS	ABNORMAL FINDINGS
Inspect **head and neck** for symmetry and movement. Observe **facial expression** (Fig. 26-2). 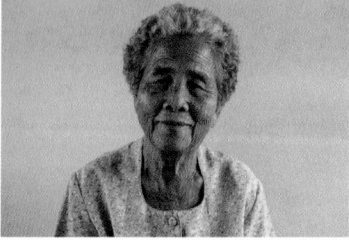 **FIGURE 26-2** Observe facial expression.	Atrophy of face and neck muscles. Reduced range of motion (ROM) of head and neck. Shortening of neck due to vertebral degeneration and development of "buffalo hump" at the top of cervical vertebrae.	Abnormalities include the following: • Asymmetry of mouth or eyes, possibly from Bell palsy or stroke (cerebral vascular accident [CVA]). • Marked limitation of movement or crepitation in back of neck from cervical arthritis. • Involuntary facial or head movements from an extrapyramidal disorder such as Parkinson disease or some medications.

MOUTH AND THROAT

ASSESSMENT PROCEDURE	NORMAL FINDINGS/VARIATIONS	ABNORMAL FINDINGS
Inspect **the gums and buccal mucosa** for color, consistency, and odor.	Slight decrease in saliva production.	Saliva-depressing medications include antihistamines, antipsychotics, and antihypertensives, and any drug with anticholinergic side effects may promote dental caries and increase the risk of pneumonia.
		Foul-smelling breath may indicate periodontal disease.
		Whitish or yellow-tinged patches in mouth or throat may be candidiasis from the use of steroid inhalers or antibiotics.
If the client is wearing dentures, inspect them for fit. Then ask the client to remove them for the rest of the oral examination.	Resorption of gum ridge commonly results in poorly fitting dentures. Tooth surfaces may be worn from prolonged use.	Loose-fitting dentures or inability to close mouth completely may also be the result of a significant weight gain or loss.
Examine the **tongue.** Observe symmetry and size.	Tongue pink and moist.	A swollen, red, and painful tongue may indicate vitamin B or riboflavin deficiency.

(Continued on following page)

MOUTH AND THROAT (*continued*)		
ASSESSMENT PROCEDURE	**NORMAL FINDINGS/VARIATIONS**	**ABNORMAL FINDINGS**
Observe the client swallowing food or fluids.	Mild decrease in swallowing ability.	Coughing, drooling, pocketing, or spitting out food are all possible signs of dysphagia. A drooping mouth, chronic congestion, or a weak or hoarse voice (especially after eating or drinking) suggests dysphagia.
Depress the posterior third of the tongue and note gag reflex.	Gag reflex may be slightly sluggish.	Absence of a gag reflex may be the result of a neurologic disorder.
NOSE AND SINUSES		
ASSESSMENT PROCEDURE	**NORMAL FINDINGS/VARIATIONS**	**ABNORMAL FINDINGS**
Inspect the **nose** for color and consistency.	Nose and nasal passages are not inflamed, and skin and mucous membranes are intact. Nose may seem more prominent on face because of loss of subcutaneous fat. Nasal hairs are coarser.	Edema, redness, swelling, or clear drainage, which may indicate allergies or rhinitis. *Note: Relocation into a newly constructed residential or long-term care facility should be investigated further as a possible cause of allergic or nonallergic rhinitis due to exposure of new carpet, fiberboard, or paint fumes.*

ASSESSMENT PROCEDURE	NORMAL FINDINGS/VARIATIONS	ABNORMAL FINDINGS
Evaluate the **sense of smell.** Have the client close the eyes and smell a common substance, such as mint, lemon, or soap.	Slightly diminished sense of smell and ability to detect odors.	Client cannot identify strong odor. This may cause a decrease in appetite and may be a safety concern.
Test **nasal patency** by asking the client to breathe while blocking one nostril at a time.	Breathes with reasonable ease.	Client reports feeling of inadequate intake of air with respirations that may result from nasal polyps, a deviated septum, or allergic or infectious rhinitis or sinusitis.
Palpate the **frontal and maxillary sinuses** to elicit possible pain. *Note: Older adults with nasogastric feeding tubes are at increased risk for sinusitis related to the obstruction.*	No lesions or pain.	Client reports pain and dryness; inflammation is evident. *Note: Older clients may self-treat sinus pain and/or nasal congestion with decongestants and antihistamines, which may further dry the nasal passages and prevent normal sinus drainage.*

(Continued on following page)

EYES AND VISION

ASSESSMENT PROCEDURE	NORMAL FINDINGS/VARIATIONS	ABNORMAL FINDINGS
Inspect **eyes, eyelids, eyelashes, and conjunctivae**. Also observe eyes and conjunctivae for dryness, redness, tearing, or increased sensitivity to light and wind.	Skin around the eyes becomes thin, and wrinkles appear normally with age. Stretched skin in eyelid may produce feeling of heaviness and a tired feeling. In lower eyelid, "bags" form. Excessive stretching of lower eyelid may cause it to droop downward, which keeps it from shutting completely and can cause dryness, redness, or sensitivity to light and wind. Eyes feel irritated or "scratchy."	A turning in of the lower eyelid (entropion) is more common and causes the eyelashes to touch the conjunctiva and cornea. Severe entropion may result in an ulcerous corneal infection. Abnormalities in blinking may result from Parkinson disease; dull or blank staring may be a sign of hypothyroidism. See Box 26-4 for age-related abnormalities of the eye.
Inspect the **corneas and lenses**. Also ask the client when they last had an eye and vision examination. **Note**: To detect glaucoma, tonometry should be performed every 1 to 2 years on everyone older than 35 years. Elevated intraocular pressure indicates referral to ophthalmologist and tonometry.	An arcus senilis, a cloudy or grayish ring around the iris, and decreased pigment in iris are age-related changes. The lens loses elasticity, which results in decreased ability to change shape (presbyopia). A loss of transparency in the crystalline lens of the eyes is a natural part of aging process. Exposure to sunlight or smoking, as well as inherited tendencies, increase risk.	Cataracts most commonly affect people after age 55 and result in a yellowish or brownish discoloration of the lens. Common symptoms include painless blurring of vision, glare and halos around lights, poor night vision, and colors that look dull or brownish. A thickening of the bulbar conjunctiva that grows over the cornea (called *pterygium*) may interfere with vision.

ASSESSMENT PROCEDURE	NORMAL FINDINGS/VARIATIONS	ABNORMAL FINDINGS
Inspect the **pupils.** With a penlight or similar device, test pupillary reaction to light.	Overall decrease in size of pupil and ability to dilate in dark and constrict in light may occur with advanced age; this results in poorer night vision and decreased tolerance to glare.	An irregularly shaped pupil may indicate removal of a cataract. Asymmetric response may be due to a neurologic condition.
Test vision. Ask the client to read from a newspaper or magazine. Use only room lighting for the initial reading. Use task lighting for a second reading. Ask about changes in vision, trouble with night vision, or differences in vision with left versus right eye. Also ask client about small specks or "clouds" that move across the field of vision.	Impaired near vision is indicative of presbyopia (farsightedness), a common finding in older adults. Also common are slight decreases in peripheral vision and difficulty in differentiating blues from greens. *Note: Older adults generally require two to three times more diffuse and task lighting.* With aging, tiny clumps of gel may develop within the eye. These are referred to as "floaters." They should occur occasionally and not increase significantly in frequency.	A significant decrease in central vision, needed for activities of daily living, may be due to *cataracts* in eyes. *Macular degeneration* (thin membrane in the center of the retina) is suspected if client has difficulty seeing with one eye (Box 26-4). This usually becomes bilateral. Related findings include blurry words in the center of the page or door frames that do not appear straight. Refer for further evaluation. A noticeable loss of vision—including cloudiness, distortion of familiar objects, and, occasionally, blind spots or floaters—is a symptom of *diabetic retinopathy.* New or increased floater frequency seen with light flashes may be sign of *retinal detachment.* Refer immediately to prevent blindness (see Box 26-4).

(Continued on following page)

EARS AND HEARING

ASSESSMENT PROCEDURE	NORMAL FINDINGS	ABNORMAL FINDINGS
Inspect the **external ear.** Observe shape, color, and hair growth. Also look for lesions or drainage.	Hairs may become coarser and thicker in the external ear, especially in men. Earlobes may elongate and pinna increases in length and width.	Inflammation, drainage, or swelling may be from infection.
Perform an **otoscopic examination** to determine quantity, color, and consistency of cerumen.	Cerumen production decreases leading to dryness and tendency toward accumulation.	Hard, dark brown cerumen signals impaction of the auditory canal that commonly causes a conductive hearing loss. A darkened hole in the tympanic membrane indicates perforation or scarring.
Perform the **voice-whisper test**, a functional examination to detect (conversational) hearing loss. Instruct the client to put a hand over one ear and to repeat the sentence you say. Stand approximately 60.96 cm (2 ft) away from the client and whisper a sentence. **Note**: *If you are facing the client, hold your hand close to your mouth so the client cannot read your lips.*	The inability to hear high-frequency sounds (presbycusis) or to discriminate a variety of simultaneous sounds and soft consonant sounds or background noises is due to degeneration of hair cells of inner ear.	Inability to hear the whispered sentence indicates a hearing deficiency and the need to refer the client to an audiologist for testing. **Note**: *Raising one's voice to someone with presbycusis usually only makes it more difficult for them to hear. Speaking more slowly will usually lower the frequency and be more therapeutic.*

THORAX AND LUNGS

ASSESSMENT PROCEDURE	NORMAL FINDINGS/VARIATIONS	ABNORMAL FINDINGS
Inspect **shape of thorax**. Note respiratory rate, rhythm, and quality of breathing.	Decreased elasticity of alveoli causes lungs to recoil less during expiration, loss of resilience that holds thorax in a contracted position, and loss of skeletal muscle strength in thorax and abdomen. Decreased vital capacity, increased residual volume, and slight barrel chest are noted.	Respiratory rate greater than 25 breaths/min may signal a pulmonary infection, respiratory diseases such as chronic obstructive pulmonary disease (COPD), congestive heart failure, pulmonary embolus, or metabolic acidosis.
	Increased reliance on diaphragmatic breathing and increased work of breathing.	Respiratory rate of less than 16 breaths/min may be a sign of neurologic impairment, which may lead to aspiration pneumonia. Significant loss of aerobic capacity and dyspnea with exertion is usually due to disease, exposure over a lifetime to pollutants, smoke, or severe or prolonged lack of exercise.
Percuss **lung tones**. Use the same technique as you would in a younger adult.	Resonant, except in the presence of structural changes such as kyphosis or a slight barrel chest, when hyperresonance may occur.	Consolidation of infection will cause dullness to percussion; alveolar retention of air, as occurs in emphysema, results in hyperresonance.

(Continued on following page)

THORAX AND LUNGS (*continued*)		
ASSESSMENT PROCEDURE	**NORMAL FINDINGS/VARIATIONS**	**ABNORMAL FINDINGS**
		Note: Pneumonia is the most common cause of infection-related deaths in older adults. Pneumonia symptoms in the elderly often vary. Along with, or without, standard symptoms of cough, fever, difficulty breathing, and chest pain, symptoms in the elderly often include reduced appetite, confusion, incontinence, delirium, poor coordination, or sudden change in day-to-day functioning (Morales-Brown, 2020).
Auscultate **lung sounds** as you would in a younger adult. *Note: Lung expansion may be diminished in older adults. It may be necessary to emphasize taking deep breaths with the mouth open during the examination. This may be very difficult for those with dementia.*	Vesicular sounds should be heard over all areas of air exchange.	Breath sounds may be distant over areas affected by kyphosis or the barrel chest of aging. Rales and rhonchi are heard only with diseases, such as pulmonary edema, pneumonia, or restrictive disorders. Diminished breath sounds, wheezes, crackles, rhonchi that do not clear with cough, and egophony are signs of consolidation.

HEART AND BLOOD VESSELS

ASSESSMENT PROCEDURE	NORMAL FINDINGS/VARIATIONS	ABNORMAL FINDINGS
Blood Pressure		
Take **blood pressure** to detect actual or potential orthostatic hypotension and, therefore, the risk for falling.	An older adult's baroreceptor response to positional changes is slightly less efficient. A slight decrease in blood pressure may occur.	More than 10 mmHg drop in systolic or diastolic pressure and an increase in heart rate of 20 beats or more per minute indicate orthostatic hypotension. A serious consequence is the potential for lightheadedness and dizziness, which may precipitate hip fracture or head trauma from a fall. *Note: Some sources of orthostatic hypotension include medications, such as antihypertensives, diuretics, and drugs with anticholinergic side effects (anxiolytics, antipsychotics, hypnotics, tricyclic antidepressants, and antihistamines).*

(Continued on following page)

HEART AND BLOOD VESSELS *(continued)*		
ASSESSMENT PROCEDURE	**NORMAL FINDINGS/VARIATIONS**	**ABNORMAL FINDINGS**
Measure **pressure with the client in lying, sitting, and standing positions.** Also measure pulse rate. Have the client lie down for 5 minutes; take the pulse and blood pressure; at 1 minute, take blood pressure and pulse after client is sitting and again at 1 minute after client stands. If dizziness occurs, instruct client to sit a few minutes before attempting to stand up from a supine or reclining position.	Blood pressure increases as elasticity decreases in arteries, with proportionately greater increase in systolic pressure resulting in a widening of pulse pressure. *Note: Any client with blood pressure greater than 160/90 mmHg should be referred to the health care provider for follow-up.*	A sudden and increasingly widened pulse pressure, especially in combination with other neurologic abnormalities and a change in mental status, is a classic sign of increased intracranial pressure (which, in older adult clients, may be due to a hemorrhagic stroke or hematoma).
Exercise Tolerance		
Measure **activity tolerance.** Evaluate either by reviewing results of stress testing or by observing the client's ability to move from a sitting to a standing position or to flex and extend fingers rapidly.	The maximal heart rate with exercise is less in a younger person. The heart rate will also take longer to return to its preexercise rate. Rise in pulse rate should be no greater than 10 to 20 beats/min. The pulse rate should return to the baseline rate within 2 minutes.	A rise in pulse rate greater than 20 beats/min and a rate that does not return to baseline within 2 minutes is an indicator of exercise intolerance. Cardiac dysrhythmias, as determined by stress testing, are also indicative of exercise intolerance.

ASSESSMENT PROCEDURE	NORMAL FINDINGS/VARIATIONS	ABNORMAL FINDINGS
Note: Poor lower body strength, especially in the ankles, may impair the ability of the frail older adult to rise from a chair to a standing position. Poor upper body strength, especially in the shoulders, may impede the ability to push up from a bed or chair or to extend and flex fingers.		
Pulses		
Determine **adequacy of blood flow** by palpating the **arterial pulses in all locations** (carotid, brachial, radial, femoral, popliteal, posterior tibial, and dorsalis pedis) for strength and quality. *Note: Palpate carotid arteries gently and one side at a time to avoid stimulating vagal receptors in the neck, dislodging existing plaque, or causing syncope or a stroke.*	Proximal pulses may be easier to palpate due to loss of supporting surrounding tissue. However, distal lower extremity pulses may be more difficult to feel or even nonpalpable. The dorsalis pedis pulse is congenitally absent in approximately 5-10% of adults.	Insufficient or absent pulses are a likely indication of arterial insufficiency. Partially obstructed blood flow increases the risk of ulcers and infection; completely obstructed blood flow is a medical emergency requiring immediate intervention to prevent gangrene and possible amputation.

(Continued on following page)

HEART AND BLOOD VESSELS *(continued)*		
ASSESSMENT PROCEDURE	**NORMAL FINDINGS/VARIATIONS**	**ABNORMAL FINDINGS**
Arteries and Veins		
Auscultate the **carotid, abdominal, and femoral arteries.**	No unusual sounds should be heard.	Bruits require prompt referral for further evaluation because of the high risk of stroke (CVA) from carotid embolism or an abdominal or femoral aneurysm.
Evaluate **arterial and venous sufficiency of extremities.** Elevate the legs above the level of the heart and observe color, temperature, size of the legs, and skin integrity.	Hair loss with advanced age (cannot be used singly as an indicator of arterial insufficiency).	Leg pain associated with walking, burning or cramping, duskiness or mottling when leg is in dependent position; paleness with elevation; cool, thin, shiny skin; thickened, brittle nails; and diminished pulses are signs of arterial insufficiency.
Inspect and **palpate veins while client is standing.**	Prominent, bulging veins are common. Varicosities are considered a problem only if ulcerations, signs of thrombophlebitis, or cords are present. Cords are nontender; palpable veins having a rubber tubing consistency.	Unilateral warmth, tenderness, and swelling may be indications of thrombophlebitis.

ASSESSMENT PROCEDURE	NORMAL FINDINGS/VARIATIONS	ABNORMAL FINDINGS
Heart		
Inspect and palpate the **precordium.**	The precordium is still and without thrills, heaves, or visible, palpable pulsations (noted exception may be the apex of the heart if close to the surface).	Heaves felt with enlarged right or left ventricular aneurysm. Thrills indicate aortic, mitral, or pulmonic stenosis and regurgitation that may originate from rheumatic fever.
		Pulsations suggest aortic or ventricular aneurysm, right ventricular enlargement, or mitral regurgitation.
Auscultate **heart sounds.** Accumulation of lipofuscin, amyloid, collagen, and fats in the pacemaker cells of heart and loss of pacemaker cells in sinus node predispose elderly to dysrhythmias, even in the absence of heart disease. ***Note:*** *Falls, dyspnea, fatigue, and palpitations are common symptoms seen with dysrhythmias in older adults.*	A soft systolic murmur heard best at the base of the heart may result from calcification, stiffening, and dilation of the aortic and mitral valve.	Abnormal heart sounds are generally considered to be disease related only if there is additional evidence of compromised cardiovascular function. However, any previously undetected extra heart sound warrants further investigation.
		S_3 and S_4 sounds may reflect cardiac and fluid overloads of heart failure, aortic stenosis, cardiomyopathy, or myocardial infarction.

(Continued on following page)

BREASTS

ASSESSMENT PROCEDURE	NORMAL FINDINGS/VARIATIONS	ABNORMAL FINDINGS
Inspect and palpate **breasts and axillae.** When viewing axillae and contour of breasts, assist a client with arthritis to raise the arms over the head. Do this gently and without force and only if it is not painful for the client.	The breasts of older women are often described as pendulous due to the atrophy of breast tissue and supporting tissues and the forward thrust of the client brought about by kyphosis. Decreases in fat composition and increase in fibrotic tissue may make the terminal ducts feel more fibrotic and palpable as linear, spoke-like strands.	Pain upon palpation may indicate an infectious process or cancer. Or breast tenderness, pain, or swelling may be side effects of hormone replacement therapy and an indication that a lower dosage is needed. Male breast enlargement (gynecomastia) may result from a decrease in testosterone.
If the breasts are pendulous, assist the client to lean slightly so the breasts hang away from the chest wall, enabling you to best observe symmetry and form.	Nipples may retract due to loss in musculature. Unlike nipple retraction due to a mass, nipples retracted because of aging can be everted with gentle pressure.	*Note: A greater percentage of older women have had radical mastectomies. If so, inquiring about pain and swelling from lymphedema is important.*
Inspect **skin under breasts.**	Skin intact without lesions or rashes.	Macerated skin under the breasts may result from perspiration or fungal infection (usually seen in an immunocompromised client).

ABDOMEN

ASSESSMENT PROCEDURE	NORMAL FINDINGS/VARIATIONS	ABNORMAL FINDINGS
Motility		
Assess **gastrointestinal (GI) motility** and auscultate **bowel sounds**. Review **fiber intake and laxative use**.	5 to 30 sounds/min are heard. A decrease in gastric emptying time occurs with aging and may cause early satiety. Intestinal motility is generally reduced from a general loss of muscle tone. Risk of constipation is increased by diminished physical activity, fluid intake, fiber in diet, and certain medications such as iron or narcotics.	Absence of bowel sounds and vomiting of undigested food. Decreased motility is exacerbated by common pathologies (e.g., Parkinson, stroke, diabetes mellitus), which increases the risk for chronic constipation and diverticula. Hiatal hernia seen with postprandial chest fullness, heartburn, or nausea.
Determine **absorption or retention problems in older adult clients receiving enteral feedings**. *Note: An abdominal radiograph, flat plate, should be taken to check for correct placement of newly inserted nasogastric tubes.*	Less than 100 mL residual is a normal finding for intermittent feedings.	More than 100 mL residual measured before a scheduled feeding is sign of insufficient absorption and excessive retention. Abdominal distention, diarrhea, fluid overload, aspiration pneumonia, or fluid/electrolyte imbalances may indicate excessive retention, although mental status changes may be the first or only sign.

(Continued on following page)

ABDOMEN (*continued*)		
ASSESSMENT PROCEDURE	**NORMAL FINDINGS/VARIATIONS**	**ABNORMAL FINDINGS**
Inspect and percuss **abdomen.** Use the same manner as you would for younger adults. ***Note:*** *The loss of abdominal musculature that occurs with aging may make it easier to palpate abdominal organs. Atrophy of intestinal villi is a common aging change.*	Liver, pancreas, and kidneys normally decrease in size, but the decrease is not generally appreciable upon physical examination.	Anorexia, abdominal pain and distention, impaired protein digestion, and vitamin B_{12} malabsorption suggest inflammatory gastritis or a peptic ulcer. Abdominal distention, cramping, diarrhea, and increased flatus are signs of lactose intolerance, which may occur for the first time in old age. Bruits over aorta suggest aneurysm. *If present, do not palpate because this could rupture the aneurysm.* Guarding upon palpation, rebound tenderness, or a friction rub (sounds like pieces of sandpaper rubbing together) suggests peritonitis, which could be secondary to ruptured diverticula, tumor, or infarct.
Palpate the **bladder.** Ask client to empty bladder before examination. If bladder is palpable, percuss from symphysis pubis to umbilicus. If client is incontinent, may need to measure postvoid residual content.	Empty bladder is not palpable or percussible.	Full bladder sounds dull. More than 100 mL drained from bladder is considered abnormal for a postvoid residual. Distended bladder with small volume urine loss may indicate overflow incontinence (see Box 26-5).

GENITALIA

ASSESSMENT PROCEDURE	NORMAL FINDINGS/VARIATIONS	ABNORMAL FINDINGS
Female		
Inspect **external genitalia.** Assist the client into the lithotomy position. Inspect the urethral meatus and vaginal opening. *Note: Arthritis may make the lithotomy position particularly uncomfortable for the elderly woman, necessitating a change in position.*	Many atrophic changes begin in women at menopause. Pubic hair is usually sparse, and labia are flattened. Clitoris is decreased in size. The size of ovaries, uterus, and cervix also decreases.	White, glistening particles attached to pubic hair may be a sign of lice. Redness or swelling from the urethral meatus indicates a possible urinary tract infection.
Ask client to **cough while in the lithotomy position.** *Note: Incontinence is not a normal part of aging. If embarrassment or acceptance is preventing the client from acknowledging the problem, the genitalia examination may be a more acceptable time to introduce the topic.*	No leakage of urine occurs.	Leakage of urine that occurs with coughing is a sign of stress incontinence and may be due to lax pelvic muscles from childbirth, surgery, obesity, cystocele, rectocele, or a prolapsed uterus. *Note: In noncommunicative clients, an excoriated perineum may be the result of incontinence.*

(Continued on following page)

GENITALIA (*continued*)

ASSESSMENT PROCEDURE	NORMAL FINDINGS/VARIATIONS	ABNORMAL FINDINGS
Test for **prolapse**. Ask the client to bear down while you observe the vaginal opening.	No prolapse is evident.	A protrusion into vaginal opening may be cystocele, rectocele, or uterine prolapse, which are common sequela of relaxed pelvic musculature in older women.
Perform a **pelvic examination**. Put on disposable gloves and use a small speculum if the vaginal opening has narrowed with age. Use lubrication on speculum and hand because natural lubrication is decreased.	Vagina narrows and shortens. A loss of elastic tissue and vascularity in vagina results in a thin, pale epithelium. Atrophic changes are intensified by infrequent intercourse. Loss of elasticity and reduced vaginal lubrication due to lower levels of estrogen can cause dyspareunia (painful intercourse). Sexual desire and pleasure are not necessarily diminished by these structural changes, nor do women lose capacity for orgasm with age. Because the ovaries, uterus, and cervix shrink with age, the ovaries may not be palpable.	Atrophic vaginitis symptoms can mimic malignancy, vulvar dystrophies, urinary tract infections, and other infections, such as *Candida albicans*, bacterial vaginosis, gonorrhea, or chlamydia (Mayo Clinic, 2019).

ASSESSMENT PROCEDURE	NORMAL FINDINGS/VARIATIONS	ABNORMAL FINDINGS
Test **pelvic muscle tone.** Ask the woman to squeeze muscles while the examiner's finger is in the vagina. Assess perineal strength by turning fingers posterior to the perineum while the woman squeezes muscles in the vaginal area.	The vaginal wall should constrict around the examiner's finger, and the perineum should feel smooth.	If the client has a cystocele, the examiner's finger in the vagina will feel pressure from the anterior surface of the vagina. In clients with uterine prolapse, protrusion of the cervix is felt down through the vagina. A bulging of the posterior vaginal wall and part of the rectum may be felt with a rectocele.

Male

Inspect the **male genital area** with the client in standing position if possible.	Decreased testosterone leads to atrophic changes. Pubic hair is thinner. Scrotal skin slightly darker than surrounding skin, smooth and flaccid in the older man. Penis and testicular size decreases, scrotum hangs lower. In addition, there is a decrease in amount and viscosity of seminal fluid. Sperm count may decrease by 50%. Orgasm may be briefer; time to obtain an erection may increase. These changes alone do not usually result in any loss of libido or satisfaction.	Scrotal edema may be present with portal vein obstruction or heart failure. Lesions on the penis may be a sign of infection. Associated symptoms frequently include discharge, scrotal pain, and difficulty with urination.

(Continued on following page)

GENITALIA (*continued*)		
ASSESSMENT PROCEDURE	**NORMAL FINDINGS/VARIATIONS**	**ABNORMAL FINDINGS**
Observe and palpate for **inguinal swelling or bulges** suggestive of hernia in the same manner as for a younger male.	No swelling or bulges are present.	Masses or bulges are abnormal, and pain may be a sign of testicular torsion. A mass may be due to a hydrocele, spermatocele, or cancer.
Auscultate the **scrotum if a mass is detected**; otherwise palpate the right and left testicles using the thumb and first two fingers.	No detectable sounds or masses are present.	Bowel sounds heard over the scrotum may suggest an indirect inguinal hernia. Masses are abnormal, and the client should be referred to a specialist for follow-up examination.

ANUS, RECTUM, AND PROSTATE		
ASSESSMENT PROCEDURE	**NORMAL FINDINGS/VARIATIONS**	**ABNORMAL FINDINGS**
Inspect the **anus and rectum**.	The anus is darker than the surrounding skin. Bluish, grape-like lumps at the anus are indicators of hemorrhoids.	Lesions, swelling, inflammation, and bleeding are abnormalities. If hemorrhoids account for discomfort, the degree to which bleeding, swelling, or inflammation interferes with bowel activity generally determines whether treatment is warranted.

ASSESSMENT PROCEDURE	NORMAL FINDINGS/VARIATIONS	ABNORMAL FINDINGS
Put on gloves to palpate the **anus and rectum.** Also palpate the **prostate** in the male client. *Note: The left side-lying position with knees tucked up toward the chest is the preferred one for comfort. Pillows may be needed for positioning and client comfort.*	Normal findings include no internal masses, polyps, hemorrhoids, rectal prolapse, or fecal impaction. The prostate is normally soft or rubbery-firm and smooth, and the median sulcus is palpable. Some degree of benign prostatic hypertrophy almost always occurs by age 85.	Palpation of internal masses could indicate polyps, internal hemorrhoids, rectal prolapse, cancer, or fecal impaction. Obliteration of the median sulcus is seen with prostatic hyperplasia. A hard, asymmetrically enlarged, and nodular prostate is suggestive of malignancy (Seymour, 2019). Tender and softer prostate is more common with prostatitis. Fever and dysuria are common with acute prostatitis. Obstructive symptoms seen with both prostate malignancy and infection.

MUSCULOSKELETAL SYSTEM		
ASSESSMENT PROCEDURE	**NORMAL FINDINGS/VARIATIONS**	**ABNORMAL FINDINGS**
Observe the **client's posture and balance when standing**, especially the first 3 to 5 seconds.	Client stands reasonably straight with feet positioned fairly widely apart to form a firm base of support. This stance compensates for diminished sense of proprioception in lower extremities. Body usually bends forward as well.	A "humpback" curvature of the spine, called *kyphosis*, usually results from osteoporosis. The combination of osteoporosis, calcification of tendons and joints, and muscle atrophy makes it difficult for the frail elderly person to extend the hips and knees fully when walking. This impairs the ability to maintain balance early enough to prevent a fall.

(Continued on following page)

MUSCULOSKELETAL SYSTEM (*continued*)

ASSESSMENT PROCEDURE	NORMAL FINDINGS/VARIATIONS	ABNORMAL FINDINGS
Note: The ability to reach for everyday items without losing balance can be assessed by asking the client to remove an object from a shelf that is high enough to require stretching or standing on the toes and to bend down to pick up a small object, such as a pen, from the floor.		Client cannot maintain balance without holding onto something. Postural instability increases the risk of falling and immobility from the fear of falling.
Observe **the client's gait** by performing the timed **TUG** test (Richardson & Podsiadlo, 1991; Box 26-6). 1. Ask client to rise from a straight-backed chair, stand momentarily, and walk about 3 m toward a wall. 2. Ask client to turn without touching wall; walk back to chair; then turn around and sit. 3. Use watch with second hand to determine how long it takes client to complete test.	Widening of pelvis and narrowing of shoulders. Client walks steadily without swaying, stumbling, or hesitating during the walk. The client does not appear to be at risk of falling. Older adult clients without impairments in gait or balance can complete the test within 10 seconds.	Shuffling gait, characterized by smaller steps and minimal lifting of the feet, increases the risk of tripping when walking on uneven or unsteady surfaces. Abnormal findings from the TUG test include hesitancy, staggering, stumbling, and abnormal movements of the trunk and arms. People who take more than 30 seconds to complete the test tend to be dependent in some activities of daily living such as bathing, getting in and out of bed, or climbing stairs.

ASSESSMENT PROCEDURE	NORMAL FINDINGS/VARIATIONS	ABNORMAL FINDINGS
Score performance (1–5): 1. Normal 2. Very slightly abnormal 3. Mildly abnormal 4. Moderately abnormal 5. Severely abnormal		
Inspect the general contour of limbs, trunk, and joints. Palpate wrist and hand joints. 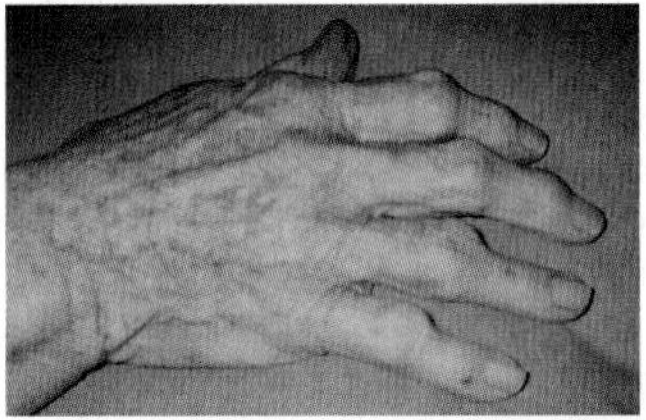 **FIGURE 26-3** Degenerative joint disease.	Enlargement of the distal, interphalangeal joints of the fingers, called *Heberden nodes*, is an indicator of degenerative joint disease (DJD), a common age-related condition involving joints in the hips, knees, and spine as well as the fingers (Fig. 26-3).	With accumulated damage and loss of cartilage, bony overgrowths protrude from bone into joint capsule, causing deformities, limited mobility, and pain. Hand deformities such as ulnar deviation, swan-neck deformity, and boutonnière deformity may cause pain, limiting activities of daily living.

(Continued on following page)

MUSCULOSKELETAL SYSTEM (*continued*)

ASSESSMENT PROCEDURE	NORMAL FINDINGS/VARIATIONS	ABNORMAL FINDINGS
Test **ROM.** Ask client to touch each finger with the thumb of the same hand, to turn wrists up toward the ceiling and down toward the floor, to push each finger against yours while you apply resistance, and to make a fist and release it.	There is full ROM of each joint and equal bilateral resistance.	Limitations in ROM or strength may be due to DJD, rheumatoid arthritis, or a neurologic disorder, which, if unilateral, suggests stroke (CVA).
		Signs of pain, such as grimacing, pulling back, or verbal messages, are indicators to perform a pain assessment (see Box 26-1).
		Grating, popping, crepitus, and palpation of fluid. Crepitus and joint pain that increases with activity and is relieved by rest in the absence of systemic symptoms may be associated with DJD.
Similarly assess **ROM and strength of shoulders and elbows**.	There is full ROM of each joint and equal strength in each joint.	Tenderness, stiffness, and pain in shoulders and elbows (and hips), aggravated by movement, are common signs of polymyalgia and rheumatica.

ASSESSMENT PROCEDURE	NORMAL FINDINGS/VARIATIONS	ABNORMAL FINDINGS
Assess **hip joint for strength and ROM.** Use the same technique as you would for a younger adult.	Intact flexion, extension, and internal and external rotation.	Hip pain that is worse with weight bearing and relieved with rest may indicate DJD. Often see crepitation, with a decrease in ROM. Hip, thigh, or groin pain; external rotation and adduction of the affected leg; and an inability to bear weight are the most common signs of a hip fracture. There is minimal shortening of leg with a complete fracture.
Inspect and palpate **knees, ankles, and feet.** Also assess comfort level, particularly with movement (flexion, extension, rotation).	The common problems associated with the aged foot, such as soreness and aching, are most frequently due to improperly fitting footwear.	A great toe overriding or underlying the second toe may be hallux valgus (bunion). Enlarged medial portion of first metatarsal head and inflammation of bursae over medial aspect of the joint are seen. May cause pain and difficulty walking.
Inspect **client's muscle bulk and tone.**	Atrophy of the hand muscles may occur with normal aging.	Muscle atrophy from rheumatoid arthritis, muscle disuse, malnutrition, motor neuron disease, or diseases of the peripheral nervous system. Increased resistance to passive ROM is classic sign of Parkinson disease, especially in clients with bradykinesia. Decreased resistance may suggest peripheral nervous system disease, cerebellar disease, or acute spinal cord injury.

(Continued on following page)

NEUROLOGIC SYSTEM

ASSESSMENT PROCEDURE	NORMAL FINDINGS/VARIATIONS	ABNORMAL FINDINGS
Observe for **tremors and involuntary movements.**	Resting tremors increase in the aged. In the absence of an identifiable disease process, they are not considered pathologic.	Tremors of Parkinson may occur when client is at rest. They usually diminish with voluntary movement, begin in the hand, and affect one side of the body early in disease and/or are accompanied by muscle rigidity.

SENSORY SYSTEM

ASSESSMENT PROCEDURE	NORMAL FINDINGS/VARIATIONS	ABNORMAL FINDINGS
Test **sensation to pain, temperature, touch position, and vibration.** Use the same assessment techniques as you would use for a younger adult.	Touch and vibratory sensations may diminish normally with aging.	Unilateral sensory loss suggests lesion in spinal cord or higher pathways; a sensory loss that is symmetrical (on both sides) suggests a neuropathy that may be associated with a condition such as diabetes.
Assess **positional sense** using **the Romberg test as presented in Chapter 21.** The exceptions to the test are clients who must use assistive devices such as a walker.	There is minimal swaying without loss of balance.	Significant swaying with appearance of a potential fall.

BOX 26-4 AGE-RELATED ABNORMALITIES OF THE EYE

Common age-related abnormalities of the eye include glaucoma, macular degeneration, retinal detachment, and diabetic retinopathy.

GLAUCOMA

The client with glaucoma is usually symptom free. In older adults, diabetes and atherosclerosis are conditions that increase the risk of glaucoma. The disorder is caused by increased pressure that can destroy the optic nerve and cause blindness if not treated properly. An acute form of glaucoma can occur at any age and is a true medical emergency because blindness can result in a day or 2 without treatment. Rainbow-like halos or circles around lights, severe pain in the eyes or forehead, nausea, and blurred vision may occur with the acute form of glaucoma.

MACULAR DEGENERATION

Macular degeneration, a gradual loss of central vision, is caused by aging and thinning of the micro-thin membrane in the center of the retina called the *macula*. Additional risk factors include sunlight exposure, family history, and White race. Most cases begin to develop after age 50, but damage may be occurring for months to years before symptoms occur. Peripheral vision is not affected, and the condition may occur initially in only one eye. Only about 10% of all age-related macular degeneration leaks occur in the small blood vessels in the retinal pigment epithelium. This type accounts for the most serious loss of vision.

RETINAL DETACHMENT

Retinal detachment occurs at a greater frequency with aging as the vitreous pulls away from its attachment to the retina at the back of the eye, causing the retina to tear in one or more places. A retinal detachment is always a serious problem. Blindness will result if the detachment is not treated.

DIABETIC RETINOPATHY

Many older adults have diabetes, which can lead to cataracts, glaucoma, and diabetic retinopathy. Of those with diabetes mellitus, about 90% will develop diabetic retinopathy to some degree. The more serious of the two forms of the disease, proliferative diabetic retinopathy, occurs most often among those who have had diabetes for more than 25 years. People with the advanced form of the disease usually experience a noticeable loss of vision, including cloudiness, distortion of familiar objects, and, occasionally, blind spots or floaters. If not treated, diabetic retinopathy will lead to connective scar tissue, which, over time, can shrink, pulling on the retina and resulting in a retinal detachment. In the early stages of the milder form of the disease, background diabetic retinopathy, the person may be unaware of problems because the loss of sight is usually gradual and mainly affects peripheral vision.

BOX 26-5 UNDERSTANDING URINARY INCONTINENCE: ASSESSMENT AND INTERVENTION

TYPES OF INCONTINENCE

The signs and symptoms associated with the involuntary loss of urine have been clustered into three categories: urge, stress, and overflow incontinence. Any one or a combination of all three types may be present in an individual. Voiding diaries are useful for determining the type of incontinence that is occurring based on the amount, timing, and associated symptoms of incontinent episodes.

Urge Incontinence

Urge incontinence is the involuntary loss of urine associated with an abrupt and strong desire to void. It is frequently caused by a neurologic disorder such as a stroke (CVA) or multiple sclerosis (MS), which impairs the ability of the bladder or urinary sphincter to contract and relax.

Stress Incontinence

Stress incontinence is the involuntary loss of urine during coughing, sneezing, laughing, or other physical activities that increase abdominal pressure. In women, stress incontinence may result from weakened and relaxed muscles from the combined effects of aging superimposed on the effects of childbirth.

Note: *Atrophic vaginitis from estrogen deficiency usually results in symptoms of urge incontinence as well as stress incontinence (mixed incontinence).*

Overflow Incontinence

Overflow incontinence is the involuntary loss of urine associated with overdistention of the bladder. Prostatic hypertrophy is a common cause in men, and diabetic neuropathy is a common cause in both sexes.

Functional Incontinence

Functional incontinence is the inability to get to the bathroom in time or to understand the cues to void due to problems with mobility or cognition.

STEPS OF ASSESSMENT

The nursing assessment varies somewhat depending on the client's general health status and whether the problem is an acute or a chronic one. In general, however, a comprehensive nursing assessment can be described as a five-step process that includes screening for an infection with a urinalysis, obtaining a voiding diary, evaluating functional status, compiling a health history, and performing a physical examination. Key features within the five steps are as follows:

- Record all incontinent and continent episodes for 3 days in a voiding diary.
- Review medication for any newly prescribed drugs that may be triggering incontinence. Follow-up with physician

regarding the need to discontinue therapy or change medication.
- Rule out constipation or fecal impaction as a source of urinary incontinence. If client has had no bowel movement within the last 3 days or is oozing stool continuously, check for impaction by digital examination or abdominal palpation. Problem should be treated if identified.
- Assess functional status along with signs and symptoms as they relate to incontinence. Contributors to incontinence may include immobility, insufficient fluid intake, and confusion. Accompanying signs and symptoms include polyuria, nocturia, dysuria, hesitancy, poor or interrupted urine stream, straining, suprapubic or perineal pain, urgency, and characteristics of incontinent episodes (precipitated by walking, coughing, getting in and out of bed, and so forth).
- Consult physician regarding physical examination and need to measure postvoid residual volume by straight catheterization (particularly if client dribbles, reports urgency, has difficulty starting stream). Components of the physical examination include direct observation of urine loss using a cough stress test; abdominal, rectal, genital, and pelvic examination; and identification of neurologic abnormalities. Abdominal and vaginal examinations are performed to detect prolapse or a palpable bladder after micturition.

INTERVENTIONS
The physician is responsible for identifying and treating the conditions causing reversible or chronic incontinence. A physical therapist may play a role in identifying specific activities that are associated with incontinent episodes. Either a nurse or physical therapist may be involved in teaching Kegel exercises to help relieve stress incontinence. When functional incontinence and urgency have been identified, the expertise of an occupational therapist in appropriate dressing and undressing and for choosing incontinence aids may be beneficial.

BOX 26-6 "TIMED UP AND GO" (TUG) TEST

Purpose: To assess mobility

Equipment: A stopwatch

Directions: Patients wear their regular footwear and can use a walking aid, if needed. Begin by having the patient sit back in a standard arm chair and identify a line 3 m, or 10 feet, away on the floor.

1. Instruct the patient:

    When I say "Go," I want you to:

    1) Stand up from the chair.

    2) Walk to the line on the floor at your normal pace.

    3) Turn.

    4) Walk back to the chair at your normal pace.

    5) Sit down again.

2. On the word "Go," begin timing.

3. Stop timing after patient sits back down.

4. Record time.

    An older adult who takes greater than or equal to 12 seconds to complete the TUG is at risk for falling.

OBSERVATIONS

Observe the patient's postural stability, gait, stride length, and sway.

Check all that apply:

☐ Slow tentative pace

☐ Loss of balance

☐ Short strides

☐ Little to no arm swing

☐ Steadying self on walls

☐ Shuffling

☐ En bloc turning

Not using assistive device properly

These changes may signify neurological problems that require further intervention.

Reprinted with permission from Richardson, S., & Podsiadlo, D. (1991). The Timed "Up & Go": A test of basic functional mobility for frail elderly persons. *Journal of the American Geriatric Society, 39*(2), 142–148. https://doi.org/10.1111/j.1532-5415.1991.tb01616.x

References

Administration on Aging. (2018). *2018 profile of older Americans.* https://acl.gov/sites/default/files/Aging%20and%20Disability%20in%20America/2018OlderAmericansProfile.pdf

Banicek, J. (2010). How to ensure acute pain in older people is appropriately assessed and managed. *Nursing Times, 106*(29), 14–17. https://insights.ovid.com/nursing-times/nrtm/2010/07/270/ensure-acute-pain-older-people-appropriately/3/00006203

Batsis, J., MacKenzie, T., Lopez-Jimenez, F., & Bartels, S. (2015). Sarcopenia, sarcopenic obesity, and functional impairments in older adults: National Health and Nutrition Examination Surveys 1999–2004. *Nutrition Research, 35*(12), 1031–1039. https://doi.org/10.1016/j.nutres.2015.09.003

Hulla, R., Vanzzini, N., Salas, E., Bevers, K., Garner, T., & Gatchel, R. (2019). Pain management and the elderly. *Practical Pain Management, 17*(1). https://www.practicalpainmanagement.com/treatments/pain-management-elderly

International Association for the Study of Pain. (2001). *Faces Pain Scale–Revised Home.* https://www.iasp-pain.org/Education/Content.aspx?ItemNumber=1519

Kim, J., & Miller, S. (2017). Geriatric syndromes: Meeting a growing challenge. *Nursing Clinics, 52*(3), ix–x. https://doi.org/10.1016/j.cnur.2017.06.001

Mayo Clinic. (2019). *Vaginal atrophy.* https://www.mayoclinic.org/diseases-conditions/vaginal-atrophy/symptoms-causes/syc-20352288

Morales-Brown, L. (2020). *What are the symptoms of pneumonia in older adults?* https://www.medicalnewstoday.com/articles/elderly-pneumonia-symptoms

National Institute on Aging. (2021). *The epigenetics of aging: What the body's hands of time tell us.* https://www.nia.nih.gov/news/epigenetics-aging-what-bodys-hands-time-tell-us

Richardson, S., & Podsiadlo, D. (1991). The Timed "Up & Go": A test of basic functional mobility for frail elderly persons. *Journal of the American Geriatric Society, 39*(2), 142–148. https://doi.org/10.1111/j.1532-5415.1991.tb01616.x

Seymour, T. (2019). *All you need to know about prostate nodules.* https://www.medicalnewstoday.com/articles/319679

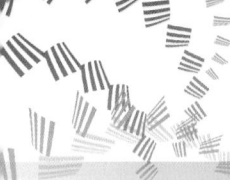

APPENDICES

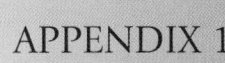

NURSING ASSESSMENT FORM BASED ON FUNCTIONAL HEALTH PATTERNS

Client Profile   **Name** _____ **Birth date** _____ **Sex** _____

Ethnic origin _____ Religion _____

Medical diagnoses _____

Present treatment _____

Past treatments _____

Past hospitalizations _____

Allergies _____

Current Medications   **Name**   **Dose**   **Purpose**   **Problems**

_____   _____   _____   _____

_____   _____   _____   _____

_____   _____   _____   _____

Health Perception–Health Management Pattern

Reason for seeking health care _____

_____

Health rating	1 Poor	2 Fair	3 Excellent

Perception of illness _____

Effect of illness on ADLs _____

Use of alcohol _____

   tobacco _____

   drugs _____

Special health habits _____

Last immunizations_____

Compliance with treatments _____

Appearance _____

Grooming _____

Posture _____

Expressions _____

Ht _____ Wt _____

P _____ R _____ T _____

(oral, axillary, rectal)

BP sitting   R _____ L _____

   standing   R _____ L _____

Nutritional–Metabolic Pattern

Daily Food and Fluid Intake

Breakfast _____

Lunch _____

Supper _____

Snacks _____

Food likes/dislikes _____

Food intolerances _____

Difficulty chewing _____

Dysphagia _____

Sore gums _____

Sore tongue _____

N and V _____

Abdominal pains _____

Antacids _____

Laxatives _____

Skin condition _____

Hair condition _____

Nail condition _____

Ideal wt. Difficulty gaining _____

Losing _____

Cold/heat intolerances _____

Voice changes _____

Difficulty with nervousness _____

Skin: Color _____

Lesions _____ Texture _____

Temp _____ Moisture _____

Turgor _____

Hair: Color _____

Amt _____ Texture _____

Scalp lesions _____ Dry _____

Nails: Color _____

Shape _____ Condition _____

Texture _____ Tenderness _____

Oral Mucosa: _____ Number of teeth _____

Condition _____

Lesions _____

Gums _____ Tongue _____

Elimination Pattern

Bowel Habits
- Frequency _____ Color _____ Pain _____
- Consistency _____ Laxatives _____
- Enemas _____ Suppositories _____
- Ileostomy _____ Colostomy _____

Bladder Habits
- Frequency _____ Amt _____ Color _____
- Pain _____ Hematuria _____
- Incontinence _____ Nocturia _____
- Retention _____ Infections _____
- Catheter _____ Type _____

Abdomen
- Contour _____
- Lesions _____ Umbilicus _____
- Striae _____ Veins _____
- Bowel sounds char. _____
- Frequency _____
- Size of liver dullness _____
- Masses palpated _____
- Liver palpated _____
- Spleen palpated _____

Rectum
- Rashes _____
- Lesions _____ Tenderness _____

Activity–Exercise Pattern

Daily Activities

Hygiene _____

Cooking _____

Shopping _____

Housework _____

Yard work _____

Eating times _____

Dyspnea _____ Palpitations _____

Chest pain _____ Stiffness _____

Weakness _____ Aching _____

Leisure activities _____

Exercise routine _____

Occupation _____

Effect of illness on activities _____

_____

Musculoskeletal

Gait _____ Posture _____

Extremity swelling _____

Symmetry _____ ROM _____

Crepitus _____ Tone _____

Strength _____

Respiratory

Thorax shape _____

Symmetry _____ Retractions _____

Tenderness _____

Diaphragmatic level _____

Breath sounds _____

Adventitious sounds _____

Cardiovascular

Jugular venous pressure _____

Pulsations _____ Heaves _____

Lifts _____

PMI _____ S_1 _____ S_2 _____

S_3 _____ S_4 _____ Murmurs _____

Peripheral Vascular Pulses

Carotid   R ____ L ____ Radial   R ____ L ____

Ulnar   R ____ L ____ Brachial   R ____ L ____

Popliteal R ____ L ____ Femoral   R ____ L ____

Pedal   R ____ L ____ Posterior tibial R ____ L ____

Bruits   R ____ L ____

Sleep–Rest Pattern

Sleep time _____ Quality _____
Difficulty falling asleep _____
Difficulty remaining asleep _____
Sleep aids _____
Sleep medications _____

Sexuality–Reproduction Pattern

Female Menstruation
Age of onset _____
Last menstrual period _____
Length _____
Problems _____
_____

Gravida _____ Para _____ Abortions_____
Current pregnancy _____
Infertility _____
Appearance _____
Irritability _____
Short attention span _____

Breasts
Last examination by primary
care provider _____
BSE? If yes, when _____
  Shape _____ Symmetry _____
  Nipples _____ Discharge _____
  Masses _____ Lymph nodes _____
Male Genitalia
Testicular examination _____ When _____
  Masses _____ Swelling _____
  Texture _____
Penile examination _____
  Masses _____ Growths _____
  Lesions _____ Discharge _____
  Foreskin retraction _____
  Urethral opening _____
Lymph nodes _____
  Inguinal masses _____

Sexuality–Reproduction Pattern (continued)

Male–Female

Contraception used _____
_____
Undesirable side effects _____
Problems with sexual activities _____
_____
_____

Effect of illness on sexuality _____
_____

Sexually transmitted diseases _____
_____

Pain _____ Burning _____
Discomfort during intercourse _____

Female Genitalia

Labia _____ Color _____
Swelling _____ Symmetry _____
Urethral opening _____
Discharge _____
Vaginal opening _____
Lesions _____ Discharge _____
Hymen _____ Inflammation _____
_____

Sensory–Perceptual Pattern

Perceptions of: Vision _____

    Hearing _____ Taste _____

    Smell _____ Sensation _____

    Pain _____

Vision aids _____

Hearing aids _____

Visual Acuity: OD _____ OS _____

    OU _____ Visual fields _____

    EOMs _____

    PERRLA _____

Funduscopic Examination: Red reflex _____

    Optic disc _____ Macula _____

    Arterioles/venules _____

Hearing: Weber _____

Rinne _____

    External canal _____

    Tympanic membrane _____

Sensations: Superficial _____ Deep pressure _____

    2-point discrimination _____

Cranial Nerves

    Olfactory _____

    Optic _____

    V. Trigeminal _____

    III, IV, VI. Oculomotor, trochlear, abducens _____

    VII. Facial _____ Acoustic _____

Cognitive Pattern

Understanding of illness _____

Understanding of treatments _____

Ability to express self _____

Ability to recall:

  Remote _____

  Recent _____

Ability to make decisions _____

Expression of feelings _____

Behavior _____

Speech _____ Vocabulary _____

Mood _____

Thought processes _____

Orientation: Person _____

  Time _____ Place _____

Attention _____ Information _____

Vocabulary _____

Abstract reasoning _____

Similarities _____ Judgment _____

Sensory perception and coordination _____

Role–Relationship Pattern

Role in family _____

Responsibility _____

Work role _____

Social role _____

Level of satisfaction _____

Effect of illness on roles _____

Communication between family members _____

Family visits _____ Length _____

Draw family genogram:

Self-Perception–Self-Concept Pattern

Identity _____
Perception of abilities _____
Body image _____
Culture or ethnic group _____
Sexual orientation _____
Tattoos _____

Coping–Stress Tolerance Pattern

Stressors _____
Coping methods _____
Support systems _____

Value–Belief Pattern

Values _____
Goals _____
Source of hope/strength _____
Significant religious person _____
Religious practices _____
Relationship with God/higher being _____
Presence of religious articles _____
Religious activities _____

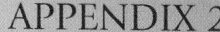

PHYSICAL ASSESSMENT GUIDE: PULLING IT ALL TOGETHER

Following is an outline guide for performing a head-to-toe physical assessment. This guide will help you pull together all your assessment skills to complete an integrated and comprehensive physical examination efficiently.

Equipment for a Head-to-Toe Assessment

- Assessment documentation forms
- Coin or key
- Cotton ball
- Cover card (for eye assessment)
- Gloves
- Goniometer
- Gown for client
- Lubricating jelly
- Magnifying glass
- Marking pencil
- Newspaper print or Rosenbaum pocket screener
- Notepad and pencil
- Ophthalmoscope
- Otoscope
- Paper clip
- Penlight
- Pillows (two small pillows)

- Platform scale with height attachment
- Reflex hammer
- Ruler with centimeter markings
- Skinfold calipers, flexible tape measure
- Small cup of water for client to drink
- Snellen chart
- Stethoscope and sphygmomanometer
- Substances for testing smell (e.g., soap, coffee)
- Substances for testing taste (e.g., salt, lemon, sugar, pickle juice)
- Supplies for collecting vaginal specimen (slides, spatula, cotton tip applicator)
- Thermometer (electronic, tympanic)
- Tongue depressor
- Tuning fork
- Vaginal speculum
- Watch

Preparing the Client

Discuss the purpose of the physical assessment with your client and acquire their permission to perform the various examinations. Ensure privacy and confidentiality. Respect the client's right to refuse any part of the assessment. Ask them to change into a gown for the examination.

General Survey

- Observe appearance including:
  - Overall physical and sexual development
  - Apparent age (compare with stated age)
  - Overall skin coloring
  - Dress, grooming, and hygiene
  - Body build, as well as muscle mass and fat distribution
  - Behavior (compare with developmental stage)
- Assess the client's vital signs:
  - Temperature
  - Pulse
  - Respiration
  - Blood pressure
  - Pain (as the fifth vital sign)
- Take body measurements:
  - Height
  - Weight

- Waist and hip circumference; mid-arm circumference
- Triceps skinfold thickness (TSF)
- Calculate ideal body weight, body mass index, waist-to-hip ratio, and mid-arm muscle area and circumference.
- Test vision using the Snellen chart.

Mental Status Examination

- In addition to data collected about the client's appearance during the general survey, observe:
  - Level of consciousness
  - Posture and body movements
  - Facial expressions
  - Speech
  - Mood, feelings, and expressions
  - Thought processes and perceptions
- Assess the client's cognitive abilities:
  - Orientation to person, time, and place
  - Concentration, ability to focus and follow directions
  - Recent memory of happenings today
  - Remote memory of the past
  - Recall of unrelated information in 5-, 10-, and 30-minute periods

- Abstract reasoning (Explain a "Stitch in time saves nine.")
- Judgment ("What would one do in case of ...?")
- Visual perceptual and constructional ability (draw a clock or shapes of square, etc.)

Ask the client to empty the bladder (give the client a specimen cup if a urine sample is needed) and change into a gown. Ask them to sit on the examination table.

Skin, Hair, and Nails

- As you perform each part of the head-to-toe assessment, assess skin for color variations, texture, temperature, turgor, edema, and lesions.
- Assess hair for distribution, color, and texture.
- Assess nails for condition, texture, and shape.
- Teach the client skin self-examination.

Head and Face

- Inspect and palpate the head for size, shape, and configuration.
- Note consistency, distribution, and color of hair.
- Observe face for symmetry, facial features, expressions, and skin condition.

- Check function of cranial nerve (CN) VII: Have the client smile, frown, show teeth, blow out cheeks, raise eyebrows, and tightly close eyes.
- Evaluate function of CN V: Using the sharp and dull sides of a paper clip, test sensations of forehead, cheeks, and chin.
- Palpate the temporal arteries for elasticity and tenderness.
- As the client opens and closes the mouth, palpate the temporo-mandibular joint for tenderness, swelling, and crepitation.

Eyes

- Determine function:
  - Test visual fields.
  - Assess corneal light reflex.
  - Perform cover and position tests.
- Inspect external eye:
  - Position and alignment of the eyeball in eye socket
  - Bulbar conjunctiva and sclera
  - Palpebral conjunctiva
  - Lacrimal apparatus
  - Cornea, lens, iris, and pupil
- Test pupillary reaction to light.
- Test accommodation of pupils.

- Assess corneal reflex (CN VII—facial).
- Use the ophthalmoscope to inspect:
  - Optic disc for shape, color, size, and physiologic cup
  - Retinal vessels for color and diameter and arteriovenous (AV) crossings
  - Retinal background for color and lesions
  - Fovea centralis (sharpest area of vision) and macula
  - Anterior chamber for clarity

Ears and Nose

- Inspect the auricle, tragus, and lobule for shape, position, lesions, discolorations, and discharge.
- Palpate the auricle and mastoid process for tenderness.
- Use the otoscope to inspect:
  - External auditory canal for color and cerumen (ear wax)
  - Tympanic membrane for color, shape, consistency, and landmarks
- Test hearing:
  - Whisper test
  - Weber test for diminished hearing in one ear
  - Rinne test to compare bone and air conduction (tuning fork on mastoid; then in front of ear)

- Inspect the external nose for color, shape, and consistency. Palpate the external nose for tenderness.
- Check patency of airflow through nostrils (occlude one nostril at a time and ask client to sniff).
- Test CN I: Ask the client to close their eyes and smell for soap, coffee, or vanilla. (Occlude each nostril.)
- Use an otoscope with a short wide tip to inspect internal nose for color and integrity of nasal mucosa, nasal septum, and inferior and middle turbinates.
- Transilluminate maxillary sinuses with a penlight to check for fluid or pus.

Mouth and Throat

Put on gloves. Use a tongue depressor and penlight as needed.
- Inspect lips for consistency, color, and lesions.
- Inspect the teeth for number and condition.
- Check the gums and buccal mucosa for color, consistency, or lesions.
- Inspect the hard (anterior) and soft (posterior) palates for color and integrity.
- Ask the client to say "aah" and observe the rise of the uvula.
- Test CN X: Touch the soft palate to assess for gag reflex.
- Inspect the tonsils for color, size, lesions, and exudates.
- Inspect the tongue for color, moisture, size, and texture. Inspect the ventral surface of the tongue for frenulum, color, lesions, and Wharton ducts.
- Palpate the tongue for lesions.
- Test CN IX and CN X: Assess tongue strength by asking the client to press the tongue against the tongue blade.
- Assess CN VII and CN IX: Have the client close their eyes. Check taste by placing salt, sugar, and lemon on the tongue.

Neck

- Inspect the neck for appearance of lesions; masses, swelling, and symmetry.
- Test range of motion (ROM).
- Palpate the preauricular, postauricular, occipital, tonsillar, submandibular, and submental nodes.
- Palpate the trachea.
- Palpate the thyroid gland for size, irregularity, or masses.
- Auscultate an enlarged thyroid for bruits.
- Palpate carotid arteries and auscultate for bruits.

Arms, Hands, and Fingers

- Inspect the upper extremities for overall skin color, texture, moisture, masses, and lesions.
- Test function of CN XI (spinal) by shoulder shrug and turning head against resistance.
- Palpate arms for tenderness, swelling, and temperature.
- Assess epitrochlear lymph nodes.
- Test ROM of the elbows.
- Palpate the brachial pulse.
- Palpate ulnar and radial pulses.
- Test ROM of the wrist.
- Inspect palms of hands and palpate for temperature.
- Test ROM of the fingers.
- Use a reflex hammer to test biceps, triceps, and brachioradialis reflexes.
- Test rapid alternating movements of hands.
- Ask the client to close the eyes; test sensation:
  - Assess light touch, pain, and temperature sensation in scattered locations over hands and arms.
  - Evaluate sensitivity of position of fingers.
  - Place a quarter or key in the client's hand to test stereognosis.
  - Assess graphesthesia by writing a number in the palm of the client's hand.
  - Assess two-point discrimination in the fingertips, forearm, and dorsal hands.

Ask client to continue sitting with arms at sides and stand behind client. Untie gown to expose posterior chest.

Posterior and Lateral Chest

- Inspect configuration and shape of scapulae and chest wall.
- Note use of accessory muscles when breathing and posture.
- Palpate for tenderness, sensation, crepitus, masses, lesions, and fremitus.
- Evaluate chest expansion at level T9 or T10.
- Percuss for tone at posterior intercostal spaces (comparing bilaterally).
- Determine diaphragmatic excursion.
- Auscultate for breath sounds, adventitious sounds, and voice sounds (bronchophony, egophony, and whispered pectoriloquy).
- Test for two-point discrimination on the client's back.
- Ask client to lean forward and exhale; use bell of stethoscope to listen over the apex and left sternal border of the heart.

Move to front of client and expose anterior chest. Allow client to maintain modesty.

Anterior Chest

- Inspect anteroposterior diameter of chest, slope of ribs, and color of chest.
- Note quality and pattern of respirations (rate, rhythm, and depth).
- Observe intercostal spaces for bulging or retractions and use of accessory muscles.
- Palpate for tenderness, sensation, masses, lesions, fremitus, and anterior chest expansion.
- Percuss for tone at apices above clavicles, then at intercostal spaces (comparing bilaterally).
- Auscultate for anterior breath sounds, adventitious sounds, and voice sounds.
- Pinch skin over sternum to assess mobility (ease to pinch) and turgor (return to original shape).

Ask client to fold gown to waist and sit with arms hanging freely.

Breasts

FEMALE BREASTS

- Inspect size, symmetry, color, texture, superficial venous pattern, areolae, and nipples of both breasts.
- Inspect for retractions and dimpling of nipples: Have the client raise her arms overhead, press her hands on her hips, press her hands together in front of her, and lean forward.
- Palpate axillae for rashes, infection, and anterior, central, and posterior lymph nodes.

MALE BREASTS

- Inspect for swelling, nodules, and ulcerations.
- Palpate the breast tissue and axillae.

Assist client to supine position with the head elevated to 30° to 45°. Stand on client's right side.

Neck

Observe and evaluate jugular venous pressure.

Assist client to supine position (lower examination table).

Complete examination of female breasts:
- Palpate breasts for masses and the nipples for discharge.
- Teach breast self-examination.

Heart

- Inspect and palpate for apical impulse.
- Palpate the apex, left sternal border, and base of the heart for any abnormal pulsations.
- Auscultate over aortic area, pulmonic area, Erb point, tricuspid area, and mitral area (apex) for:
  - Heart rate and rhythm (with diaphragm of stethoscope). If irregular, auscultate for a pulse rate deficit.
  - S_1 and S_2 (with diaphragm of stethoscope)
  - Extra heart sounds, S_3 and S_4 (with diaphragm and bell of stethoscope)
  - Murmurs (using bell and diaphragm of the stethoscope)
- *Ask the client to lie on left side;* use bell of stethoscope to listen to apex of the heart.

Cover chest with gown and arrange draping to expose abdomen.

Abdomen

- Inspect for:
  - Overall skin color
  - Vascularity, striae, lesions, and rashes
  - Location, contour, and color of umbilicus
  - Symmetry and contour of abdomen
  - Aortic pulsations or peristaltic waves
- Auscultate for:
  - Bowel sounds (intensity, pitch, and frequency)
  - Vascular sounds and friction rubs (over spleen, liver, aorta, iliac artery, umbilicus, and femoral artery)
- Percuss for:
  - Tone over four quadrants
  - Liver location, size, and span
  - Spleen location and size
- Lightly palpate:
  - Abdominal reflex
  - Four quadrants to identify tenderness and muscular resistance

- Deeply palpate:
  - Four quadrants for masses
  - Aorta
  - Liver, spleen, and kidneys for enlargement or irregularities

Replace gown and position draping so lower extremities are exposed.

Legs, Feet, and Toes

- Inspect the lower extremities for overall skin coloration, texture, moisture, masses, lesions, and varicosities.
- Observe muscles of the legs and feet.
- Note hair distribution.
- Palpate joints of hips and test ROM. Palpate the femoral pulse.
- Palpate for:
  - Edema, skin temperature
  - Muscle size and tone of legs and feet
- Palpate knees including popliteal pulse.
- Palpate the ankles; assess dorsalis pedis and posterior tibial pulses. Test ROM.
- Assess capillary refill.
- Test:
  - Sensation to dull and sharp sensations
  - Two-point discrimination (on thighs)
  - Patellar reflex, Achilles reflex, and plantar reflex
  - Position sense
  - Vibratory sensation on bony surface of big toe
- Perform heel-to-shin test.
- As warranted, perform special tests:
  - Position change for arterial insufficiency
  - Manual compression test
  - Trendelenburg test
  - Bulge knee test
  - Ballottement test
  - McMurray test

Secure gown and assist client to standing position.

Musculoskeletal and Neurologic Examination

Note: Parts of these systems have already been assessed throughout the physical examination.

- Check for spinal curvatures and scoliosis.
- Observe gait including base of support, weight-bearing stability, foot position, stride, arm swing, and posture.

- Observe as the client:
  - Walks heel to toe (tandem walk)
  - Hops on one leg, then the other
  - Performs Romberg test
  - Performs finger-to-nose test

Perform the female and male genitalia examination last, moving from the less private to more private examination for client comfort.

Genitalia

FEMALE GENITALIA

Have female client assume the lithotomy position. Apply gloves. Apply lubricant as appropriate.

- Inspect:
  - Distribution of pubic hair
  - Mons pubis, labia majora, and perineum for lesions, swelling, and excoriations
  - Labia minora, clitoris, urethral meatus, and vaginal opening for lesions, swelling, or discharge
- Palpate:
  - Bartholin glands, urethra, and Skene glands
  - Size of vaginal opening and vaginal musculature

- Insert speculum and inspect:
  - Cervix for lesions and discharge
  - Vagina for color, consistency, and discharge
- Obtain cytologic smears and cultures.
- Perform bimanual examination; palpate:
  - Cervix for contour, consistency, mobility, and tenderness
  - Uterus for size, position, shape, and consistency
  - Ovaries for size and shape

Discard gloves and apply clean gloves and lubricant.

- Perform the rectovaginal examination; palpate rectovaginal septum for tenderness, consistency, and mobility.

MALE GENITALIA AND RECTUM

Sit on a stool. Have client stand and face you with gown raised. Apply gloves.

- Inspect the penis, including:
  - Base of penis and pubic hair for excoriation, erythema, and infestation
  - Skin and shaft of penis for rashes, lesions, lumps, or hardened or tender areas
  - Color, location, and integrity of foreskin in uncircumcised men
  - Glans for size, shape, lesions, or redness and location of urinary meatus

- Palpate for urethral discharge by gently squeezing glans.
- Inspect scrotum, including:
  - Size, shape, and position
  - Scrotal skin for color, integrity, lesions, or rashes
  - Posterior skin (by lifting scrotal sac)
- Palpate both testis and epididymis between thumb and first two fingers for size, shape, nodules, and tenderness. Palpate spermatic cord and vas deferens.
- Transilluminate scrotal contents for red glow, swelling, or masses. If a mass is found during inspection and palpation, have the client lie down and inspect and palpate for scrotal hernia.
- As client bears down, inspect for bulges in inguinal and femoral areas and palpate for femoral hernias.
- While client shifts weight to each corresponding side, palpate for inguinal hernia.
- Teach testicular self-examination.

Ask the client to remain standing and to bend over the examination table. Change gloves.

- Inspect:
  - Perianal area for lumps, ulcers, lesions, rashes, redness, fissures, or thickening of epithelium
    - Sacrococcygeal area for swelling, redness, dimpling, or hair
- While client bears down or performs Valsalva maneuver, inspect for bulges or lesions.
- Apply lubrication and use finger to palpate:
  - Anus
  - External sphincter for tenderness, nodules, and hardness
  - Rectum for tenderness, irregularities, nodules, and hardness
  - Peritoneal cavity
  - Prostate for size, shape, tenderness, and consistency
- Inspect stool for color and test feces for occult blood.

Abbreviated Physical Assessment Format

The following is a brief "Head-to-Toe Physical Assessment Guide" that may be used to establish the client's physical status. This type of assessment is frequently used by nurses at the beginning of a hospital shift when the nurse has multiple clients to whom she will provide nursing care. Often a total physical examination is done upon admission to the hospital by the physician or nurse practitioner. Therefore, this shorter format is more practical for ongoing client assessments.

ASSESSMENT PROCEDURE	NORMAL FINDINGS	ABNORMAL FINDINGS
General Survey		
Assess level of consciousness (LOC)	Awake, alert, and oriented to person, place, and time.	If altered LOC, consider the Glasgow Coma Scale.
Assess speech	Speech clear. Makes and maintains conversation appropriately.	
Assess comfort level	Denies c/o pain/discomfort.	If the patient reports or c/o pain: rate the pain using the 0 to 10 pain scale, intervene to provide comfort measures, and evaluate the effectiveness of such interventions.
Skin color, temperature, moisture, turgor	Skin: pink, warm, and dry. Immediate recoil noted at the clavicle.	Pale, pallor ← anemia Erythema ← infection Warmth ← infection Increased tenting ← dehydration
Eyes		
Assess pupils	Pupils equal, round, react to light and accommodation (PERRLA).	Pupils unequal or nonreactive to light.

ASSESSMENT PROCEDURE	NORMAL FINDINGS	ABNORMAL FINDINGS
Chest		
Assess breath sounds	Lungs: clear to auscultation (CTA) anterior and posterior (A & P), bilaterally. Respiratory rate 18, no reports of dyspnea.	Note any wheezes or crackles and identify their location (anterior or posterior, upper or lower lobes, right or left).
Assess heart sounds Note if rhythm is irregular	Heart: S_1 and S_2 present, regular rate (82) and rhythm. No S_3 or S_4 appreciated. No murmur, rub, or gallop (MRG).	Heart sounds irregular or irregularly irregular. Murmurs, rub, or gallop—if present.
Abdomen		
Assess contour and firmness Assess bowel sounds	Nondistended, soft, and nontender Active bowel sounds noted in all four quadrants ($+$ABS $\times$ 4Q).	Distended and firm, visible palpations. Absence of bowel sounds in one or more quadrants. One must listen for 5 minutes to document absent bowel sounds. Normal bowel sounds 5 to 35 per minute.
Extremities		
Assess mobility of extremities, strength of extremities, and peripheral pulses	Able to actively move all extremities. Equal strength, 5/5. Radial, dorsalis pedis, and posterior tibia pulses 2$+$. No peripheral edema.	Unable to actively or passively move one or more extremities.

(Continued on following page)

ASSESSMENT PROCEDURE	ABNORMAL FINDINGS
Other	
Note any wounds or lesions.	Describe: size, shape, location, color, characteristics of any drainage, type of dressing.
Note any drains: Jackson–Pratt, Foley catheter, Hemovac, nasogastric tube.	Describe insertion site: color, consistency, and/or odor of any drainage.
Note any venous access devices.	Describe the location, appearance, type and size of device, type of intravenous fluids and rate of infusion, and infusion device(s).
Note any other therapies: external ice/heat devices, continuous passive motion devices, transcutaneous electrical nerve stimulation (TENS) unit, etc.	Describe the presence of correct functioning of any of these devices.

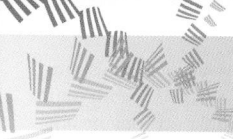

APPENDIX 3

SAMPLE ADULT NURSING HEALTH HISTORY AND PHYSICAL ASSESSMENT

Health History

CLIENT PROFILE

S.L. is a 72-year-old White female, born on a small farm in southern Missouri. Appears younger than stated age. English speaking, with a German ethnic origin. High school graduate and presently retired from restaurant work. Lives in a one-bedroom apartment on the first floor. Drives own car. Seeks health care in local community hospital 4 miles from home. Major reason for seeking health care is for routine checkup—has not had one since 2010. Understands that she has adult-onset diabetes mellitus (type 2), which is controlled with 1,800-calorie diet and moderate amount of exercise. Also has "mild rheumatoid arthritic" pains in the right hip and finger joints in early mornings; relieved with exercise, warm baths, and ASA.

Treatments/Medications

1. Prescribed: none
2. OTC
   a. ASA gr at H.S. for "arthritis aches." Takes about 2×/month. Denies nausea, abdominal pains, or evidence of bleeding while taking
   b. Mylanta at H.S. for "gas pains"

c. Dulcolax suppository 3×/week for past 4 years
d. Multivitamin 1 qd, for past 4 years

Past Illnesses/Hospitalizations

1. Appendectomy age 18
2. Left arm fracture age 20
3. Cholecystectomy age 56, performed for complaint of gas pains after eating fatty foods. Satisfied with care received at local hospital

Allergies

Denies food, drug, and environmental allergies

DEVELOPMENTAL HISTORY

Developmental Level: Integrity vs. Despair

Describes childhood as a very happy time for her. Becomes excited and smiles as she relates stories of her childhood on the farm. States she was an average child and ran and played like all the others. Companions were brothers and sisters. Has been married for 55 years. Describes relationship with husband as close and sharing. Owned and operated a restaurant for 30 years with husband and was a waitress at another restaurant after they retired from their own. Lived in a large house until 1988. Currently lives in a one-bedroom apartment. Active in church and society. Volunteers at community functions. She and her husband are active in their church. States she enjoys being retired and lives a "comfortable" life. Does not voice financial concerns. Has begun to write will and distribute personal heirlooms to son and grandchildren. States she is not afraid of death and wishes to have the "business part taken care of" in order to enjoy the rest of her life together with her husband.

HEALTH PERCEPTION–HEALTH MANAGEMENT PATTERN

1. Client's rating of health:
   Scale: 10—best; 1—worst
   5 years ago: 10
   Now: 8
   5 years from now: 6
   Sees health deterioration as normal aging process and states, "I feel really good when I look at a lot of people my age with all their problems and the medicine they take."

2. Health does not interfere with self-care or other desired activities of daily living. Unaware of signs, symptoms, and Tx of hyperglycemia and hypoglycemia. Denies use of alcohol, tobacco, and drugs.
3. Client seeks health care only in emergencies. Last medical examination September 2010. Keeps active and feels well. Feels lifestyle and faith "keep her going." Does not check own blood sugar or do breast self-examinations.

NUTRITIONAL–METABOLIC PATTERN

States she is on a "no concentrated sweet" meal pattern as follows: Eats breakfast of whole wheat toast, one boiled egg, orange juice, and decaf coffee at 7 AM. Eats lunch at noon. Today had tuna, lettuce salad, apple, and milk. Eats light supper around 6 PM. Typical dinner includes small serving broiled meat, green vegetables, piece of fruit, and glass of milk. Tries not to snack but will have fruit if she feels the urge. Drinks two 8-oz glasses of water a day. Drinks decaf coffee—no tea or colas. Voices no dislikes or food intolerances.

Wears dentures. Last dental examination October–November 2017. Denies problems with proper fit, eating, chewing, swallowing, sore throat, sore tongue, or colds. Complains of "canker sore" if she eats strawberries. Denies n/v, abdominal pain, or excessive gas. Complains of dyspepsia approx. 2×/month, relieved by Mylanta. Does not associate this with the time she takes ASA.

Describes skin and scalp as dry. Uses lotions frequently. Denies easy bruising, pruritus, or nonhealing sores. Nails are hard and brittle. Hair is fine and soft.

Current weight: 120 lb; height: 5'4"

Previous weight: 150 lb 10 years ago. Desires to maintain current weight.

Weight fluctuates ±5 lb/month. Client states, "I've always had to watch what I eat because I gain so easily." Denies intolerance to heat or cold, or voice changes.

ELIMINATION PATTERN

Bowel habits: Soft, formed, med. brown bowel movement (BM) every third day after Dulcolax suppository. States she becomes constipated without use of laxative. Denies mucous, bloody, or tarry stools. States discomfort with BMs starting 6 weeks ago. When having to strain with BMs felt "some kind of mass" prolapsing from rectum. Consulted her doctor, who explained to her "it was a piece of my colon slipping out." No surgical treatment or exercises prescribed. Gently reinserts tissue when this happens. Denies rectal bleeding, change in color, consistency, or habits.

Bladder habits: Voids 4 to 5×/day, clear yellow urine. Denies current problems with dysuria, hematuria, polyuria, hesitancy, incontinence, or nocturia. Complaint of urgency during the colder months with no increase in frequency. Had polyuria and polydipsia prior to diagnosis of diabetes type 2. Developed UTI at age 60, at which time she sought medical advice and was diagnosed with type 2 diabetes mellitus.

ACTIVITY–EXERCISE PATTERN

1. ADLs on an average day: Arises at 6 AM. Eats breakfast and does housekeeping. In early afternoon goes to the community center to eat lunch, quilt, and visit. Goes home around 2 PM. Walks about four blocks with a friend every day. Cleans own house daily for one 2-hour period (includes dusting, vacuuming, washing). Denies palpitations, chest pain, SOB, fatigue, wheezing, claudication, cramps, stiffness, or joint pain or swelling with activity. Walking relieves ache in hips and makes her feel good. After walking, returns home and relaxes with crafts and visiting with husband. During evenings attends church-related activities. Expresses satisfaction with activity and believes she functions above the level of the average person her age.
2. Hygiene: Showers and washes hair every day.
3. Occupational activities: Retired from being a cook and waitress. Volunteers to cook for church group. Occasionally has lower back pains when carrying large amounts of food or when carrying large trays.

SEXUALITY–REPRODUCTION PATTERN

Menstrual history: Age of menarche: approx. 12 years; age of menopause: 50 years. States, "going through my change of life wasn't difficult for me physically or emotionally." Described menstrual period as regular, lasting 4 days with moderate flow. Denies postmenopausal spotting at this time.

Obstetric history: Gravida 1, Para 1. No complications with pregnancy or childbirth.

Contraception: Never used any form.

Sexual activities: Sexually active. States, "My husband and I have good relations." Denies pain, discomfort, or postcoital bleeding.

Special problems: Denies history of any sexually transmitted diseases. Denies problem with vaginal itching. Last Pap smear: negative in 1988.

SLEEP–REST PATTERN

Goes to bed at 10 PM. Denies difficulty falling asleep or sleeping. Feels well rested when she arises at 6 AM. Never used sleep medications. Denies orthopnea and nocturnal dyspnea. Enjoys reading 1 to 2 pages of Bible history each evening.

SENSORY–PERCEPTUAL PATTERN

1. *Vision:* Has worn glasses "all of my life." Cannot recall age at which they were prescribed. Prescription change from bifocals to trifocals August 2010. Complains of blurred vision without glasses. Denies diplopia, itching, excessive tearing, discharge, redness, or trauma to eyes.
2. *Hearing:* Believes she is "a little slow to grasp, and I think it may be because of my hearing." Does not wear hearing aid. Cannot recall last hearing test. Denies tinnitus, pain, discharge, or trauma to ears. Does not ask for questions to be repeated when asked at normal voice tone and level.
3. *Smell:* Denies difficulty with smell, pain, postnasal drip, sneezing, or frequent nosebleeds.
4. *Touch:* States "occasionally my feet feel numb"; subsides on own.
5. *Taste:* No difficulty tasting foods.

COGNITIVE PATTERN

Speech clear without slur or stutter. Follows verbal cues. Expresses ideas and feelings clearly and concisely. States she has had a gradual loss of memory over past 5 to 6 years. Believes long-term memory is better than short-term. She can recall past weekly events but has trouble recalling dates, times, and places of events. Learns best by writing information down and then reviewing it. Makes major decisions jointly with husband after prayer.

ROLE–RELATIONSHIP PATTERN

Client has been married 55 years. Describes relationship as the best part of her life right now. Only son lives in Minnesota, and they visit one to two times a year. Is very fond of three grandchildren. Expresses desire to visit more often but states, "He has his own life and family now." Communicates once a month by phone. Explains her relationship with other members of the church and community groups as friendly and "family like." Lives with husband in first-floor apartment. Has casual relationship with apartment neighbors—friendly but distant. Was the oldest of five children. See family genogram.

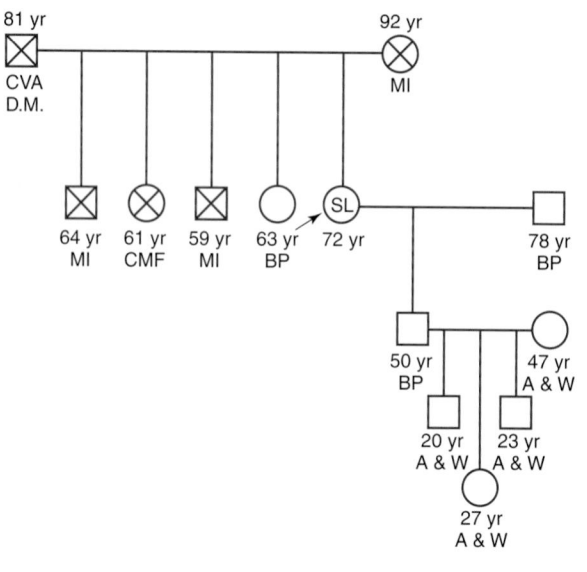

SELF-PERCEPTION–SELF-CONCEPT PATTERN

Describes self as a normal person. Talkative, outgoing, and likes to be around people but hates noisy environments. Happy with the person she has become and states, "I can definitely live with myself." States a weakness is that she worries about "little things" more now than she used to and tends to be irritated more easily. Cannot place specific onset of these feelings. Feels good about self-control of diabetes.

COPING–STRESS TOLERANCE PATTERN

States husband's high blood pressure has never been a source of stress to her. Shares confidences with husband and with a few close friends. Most stressful time in life was losing two brothers and a sister, all in 1994. States with the support of husband and church she handled it "better than most people would have." States she prays and eats when under stress. Cannot identify any major stresses that have occurred in the last year.

VALUE–BELIEF PATTERN

Religious preference is Lutheran. Values relationship with husband, family, and God. Enjoys helping others in the church and community. Believes God is loving, supportive, and forgiving.

Places God as first priority in life. States prayer is extremely important to her and practices it daily. States this personalizes her relationship with God. Has been Lutheran all her life and states she and her husband share in church activities together.

Physical Assessment

GENERAL PHYSICAL SURVEY

Ht: 5'4"; Wt: 120 lb; Radial pulse: 71; Resp: 16; BP: R arm—120/72; L arm—120/70; Temp: 98.6°F. Client alert and cooperative. Sitting comfortably on table with arms crossed and shoulders slightly slouched forward. Smiling with mild anxiety. Dress is neat and clean. Walks steadily with posture slightly stooped.

SKIN, HAIR, AND NAIL ASSESSMENT

1. *Skin:* Pale pink, warm and dry to touch. Skinfold returns to place after 1 second when lifted over clavicle. Tan "age spots" on posterior hands bilaterally in clusters of four to five and evenly distributed over lower extremities. A 3-cm nodule with 2-mm macule in center noted in right axilla; indurated, nontender, and nonmobile. No evidence of vascular or purpuric lesions. No edema.

2. *Hair:* Chin length, gray, straight, clean, styled, medium-textured, evenly distributed on head. No scalp lesions or flaking. Fine blond hair evenly distributed over arms bilaterally and sparsely on legs bilaterally. No hair noted on axilla or on chest, back, or face.

3. *Nails:* Fingernails medium length, and thickness, clear. Splinter hemorrhages noted on right thumb near fingertip in midline. No clubbing or Beau lines.

HEAD AND NECK ASSESSMENT

Head symmetrically rounded, neck nontender with full ROM. Neck symmetrical without masses, scars, pulsations. Lymph nodes nonpalpable. Trachea in midline. Thyroid nonpalpable. Carotid arteries equally strong without bruits. Identifies light and deep touch to various parts of face.

CN V: Identifies light touch and sharp touch to forehead, cheek, and chin. Bilateral corneal reflex intact. Masseter muscles contract equally and bilaterally. Jaw jerk + 1.

CN VII: Identifies sugar and salt on anterior two-thirds of tongue. Smiles, frowns, shows teeth, blows cheeks, and raises eyebrows as instructed.

EYE ASSESSMENT

Eyes 2 cm apart without protrusion. Eyebrows sparse with equal distribution. No scaliness noted. Lids pink without ptosis, edema, or lesions, and freely closeable bilaterally. Lacrimal apparatus nonedematous. Sclera white without increased vascularity or lesions noted. Palpebral and bulbar conjunctiva slightly reddened without lesions noted. Irises uniformly blue. PERRLA, EOMs intact bilaterally. Peripheral vision equal to examiner's.

Visual acuity: With glasses off vision is blurred at 14" away, but can identify number of fingers held up. With glasses on reads newspaper print at 14".

Funduscopic examination: Red reflex present bilaterally. Optic disc round with well-defined margins. Physiologic cup occupies disc. Arterioles smaller than venules. No A-V nicking, no hemorrhages, or exudates noted. Macula not seen. (CNs II, III, IV, and VI intact.)

EAR ASSESSMENT

Auricle without deformity, lumps, or lesions. Right auricle with tag at top of pinna. Auricles and mastoid processes nontender. Bilateral auditory canals contain moderate amount of dark-brown cerumen. Tympanic membrane difficult to view due to wax.

Whisper test: Client identifies one out of two words in four attempts. Weber test: No lateralization of sound to either ear. Rinne test: AC is greater than BC both ears (CN VIII).

NOSE AND SINUSES ASSESSMENT

External structure without deformity, asymmetry, or inflammation. Nares patent. Turbinates and middle meatus pale pink, without swelling, exudate, lesions, or bleeding. Nasal septum midline without bleeding, perforation, or deviation. Frontal and maxillary sinuses nontender. Identifies smells of coffee and soap (CN I).

MOUTH AND PHARYNX ASSESSMENT

Lips moist with peach lipstick. No lesions or ulcerations. Buccal mucosa pink and moist without discoloration or increased pigmentation. No ulcers or nodules. Upper and lower dentures secure. Gums pink and moist without inflammation, bleeding, or discoloration. Hard and soft palates smooth without lesions or masses. Tongue midline when protruded without fasciculations (CN XII intact), lesions, or masses. No lesions, discolorations, or ulcerations on floor of mouth, oral mucosa, or gums. Gag reflex intact, and client identifies sugar and salt on posterior tongue. Uvula in midline and elevates on phonation. (CNs IX and X intact.) Tonsils present without exudate, edema, ulcers, or enlargement.

CARDIAC ASSESSMENT

No pulsations visible. No heaves, lifts, or vibrations. PMI: fifth ICS to LMCL. Clear, brief heart sounds throughout. Physiologic S_2. No gallops, murmurs, or rubs. AP = 72/min and regular.

PERIPHERAL VASCULAR SYSTEM ASSESSMENT

Arms: Equal in size and symmetry bilaterally; pale pink; warm and dry to touch without edema, bruising, or lesions noted. Radial pulses equal in rate and amplitude, and strong. Allen test: Right equal 2-second refill, left equal 2-second refill. Brachial pulses strong, equal, and even. Epitrochlear nodes nonpalpable.

Legs: Legs large in size and bilaterally symmetrical. Skin intact, pale pink; warm and dry to touch without edema, bruising, lesions, or increased vascularity. Superficial inguinal, horizontal, and vertical lymph nodes nonpalpable. Femoral pulses strong and equal without bruits. Popliteal pulse nonpalpable with client supine or prone. Dorsalis pedis and posterior tibial pulses strong and equal. No edema palpable. Homans negative bilaterally. No retrograde filling noted when client stands. Toenails thick and yellowed. Special maneuver for arterial insufficiency: feet regain color after 4 seconds and veins refilled in 5 seconds.

THORAX AND LUNG ASSESSMENT

Skin pale pink without scars, pulsations, or lesions. No hair noted. Thorax expands evenly bilaterally without retractions or bulging. Slope of ribs = 40°. No use of auxiliary respiratory muscles and no nasal flaring. Mild kyphosis. Respirations even, unlabored, and regular (16/min). No cough noted. No tenderness, crepitus, or masses. Tactile fremitus decreases below T5 bilaterally posteriorly, and fourth ICS anteriorly bilaterally. Thorax resonance throughout. Diaphragmatic excursion: Left—on inspiration diaphragm descends to T11, and on expiration diaphragm ascends to T9. Right—on inspiration diaphragm descends to T12, and on expiration diaphragm ascends to T9. Vesicular breath sounds heard in all lung fields. No rales, rhonchi, friction rubs, or abnormal whispered pectoriloquy, bronchophony, or egophony noted.

BREAST ASSESSMENT

Breasts moderate in size, round, and symmetrical bilaterally. Skin pale pink with light-brown areola. No dimpling or retraction.

Free movement in all positions. Engorged vein noted running across UOQ to areola in the right breast. Nipples inverted bilaterally. No discharge expressed. No thickening or tenderness noted. A 2-cm, hard, immobile round mass noted in the left breast in LUOQ. Client denies ever noticing this. Nontender to palpation. Lymph nodes nonpalpable. Client does not know how to do breast self-examination.

ABDOMINAL ASSESSMENT

Abdomen rounded, symmetrical without masses, lesions, pulsations, or peristalsis noted. Abdomen free of hair, bruising, and increased vasculature. Healed with appendectomy scar. Umbilicus in midline, without herniation, swelling, or discoloration. Bowel sounds low pitched and gurgling at 22/minute × four quads. Aortic, renal, and iliac arteries auscultated without bruit. No venous hums or friction rubs auscultated over liver or spleen. Tympany percussed over all four quads. An 8-cm liver span percussed in RMCL. Area of dullness percussed at ninth ICS in left postaxillary line. No tenderness or masses noted with light and deep palpation in all four quadrants. Liver and spleen nonpalpable.

GENITOURINARY–REPRODUCTIVE ASSESSMENT

No bulging or masses in inguinal area. A 1-cm nodule palpated in the right groin. Labia pink with decreased elasticity and vaginal secretions. No bulging of vaginal wall, purulent foul drainage, or lesions. Skene gland not visible. Anal area pink with small amount of hair. Rectal mucosa bulges with straining.

MUSCULOSKELETAL ASSESSMENT

Posture slightly stooped with mild kyphosis. Gait steady, smooth, and coordinated with even base. Limited ROM of lateral flexion and extension of spine. Paravertebrals equal in size and strength. Shrugs shoulders and moves head to right and left against resistance (CN XI intact); upper extremities and lower extremities have full ROM. Muscles moderately firm bilaterally. No deviations, inflammations, or bony deformities. Small callus on left heel. Moves upper and lower extremities freely against gravity and against resistance. Rheumatoid nodule noted on dorsal surface of left hand.

NEUROLOGIC ASSESSMENT

Mental status: Pleasant and friendly. Appropriately dressed for weather with matching colors and patterns. Clothes neat and clean. Facial expressions symmetrical and correlate with mood and topic discussed. Speech clear and appropriate. Follows through with train of thought. Carefully chooses words to convey feelings and ideas. Oriented to person, place, time, and events. Remains attentive and able to focus on examination during entire interaction. Short-term memory intact, long-term memory before 2015 unclear—especially cannot recall dates and sequencing of events. General information questions answered correctly 100% of the time. Vocabulary suitable to educational level. Explains proverb accurately. Gives semiabstract answers and enjoys joking. Is able to identify similarities 5 seconds after asked. Answers to judgment questions in realistic manner.

Cranial nerves: I–XII intact (integrated throughout examination).

Cerebellar and motor function: Alternates finger to nose with eyes closed; occasionally tends to hit opposite side of nose. Rapidly opposes fingers to thumb bilaterally without difficulty. Alternates pronation and supination of hands rapidly without difficulty. Heel to shin intact bilaterally. Romberg: minimal swaying. Tandem walk: steady. No involuntary movements noted.

Sensory status: Superficial light- and deep-touch sensation intact on arms, legs, neck, chest, and back. Position sense of toes and fingers intact bilaterally. Identifies point localization correctly. Identifies coin placed in hand and number written on palm of hand correctly.

Two-Point Discrimination (in mm)	Right	Left
Fingertips	6	6
Dorsal hand	15	15
Chest	45	49
Forearm	39	35
Back	45	45
Upper arm	40	45

Reflexes	Right	Left
Biceps	2+	2+
Triceps	2+	2+
Patellar	3+	3+
Achilles	2+	2+
Abdominal	1+	1+
Babinski	neg	neg

Motor status: Muscle tone firm at rest, abdominal muscles slightly relaxed. Muscle size adequate for age. No fasciculations or involuntary movements noted. Muscle strength moderately strong and equal bilaterally.

CLIENT'S STRENGTHS

- Positive attitude and outlook in life
- Motivation to comply with prescribed diet
- Strong support systems: husband and spiritual beliefs
- No physical limitations

CLIENT CONCERNS

- Poor health care habits associated with a lack of knowledge concerning importance of regular medical checkups, re: lesion in UOQ of left breast not seen by physician, no Pap smear, no follow-up with diabetes, and lack of knowledge of BSE
- Constipation associated with lack of bowel routine and lack of knowledge regarding laxative overuse and causes of constipation
- Opportunity to improve health associated with interest in learning the signs of hyperglycemia/hypoglycemia and the importance of self-blood glucose monitoring

COLLABORATIVE PROBLEMS

- Risk for complication: hyperglycemia, hypoglycemia
- Risk for complication: hypertension

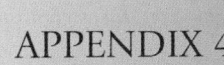

ASSESSMENT OF FAMILY FUNCTIONAL HEALTH PATTERNS

The nurse obtains data about the family's functional health patterns by interviewing the family as a group or by interviewing one or two family members who are reliable historians and seem knowledgeable about their family's health patterns. If data reveal a particular problem identified with an individual family member, the nurse can then focus attention on obtaining more data from that individual.

Family Profile

The purpose of the family profile is to obtain biographical family data (e.g., age, sex, and current health status of each family member). A genogram may be used to illustrate this information.

Health Perception–Health Management Pattern

SUBJECTIVE DATA

- Describe your family's general health during the past few years.
- Has your family been able to participate in their usual activities (i.e., at work, school, sports)?

- Describe what your family does to try to stay healthy (diet, exercise, etc.).
- From whom does your family seek health care? When?
- Describe how your family members check their health status (e.g., eye exams, dental exams, breast exams, testicular exams, medical checkups).
- Describe any behaviors in your family that are considered unhealthy.
- Who cares for family members who are or who become ill?
- How would you know if a family member were ill?

OBJECTIVE DATA

1. Observe the appearance of family members.
2. Observe the home (hazards and safety devices, storage facilities, cooking facilities).

Nutritional–Metabolic Pattern

SUBJECTIVE DATA

- Describe typical breakfast, lunch, supper, and snacks that you eat as a family.
- What type of drinks do you usually have during the day and at night?

- How would you describe your family's appetite in general?
- How often does your family seek dental care? Are there any dental problems in your family?
- Does anyone in your family have skin rashes or problems with sores healing? Explain.
- Who usually prepares the family meals? Who shops for groceries?

OBJECTIVE DATA

1. Observe kitchen appliances, availability of food, and types of foods kept in the home, if possible.
2. Observe preparation of a family meal, if possible.
3. Observe family members for obvious signs of malnutrition or obesity.

Elimination Pattern

SUBJECTIVE DATA

- How often do family members have bowel movements? Urinate?
- Are laxatives used in your family? Explain.
- Are there problems with disposing of waste or garbage?
- Describe any recycling you do.

- Does your family have pets (indoor or outdoor)? How are their wastes disposed?
- Do you have problems with insects in your home? Explain.

OBJECTIVE DATA

1. Observe bathroom facilities.
2. Inspect home for insects.
3. Observe garbage and waste disposal.

Activity–Exercise Pattern

SUBJECTIVE DATA

- Describe how your family exercises. Frequency?
- How does your family relax?
- What does your family do for enjoyment?
- Describe a typical day of activities in your family (work, school, play, games, meals, hobbies, house cleaning, yard work, cooking, exercise).

OBJECTIVE DATA

1. Observe the pace of family activities.
2. Observe any exercise equipment kept in home.

Sleep–Rest Pattern

SUBJECTIVE DATA

- When does your family generally go to bed and awaken? Do family members go to bed and arise at different times? Explain.
- Does your family seem to get enough time to sleep? To rest and relax?
- Do any family members work at night? How does this affect other family members?

OBJECTIVE DATA

1. Observe sleeping areas.
2. Observe temperament and energy level of family members.

Sensory–Perceptual Pattern

SUBJECTIVE DATA

- Are there any hearing or visual problems that affect your family members?
- Are there any deficits in a family member's ability to taste and smell that affect how food is prepared for the family?

- Does pain seem to be a family problem? Explain. How is this managed?
- What is the usual form of pain relief used by family members?

OBJECTIVE DATA

1. Observe any visual or hearing aids used by family members.
2. Observe medications kept on hand to relieve pain.

Cognitive Pattern

SUBJECTIVE DATA

- Who makes the major family decisions? How?
- Describe the highest educational level of all family members.
- Does your family understand any illnesses and treatments that affect any of your family members?
- How does your family enjoy learning (e.g., reading, watching television, attending classes)?
- Are there any problems with memory in the family? Explain.

OBJECTIVE DATA

1. Observe language spoken by all family members.
2. Observe use of words (vocabulary level) and ability to grasp ideas and express self.

3. Are family decisions present or future oriented? Observe family decision-making strategies.
4. Observe school attended by children.

Self-Perception–Self-Concept Pattern

SUBJECTIVE DATA

- Describe the general mood of your family (e.g., sad, happy, eager, depressed, anxious, relaxed).
- Do you consider yourselves to be a close family? How do you spend time together? Is this time satisfying?
- Do family members share any common goals? Explain.
- What does the family enjoy doing most together?
- How does your family deal with disagreements?
- How do your family members express their affection, feelings, and/or concerns? Are they allowed to do so freely? Explain.
- Does your family seem to discuss problems that affect individual members?
- How does your family deal with change?

OBJECTIVE DATA

1. Observe family discussions.
2. Observe mood and temperament of family.

3. Observe how family members deal with conflict.
4. How do family members show concern and consideration for each other's needs and desires?

Role–Relationship Pattern

SUBJECTIVE DATA

- Describe how your family members support each other, show affection, and express concerns.
- Describe any problems with relationships between family members.
- Describe your family resources (financial, community support systems, family support systems).
- How active is your family in your neighborhood and/or community?
- Explain family responsibilities for various household chores (washing, cooking, driving, lawn maintenance, etc.).
- Explain how discipline is used in your family. How are family members rewarded? Describe any aggression and/or violence that occurs in your family.

OBJECTIVE DATA

1. Observe family interaction patterns (verbal and nonverbal).
2. Explore which family members take responsibility for managing and leading family activities.
3. Observe living space and ownership of rooms by family members.

Sexuality–Reproductive Pattern

SUBJECTIVE DATA

If appropriate: Are sexual partners within home satisfied with sexual relationship and activities? Describe any problems.

- Are contraceptives used?
- Is family planning used? How?
- Are parents comfortable answering questions and explaining topics related to sexuality to their children?

Coping–Stress Tolerance Pattern

SUBJECTIVE DATA

- What major changes have occurred in your family during the past year (e.g., divorce, marriage, family members leaving

home, new members coming into home, death, illness, births, accidents, change in finances and/or occupation)?
- How does your family *cope* with major stressors (e.g., exercise, discussion, prayer, drugs, alcohol, violence)?
- Who in the family copes best with stressors?
- Who has the most difficult time coping with stress?
- Who outside the family (e.g., friends, church, support groups) seems to help your family most during difficult times?

OBJECTIVE DATA

- Observe effect and pace of family interactions.

Value–Belief Pattern

SUBJECTIVE DATA

- What does your family consider to be most important in life?
- What does your family want from life?

- What rules does your family hold most important?
- Is religion important in the family? What religion are family members? What religious practices are important to the family? Is a relationship with God important to the family?
- What does your family look forward to in the future?
- From where do the family's hope and strength come?

OBJECTIVE DATA

1. Observe family rituals and/or traditions.
2. Observe pictures and other articles (religious or other) in home.
3. Listen to general topics discussed in home by family members.
4. Observe the type of television programs viewed by family members and the type of music to which family members listen.

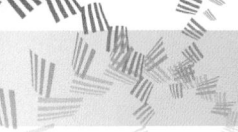

CHILD COGNITIVE (PIAGET) AND PSYCHOSOCIAL (ERICKSON) DEVELOPMENT (BIRTH TO 18 YEARS)

Age	Physical Development	Language (Cognitive) Development (Based on Piaget)	Psychosocial Development (Based on Erikson)	Nurse's Approach to Assessment
Overview of birth to 1 year		*Sensorimotor stage of development*	*Developmental task: trust vs. mistrust.* Learns to trust and to anticipate satisfaction. Sends cues to mother/caretaker. Begins understanding self as separate from others (body image).	Involve caretaker in assessment (e.g., allow them to hold child in lap for parts of examination).

Age	Physical Development	Language (Cognitive) Development (Based on Piaget)	Psychosocial Development (Based on Erikson)	Nurse's Approach to Assessment
1–2 months	Lifts chin and chest off bed. Holds extremities in flexion and moves at random; weak neck muscles. Activity varies from quiet sleep to drowsiness to alert activity.	Can discriminate between various sensations and prefers certain ones. Follows moving objects with eyes.	Begins to bond with mother during alert periods.	Conserve infant's body heat. Assess while asleep or quiet. Place infant on table or in caretaker's arms. Give bottle if awake.
3–4 months	Head and back control developing. Holds rattle. Looks at own hands. Infant reflexes begin to disappear. Able to sit propped. Props self on forearm in prone position. Rolls from side to back and vice versa and from back to abdomen. Takes objects to mouth. Drools with eruption of lower teeth.	Responds to parent. Social smile. Begins to vocalize; coos, babbles. Locates sounds by turning head, looking.	Learns to signal displeasure. Shows excitement with whole body. Begins to discriminate strangers. Squeals.	Speak softly to infant. Use brightly colored toys, bells, rattles to elicit necessary responses and to distract. Assess ears, mouth, nose last. Assess lungs and heart when quiet.

Age	Physical Development	Language (Cognitive) Development (Based on Piaget)	Psychosocial Development (Based on Erikson)	Nurse's Approach to Assessment
5–8 months	Begins to develop teeth. Birth weight doubled. Grasps objects. Sits unsupported.	Begins to imitate sounds, two-syllable words ("dada," "mama"). Responds to own name.	Increased fear of strangers. Definite likes/dislikes. Responds to "no."	Place on caretaker's lap (same as above).
9–12 months	Birth weight tripled. Anterior fontanelle nearly closed. Learns to pull in order to stand, creep, and crawl.	Says two-syllable words besides "dada," "mama." Understands simple commands. Imitates animal sounds.	Looks for hidden objects. Unceasing determination to move about. Clings to mother. Shows emotion. Plays peek-a-boo and pat-a-cake.	
1–3 years	Begins to walk and run well. Drinks from cup, feeds self. Develops fine motor control. Climbs. Begins self-toileting. Kneels without support.	*Preoperational stage of development.* Has poor time sense. Increasing verbal ability. Formulates sentences of 4–5 words by age 3. Talks to self and others. Has misconceptions about cause and effect. Interested in pictures.	*Developmental task: autonomy vs. shame and doubt.* Establishes self-control, decision-making, independence (autonomy). Extremely curious and prefers to do things by self. Demonstrates independence through negativism. Very egocentric; believes they control the	Be flexible. Begin assessment with play period to establish rapport. Be honest. Praise for cooperation. Begin slowly; speak to child. Involve caretaker/parent in holding on examination table. Let child hold security object.

(*Continued on following page*)

Age	Physical Development	Language (Cognitive) Development (Based on Piaget)	Psychosocial Development (Based on Erikson)	Nurse's Approach to Assessment
	Steady growth in height/ weight. Adult height will be approximately double the height at age 2. Dresses self by age 3.	*Fears:* • Loss/separation from parents—peak • Dark • Machines/equipment • Intrusive procedures • Bedtime Speaks to dolls and animals. Increasing attention span. Knows own sex by age 3.	world. Attempts to please parents. Participates in parallel play; able to share some toys by age 3.	Allow child to play with stethoscope, tongue blade, flashlight before using on child if possible. Assess face, mouth, eyes, ears last. May need to restrain when lying prone. If resistant, save that part of the assessment for later.
4–6 years	Growth slows. Locomotion skills increase and coordination improves. Tricycle/ bicycle riding. Throws ball but has difficulty catching. Constantly active, increasing dexterity. Eruption of	Preoperational stage of development continues. Language skills flourish. Generates many questions (e.g., How, Why, What?) Simple problem	*Developmental tasks: initiative vs. guilt.* Attempts to establish self like their parents, but independent. Explores environment on own initiative. Boasts, brags, has feelings of indestructibility.	Establish rapport through talking and play. Introduce self to child. Have parent present but direct conversation to child. Games such as "follow the leader" and

Age	Physical Development	Language (Cognitive) Development (Based on Piaget)	Psychosocial Development (Based on Erikson)	Nurse's Approach to Assessment
	permanent teeth. Skips, hops, jumps rope.	solving. Uses fantasy to understand and problem-solve. *Fears:* • Mutilation • Castration • Dark • Unknown • Inanimate • Unfamiliar objects Causality related to proximity of events. Enjoys mimicking and imitating adults.	Family is primary social group. Peers increasingly important. Assumes sex roles. Aggressive, very curious. Enjoys activities such as sports, cooking, shopping. Cooperative play. Likes rules. May stretch the truth and tell large stories.	"Simon says" can be used to elicit necessary behaviors. Explain each assessment in simple language. Ask for child's help and use flattery. Use pictures, models, or items they can see or touch. Reserve genital examination for last; drape accordingly.
6–11 years	Moves constantly. Physical play prevalent; sports, swimming, skating, etc. Increased smoothness of	*Concrete operations stage of development.* Organized thought; memory concepts more complicated.		Explain all procedures and impact on body. Encourage questioning and active participation in care. Be direct

(*Continued on following page*)

Age	Physical Development	Language (Cognitive) Development (Based on Piaget)	Psychosocial Development (Based on Erikson)	Nurse's Approach to Assessment
	movement. Grows at rate of 2 in/7 lb a year. Eyes/hands well-coordinated.	Reads, reasons better. Focuses on concrete understanding. *Fears*: • Mutilation • Death • Immobility • Rejection • Failure	*Developmental task: industry vs. inferiority.* Learns to include values and skills of school, neighborhood, peers. Peer relationships important. Focuses	about explanation of procedures, based on what child will hear, see, smell, and feel. (In addition, explain body part involved and use anatomic names and pictures to explain step by step.) Be honest. Reassure child that they are liked. Provide privacy. Involve parents, but give child choice as to whether parent will stay during

Age	Physical Development	Language (Cognitive) Development (Based on Piaget)	Psychosocial Development (Based on Erikson)	Nurse's Approach to Assessment
		more on reality, less on fantasy. Family is main base of security and identity. Sensitive to reactions of others. Seeks approval and recognition. Enthusiastic, noisy, imaginative, desires to explore. Likes to complete a task. Enjoys helping others.		examination. Reason and explain. Allow child some choice as to direction of assessment. May be able to proceed as if assessing adult. Praise cooperation.
12–18 years	Well developed. Rapid physical growth (early adolescence: maximum growth). Secondary sex characteristics. (See Chapters 22 and 23.)	*Formal operations stage of development.* Abstract reasoning, problem solving. Understanding of multiple cause-and-effect relationships. May plan for future career.	*Developmental task: identity vs. role confusion.* Predominant values are those of peer group. Early adolescence: outgoing and enthusiastic. Emotions are extreme, with mood swings. Seeking self-identity, sexual identity.	Respect privacy. Accept expression of feelings. Direct discussions of care and condition to child. Ask for child's opinions and encourage questions. Allow input into decisions. Be

(*Continued on following page*)

Age	Physical Development	Language (Cognitive) Development (Based on Piaget)	Psychosocial Development (Based on Erikson)	Nurse's Approach to Assessment
		Fears: • Mutilation • Disruption of body image • Rejection by peers	Wants privacy and independence. Develops interests not shared with family. Concern with physical self. Explores adult roles.	flexible with routines. Explain all procedures/ treatments. Encourage continuance of peer relationships. Listen actively. Identify impact of illness on body image, future, and level of functioning. Correct misconceptions. Involve parent in assessment only if child requests presence.

Information adapted from Erikson, E. H. (1991). *Erikson's stages of personality development. Childhood and society.* W. W. Norton & Company; Piaget, J. (1981). *The psychology of intelligence* (M. Piercy & D. E. Berlyne, Trans.). Littlefield & Adams.

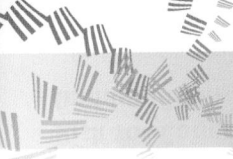

COLLABORATIVE PROBLEMS[‡]

Risk for Complications of Cardiac/Vascular Dysfunction

RC of Decreased Cardiac Output
RC of Dysrhythmias
RC of Pulmonary Edema
RC of Cardiogenic Shock
RC of Thromboembolic/Deep Vein Thrombosis
RC of Hypovolemia
RC of Peripheral Vascular Insufficiency
RC of Hypertension
RC of Congenital Heart Disease
RC of Angina
RC of Endocarditis
RC of Pulmonary Embolism
RC of Spinal Shock
RC of Ischemic Ulcers

Risk for Complications of Respiratory Dysfunction

RC of Hypoxemia
RC of Atelectasis/Pneumonia
RC of Tracheobronchial Constriction
RC of Pleural Effusion
RC of Tracheal Necrosis
RC of Ventilator Dependency
RC of Pneumothorax
RC of Laryngeal Edema

Risk for Complications of Renal/Urinary Dysfunction

RC of Acute Urinary Retention
RC of Renal Failure
RC of Bladder Perforation
RC of Renal Calculi

Risk for Complications of Gastrointestinal/Hepatic/Biliary Dysfunction

RC of Paralytic Ileus/Small Bowel Obstruction
RC of Hepatic Failure
RC of Hyperbilirubinemia
RC of Evisceration
RC of Hepatosplenomegaly
RC of Curling's Ulcer
RC of Ascites
RC of Gastrointestinal Bleeding

Risk for Complications of Metabolic/Immune/Hematopoietic Dysfunction

RC of Hypoglycemia/Hyperglycemia
RC of Negative Nitrogen Balance

RC of Electrolyte Imbalances
RC of Thyroid Dysfunction
RC of Hypothermia (Severe)
RC of Hyperthermia (Severe)
RC of Sepsis
RC of Acidosis (Metabolic, Respiratory)
RC of Alkalosis (Metabolic, Respiratory)
RC of Hypo/Hyperthyroidism
RC of Allergic Reaction
RC of Donor Tissue Rejection
RC of Adrenal Insufficiency
RC of Anemia
RC of Thrombocytopenia
RC of Opportunistic Infection
RC of Polycythemia
RC of Sickling Crisis
RC of Disseminated Intravascular Coagulation

Risk for Complications of Neurological/Sensory Dysfunction

RC of Increased Intracranial Pressure
RC of Stroke
RC of Seizures
RC of Spinal Cord Compression

RC of Meningitis
RC of Cranial Nerve Impairment (Specify)
RC of Paralysis
RC of Peripheral Nerve Impairment
RC of Increased Intraocular Pressure
RC of Corneal Ulceration
RC of Neuropathies

Risk for Complications of Muscular/ Skeletal Dysfunction

RC of Osteoporosis
RC of Joint Dislocation
RC of Compartment Syndrome
RC of Pathologic Fractures

Risk for Complications of Reproductive Dysfunction

RC of Fetal Distress
RC of Postpartum Bleeding
RC of Gestational Hypertension
RC of Hypermenorrhea
RC of Polymenorrhea

RC of Syphilis
RC of Prenatal Bleeding
RC of Preterm Labor

Risk for Complications of Medication Therapy Adverse Effects

RC of Adrenocorticosteroid Therapy Adverse Effects
RC of Antianxiety Therapy Adverse Effects
RC of Antiarrhythmic Therapy Adverse Effects
RC of Anticoagulant Therapy Adverse Effects
RC of Anticonvulsant Therapy Adverse Effects
RC of Antidepressant Therapy Adverse Effects
RC of Antihypertensive Therapy Adverse Effects
RC of Beta-Adrenergic Blocker Therapy Adverse Effects
RC of Calcium-Channel Blocker Therapy Adverse Effects
RC of Angiotensin-Converting Enzyme Therapy Adverse Effects
RC of Antineoplastic Therapy Adverse Effects
RC of Antipsychotic Therapy Adverse Effects
RC of Diuretic Therapy Adverse Effects

† Frequently used collaborative problems are represented on this list. Other situations not listed here could qualify as collaborative problems.

Reprinted from Carpenito, L. J. (2021). *Handbook of nursing diagnosis* (16th ed.). Burlington, MA: Jones and Bartlett, with permission from Lynda Carpenito.

SPANISH TRANSLATION FOR NURSING HEALTH HISTORY AND PHYSICAL EXAMINATION

Biographic Data

English	Spanish
What is your name?	¿Cómo se llama Ud.? ¿Cómo te llamas? (For child)
How old are you?	¿Cuántos años tiene?
Where do you live?	¿Dónde vive Ud.?
Are you allergic to anything?	¿Tiene Ud. alérgias a algún medicamento?
Do you have any handicaps?	¿Tiene Ud. alguna discapacidad? ¿Incapacidad física?
Do you have any illnesses that you know of?	¿Padece Ud. de alguna enfermedad? ¿Más de una?
Have you had any past surgeries?	¿Ha sido operado?

Functional Health Pattern History

HEALTH PERCEPTION/HEALTH MANAGEMENT PATTERN

English	Spanish
Rate your health on a scale of 1–10 (1 being poor, 10 being good).	Estime su salud en una escala de uno a diez (cuando uno significa malo y diez bueno).
Describe your current health.	Describa cómo está su salud actual.
When was your last tetanus shot?	¿Ha tenido inyección de tétano? ¿Cuándo fue la última?
Do you use drugs? If yes, explain.	¿Toma Ud. medicamentos? ¿drogas? Si 'si,' ¿cuales son?
Do you use alcohol? If yes, explain.	¿Toma alcohol? Si 'si,' ¿de qué clase y cuánto toma?
Do you use caffeine? If yes, explain.	¿Toma cafeína? ¿En qué forma y cuánto por dia?

NUTRITIONAL/METABOLIC PATTERN

English	Spanish
What do you eat for breakfast? For lunch? For supper? For snacks?	¿Qué come en el desayuno? ¿en el almuerzo? ¿en la cena? ¿bocaditos? ¿tapas?
Describe the condition of your: • Skin • Hair • Nails	Por favor, describa la condición • de la piel • del pelo • de las uñas
Have you recently gained or lost weight? How much?	Ha aumentado o bajado su peso recientemente

ELIMINATION PATTERN

English	Spanish
Describe your bowel pattern. How often? Color and consistency?	¿Cuándo hizo la defecación/evacuación la última vez? (¿Cuándo fue al bano la última vez?) ¿Puede describer el patrón de la defecación? ¿Cuántas veces al día/a la semana? ¿Color? ¿Textura?
Describe your urinary pattern. How often? Color?	Puede describer el color de la orina? ¿Cuántas veces al dia orina? (hace pi pi)
Do you need to urinate at night?	¿Tiene necesidad de orinar de noche?
Is there a sense of urgency?	¿Hay un sentido de urgencia?

ACTIVITY/EXERCISE PATTERN

English	Spanish
What activities do you do in a normal day?	Describa un dia usual. ¿Cuáles actividades hace?
What do you do to relax?	¿Qué hace para descansar?
Do you physically exercise? Explain.	¿Hace ejercicio? Descríbalo, por favor.

SEXUAL/REPRODUCTION PATTERN

English	Spanish
How old were you when you started menstruating? Or when you stopped menstruating?	¿Cuántos años tenía cuando comenzó la menstruación? (a menstruar) ¿Cuándo paró la menstruación?
How many times have you been pregnant?	¿Cuántos embarazos ha tenido?
How many children do you have?	¿Cuántos ninos/hijos tiene?
Do you do anything to prevent pregnancy?	¿Hace algo por evitar el embarazo?
Do you have any sexually transmitted diseases?	¿Padece de enfermedades sexuales/transmitidos por el sexo?

SLEEP/REST PATTERN

English	Spanish
What time do you go to bed at night?	¿A qué hora se aquesta?
How long do you sleep each night?	¿Cuántas horas duerme en la noche?
Does anything wake you?	¿Hay algo que lo despierte?
What helps you fall asleep?	¿Qué le ayuda a dormir?
Do you take naps? How often?	¿Toma siestas? ¿Con que frecuencia?

SENSORY/PERCEPTUAL PATTERN

English	Spanish
When was your last eye examination?	¿Cuándo fué el último examen de los ojos?
Do you have any problems: • Seeing? • Hearing? • Smelling? • Tasting? • Feeling?	¿Padece de problemas de • la vista? • oir? escuchar? • oler? • saber? • sentir sensaciones?
Do you have any pain now? Show me on this picture. • What causes it? • What relieves it? • When does it occur? • How often? • How long does it last? • Show me on this scale how bad it hurts (use facial scale).	¿Tiene dolor ahora? ¿Dónde le duele? Muéstramelo en este dibujo. • ¿Qué cree que causa el dolor? • ¿Qué reduce o quita el dolor? • ¿Cuándo ocurre el dolor? • ¿y la frecuencia del dolor? • ¿Cuánto tiempo dura el dolor? • Muéstreme la intensidad del doloren esta escala.

COGNITIVE PATTERN

English	Spanish
What did your doctor tell you?	¿Qué le dijo el medico?
Do you have questions about your illness? Or treatments?	¿Quiere preguntar algo sobre la enfermedad? ¿sobre los tratamientos?

ROLE/RELATIONSHIP PATTERN

English	Spanish
Who do you live with?	¿Con quién vive Ud.?
Are you married?	¿Está Ud. casado? casada (fem.)
Does your family get along well?	¿Se lleva bien la familia?
What is your role in your family?	¿Cuál es el papel que juega en la familia?

SELF-PERCEPTION/SELF-CONCEPT PATTERN

English	Spanish
What are your strengths?	¿Cuáles son sus fortalezas que tiene en cuanto a la salud?
What are your weaknesses?	¿Cuáles son sus debilidades?

COPING/STRESS-TOLERANCE PATTERN

English	Spanish
What is stressful in your life?	¿Cuáles son los estreses de su vida?
What or who helps you most when you have a problem?	Cuándo tiene un problema, ¿quién o qué lo ayuda más?

VALUE/BELIEF PATTERN

English	Spanish
What is very important to you in life?	¿Qué es muy importante en su vida?
What religion are you?	¿A qué religion pertenece?
Are there certain foods you cannot have?	¿Hay comidas o ingredientes que no puede comer?
Do you want a priest or hospital chaplain to visit you?	¿Quiere que el padre, el capillán del hospital le haga una visita?

Phrases to Use to Help the Client Through the Physical Assessment

English	Spanish
Please	Por favor
Take off all your clothes and put on this gown.	Quitese toda la ropa y póngase esta bata.
Urinate in this cup.	Orine (hace pi pi) en este recipiente.
Lie down.	Acuéstese, por favor.
Stand up.	Póngase de pie, por favor.
Sit up.	Siéntese.
Get up and sit again.	Levántese y siéntese de nuevo.
Roll over to your right.	Voltéese a la derecha.
Roll over to your left.	Voltéese a la izquierda.
Take a deep breath.	Respire profundo.
Hold it.	Manténgalo.
Breathe out.	Respire de nuevo.
Cough.	Tosa.
Bend your leg.	Doble la pierna.
Bend your arm.	Doble el brazo.
Look up.	Mire hacia arriba.
Look down.	Mire hacia abajo.
Look to your right.	Mire al lado derecho.
Look to your left.	Mire al lado izquierdo.

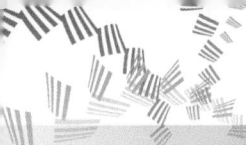

INDEX